Case Documentation in Counseling and Psychotherapy

A Theory-Informed, Competency-Based Approach

DIANE R. GEHART, Ph.D.
California State University, Northridge

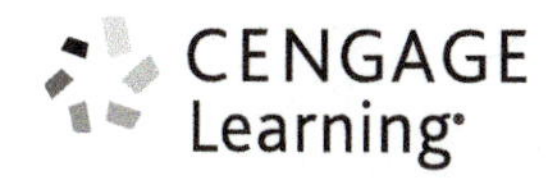

Australia • Brazil • Mexico • Singapore • United Kingdom • United States

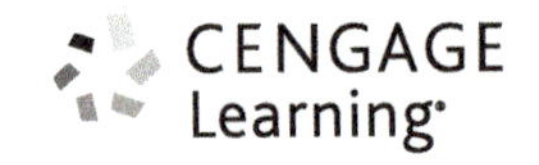

Case Documentation in Counseling and Psychotherapy: A Theory-Informed, Competency-Based Approach
Diane R. Gehart

Product Director: Jon-David Hague

Product Manager: Julie Martinez

Product Assistant: Nicole Richards

Media Developer: Sean Cronin

Marketing Manager: Shanna Shelton

Production Management, and Composition: Manoj Kumar, MPS Limited

Art Director: Carolyn Deacy, MPS Limited

Manufacturing Planner: Judy Inouye

IP Analyst: Deanna Ettinger

IP Project Manager: Brittani Morgan

Text Researcher: Pinky Subi, Lumina Datamatics

Cover Designer: Ellen Pettengell

Cover Image: kyoshino/E+/Getty Images

WCN: 01-100-101

Library of Congress Control Number: 2015931698

ISBN: 978-1-305-40521-9

Cengage Learning
20 Channel Center Street
Boston, MA 02210
USA

Cengage Learning is a leading provider of customized learning solutions with employees residing in nearly 40 different countries and sales in more than 125 countries around the world. Find your local representative at **www.cengage.com.**

Cengage Learning products are represented in Canada by Nelson Education, Ltd.

To learn more about Cengage Learning Solutions, visit **www.cengage.com.**

Purchase any of our products at your local college store or at our preferred online store **www.cengagebrain.com.**

Printed at CLDPC, USA, 02-20

Dedication

This book is dedicated to the counselors and therapists who dedicate their lives to reducing the suffering of others. Your efforts are a gift to us all.

Brief Contents

Contents

Preface

Text Overview

Part of the *Mastering Competencies* series, *Case Documentation in Counseling and Psychotherapy* teaches counselors and psychotherapists how to apply counseling theories in real-world settings. The text provides a comprehensive introduction to case documentation using four commonly used clinical forms: case conceptualization, clinical assessment, treatment plan, and progress note. These documents are uniquely designed to incorporate counseling theory and help new practitioners understand how to use theory in everyday practice. Seven comprehensive case studies with diverse clients illustrate how to complete documentation using a single counseling model: psychodynamic, Adlerian, humanistic, cognitive-behavioral, family systemic, solution-focused, and postmodern/feminist. Furthermore, readers learn about the evidence base for each theory as well as applications for specific diverse populations. Unlike a typical textbook, this book can be used as a clinical reference manual to assist mental health professionals in their practice settings for years to come, providing practical overviews of theories, conceptualization, treatment planning, and documentation.

Using state-of-the-art pedagogical methods, *Case Documentation in Counseling and Psychotherapy* is part of a new generation of textbooks designed to produce measurable results that have value beyond the classroom. The text employs a learning-centered, outcome-based pedagogy to engage students in an active learning process that enables them to apply theory using case documentation. These case documents were created using national standards for counseling, family therapy, psychology, and social work. Students demonstrate their learning using these forms, which instructors can then use to easily measure educational outcomes. These assignments empower students to apply theoretical concepts and develop professional skills as early as possible in their training, resulting in faster mastery of the material.

The author uses a down-to-earth style to explain concepts in clear and practical language that contemporary students appreciate. Instructors will enjoy the simplicity of having the text and assignments work seamlessly together, thus requiring less time in class preparation and grading. The extensive set of instructor materials—which include syllabi templates, detailed PowerPoints, test banks, online lectures, and scoring rubrics designed for accreditation assessment—further reduce educators' workloads. In summary, the book employs the most efficient and effective pedagogical methods available to teach case documentation and counseling theories, resulting in a win-win for instructors and students alike.

Text Features

- *Clinical Forms:* The book provides a comprehensive set of four clinical forms that can be used in practice environments, either in university training clinics or community agencies:
  - Theory-informed case conceptualization
  - Clinical mental health assessment and DSM-5 diagnosis

    - Treatment plan that includes theory, diversity, and evidence-based practice
    - HIPAA-compliant progress notes
- *Outcome-Based Pedagogy:* This text teaches the skills and knowledge outlined in accreditation standards for counselors, psychologists, social workers, and family therapists.
- *Assessment of Student Learning:* Using four clinical documentation forms, this text enables faculty to easily measure students' mastery of competencies and learning outcomes, which are now required for both regionally accredited university boards (WASC, SACS, etc.) and professional accrediting bodies (APA, CACREP, COAMFTE, and CSWE). Assessments with scoring rubrics correlated to each discipline's competencies are part of the ancillary materials.
- *Comprehensive Treatment Model:* A comprehensive five-step model for competent treatment provides students with a clear map for their work. The model includes (a) theory-informed case conceptualization, (b) clinical assessment (diagnosis) and case management, (c) treatment planning, (d) evaluation of progress, and (e) progress note documentation.
- *Theory-Based Case Conceptualizations:* A cross-theoretical case conceptualization form enables counselors to do a comprehensive case conceptualization for clients; the form can also be used in segments to create theory-specific conceptualizations.
- *DSM-5 Clinical Assessment:* A clinical assessment form uses the DSM-5 diagnosis format and includes mental status exam, crisis assessment, safety plan, and case management.
- *Theory-Specific Treatment Plan Templates:* Each theory chapter provides practical treatment plan templates for use with individuals struggling with depression or anxiety. These templates will better enable therapists to develop thoughtful, theory-based treatment plans for their clients.
- *Theory-Specific Progress Note:* Detailed introduction to HIPAA-compliant progress note format, including CPT codes.
- *Theory Considerations and Adaptations with Diversity Clients:* The diversity sections in each theory chapter include specific, practical applications of the theory with specific populations. Each chapter contains a discussion of ethnic/racial diversity and sexual identity diversity. Expanded sections on specific populations provide students with detailed suggestions, adaptations, and cautions for using a given theory with a specific population, including African Americans, Hispanic/Latinos, Asian Americans, Native Americans/First Nation/Aboriginals, and LGBTQ individuals.
- *Practical Applications to Diversity:* Each clinical form requires students to identify specific ways that the treatment will be adjusted to address diversity issues, including the formation of a counseling relationship, assessment, and intervention.
- *Research and the Evidence Base:* The evidence base and research foundations for each theory are reviewed, and numerous evidence-based treatments are highlighted throughout the book.
- *Practice and Reflection:* Throughout the text, readers are provided instructions and prompts for practicing clinical skills, with or without a partner. In addition, reflection and discussion questions invite readers to engage thoughtfully with the material.
- *Readable:* The author uses an engaging writing style that speaks to—and at times may even entertain—today's students.

Organization

This book is organized into three parts:
Part I: Introduction to Case Documentation details the five steps to competent therapy described at the beginning of this chapter:

- Case conceptualization
- Clinical assessment

- Treatment planning
- Evaluating progress
- Progress notes

Part II: Theory-Informed Case Documentation: The next section of the text reviews key concepts of each of the major counseling theories and provides a detailed case study with all four elements of case documentation presented in the book: counseling case conceptualization, clinical assessment with DSM-5 diagnosis, treatment plan, and progress note. Case documentation is presented for the following theories:

- Psychodynamic
- Adlerian
- Humanistic
- Cognitive-behavioral
- Family systems
- Solution-focused therapies
- Postmodern/Feminist

Part III: The Competent Supervisee: The last chapter introduces you to the paradigm of the competent supervisee and provides guidance for how to approach the supervisory relationship. If you have already started seeing clients, you might want to begin here; otherwise, this chapter will get you ready for doing so. This chapter includes elements such as:

- Managing initial anxiety
- Your role as supervisee
- Your supervisor's role
- Getting the most out of supervision
- What to do if things get bumpy

Appropriate Courses

A versatile book that serves as a reference across the curriculum, this text is specifically designed for use as a primary or secondary textbook in the following courses:

- Introductory or advanced counseling theories courses
- Pre-practicum skills classes
- Practicum or fieldwork classes

Assessing Student Learning

The learning assignments in the text are designed to simplify the process of measuring student learning for regional and national accreditation. Each case document in the book comes with scoring rubrics, which are available on the student and instructor websites for the book at www.CengageBrain.com. Scoring rubrics are available for all major mental health disciplines using the following sets of competencies:

- *Counseling:* Council on the Accreditation of Counseling and Related Educational Programs (CACREP) standards
- *Marriage and Family Therapy:* MFT core competencies
- *Psychology:* Psychology competency benchmarks
- *Social work:* Council for Social Work Education accreditation standards

Rubrics are provided correlating competencies for each profession to the skills demonstrated on the four learning assignments: case conceptualization, clinical assessment, treatment planning, and progress notes.

Instructor's Supplements

Instructors will find numerous resources for the book online on the Cengage website (www.cengage.com) or the author's websites (www.masteringcompetencies.com; www.dianegehart.com).

- Online lectures by the author
- Sample syllabi for how to use this book in pre-practicum skills class, practicum, or fieldwork class
- PowerPoints for all of the chapters
- Digital forms for the case conceptualization, clinical assessment, treatment plan, and progress note
- Test bank (available from your Cengage representative)
- Webquizzes
- Scoring rubrics precorrelated for national accreditation bodies
    - *Counseling:* Council on the Accreditation of Counseling and Related Educational Programs (CACREP) standards
    - *Marriage and Family Therapy:* MFT core competencies
    - *Psychology:* Psychology competency benchmarks
    - *Social Work:* Council for Social Work Education accreditation standards

Instructors can access these materials through their "Instructor Bookshelf" at Cengage Learning (https://login.cengage.com/cb), which can be created by completing a brief online registration form. Instructors can add the ancillaries for this title, and others, to their virtual bookshelves at any time.

Student Supplements

Students will find numerous useful resources for the text on the Cengage website (www.CengageBrain.com) and author websites (www.masteringcompetencies.com). These include:

- Online lectures: mp4 recordings of yours truly discussing content of select chapters
- Digital forms for the case conceptualization, clinical assessment, treatment plan, and progress note
- Scoring rubrics for each assignment
- Links to related websites and readings
- Glossary of key terms

Acknowledgements

I would like to thank the following content experts who gave their time and energy to ensure that the information in this textbook is accurate and current:

Rie Rogers Mitchell: Jungian sand play, psychodynamic theories
Luis Rubalcava: Psychodynamic theories
Stan Charnofsky: Humanistic, person-centered, Gestalt, existential
Wendel Ray and his doctoral students, Todd Gunter and Allison Lux: Systemic theories
Marion Lindblad-Goldberg: Systemic theories
Scott Woolley: Emotionally focused therapy
Bill O'Hanlon: Solution-based therapies
Harlene Anderson: Collaborative therapy
Gerald Monk: Narrative therapy
Ron Chenail: Competencies Assessment System
Thorana Nelson: Competencies Assessment System
William Northey: Competencies Assessment System

Instructor and student materials:

Diana Pantaleo
Rena Jacobs
Kayla Caceres

I would also like to thank the following people for their assistance:

Kayla Caceres: Research assistant
Eric Garcia: Librarian extraordinaire
Julie Martinez: My amazing and inspiring editor
Lori Bradshaw: Editorial guidance and instructor materials development
Anna and Guenther Gehart: For the extra hours taking care of Michael and Alex
Joseph McNicholas: For watching kids when I needed to write and for being my best friend
Michael McNicholas: For making each day a new adventure, for the best hugs ever, and for decorating my office with your art
Alexander McNicholas: For melting my heart each day with your "crazy cute" baby ways

Finally, I would like to thank the following reviewers and survey respondents who provided invaluable feedback on making this book work for faculty:

Stephan Demanchick, Nazareth College
Lori Longs Painter, Jack, Joseph and Morton Mandel School of Applied Social Sciences and Case Western Reserve University
Elizabeth Richardson, University of Massachusetts, Dartmouth
Mary Ballou, Northeastern University

Lisa Wilson, Hope International University
Claudia Sadler-Gerhardt, Ashland University/Ashland Seminary
Donna Dockery, Virginia Commonwealth University
Eric Nath, California State University, Stanislaus
Ginger Welch, University of Oklahoma, Norman
Neil Castronovo, Assumption College, Worcester
Patricia Cardner, Park University, Austin
Patricia Robey, Governors State University
Yvonne Barry, John Tyler Community College

About the Author

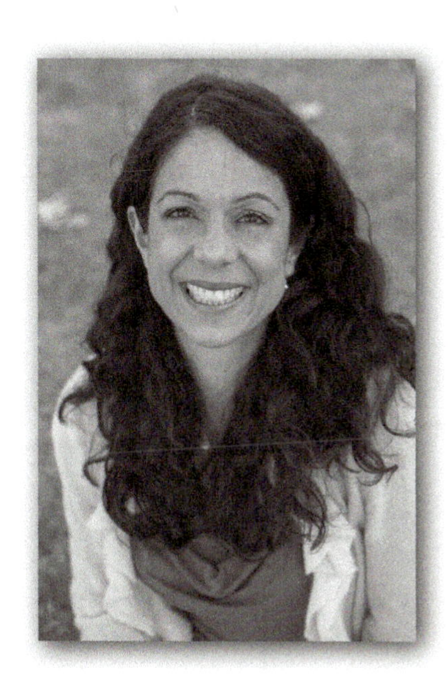

DR. DIANE R. GEHART is a professor in the Marriage and Family Therapy and Counseling Programs at California State University, Northridge. Having practiced, taught, and supervised for over 20 years, she has authored/edited the following:

- *Theory and Treatment Planning in Counseling and Psychotherapy*
- *Mastering Competencies in Family Therapy*
- *Theory and Treatment Planning in Family Therapy*
- *Mindfulness and Acceptance in Couple and Family Therapy*
- *Collaborative Therapy: Relationships and Conversations That Make a Difference* (coedited with Harlene Anderson)
- *The Complete MFT Core Competency Assessment System*
- *The Complete Counseling Assessment System*
- *Theory-Based Treatment Planning for Marriage and Family Therapists* (coauthored)

She has also written on postmodern therapies, mindfulness, mental health recovery, sexual abuse treatment, gender issues, children and adolescents, client advocacy, qualitative research, and counselor and marriage and family therapy education. She speaks internationally, having given workshops to professional and general audiences in the United States, Canada, Europe, and Mexico. Her work has been featured in newspapers, radio shows, and television worldwide, including the BBC, National Public Radio, Oprah Winfrey's *O* magazine, and *Ladies' Home Journal*. She is an associate faculty member at three international postgraduate training institutes: the Houston Galveston Institute, the Taos Institute, and the Marburg Institute for Collaborative Studies in Germany. Additionally, she is an active leader in state and national professional organizations. She maintains a private practice in Agoura Hills, California, specializing in couples, families, women's issues, trauma, life transitions, and difficult-to-treat cases. For fun, she enjoys spending time with her family, hiking, swimming, yoga, meditating, and savoring all forms of dark chocolate. You can learn more about her work at www.dianegehart.com

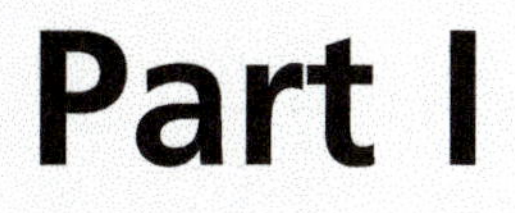

Part I

Introduction to Case Documentation

CHAPTER 1

Introduction to Case Documentation

Making a Difference—Competently

"I want to help others."
"I want to give back to my community."
"I want to make a difference."

Those who seek to become counselors and psychotherapists typically say they are drawn to the profession to help others with their struggles and to do something that makes the world a better place (Bager-Charleson, Chatterjee, Critchley, Lauchlan, McGrath, & Thorpe, 2010; Barnett, 2007; Hill et al., 2013). Many want to give back what they themselves have found life-transforming. Most envision days spent in meaningful conversations that are reflective, intimate, and life-altering.

Often, those drawn to the field find inspiration for this profound form of altruism and caring in the work of Carl Rogers (1961). Rogers proposed that accurate empathy, unconditional positive regard, and counselor genuineness were necessary and sufficient conditions for promoting change in clients. Although research over the years has not substantiated his proposition that these conditions alone are sufficient to promote change in all clients, mounting research suggests that they are typically necessary for virtually any form of counseling or psychotherapy to be successful (Kirschenbaum & Jourdan, 2005). In fact, the quality and strength of the counseling relationship is one of the best predictors of change in the counseling process (Miller, Duncan, & Hubble, 1997). However, an empathetic and caring relationship is only one piece of the puzzle; more is required to be considered *competent*, especially in contemporary mental health practice.

Over the past decade, mental health professionals have witnessed a transformation in their approach to training and conceptualizing what they do. External third parties, such as insurance companies, regulatory boards, and client families, want to more precisely understand what all counselors and therapists are expected to know and do. To address these demands, mental health professionals have develop detailed lists of competencies: specific areas of knowledge and skill sets that one must possess in order to be considered "competent" to practice independently (Gehart, 2011; Hoge et al., 2005; Nelson, Chenail, Alexander, Crane, Johnson, & Schwallie, 2007; Urofsky, 2013). Although each mental health profession has its own set of competencies—counselors, family therapists, clinical and counseling psychologists, clinical social workers, psychiatric nurses, and psychiatrists—the core features are, thankfully, more similar than different. This book helps readers understand and ultimately master mental health competencies that relate specifically to the counseling and psychotherapy process: *what competent counselors do, think, and say in session with clients*. These competencies are based on the foundational theories of the field, which provide a road map for professional counseling and psychotherapy.

The Other Half of Competence

To those less familiar with the field, it appears that competent counseling primarily involves good in-session skills: building a relationship, listening well, and offering helpful and well-timed interventions. However, those with more practical experience know the other half of the story: all of those subtle in-session assessments and interventions need to be carefully documented in writing. In fact, from the perspective of third-party stakeholders—insurance companies, clinic directors, and in some cases even supervisors—the written half of the job often trumps the verbal elements in terms of importance. Without clear, written documentation of one's work, there is no evidence that competent care was rendered—or that payment is due. In fact, in modern practice environments, documentation is the primary means of demonstrating proficient counseling. Thus, to be considered competent one needs to know not only what to think, say, and do with clients but also how to document what transpired.

Historically, these two sets of competencies have been thought of and taught separately (Wiger, 2005). However, in this book, we are going to explore these skills as two halves of the same process. The experience of my students is that the two sets of competencies—in-session skills and documentation—are interrelated and work synergistically together. The more competent you are in-session, the better able you are to document what you do. The clearer you document what you do, the clearer you become with words and actions in session. It becomes a virtuous cycle that leads to greater and greater competence. The case documentation presented in this book has evolved over the past two decades and has been constantly revised to simultaneously and efficiently develop both in-session counseling and documentation skills. So, you will be traversing a relatively new yet well-traveled bridge between two formerly separate worlds.

The Road to Competent Counseling

To conceptualize the numerous and sometimes seemingly contradictory elements of competent counseling, we will use a five-step map to competent counseling. This map provides a compact yet comprehensive guide to navigating the often-bumpy road of the 50-minute psychotherapy hour. Each step is solidly grounded in an essential clinical case document. Using this map, you will learn to link what you think, do, and say in session directly to what you write in your formal case files. Although they may seem like several complex steps in the beginning, with a little practice you will be zooming along from the first step to the last.

The Five Steps to Competent Counseling

The Five Steps to Competent Counseling: Mapping a Successful Counseling Journey

Step 1: Map the Territory: Conceptualize the situation using counseling and psychotherapy theories.

Step 2: Identify Oases and Obstacles: Assess client's mental status and strengths and provide case management.

Step 3: Chart a Course: Develop a treatment plan with treatment tasks—including how to build a working counseling relationship—and measurable client goals.

Step 4: Leave a Trail: Document your work with progress notes.

Step 5: Track Your Progress: Evaluate client response to the counseling process.

The five steps above follow a classic method used by all explorers in uncharted territory. And that's what each new counseling process is: uncharted territory, an unknown region, a *terra incognita*. It may seem at first that clients can be easily lumped into groups—anxious clients, divorcing couples, conduct-disordered children, for example—but any experienced counselor can tell you that each counselee's journey is unique. The excitement—and secret—to competent counseling is mapping the distinctive terrain of each client's life and charting a one-of-a-kind journey through it.

The first step is to delineate as much of the terrain as possible: to get the big picture. What are the contours of early development? Where are the comfort zones? Where is the well-traveled terrain? Is there a page marked "Here Be Dragons"? As with all maps, the more accurate and detailed the record, the easier it is to move through the actual territory. In counseling and psychotherapy, our maps are our *theoretical case conceptualizations*, assessments of the client using mental health theories. Although considered the most essential part of most approaches, in one study over 94% of practitioners failed to include a well-developed conceptualization in their formal case reports (Abbas, Premkumar, Goodarzi, & Walton, 2013). Now that you have this book in hand, you have a good chance of being in the most competent 6%.

Once you have a map, you identify the significant landmarks, the oases and the obstacles. Notice where the rest stops are and identify what dangers lie ahead. In counseling, you can recognize the *oases* as *client resources*: anything that can be used to strengthen and support the client. The *obstacles* appear as those potential or existing hindrances to creating change in the client's life. Are there really dragons in that region, or is the region just unfamiliar? Like a cartographer surveying the landscape, counselors assess potential obstacles carefully, ruling out potential medical issues in consultation with physicians, identifying psychiatric issues by conducting a *mental status exam*, and considering basic life needs such as a lack of financial and/or social resources through *case management*. By addressing actual or probable impediments early in counseling through a process called *clinical assessment*, the therapeutic journey is likely to proceed more easily and smoothly.

Once you have your conceptual map with oases and obstacles clearly identified, you can confidently chart a course toward the client's chosen destination or *goal*. If you have done a good job mapping, you will be able to choose from among several different courses, depending on what works best for those on the journey: namely, you and the client. This translates to being able to choose a counseling theory and style that suits all involved and that research indicates is likely to be helpful given the client's situation. Seasoned clinicians distinguish themselves from newer counselors in their ability to identify and successfully navigate through numerous terrains: forests, seas, deserts, plains, paradises, and wastelands. The greater a counselor's repertoire of skills, the better able the counselor is to move through each terrain. Once a preferred path is chosen, the counselor generates a *treatment plan*, a general set of directions for how to address client concerns. Like any set of travel plans, treatment plans are subject to change due to weather, natural disaster, human error, and other unforeseeable events, otherwise known as "real life." Counselors should be aware that unexpected detours, delays, and shortcuts (yes, unexpected good stuff happens, too) will be part of any counseling journey.

Once you select a course of action, you need to leave a trail to track where you have been. Leaving a trail always helps you find your way back if you get lost. It allows others (as well as yourself) to see why and how you proceeded. Counselors leave a trace of their path with *progress notes*, formal documentation of what happened in a given session. In addition to being the essential travel log, progress notes are also helpful with three highly prized aspects of professional counseling and psychotherapy: getting paid by third-party payers (i.e., insurance), avoiding lawsuits (i.e., the state lets you practice), and maintaining a license. By making it clear where you have been, you can help others—as well as you and the client—better understand your specific route of treatment.

Finally, you need to check frequently to make sure that you are on the right road. In counseling, this translates to *assessing client progress* along the way. If the client is not making progress, the counselor needs to go back and reassess (a) the accuracy of the map (conceptualization and clinical assessment) and (b) the wisdom of the plan.

Most always, it is easy to make improvements in one or both areas that will get things back on course again. The key is assessing client progress often enough to notice when you are off course as soon as possible.

These five steps of competent counseling cover quite a bit of terrain; so it will take some time to get comfortable with all the steps, and even longer to become nimble with linking the steps together. However, as you practice putting these steps together, you will find that working with clients becomes increasingly easier: you will become clearer about what to focus on, what to say, and what to do. This book is designed to help you move through these five steps more effectively, whether you are just starting out or have been counseling for years.

Engaging Case Documentation Mindfully

The five steps of competent counseling are organized around essential case documentation forms for a simple reason: these are the only concrete evidence of the counseling and therapeutic journey. However, for numerous reasons, many clinicians and educators would prefer to avoid them. In fact, clinical case documentation is readily identified as one of the most neglected educational tasks in the field, and also as a correlate to professional counselor burnout after graduation (Cianfrini, 1997; Elliott & Schrink, 2009; Prieto & Scheel, 2002). Completing long forms that require numeric codes, austere language, and painful detail leaves most warm-hearted counselors frozen with dread. Those who have not learned how to make documentation clinically relevant complain that the burden of paperwork detracts from their true mission: to help real people with real-life problems: "How can completing a form help a client? In no way can it possibly help me do my *real* job." This book will teach you to have a more productive and enjoyable relationship to case documentation—and learn to use it as a tool to support and further your true mission.

When mindless paperwork is completed as part of an endless churning bureaucracy, it can easily detract from being a good counselor. However, I propose that when approached mindfully and thoughtfully, case documentation paperwork can significantly enhance not only counselors' effectiveness but it can ultimately—once they have enough practice to do it quickly—make their jobs easier. How? Essentially, well-done case documentation helps clinicians think more clearly and precisely about that they are doing, which translates to being more focused and on-target in the counseling room (Abbas et al., 2013; Prieto & Scheel, 2002). So, my humble goal with this book is to help you befriend case documentation—if not for the idealistic goal of being a highly competent counselor, at minimum for the more realistic practicalities that involve getting paid and staying out of trouble.

Clear Writing=Clear Thinking

Writing skills have repeatedly been linked to better analytical and reasoning skills (Flateby, 2011; Hunter & Tse, 2013; Preiss, Castillo, Flotts, & Martín, 2013). Through writing, one has a chance to "see" one's own thinking more clearly and precisely. Often patterns and insights emerge on the page that are not imaginable when the same information stays in the head. This is the reason so many clients benefit from journaling, especially when the writing is focused on cognition and facts in addition to emotions (Borkin, 2014; Ullrich & Lutgendorf, 2002).

For counselors and psychotherapists, the particular gift of writing is enabling the practitioner to link in-session experiences to theory, research, and the knowledge base of the field. Case documentation is the one place where all of these worlds have the possibility to come together. When done well, case documentation quickly becomes a form of self-supervision, a reflective process that provides the type of insight and guidance one might expect from a clinical supervisor (Morrissette, 2001).

I would be the first to agree that not all case documentation achieves this end: some forms of documentation are too far removed from what is actually happening in session and others are too heavily weighed down in bureaucratic minutia that the larger clinical parts get lost (e.g., productivity logs). In this text, I introduce readers to a set of four clinical documents that have significant clinical utility and also meet contemporary documentation standards. This documentation aims to closely integrate theoretical and research findings of the field with real-world practice to create a system of documentation that enables counselors to meaningfully reflect upon and focus their work.

Documentation Practicalities

If clearer thinking does not inspire your enthusiasm for mastering case documentation competencies, then perhaps you will appreciate more traditional reasons. The first reason most clinicians cite for doing paperwork is the legal and ethical requirement (Wiger, 2005). Increasingly, "standard care" has come to mean maintaining specific written records that document client concerns and the course of action counselor's take to address them. When counselors do not maintain such records, they are increasingly found "negligent" when ethics review boards or legal entities become involved. In the past, the legal and ethical requirement for case documentation was less clear. However, after the implementation of the federal HIPAA privacy act in 2004, more systematic requirements have been established (see progress notes in Chapter 6). Although there is still wide variability in the form and level of detail and complexity of case documentation, increasingly the basic content is similar across clinicians and worksites, with greater consistency across the mental health disciplines in general—which is all a good thing for those learning case documentation.

The other common motivation for doing progress notes is financial. If you hope to be paid for your work, you will find that most employers and third-party payers require a significant amount of case documentation in order to pay you (Wiger, 2005). Although most in the field are motivated largely by compassion and selflessness, in the end counselors need to eat and pay their bills like everybody else. Employers need to document to third-party payers the fact that competent and appropriate services were provided.

Finally, short of observing sessions, case documentation is the easiest way to ensure competent care is being rendered. Rather than ask for videos of our sessions to prove our competence, third-party payers such as insurance companies instead verify our competence with our written case documentation. Clinical case documents, such as treatment plans and progress notes and assessments, are used to efficiently provide evidence that counselors are doing something worthy of reimbursement.

Developing In-Session Competencies Using Case Documentation

The majority of my students agree that the most cringe-inducing and humility-inspiring training technique is watching your own counseling videos: personally witnessing your awkward expressions, reexperiencing the uncomfortable silences, and hearing your rambling or off-target responses. A close second is transcribing and then analyzing those same videos. Both are excellent for developing humbleness and a greater understanding of the counseling process. I am hoping that writing the theory-informed case documentation in this book will provide similar learning outcomes without the humbleness factor. By taking the time to write a theory-informed case conceptualization, counselors more quickly develop a sophisticated clinical picture and a clear sense of where and how to best intervene with the client. Similarly, by taking time to identify the theory-specific interventions used in each session and the client's response to these interventions, counselors can quickly adjust what they say and do in session to help clients.

How This Book Is Different and What It Means to You

Case Documentation in Counseling and Psychotherapy is a different kind of textbook. Based on a new pedagogical model, learning-centered teaching (Killen, 2004; Weimer, 2002), this book is designed to help you *actively learn* the content and develop real-world competencies, rather than simply to provide information to be memorized. This book teaches real-world skills that you can immediately use to better serve your clients. Thus, learning activities are a central part of the text so that you have opportunities to apply and use the information in ways that facilitate learning. The specific learning activities in this book are (a) case conceptualization, (b) clinical assessment, (c) treatment planning, and (d) progress notes. These activities translate the theory learned in each chapter to practical client situations.

This book is different in another way: it is organized by key concepts rather than general headings with long narrative sections. This organization—which evolved from my personal study notes for my university and licensing exams—facilitates the retention of vocabulary and terms because of the visual layout. Each year I receive numerous emails from enthusiastic newly licensed counselors and therapists thanking me for helping them to pass their licensing exams—they all say that the organization of the book made the difference. So, spending some time with this text should better prepare you for the big exams in your future (and if you have already passed these, you should be all the more impressed with yourself for doing it the hard way).

Lay of the Land

This book is organized into three parts:

Part I: Introduction to Case Documentation: The first section details the five steps to competent counseling described at the beginning of this chapter:

- Case conceptualization
- Clinical assessment
- Treatment planning
- Progress notes
- Evaluating progress

Part II: Theory-Informed Case Documentation: The next section of the text reviews key concepts of each of the major counseling theories and provides a detailed case study with all four elements of case documentation presented in the book: counseling case conceptualization, clinical assessment with DSM-5 diagnosis, treatment plan, and progress notes. Case documentation is presented for the following theories:

- Psychodynamic
- Adlerian individual psychology
- Humanistic-existential: Person-centered, Gestalt, and existential
- Cognitive-behavioral
- Family systemic-structural
- Solution-focused
- Postmodern: Collaborative, narrative, and feminist

Part III: The Competent Supervisee: The last chapter introduces you to the paradigm of the competent supervisee and provides guidance for how to approach the supervisory relationship. If you have already started seeing clients, you might want to begin here; otherwise, this chapter will get you ready for doing so. This chapter includes elements such as:

- Managing initial anxiety
- Your role as supervisee
- Your supervisor's role
- Getting the most out of supervision
- What to do if things get bumpy

Where to Start Reading

This book is designed to be a versatile text for use in different class settings or for use by those in clinical practice. Thus, depending on a person's needs and primary learning goals, it can be read in different order. Some options include:

Pre-Practicum Course with Case Documentation as Primary Focus
- Part I: Introduces students to case documentation
- Part II: Provides review of documentation for each theory
- Part III: Prepares students for transition to seeing clients

Pre-Practicum Course with Skills as Primary Focus

- Part II: Provides review of assessment and intervention for each theory
- Part I: Introduces students to case documentation
- Part III: Prepares students for transition to seeing clients

Fieldwork Course

- Part III: Provides practical framework for conceptualizing supervisee role and for managing common problems
- Part I: Teaches foundational case documentation skills
- Part II: Provides examples of how to write case documentation for student's theory (ies) of choice

Counseling Theories Course

- Part II: Provides foundational instruction in counseling theories and methods
- Part I: Provides overview of case documentation
- Part III: Prepares students for transition to seeing clients

Theory Review

The chapters in Part II are designed to *briefly review* key concepts from each theory that are most applicable to case documentation; more thorough discussions of the theories are provided in *Theory and Treatment Planning in Counseling and Psychotherapy* (Gehart, 2013). These theory-review chapters are organized in a user-friendly way to maximize your ability to use the book to support you when developing case conceptualizations, writing treatment plans and progress notes, and designing interventions with clients. Theory chapters follow this outline:

Anatomy of a Theory

In a Nutshell: The Least You Need to Know

The Juice: Significant Contributions to the Field: If there is one thing to remember from this chapter it should be...

The Big Picture: Overview of the Therapy Process

Making Connection: The Therapy Relationship

The Viewing: Case Conceptualization

Targeting Change: Goal Setting

The Doing: Interventions

Try It Yourself: Exercises for Practicing Clinical Skills

Putting It All Together: Treatment Plan Template

- Treatment Plan Template for Individuals with Depression/Anxiety Symptoms

Tapestry Weaving: Working with Diverse Populations

- Ethnic, Racial, Gender, and Cultural Diversity
- Sexual Identity Diversity

Research and Evidence Base

Online Resources

Reference List

Case Example: Vignette with a complete set of clinical paperwork described in Part I, including case conceptualization, clinical assessment, treatment plan, and a progress note.

In a Nutshell: The Least You Need to Know: The chapters begin with a brief summary of the key features of the theory. Although it may not be the absolute least you need to know to get an A in a theory class or help a client, it is the basic information you should have memorized and be able to quickly articulate with a supervisor or colleague.

The Juice: Significant Contributions to the Field: In the next section, I use the principle of primacy (first information introduced) to help you remember one of the theory's most significant contributions to the field. In most cases, well-trained clinicians who generally use another approach to counseling are likely to use this particular concept because it has shaped standard practice in the field. This section is your red flag to remember a seminal concept or practice for the theory. Feedback from students indicates that this is often one of their favorite sections (I only hope that isn't because they skim the rest of the chapter).

Big Picture: Overview of Therapy Process: The big picture provides an overview of the flow of the therapy process: what happens in the beginning, middle, and end, and how change is facilitated across these phases.

Making Connection: Counseling Relationship: All approaches start by establishing a working relationship with clients, but each approach does it differently. In this section you will read about the unique ways that counselors of various schools build relationships that provide the foundation for change.

The Viewing: Case Conceptualization: The case conceptualization section will identify the signature theory concepts that counselors use to identify and assess clients and their problems. This really is the heart of the theory and where the real differences between theories emerge: I encourage you to spend extra time with these concepts.

Note: Theory-Specific Case Conceptualization: In the companion text, *Theory and Treatment Planning in Counseling and Psychotherapy* (Gehart, 2013), I provide templates and examples of *theory-specific* case conceptualizations: a narrative approach to case conceptualization using only one theory. To avoid confusion with the cross-theoretical conceptualization in this book, I have not included these templates in this text; however, you can use the concepts presented in the Case Conceptualization section of each chapter to develop a theory-specific case conceptualization.

Targeting Change: Goal Setting: Based on the areas assessed in the case conceptualization and the overall therapy process, each approach has a unique strategy for identifying client goals that become the foundation for the treatment plan.

The Doing: Interventions: Probably the most exciting part for most new counselors, the doing section outlines the common techniques and interventions for each theory. In some cases, a section for techniques used with special populations is included if these are notably different from those in standard practice.

Putting It All Together: Treatment Plan Templates: After graduation, you will probably thank me most for this section, which provides templates for a treatment plan that can be used for addressing depression, anxiety, or trauma with individual clients. These plans tie everything in the chapter together.

Tapestry Weaving: Working with Diverse Populations: This section reviews specific approaches for working with diverse populations using the theories covered in the chapter. Each chapter includes sections on (a) ethnic and (b) sexual identity diversity issues.

Research and Evidence Base: Finally, the chapters end with a brief review of the research and evidence base for each theory to offer a general sense of empirical foundations for the theory. In some cases, influential evidence-based treatments are highlighted.

Online Resources: A list of web pages and web documents are included for those who want to pursue specialized training or conduct further research on the theory.

Reference List: Many students pass right over reference lists and forget all about them. But if you have to do an academic paper or literature review on any of these theories, this should be your first stop. I used several hundred books and articles go through while writing this book. Thus, you can certainly shorten the time it takes to locate key resources by pursuing these before you hit the library yourself (oh, I forgot, no one steps foot in these places anymore; I meant "surf" the library's web page from your favorite couch or coffee house).

Case Example: Finally, each chapter ends with a case vignette, case conceptualization, clinical assessment, treatment plan, and progress note to give you a sense of how the theory looks in action and how to put it down on paper.

Voice and Tone

You have probably noticed that the voice and tone of this textbook is a bit different than your average college read. At times, I am talking right at ya'. I also like to add a touch of humor and fun. Why? I want to engage you as if you were one of my students or supervisees learning about how to apply these ideas for the first time. Counseling is a relationship-based practice, one in which the parties co-construct knowledge together. Thus, it is hard for me to write about these ideas as a detached, faceless author, thereby perpetuating the myth of objectivity in knowledge construction. So, as I write, I am imagining you as a full and real person eager to learn about how to use these ideas to help others. I am going to try to reach out to you, answer questions I imagine you have, and periodically tap you on the shoulder to make sure you are still awake.

Suggested Uses for This Text

Suggestions for Thinking about Theories

As you read the chapters in this book, you are going to be tempted to identify which ones you like the best and deemphasize the ones to which you are less attracted. This may seem like a great idea at first, but here are some points to consider:

Favorite versus Useful: The theories that the average counselor finds personally useful are probably not the same ones that the average client of a new counselor is likely to find useful. Many counselors are psychologically minded, meaning that they enjoy thinking about the inner world and how it works. However, most new counselors begin working with lower-fee clients that serve diverse, multi-problem clients and families, many (but not all) of whom are not psychologically minded because they are often struggling with issues of survival and/or they come from cultural traditions that place less value on cognitive analysis and insight into an inner world (Greenfield, 2013; Saravanan, Jacob, Prince, Bhugra, & David, 2004). So, the theory you find most useful to you personally may not be a good fit for your first client.

Appreciative: Regarding counseling theories, I also encourage a broad and generous attitude of appreciative inquiry, a solution-focused approach that identifies what is working and strives to build upon it (Cooperrider, Whitney, & Stavros, 2008). The theories in this book are not casually chosen; each has wisdom worthy of study. They have become part of the standard canon of theories because generations of counselors have found them uniquely helpful. The one lesson I have learned over the years is that the more theories counselors understand, the better able they are to serve their clients, because their understanding of the human condition and its concomitant problems is broader. Thus, I recommend approaching each theory with an attitude of searching for its most wide and useful parts. I facilitate this for you in the "Juice" section of each chapter that identifies the one concept I believe has near-universal utility from the particular theory.

Common Threads: Counseling theories are somewhat paradoxical: in one sense they are very different and inform distinct and mutually exclusive behaviors and attitudes. However, the better you understand one, the better you understand them all. In fact, some counselors, the common factors proponents, argue that theories are generally equally effective because they are simply different modes for delivering the same factors (Miller et al., 1997). So, it is quite possible that commonalities across theories are *more important* than their differences. As you read, you may want to watch for these common threads.

Suggestions for Using this Book to Learn Theories

First, I recommend that you set aside an hour or two to read about a single theory from beginning to end (from the In a Nutshell to Putting It All Together) to help get the full sense of the theory. Some chapters cover two theories, so for these it is fine to read the chapter in chunks. Additionally, some learners may find it helpful to scan the treatment plan (either the template or example at the end of the chapter) or some other section first to provide a practical overview; that said, I have tried to organize the ideas in the way most people seem to prefer. I encourage you to discover what works best for you, since different learners have different strategies that work best for them. When you are done with a chapter, you might want to try completing a case conceptualization and treatment plan for yourself (you may have to make up a problem if you are nearly perfect) or for someone else, to get a sense of how this would work.

Finally, I strongly recommend that either after reading the chapter or after going to class you take good old-fashioned notes. Yes, I mean it. I recommend that you type up (or if you prefer, handwrite) a complete outline of the key concepts in your own words. Why do I advocate for such a laborious task? All of us, myself included, when we read long, dense books such as this one, fade in and out of alert attentiveness to what we are reading—often lapsing into more interesting fantasies or less interesting to-do lists—and, gasp!—sometimes even skim large sections of the text (no, I am not surprised or offended). The only way to make sure that you really understand the concepts you read about is to put them in your own words and organize them in a way that make sense to you. If you need to take culminating exams or plan to pursue licensure, you will have to log the concepts in this book into your long-term memory, which requires more than cramming for a final exam. Being a mental health professional requires that you master what you learn. You will be expected to know what is in this book for the entire time you are active in the profession (and if you think that is bad, just wait until you see the text you're assigned in your diagnosis class). Thus, if your former study habits included all-night cramming, gallons of espresso (or another favorite caffeine delivery system), and little recall after the exam, you might want to try my note-taking tip or some other strategy as you move forward.

Suggestions for Writing Assessments, Treatment Plans, and Notes

I want to be the first to inform you that each agency and counseling center will have its unique set of forms for clinical assessment, treatment planning, and progress notes. Some will look nothing like what is in this book. Many of my readers find this distressing at first. However, if you look closely, you will notice that regardless of the vastly different forms, the basic ingredients are very similar—if not identical. The documents in this text are likely more detailed and with more prompts than what you will find in the field: this is intended to make the micro-steps clear for those in the early process of learning. You may find it helpful to take the time to label the items on the forms at your practice site with the various elements of the forms in the text to help you see the connections. If that is still a struggle, you may contact me via masteringcompetencies.com or YouTube.com, and I will personally help you translate. Additionally, the chapters in Part I of the book include resources to help with completing forms at any site, such as the list of mental status exam terms in Chapters 3 and 4.

Similarly, I want to emphasize that the treatment plan templates and examples in this book are just that: templates and examples. They do not represent the only approach or the only right approach, simply a solid approach based on the common standards and expectations. Feel free to modify the goal statements and techniques to fit the unique needs of your client. I have provided some relatively specific goals as an example of what might work, and I encourage you to radically tailor these for each client's unique needs. You will notice that treatment plans in the case study do not rigidly follow the templates; I encourage you to do the same.

Suggestions for Use in Internships and Clinical Practice

When working as an intern or licensed mental health professional, this book can be useful for teaching yourself theories and techniques in addition to learning how to complete clinical documentation. You will likely find that when you work with new populations and problems, you may be interested in considering how other therapy models might approach these situations. This book is designed to be a prime resource for quickly scanning to identify other possibilities. Alternatively, you might have a colleague or supervisor who uses a theory with which you are not familiar. You can use this book to quickly review that theory and avoid looking uneducated. In addition, this book is written to help you appreciate and find common ground across theories, which can be of particular benefit when working in a "mixed theory" context. However, to actually learn to practice any of these theories well, I strongly urge you to take advanced training from experts in that approach.

Suggestions for Studying for Licensing Exams

Licensing exams are not designed to be unnecessarily tricky or scary, simply to ensure that you have knowledge necessary to practice without supervision *and not harm anybody*. If you have honestly engaged your classes, done your homework, avoided cramming for tests and papers, and made it a priority to get decent supervision, you should have a strong foundation for taking your licensing exam. You should already have in your possession books (such as this) that cover all of the content to be studied for the exam. If your exam is to be taken upon finishing a lengthy post-Masters internship, you should use the entire two- to four-year period to read as many books as possible on the theories and materials covered by the exam (no novels for a few years).

I do not recommend that all of my students take long, expensive "review courses," because such courses are not necessary for those who are proactive in mastering the material on the exam long before they sign up to take it. If you start studying only after you are approved to take the test, you are starting about two to four years too late—and then, yes, you will need to take a crash course. My basic suggestion for studying for the mental health licensing exam is this: Read an original text on each major theory during your post-degree internship, use the DSM, and keep up with laws and ethics; then buy the practice exams (without the study guides) and take them until you consistently get 5% above the required passing score (e.g., 75% if the passing score is 70%). If you find that you are weak in a particular area, such as theory or DSM, use a text such as this, which is designed with the license review in mind. Once you consistently get 75%, you are ready to take the test with the most learning and the least expense.

Suggestions for Faculty to Measure Competencies and Student Learning

This book is specifically designed to help faculty and supervisors simplify and streamline the onerous task of measuring student competencies as required by the various accreditation bodies. The forms and scoring rubrics for assessing student learning using counseling, psychology, social work, and family therapy competencies are available on the book's web page for instructors (see www.CengageBrain.com and www.masteringcompetencies.com). On this website, instructors will also find free online lectures, PowerPoints, sample syllabi, and a test bank (test banks are available only from your Cengage sales representative to maintain security of the questions). This text may be used as the primary or secondary text in a counseling therapy theories class or as a primary text in a pre-practicum or practicum/fieldwork class. Because of its combination of solid theory and practical skills, it can easily be used across more than one class to develop students' abilities to conceptualize theory and complete clinical documentation, skills that are not likely to be mastered in a single class.

When designing a class to measure competencies and student learning using these case documents, I recommend initially going over the scoring rubrics with students so that they understand how these are used to clearly define what needs to be done and the expectations for the final product. I have found that it is most helpful to provide two to three opportunities to practice case conceptualization and treatment planning over a semester to provide feedback and enable students to improve and build upon these skills in a systematic fashion. Specifically, I have a small group present a case conceptualization and treatment plan with each theory studied, based on a video the class watches on the theory; that way students have enough information to actually conceptualize the client dynamics and treatment. Then, the entire class can see an example and discuss the thought process of developing the plan. A later or final assignment for the class can be to independently develop a treatment plan for a case (either one assigned by the instructor, from a popular movie, personal life, or actual client). By the end of a semester with these activities, students will have developed not only competence but also confidence in their case conceptualization and treatment planning abilities.

Questions for Personal Reflection and Class Discussion

1. How would you define professional "competence"?
2. What is the relative importance of in-session skills versus written documentation skills in defining a counselor's or psychotherapist's professional competence?
3. What are your thoughts on the relationship between writing and thinking?
4. Of the five steps to competent counseling—case conceptualization, clinical assessment, treatment planning, progress notes, and evaluation—which are you most excited about? Which is the least intriguing? Why?
5. What personal strengths do you bring to the five steps of competent counseling? What limitations might you have?

Online Resources for Students

Students will find numerous useful resources for the text on the Cengage (www.CengageBrain.com) and author websites (www.dianegehart.com; www.masteringcompetencies.com) and YouTube.com. These include:

- Online lectures: mp4 recordings of "yours truly" discussing content of select chapters
- Digital forms for all assignments: case conceptualization, clinical assessment, treatment plan, and progress note
- Scoring rubrics for each assignment
- Links to related websites and readings
- Glossary of key terms

Online Resources for Instructors

Instructors will find numerous resources for the book online on the Cengage site (www.CengageBrain.com) or the author's sites (www.masteringcompetencies.com; www.dianegehart.com):

- Online lectures by the author
- Sample syllabi for how to use this book in a theory class, pre-practicum skills class, or practicum class
- PowerPoints for all of the chapters
- Digital forms for all assignments: case conceptualization, clinical assessment, treatment plan, and progress note
- Scoring rubrics for each assignment correlated to each profession's competencies: counseling, family therapy, psychology, and social work
- Test bank
- Webquizzes

References

Abbas, M., Premkumar, L., Goodarzi, A., & Walton, R. (2013). Lost in documentation: A study of case-formulation in letters after outpatient assessment. *Academic Psychiatry*, *37*(5), 336–338. doi:10.1176/appi.ap.12060114

Bager-Charleson, S., Chatterjee, S., Critchley, P., Lauchlan, S., McGrath, S., & Thorpe, F. (2010). *Why therapists choose to become therapists: A practice-based inquiry*. London: Karnac Books.

Barnett, M. (2007). What brings you here? An exploration of the unconscious motivations of those who choose to train and work as psychotherapists and counsellors. *Psychodynamic Practice: Individuals, Groups and Organisations*, *13*(3), 257–274. doi:10.1080/14753630701455796

Borkin, S. (2014). *The healing power of writing: A therapist's guide to using journaling with clients*. New York: W. W. Norton.

Cianfrini, C. (1997, March). A comparison of university academic and psychological counselors: Burnout and its relationship with social support, coping, and job satisfaction. *Dissertation Abstracts International Section A*, *57*, p. 3824.

Cooperrider, D. L., Whitney, D., & Stavros, J. M. (2008). *Appreciative inquiry handbook: For leaders of change* (2nd ed.). San Francisco, CA: Berrett-Koehler Publishers.

Elliott, W. N., & Schrink, J. L. (2009). Understanding the special challenges faced by the correctional counselor in the prison setting. In P. Van Voorhis, M. Braswell, & D. Lester (Eds.), *Correctional counseling and rehabilitation* (7th ed.) (pp. 23–40). Cincinnati, OH: Anderson Publishing.

Gehart, D. (2011). The core competencies in marriage and family therapy education: Practical aspects of transitioning to a learning-centered, outcome-based pedagogy. *Journal of Marital and Family Therapy*, *37*, 344–354. doi:10.1111/j.1752-0606.2010.00205.x

Gehart, D. (2013). *Theory and treatment planning in counseling and psychotherapy: A competency-based approach for applying theory in clinical practice*. Pacific Grove, CA: Brooks/Cole.

Greenfield, P. M. (2013). The changing psychology of culture from 1800 through 2000. *Psychological Science*, *24*(9), 1722–1731.

Hill, C. E., Lystrup, A., Kline, K., Gebru, N. M., Birchler, J., Palmer, G., et al. (2013). Aspiring to become a therapist: Personal strengths and challenges, influences, motivations, and expectations of future psychotherapists. *Counselling Psychology Quarterly*, *26*(3–4), 267–293. doi:10.1080/09515070.2013.825763

Flateby, T. L. (2011). *Improving writing and thinking through assessment.* Charlotte, NC: IAP Information Age Publishing.

Hoge, M. A., Paris, M., Jr., Adger, H., Jr., Collins, F. L., Jr., Finn, C. V., Fricks, L., et al. (2005). Workforce competencies in behavioral health: An overview. *Administration and Policy in Mental Health and Mental Health Services Research*, *32*, 593–631.

Hunter, K., & Tse, H. (2013). Making disciplinary writing and thinking practices an integral part of academic content teaching. *Active Learning in Higher Education*, *14*(3), 227–239. doi:10.1177/1469787413498037

Killen, R. (2004). *Teaching strategies for outcome-based education*. Cape Town, South Africa: Juta Academic.

Kirschenbaum, H., & Jourdan, A. (2005). The current status of Carl Rogers and the Person-Centered Approach. *Psychotherapy: Theory, Research, Practice, Training*, *42*, 37–51.

Miller, S. D., Duncan, B. L., & Hubble, M. (1997). *Escape from Babel: Toward a unifying language for psychotherapy practice*. New York: Norton.

Morrissette, P. J. (2001). *Self-supervision: A primer for counselors and helping professionals*. New York: Brunner-Routledge.

Nelson, T. S., Chenail, R. J., Alexander, J. F., Crane, R. Johnson, S. M., & Schwallie, L. (2007). The development of the core competencies for the practice of marriage and family therapy. *Journal of Marital and Family Therapy*, *33*, 417–438.

Preiss, D. D., Castillo, J., Flotts, P., & Martín, E. (2013). Assessment of argumentative writing and critical thinking in higher education: Educational correlates and gender differences. *Learning and Individual Differences*, *28*, 193–203. doi:10.1016/j.lindif.2013.06.004

Prieto, L. R., & Scheel, K. R. (2002). Using case documentation to strengthen counselor trainees' case conceptualization skills. *Journal of Counseling & Development*, *80*(1), 11–21. doi:10.1002/j.1556-6678.2002.tb00161.x

Rogers, C. (1961). *On becoming a person: A counselor's view of psychocounseling*. London: Constable.

Saravanan, B. B., Jacob, K. S., Prince, M. M., Bhugra, D. D., & David, A. S. (2004). Culture and insight revisited. *British Journal of Psychiatry*, *184*(2), 107–109. doi:10.1192/bjp.184.2.107

Ullrich, P. M., & Lutgendorf, S. K. (2002). Journaling about stressful events: Effects of cognitive processing and emotional expression. *Annals of Behavioral Medicine*, *24*(3), 244–250. doi:10.1207/S15324796ABM2403_10

Urofsky, R. I. (2013). The council for accreditation of counseling and related educational programs: Promoting quality in counselor education. *Journal of Counseling & Development*, *91*(1), 6–14. doi:10.1002/j.1556-6676.2013.00065.x

Weimer, M. (2002). *Learner-centered teaching: Five key changes to practice*. New York: Jossey-Bass.

Wiger, D. E. (2005). *The psychotherapy documentation primer* (2nd ed.). New York: Wiley.

CHAPTER

2

Case Conceptualization

Map the Territory: Case Conceptualization

Only one thing separates a great counselor from a caring friend, bartender, or hairdresser who listens well—what each does with the information that is shared. After hearing a heartfelt story of struggle, friends, bartenders, and hairdressers tend to do one of two things: give advice or offer sympathy. Counselors do something different. They use what they have heard to develop a deeper understanding of clients, often a more sensible and compassionate story than clients tell themselves. When counselors listen to clients, they take the information that they are hearing to develop a map of the person's experience and inner world. This map is called case conceptualization, and it is the key to skillful, competent counseling. If you can develop a clear and accurate case conceptualization, the counseling journey is quick and smooth. If you miss the boat with this first step, you won't get very far.

Case Conceptualization is the technical term for the counseling art of viewing; it is also sometimes referred to as *assessment.* Assessment is a tricky term because it can refer to two different counseling tasks: either a case conceptualization approach to assessing individual and family dynamics (covered in this chapter) or a diagnostic approach to assess client symptoms (which will be covered in Chapter 3, Introduction to Clinical Assessment and Diagnosis). To reduce confusion, I refer to a theory-informed assessment as *case conceptualization* and to a diagnostic assessment as *clinical assessment.*

Counseling theories provide counselors with unique lenses through which they may view the problems clients bring to them. Much like a detailed map, theories allow counselors to view clients and their problems in a broader and more comprehensive context. This broad view allows counselors to see how the pieces fit together in a client's life and provides clues as to the best path out of a sticky situation.

Realistic Expectations

After forming a strong working relationship with clients, case conceptualization is the second most important skill in counseling. However—and I will tell this to you without sugercoating—case conceptualization is one of the hardest skill to learn. In short, case conceptualization requires that you understand and apply most of what is in the second half of this book. That said, case conceptualization is also the most empowering and liberating counseling competency—because once you can do this, you will know how to handle almost every situation. So, roll up your sleeves and get ready for intense work.

In most cases, the first time you complete the case conceptualization in this text, it will take several hours over the course of a week or more (this is one assignment you cannot cram the night before it is due). However, each time you do another one, you will find you can complete it more quickly and easily because you are learning how to integrate and use the theoretical concepts. By doing this once, you learn what to listen for and ask about in session with clients. The next time you do it, you begin to better understand how dynamics in one section correlate with dynamics in another. After you do 10–20 of these, your ability to conceptualize will significantly increase your counseling abilities in both in-session interventions and out-of-session communications with your supervisor and other professionals.

Elements of Case Conceptualization

As counselors become more experienced, case conceptualization takes place primarily in their heads—while clients are talking. It happens so fast that often they have a hard time tracing their steps. However, new counselors need to take things more slowly. Similar to learning a new dance step, the new move needs to be broken down into small pieces with specific instructions for where the hands and feet go; with practice, the dancer is able to put the pieces together more quickly and smoothly until it becomes "natural" to them. That is what we are going to do here with case conceptualization.

So, let's start with identifying the components of a counseling case conceptualization for working with an individual (for those who are interested, a separate case conceptualization for working with couples and families is presented in *Mastering Competencies in Family Therapy*):

1. **Introduction of Client:** Identify the client's and his/her significant others' most salient demographics (e.g., age, ethnicity, language, job, grade, etc.).
2. **Presenting Concern:** Specify how all parties involved are defining the problem: client, family, friends, school, work, legal system, society, etc.
3. **Background Information:** Summarize recent changes including precipitating events as well as related historical background.
4. **Strengths and Diversity:** Identify personal, relational, and spiritual strengths as well as resources and limitations related to diversity issues.
5. **Theoretical Case Conceptualization(s)**
   Use one or more of the following to develop an initial theoretical understanding of the client's personal and relational dynamics:
   - *Psychodynamic/Adlerian Conceptualization:* Includes defense mechanisms, object relations patterns, Erickson's psychosocial development stages, and Adlerian style of life and basic mistake
   - *Humanistic-Existential Conceptualization:* Expression of authentic self, existential analysis, and Gestalt contact boundary disturbances
   - *Cognitive-Behavioral Conceptualization:* Behavioral Baseline, ABC analysis, and schema analysis
   - *Family Systemic:* Family life-cycle stage, boundaries, triangles, hierarchy, complementarity, intergenerational patterns
   - *Solution-Based and Cultural Discourse Conceptualization:* Previous solution, unique outcomes, miracle question, dominant discourses, identity narratives, and preferred discourses.

Alternatively, you can use the "case conceptualization" section of your preferred theory to develop a shorter, theory-specific case conceptualization for your client. The complete form for case conceptualization is at the end of this chapter and is also available on the publisher's and book's websites (www.CengageBrain.com; www.masteringcompetencies.com). Below you will find basic instructions for completing each section; you will find the concepts in the "theoretical conceptualization" sections described in more depth in the corresponding theory chapter later in the book. *Examples of how to complete a case conceptualization are found at the end of each of the theoretical chapters of this text.*

Digital Download

Introduction to Client

Client				
Select Client Type Age: ____	Select Ethnicity	Select Relational Status	Occupation/Grade: ____	Other: ______
Significant Others				
Select Person Age: ______	Select Ethnicity	Select Relational Status	Occupation/Grade: ______	Other: ______
Select Person Age: ______	Select Ethnicity	Select Relational Status	Occupation/Grade: ______	Other: ______
Select Person Age: ______	Select Ethnicity	Select Relational Status	Occupation/Grade: ______	Other: ______
Select Person Age: ______	Select Ethnicity	Select Relational Status	Occupation/Grade: ______	Other: ______

Case conceptualization starts by identifying the most salient demographic features that relate to treatment. Common demographic information includes:

- gender,
- age,
- ethnicity,
- current occupation/work status or grade in school,
- family status, sexual orientation, and so on.

This initial introduction provides the reader with a basic sketch of the client that will be elaborated upon as the case conceptualization unfolds.

Symbols:

AF = Adult Female   CF = Child Female

AM = Adult Male   CM = Child Male

Presenting Concern

II. Presenting Concern(s)

Client Description of Problem(s): ______________________________

____

____

Significant Other/Family Description(s) of Problems: ______________________________

____

____

Broader System Problem Descriptions: Description of problem from referring party, teachers, relatives, legal system, etc.:

Name: ______________________________

Name: ______________________________

Often, new and even experienced counselors assume that the "presenting concern" is a straightforward and clear-cut matter. Once in a while it is, but most of the time it is surprisingly complex. Anderson and Goolishian (Anderson, 1997; Anderson & Gehart, 2007) developed a unique way of conceptualizing the presenting problem in their Collaborative Language Systems Approach, also referred to as Collaborative Therapy (Chapter 14). This postmodern approach maintains that each person who is talking about the problem is part of the *problem-generating system*, the set of relationships that generated the perspective or idea that there is a problem. Each person who is talking about the problem has a different definition of the problem; sometimes the difference is slight and sometimes stark. For example, when parents bring a child to counseling, the mother, father, siblings, grandparents, teachers, school counselors, doctors, and friends have different ideas as to what the problem *really* is. The mother may think it is a medical problem, such as ADHD; the father may believe it is related to his wife's permissiveness; the teacher may say it is poor parenting; and the child may think there really is not a problem at all.

Historically, counselors move rapidly to define the problem in a way that fits with their theoretical worldview: either a formal diagnosis (ADHD, depression, etc.) or another mental health category (such as parenting style, defense mechanism, family dynamics, etc.), with little reflection on the contradictory opinions and descriptions of the problem by the various people involved. Having a single problem definition helps focus the treatment. However, if adhered to too rigidly, having a single problem definition can quickly become a liability rather than an asset. The more a counselor can remain open to the alternative descriptions of the problem, the more maneuverability, adaptability, and creativity can be infused in treatment. In addition, remaining cognizant of the variability of understanding throughout treatment allows the counselor to maintain stronger rapport with each person involved, because each person's perspective is honored and referred to throughout the treatment.

A description of the presenting problem should include:

a) the reason(s) each client states he/she is seeking counseling or has been referred,
b) any information from the referring agent (teacher, doctor, psychiatrist, etc.) and his/her description of the problem,
c) a brief history of the problem and family (if applicable),
d) descriptions of the attempted solutions and the outcome of these attempts, and
e) perspectives from significant persons and institutions in the client's broader social network, including professional associates, religious organizations, close friends, etc.

Background Information

III. Background Information

Trauma/Abuse History (recent and past): ______________________

____

Substance Use/Abuse (current and past; self, family of origin, significant others): ______

____

____

Precipitating Events (recent life changes, first symptoms, stressors, etc.): ____________

____

____

(continued)

Related Historical Background (family history, related issues, previous counseling, medical/mental health history, etc.):________________________________

____

____

Obtaining background information about the problem is the next step. Traditionally, counselors include information such as:

- history of childhood and adulthood abuse and trauma, including childhood abuse, rape, domestic violence, natural disasters, war, witnessing violence, etc.
- history of substance abuse by client, client's family, and significant others,
- precipitating events that are associated with the onset of the problem, such as recent life changes, breakups, losses, developmental milestones, career moves, etc.
- related historical background, including history of mental disorders, previous counseling, significant health concerns, etc.

Often, this background information is considered the "facts" of the case. However, as counselors have historically cautioned, how we "language" the facts makes all the difference (Anderson, 1997; O'Hanlon & Weiner-Davis, 1989; Watzlawick, Weakland, & Fisch, 1974). For example, whether you begin by saying that the client "recently won a state-level academic decathlon" or begin with "her mother recently divorced her alcoholic father," you paint two very different pictures of the same client for both you and anyone else who reads the assessment. Therefore, although this may seem like the "factual" part of the report where you as a professional are not imposing your bias, in fact, you impose bias by the subtle choice of words, ordering of information, and emphasis on particular details.

Based on research about the importance of the counseling relationship and of hope (Lambert & Ogles, 2004; Miller, Duncan, & Hubble, 1997), I recommend that counselors write the background section in such a way that the counselor and anyone reading the report, including potentially the client, would have a positive impression of and hope for the client because these two factors have an effect on the outcome of treatment.

Assessment of Strengths and Diversity

Everything up to this point has been an introduction that provides a context and framework for understanding the actual assessment elements of the case conceptualization. In the following areas of assessment, counselors assess their clients using theoretical constructs from the major counseling theories to paint a multidimensional picture of clients and their life situation.

Client Strengths

Client Strengths

Personal: ____

____

Relational/Social: ____

____

Spiritual: ____

____

Client strengths and resources should be the first thing assessed. This is a lesson I learned the hard way. When I began teaching case conceptualization, I put the client strength section at the end because it is more clearly associated with solution-based and postmodern approaches (Chapters 13 and 14; Anderson, 1997; de Shazer, 1988; White & Epston, 1990), which were developed later historically. What I discovered is that after reading about the presenting problem, history, and problematic family dynamics, I was often feeling quite hopeless about the case. However, often upon reading the strengths section at the end, I would immediately perk up and find myself having hope, deep respect, and even excitement about the clients and their future. I have since decided to *start* by assessing strengths and I believe it puts the counselor in a more resourceful mind-set.

Emerging research supports the importance of identifying client strengths and resources. Researchers who developed the *common factors model* (Lambert & Ogles, 2004; Miller et al., 1997) estimate that 40% of outcome variance can be attributed to client factors, such as severity of symptoms, access to resources, support system, and so on; the remaining factors include the quality of the counseling relationship (30%), counseling interventions and treatment models (15%), and the client's sense of hope (15%). Counselors can leverage client factors best by assessing for resources. Furthermore, assessing for strengths also strengthens the counseling relationship (30%) and can be done in such a way as to instill hope (15%), thus drawing on three of the four common factors. The potential impact of assessing strengths is hard to overestimate.

To conceptualize a full spectrum of client strengths and resources, counselors can include strengths at several levels:

- Personal/individual strengths
- Relational/social strengths and resources
- Spiritual resources

Personal/Individual Strengths

When assessing for personal/individual strengths and resources, you can begin by reviewing two general categories of strengths: abilities and personal qualities.

- **Abilities:** Where and how are clients functioning in daily life? How do they get to session? Are they able to maintain a job, a hobby, or a relationship? Are there any special talents, either now or in the past? If you look, you will always find a wide range of abilities with even the most "dysfunctional" of clients, especially if you consider the past as well as present and future.

  Naming the abilities can increase clients' sense of hope and confidence to address the problem at hand. I find this especially helpful with children. If a child is having academic problems at school, the family, teachers, and child may not notice how the child is excelling in an extracurricular activity such as karate, soccer, or piano. Often noticing these areas of accomplishment makes it easier for all involved to find hope for improving the situation.

  Identifying the abilities may give clients or counselors creative ideas about how to solve a current problem. For example, I worked with a recovering alcoholic who hated the idea of writing but spoke often of how music inspired her. By drawing on this strength, we developed the idea of creating a special "sobriety mix" of favorite songs to help maintain sobriety and prevent relapse, an activity that had deep significance and inspiration for her.
- **Personal Qualities:** Another area where counselors can identify client strengths is personal qualities. Ironically, the best place to find these is embedded within the presenting problem or complaint. Usually, the thing that brings them to see a counselor is the flip side of another strength. For example, if a person complains about worrying a lot, that person is equally likely to be a diligent and productive worker. Persons who argue with a spouse or child are more likely to speak up for themselves and are generally invested in the relationship in which they are arguing. In virtually

all cases, the knife cuts both ways: each liability contains within it a strength in another context. Conversely, a strength in one context is often a problem in another. Here is a list of common problems and the strengths that may be found in clients with the presenting problems.

Problem	Possible Associated "Shadow Strengths"
Depression	• Awareness of what others think and feel • Connected to others and/or desires connection • Has dreams and hopes • Has had the courage to take action to realize dreams • Realistic assessment of self/others (according to recent research; Seligman, 2002)
Anxiety	• Pays attention to details • Desires to perform well • Careful and thoughtful about actions • Able to plan for future and anticipate potential obstacles
Arguing	• Stands up for self and/or beliefs • Fights injustice • Wants the relationship to work • Has hope for better things for others/self
Anger	• In touch with feelings and thoughts • Stands up against injustice • Believes in fairness • Able to sense their boundaries and when they are crossed
Overwhelmed	• Concerned about others' needs • Thoughtful • Able to see the big picture • Sets goals and pursues them

As you can see, identifying strengths relies heavily on the counselor's viewing skills. A skilled counselor is able to "see" the strengths that are the flip side of the presenting problem while remaining aware of the problem tendencies that are the inverse of a particular strength.

Relational/Social Strengths and Resources

- **Social support network:** Family, friends, professionals, teachers, coworkers, bosses, neighbors, church members, salespeople, and numerous others in a person's life can be part of a network of social support that helps the client in physical, emotional, and spiritual ways.
    - *Physical forms of support* include people who may help with errands, picking up the children, or doing tasks around the house.
    - *Emotional support* may take the form of listening or helping resolve relational problems.
    - *Community support* includes friendships and acceptance provided by any community, and it is almost always there in some form with a person who may be feeling marginalized due to culture, sexual orientation, language, religion, or similar factors. These communities are critical for coping with the inherent stress of marginalization.

Simply naming, recognizing, and appreciating that there is support can immediately increase a client's sense of hope and reduce feelings of loneliness.

Spiritual Resources

- **Spiritual:** Increasingly, counselors are increasing their awareness of how clients' spiritual resources can be used to address the problems they bring to counseling (Morgan, 2006; Sperry, 2001; Walsh, 2003). Counselors should become familiar with the major religious traditions in their community, such as Protestantism, Catholicism, Judaism, Islam, New Age religions, Native American practices, or others as needed.

  Drawing on the epistemological foundations of Bateson (1972, 1979/2002) and more recent postmodern philosophies (Gergen, 1999), I have developed a definition of spirituality that I find particularly helpful for work as a counselor:

Spirituality: How a person conceptualizes his/her relationship to the universe or God (or however he/she constructs that which is larger than the self). In short, how a person relates to Life (in the largest sense of the word).

Using this definition, everyone has some form of spirituality, which ultimately relates to how a person believes the universe operates. The rules of "how life should go" inevitably inform (a) what the person perceives to be a problem, (b) how a person feels about it, and (c) what that person believes can "realistically" be done about it, all of which a counselor wants to know about in order to help develop an effective treatment plan.

Questions to Assess Spirituality

A counselor can use some of the following questions to assess a client's spirituality, whether traditional or nontraditional:

- Do you believe there is a God or some form of intelligence that organizes the universe? If so, what types of things does that being/force have control over?
- If there is not a God, by what rules does the universe operate? Why do things happen? Or is life entirely random?
- What is the purpose and/or meaning of human existence? How does this inform how a person should approach life?
- Is there any reason to be kind to others? To one's self?
- What is the ideal versus realistic way to approach life?
- Why do "bad" things happen to "good" people?
- Do you believe things happen for a reason? If so, what reason?
- Does the client belong to a religious community or spiritual circle of friends that provides spiritual support, inspiration, and/or guidance in some way?

Digital Download Download from CengageBrain.com

With the answers to these questions, counselors can create a map of the client's world, which can then be used to develop conversations and interventions that are deeply meaningful and a good "fit" for the client. An accurate understanding of a client's "map of the life" reveals what logic and actions will motivate the client to make changes, providing counselors with invaluable resources for changes. For example, I have often found that many clients from traditional religious backgrounds as well as more New Age groups believe that "things happen for a reason." I have had numerous clients use this one belief to radically and quickly transform how they feel, think, and respond to difficult situations.

Diversity

Diversity: Resources and Limitations

Identify potential resources and limitations available to clients based on their age, gender, sexual orientation, cultural background, socioeconomic status, religion, regional community, language, family background, family configuration, abilities, and so on.

Unique Resources: ______________________________

Potential Limitations: ______________________________

Related to strengths, diversity issues refer to characteristics such as age, gender, sexual orientation, cultural background, immigration status, socioeconomic status, religion, regional community, language, family background, family configuration, or ability. Much like strengths and symptoms, in most cases, each form of diversity brings with it both unique resources and limitations. For many clients, traumatic and oppressive experiences related to being in a minority or being simply "different" are at the core of their problematic situation, if not an exacerbating factor. Some counseling theories, such as feminist theory, narrative, and collaborative, consider these at the heart of the case conceptualization process (see Chapter 2). But in all cases, counselors need to take time to think about how the client's situation is affected by limitations created by diversity issues, such as living in poverty or being an immigrant, and consider these when conceptualizing the client's situation. As silly as it may sound to new counselors, it is *very* easy to not adjust the conceptualization assessment based on theory. For example, how to adjust what a secure attachment looks like in a Japanese versus Italian family? What happens when you consider generation of immigration and socioeconomic status? What is normal then? Quickly, things become murky.

Furthermore, in most cases, each limitation that arises from being different has a correlating resource. For example, gay men and lesbians are marginalized in numerous ways in our society and are often targeted for abuse, resulting in various levels of trauma; these experiences add significantly to their overall level of psychological stress. However, because of this marginalization, they tend to develop unusually strong social and friendship networks that help them not only to cope but to thrive. Similarly, many cultural and ethnic groups are marginalized in dominant society, but they also tend to have stronger-than-average social and religious networks that provide them a sense of belonging and support.

Theoretical Conceptualizations

The remainder of this form includes five potential areas of conceptualization using the major schools of theory covered in this book:

- Psychodynamic/Adlerian
- Humanistic-Existential
- Cognitive-Behavioral
- Family Systemic
- Postmodern and Feminist

Using one or more of these allows for a slightly more integrative approach. Alternatively, you can use the "case conceptualization" section of a single theory to develop a theory-specific conceptualization.

Psychodynamic and Adlerian Conceptualization

Psychodynamic Defense Mechanisms

Psychodynamic Defense Mechanisms

Check 2–4 most commonly used defense mechanisms

- ❑ Acting Out: *Describe:* ____________________
- ❑ Denial: *Describe:* ____________________
- ❑ Displacement: *Describe:* ____________________
- ❑ Help-rejecting Complaining: *Describe:* ____________________
- ❑ Humor: *Describe:* ____________________
- ❑ Passive Aggression: *Describe:* ____________________
- ❑ Projection: *Describe:* ____________________
- ❑ Projective Identification: *Describe:* ____________________
- ❑ Rationalization: *Describe:* ____________________
- ❑ Reaction Formation: *Describe:* ____________________
- ❑ Repression: *Describe:* ____________________
- ❑ Splitting: *Describe:* ____________________
- ❑ Sublimation: *Describe:* ____________________
- ❑ Suppression: *Describe:* ____________________
- ❑ Other: ____________________

Psychodynamic defense mechanisms refer to automatic psychological processes that a person uses to ward off anxiety and external stressors and thus describe strategies the person frequently uses to handle problems. A person may be conscious or unconscious about using a defense mechanism; generally, the more aware one is of using a defense mechanism, the more functional he/she is. In addition, certain defense mechanisms are considered more functional than others. For example, humor, sublimation, and suppression are considered more functional than mechanisms that require image distortion or disavowal, such as idealization, denial, and projection.

Originally described in early psychoanalytic writing, these defense mechanisms are widely recognized by counselors practicing from a variety of theoretical perspectives. The purpose of identifying defense mechanisms is to better understand the client's internal dynamics, particularly those that are contributing to the presenting problem. That said, not all defenses are bad, and in fact, they can be quite helpful at times. For example, at the beginning of Chapter 4, I share how my career in writing began as a type of sublimation. Similarly, I encourage new counselors to master the art of suppression: putting difficult ideas out of one's mind. Sublimation is an important skill that enables them to continue to focus on their clients during work hours even when they are dealing with difficult matters in their personal life (disappointing side note: life still happens to professional counselors and therapists). Thus, you should carefully reflect on what defense mechanisms your clients use, considering how they may be helpful in certain contexts.

Acting Out

A common term that has trickled into the vernacular, the technical meaning of acting out as a defense mechanism refers to dealing with inner emotional conflict through action rather than reflecting on feelings. These actions may or may not translate to "bad behavior," but rather to a pattern of engaging in a behavior (e.g., such as physically fighting, starting verbal fights, etc.) to deal with inner conflict.

Denial

One of the more famous defense mechanisms ("Denial is not just a river in Egypt") and one of the more difficult to assess initially (because your client probably won't mention it), denial refers to refusing to acknowledge a painful reality that is readily apparent to others. Denial is commonly seen in families with substance and alcohol abuse as well as people in dead-end jobs and relationships.

Displacement

Most frequently observed in family dynamics, displacement refers to transferring feelings about one person (or situation) to another, less threatening substitute object. For example, if a person is angry at a spouse but afraid to raise the issue, it is usually easier to displace this anger onto one's young children, with whom a person is more likely to win an argument.

Help-Rejecting Complaining

Commonly observed in counseling sessions, help-rejecting complaining is just like it sounds: a person deals with stress by complaining but invariably rejects suggestions, advice, or help that others offer. I'd offer an example here, but I am confident you just came up with five examples from your personal list of friends, family, and acquaintances.

Humor

All joking aside, humor can be used as a defense mechanism whereby a person manages emotional conflict by identifying the amusing or ironic qualities of the situation. Humor can be used in a highly adaptive way, and it can also be used so rigidly that it almost becomes a form of denial.

Passive Aggression

Another of the more frequently cited defense mechanisms, passive aggression refers to when a person portrays a facade of cooperation but then covertly resists, resents, or undermines, thus indirectly expressing aggression. Sometimes this is easy to detect, as in a classic case of "backstabbing," and other times it is more subtle, such as endless procrastination or "forgetting."

Projection

Projection refers to falsely attributing one's own unacceptable feelings, impulses, or wishes onto another, typically without being aware of what is going on. In clinical practice, this is often seen in the case where one partner has cheated and then projects similar actions onto the faithful partner; this can happen whether or not the infidelity has been discovered.

Projective Identification

Projective identification takes simple projection to a whole new level. Similar to simple projection, projective identification involves falsely attributing one's own unacceptable feelings to another. However, in this case, the person is aware of having the unacceptable feelings but inappropriately justifies them by claiming they are reasonable reactions to the other person, which often results in the other person acting in such a way as to confirm the projection, making it difficult to clarify who did what to whom first. The classic example of this is jealousy: a person is jealous of his partner's relationship with other men, but claims that is because of her behavior. His jealousy causes her to be more secretive to avoid conflict, which further confirms his hypothesis about her, quickly creating a negative, downward spiral.

Rationalization

A favorite of the educated, rationalization refers to dealing with emotional conflict by concealing true motivations by developing elaborate reassuring but incorrect explanations for thoughts, feelings, and emotions. For example, a person may offer intricate and convoluted explanations for excessive drinking behavior, staying in a bad relationship, or failing to take needed action.

Reaction Formation

Often linked with repression, reaction formation refers to dealing with difficult inner conflict by engaging in actions that are diametrically opposed to the denied thought, feelings, and behaviors. A frequent example of this is someone who becomes a rigid religious adherent to cope with unacceptable sexual or materialistic desires; often this backfires, and the person makes headlines when they are caught in a sex or financial scandal.

Repression

More pathological than suppression, repression refers to eliminating unacceptable desires, thoughts, or experiences from conscious awareness to the extent that the person is unaware of the inner conflict. Often the repression is used to describe how traumatized persons will sometimes repress memories associated with the event as a means of coping; the memory may later be triggered by another event, conversation, or other reminder.

Splitting

A term from object relations theory, splitting refers to the inability to see an individual—self included—as having both positive and negative qualities. Instead, the person swings from seeing people as all-good or all-bad: idealizing or villainizing. In some cases, they can rapidly alternate between an all-good or all-bad view of the same person, creating significant chaos in relationships.

Sublimation

One of the more functional defenses, sublimation refers to dealing with internal conflict by channeling potentially inappropriate feelings or impulses into socially acceptable activities, such as challenging aggression through sports or sadness through art. This defense can be developed to help people find creative ways to use difficult emotions, such as sadness, anger, rage, fear, and such.

Suppression

Unlike repression, suppression is the *intentional* avoidance of difficult inner thoughts, feelings, and desires. When thoughtfully chosen, this defense can be very useful when facing difficult emotions over extended periods of time, such as grief, complicated loss, and others.

Object Relational Patterns

Object Relational Patterns

Describe relationship with early caregivers in past: ____________________

Was the attachment with the mother (or equivalent) primarily: ❑ Generally Secure
❑ Anxious and Clingy ❑ Avoidant and Emotionally Distant ❑ Other: __________

Was the attachment with the father (or equivalent) primarily: ❑ Generally Secure
❑ Anxious and Clingy ❑ Avoidant and Emotionally Distant ❑ Other: __________

Describe present relationship with these caregivers: ____________________

Describe relational patterns with partner and other current relationships: __________

____

Object relations theorists examine the client's relationship with early caregivers to understand the dynamics that are creating current difficulties (Bowlby, 1988; Johnson, 2004; St. Clair, 2000). In general, these patterns can be described in three ways:

- **Secure:** Client feels safe in relationships; is comfortable with intimacy; does not have unreasonable fears of abandonment or losing self in a relationship; generally, people with secure relationships seek counseling in response to a specific trauma or event.
- **Anxious:** Client unnecessarily worries about abandonment or rejection, often displaying jealously and feeling insecure with the slightest criticism (or even without significant praise). The anxiety such a person experiences in relationships frequently brings them to counseling for help.
- **Avoidant:** Clients with avoidant relational patterns often fear being swallowed or lost in a relationship and therefore remain emotionally unavailable and distant to help them preserve a sense of self.

These early childhood patterns typically repeat like variations on a theme in adulthood, both with the primary caregiver and in other relationships. By tracing these patterns, counselors can help clients more quickly identify core dynamic patterns that are affecting all areas of life.

Erickson's Psychosocial Developmental Stage

Describe development at each stage up to current stage:

Trust vs. Mistrust (Infant stage): ______________________

Autonomy vs. Shame and Doubt (Toddler stage): ______________________

Initiative vs. Guilt (Preschool age): ______________________

Industry vs. Inferiority (School age): ______________________

Identity vs. Identity Confusion (Adolescence): ______________________

Intimacy vs. Isolation (Young adulthood): ______________________

Generativity vs. Stagnation (Adulthood): ______________________

Integrity vs. Despair (Late Adulthood): ______________________

Erickson's eight stages of psychosocial development are one of the more useful developmental theories in applied clinical counseling. These stages provide a template for understanding the larger developmental concerns that may be underlying the problems clients bring to session. When viewed through a developmental lens, client problems often make more sense, and typically this insight informs more resourceful direction for counseling. For example, if a middle-aged man presents with depressive symptoms, examining these symptoms in the context of the struggle for generativity versus stagnation can help focus counseling at the deeper underlying issues that may be fueling the depression. In this case, rather than simply trying to relieve symptoms, the focus of counseling can be to help him achieve a sense of purpose and contribution.

Chapman (2006) explains that the developmental challenge at each stage of development is to achieve an effective *ratio* between the two counterbalancing dispositions, such as trust and mistrust, rather than maximize one at the expense of the other. Ideally, a person will develop a tendency toward trust yet also know when it is appropriate to distrust; having blind trust in everyone and everything is not adaptive. Thus, a person strives to find a healthy balance between the two propensities at each stage. Development issues arise when a person develops an extreme tendency toward one of the two dispositions, such as being overly trusting *or* overly distrustful. When one tends toward the first, more positive-sounding disposition, this is referred to as a *maladaptation*; if one tends toward the second, this is referred to as a *malignancy*.

Trust versus Mistrust: Infant Stage

Maladaptation (overemphasize trust): Unrealistic, spoiled, deluded
Malignancy (overemphasize mistrust): Withdrawal, neurotic, depressive, afraid

Applicable to the first year or two of life, infants in this stage develop a healthy balance of trust or mistrust based on their experiences with early caregivers. A healthy balance of trust translates to a general sense of hope and safety in the world while simultaneously knowing when caution is warranted. Persons who have had traumatic childhoods or whose parents overly protected them often have confusion over when, where, and whom to trust, resulting in a sense of being either unrealistically entitled or needlessly afraid.

Autonomy versus Shame and Doubt: Toddler Stage

Maladaptation (overemphasis of autonomy): Impulsivity, recklessness, inconsiderate, thoughtless
Malignancy (overemphasis of shame/doubt): Compulsion, constrained, self-limiting

During toddlerhood, children develop a sense of autonomy and having an impact in their lives while also learning the limits of their abilities. If caretakers are either neglectful or overly protective, children become overburdened with a sense of shame and may grow up to have lingering issues that manifest as extreme self-doubt or debilitating shame and/or shyness. Alternatively, if parents do not allow their children to experience shame and self-doubt, these children tend to become impulsive and inconsiderate of others.

Initiative versus Guilt: Preschool and Kindergarten Age

Maladaptation (overemphasis of initiative): Ruthless, exploitative, uncaring, dispassionate
Malignancy (overemphasis of guilt): Inhibition, risk-aversive, unadventurous

During preschool and kindergarten, children transition through a developmental stage in which they develop a sense of initiative and purpose tempered by guilt when their actions hurt others. Children who have either overly protective or neglectful parents may develop a strong sense of guilt and insecurity about making their own choices, leading to risk avoidance and inhibition. Alternatively, children who have an underdeveloped awareness of guilt and how their actions affect others become overly aggressive and even ruthless.

Industry versus Inferiority: School Age

Maladaptation (overemphasis of industry): Narrowly virtuous, workaholic, obsessive specialist
Malignancy (overemphasis of inferiority): Inertia, lazy, apathetic, purposeless

In the early years in school, children learn new skills, developing a sense of competence from which they build their sense of self-worth; thus, the task at this stage is to engage in industrious activities to build confidence in their abilities. Children who are frequently criticized or compared to others and found to be lacking develop a pervasive sense of inferiority. Recent research also shows that overly praised children who are protected from experiencing failure and obstacles also develop a sense of inferiority because they are thwarted from developing a genuine sense of mastery (Seligman, 2002). Thus, contrary to their parents' intentions, children who are constantly sheltered from the feelings of losing a game, getting bad grades, being left out, and similar feelings of inferiority are actually likely to develop a lingering sense of inadequacy as they get older that can manifest as "underachieving" down the road. Alternatively, overly identifying with one's industriousness can result in obsessiveness in their activities.

Identity versus Identity Confusion: Adolescence

Maladaptation (overemphasis of identity): Fanaticism, self-important, extremist
Malignancy (overemphasis of identity confusion): Repudiation, socially disconnected, cut-off

Few developmental stages are more fabled—or as well researched—as adolescence. Erickson saw this as a time of identity development when a person first begins to answer questions, such as who am I, and how do I fit in? Developmentally, this is a time of exploring possible identities and social roles, which often takes the form of wild outfits, colorful hair, rebellious music, rotating social groups, and other ways to magnificently annoy one's parents. Teens who are not allowed to explore their identity or are made to feel guilty for not pursuing certain life paths may experience role confusion, failing to identify a clear or viable sense of identity. Alternatively, role confusion can also take the form of failing to adopt a viable social role and instead developing a reactive identity that is based on a rebellious need to "not be" what someone wants, often taking the form of drug use, a radical social group, gang membership, or dropping out of high school. In such cases, teens are not able to conceive of themselves as productive members of one's family or society.

Intimacy versus Isolation: Young Adulthood

Maladaptation (overemphasis of intimacy): Promiscuous, needy, vulnerability
Malignancy (overemphasis of isolation): Exclusivity, loner, cold, self-contained

In recent generations, young adulthood has become much longer than in years prior, as more people seek higher education and views of marriage and "settling down" change. During this time, people establish intimate relationships in their personal, social, and work lives, developing their own families and social networks. People who struggle with this stage can become either overly focused on their relationships, possibly becoming sexual promiscuous or overly identified with being in a relationship, or increasingly socially isolated.

Generativity versus Stagnation: Adulthood

Maladaptation (overemphasis of generativity): Overextension, do-gooder, busy-body, meddling
Malignancy (overemphasis of stagnation): Rejecting, disinterested, cynical

The developmental tasks of adulthood focus on feeling as though one meaningfully contributes to society and the succeeding generations, and this is often measured by whether one is satisfied with life accomplishments. A midlife crisis refers to feeling that one's life is stagnant, off course, and/or in need of fixing, which some pursue by trying to make radical life changes—sometimes these help, and at other times these get a person even more off course. Often, the consequences of developmental deficiencies from prior stages come to a head during this time and can now be worked through and more readily addressed. Additionally, developmental issues at this stage can take the form of being overly involved and extended in one's social or work world or, alternatively, becoming cynical and disconnected.

Integrity versus Despair: Late Adulthood

Maladaptation (overemphasis of integrity): Presumption, conceited, pompous, arrogant
Malignancy (overemphasis of despair): Disdain, miserable, unfulfilled, blaming

The final developmental stage is an increasingly important one for counselors to understand as more elderly are receiving professional services. During this stage, people balance a sense of integrity with a sense of despair as they look back over their lives and face the inevitability of death. Those who are able to face the end of life with a greater sense of integrity and wisdom are able to integrate the experiences of their life to make meaning and to accept what and who they have been. In contrast, others struggle to make peace with their lives and with life more generally and experience inconsolable sadness and loss or, alternatively, develop a false sense of self-importance that is conveyed as arrogance and self-righteousness.

Adlerian Style of Life Theme

Adlerian Style of Life Theme

❑ Control: ______________________________

❑ Superiority: ______________________________

❑ Pleasing: ______________________________

❑ Comfort: ______________________________

Basic Mistake Misperceptions: ______________________________

____

____

When working with clients, one of the most important areas Adlerian counselors assess is a person's *style of life*, which can be described as a person's characteristic way of thinking, doing, feeling, living, and striving: one's road map for life. This "style" or map of life both shapes and is shaped by the goals we choose for our lives and becomes the thread that runs through all aspects of our lives. Eckstein (2009) identifies four general patterns that are commonly adopted as a style of life: control, superiority, pleasing, and comfort. Although these are not the only way to assess a client's style of life, they are an easy way to begin. A person may have more than one of these themes in their style of life.

Control

Persons whose lifestyle is characterized by control frequently seek to control others, themselves, and/or the situation in order to create a sense of safety and security. However, you have no doubt lived long enough to realize that total control over anyone, including oneself, is not humanly possible. Thus, those whose life theme includes elements of control are frequently frustrated, often perceiving others as being resistant or difficult. These people tend often to be drawn into power struggles and distancing themselves from people and situations over which they have no control. Counseling can help people with a controlling lifestyle accept what they cannot change and develop greater tolerance for others.

Superiority

Not be confused with control, those whose life theme is characterized by superiority are commonly referred to as "perfectionists." They need to be better than others, as well as "right," useful, and competent. However, underneath an outer layer of what appears to be superiority, they tend to have an ongoing inner doubt about whether they are "good enough." Inside they tend to be hard on themselves, often taking on more than they can reasonably handle. Sometimes this standard of superiority gets projected onto others, especially children, and the person becomes impossible to please. Counselors can help those with superiority life themes develop more realistic expectations for themselves and others.

Pleasing

One of the easiest to work with and most commonly seen in counseling settings, those clients whose life theme involves pleasing focus their energies on understanding the needs of others and finding ways to meet them. They often need everyone else to be happy before they can be happy, thus making their happiness dependent on how they are treated by others. Typically, a person with a pleasing lifestyle gives and gives and gives and then at a certain point becomes resentful. In some cases, others take advantage of them or abuse them; in other cases, those around them are unaware of the sacrifices they are making. Their fear of rejection and habit of pleasing others at the expense of their own integrity can cause significant hardship in their lives. In counseling, they can learn to set health boundaries and find ways to assert their needs in relationships while still respecting those of others.

Comfort

Those whose life theme involves comfort seek comfort at the expense of taking the risks involved with pursuing life goals and achievement. They tend to avoid the stress of responsibility and delayed reward, often due to a sense of inadequacy or fear of failure. In moderation, seeking comfort leads to underachieving, while in its extreme may take the form of addiction. Counselors can help those with this theme to take small steps toward their goals, emphasizing small successes along the way.

Basic Mistake Perceptions

Each person's style of life reveals their *private logic* about how life and the world work. Children begin developing their personal map of the universe—their private logic—from their earliest experiences. Thus, virtually everyone ends up with a system of private logic that has some *basic mistakes*, perceptions about the world that are inaccurate. Basic mistakes are similar to what cognitive counselors call *irrational beliefs*, but they refer to the core and most general irrational beliefs that inform one's view of life, self, and others. Adlerian counseling involves helping people identify these often unconscious or semiconscious erroneous assumptions about life, to enable those people to develop a system of private logic that supports them in pursuing their life goals.

Basic mistakes are individual and unique. Thus, assessing them requires carefully listening to what clients say and asking about their thinking process in situations related to the presenting problem: "What did you find so offensive in what your husband said?" or "What motivated you to take such a desperate action?" With careful listening, astute observations, and probing questions, counselors can help clients identify basic mistake misperceptions that contribute to their current concerns. Examples include:

- Overgeneralizations: "People cannot be trusted"; "No one cares about me."
- Unrealistic expectations: "I should always be happy"; "Life should be easy."
- Unsustainable goals: "Everyone must be happy for me to be happy"; "I must always be the best at what I do."
- Misperceptions about life/god: "Life should be fair"; "God will give me what I want."
- Denying one's worth: "I will never be good enough"; "I am not worth loving."
- Problematic values: "I must get to the top at any cost"; "I do not apologize for my actions."

Humanistic-Existential Conceptualization

Expression of Authentic Self

Humanistic Assessment: Expression of Authentic Self

Problems: Are problems perceived as internal or external (caused by others, circumstance, etc.)? ❑ Predominantly internal ❑ Mixed ❑ Predominantly external

Agency and Responsibility: Is self or other discussed as agent of story? Does client take clear responsibility for situation? ❑ Strong sense of agency and responsibility ❑ Agency in some areas ❑ Little agency; frequently blames others/situation ❑ Often feels victimized

Recognition and Expression of Feelings: Are feelings readily recognized, owned, and experienced? ❑ Easily expresses feelings ❑ Identifies feelings with prompting ❑ Difficulty recognizing feelings

(continued)

Here-and-Now Experiencing: Is the client able to experience full range of feelings as they are happening in the present moment? ❑ Easily experiences emotions in present moment ❑ Experiences some present emotions with assistance ❑ Difficulty with experiencing present moment

Personal Constructs and Facades: Is the client able to recognize and go beyond roles? Is identity rigid or tentatively held? ❑ Tentatively held; able to critique and question ❑ Some awareness of facades and construction of identity ❑ Identity rigidly defined; seems like "fact"

Complexity and Contradictions: Are internal contradictions owned and explored? Is client able to fully engage the complexity of identity and life? ❑ Aware of and resolves contradictions ❑ Some recognition of contradictions ❑ Unaware of internal contradictions

Shoulds: Is client able to question socially imposed shoulds and oughts? Can client balance desire to please others and desire to be authentic? ❑ Able to balance authenticity with social obligation ❑ Identifies tension between social expectations and personal desires ❑ Primarily focuses on external shoulds

List shoulds: ______________________________

Acceptance of Others: Is client able to accept others and modify expectations of others to be more realistic? ❑ Readily accepts others as they are ❑ Recognizes expectations of others are unrealistic but still strong emotional reaction to expectations not being met ❑ Difficulty accepting others as they are; always wanting others to change to meet expectations

Trust of Self: Is client able to trust self as a process (rather than as a stable object)? ❑ Able to trust and express authentic self ❑ Trust of self in certain contexts ❑ Difficulty trusting self in most contexts

In humanistic approaches to counseling, such as person-centered and Gestalt, assessment focuses on the person's ability to experience and express their authentic self. As you can imagine, this is a subtle process that is difficult to assess. Carl Rogers (1961) identifies several telltale signs of authenticity, which include the following:

Problems

Rogers noticed that as people move toward greater authenticity, they begin to see problems and solutions to problems primarily as an internal rather than external matter. People early in the growth process tend to see problems as caused by others or attributable to external circumstances, such as someone not doing what they want or an unfortunate event. In contrast, as persons move toward greater authenticity, they begin to describe problems in terms of their needing to take some action or respond differently to a situation; they no longer see others or situations as the problem—rather, they see that the problem is that they need to change their role in the situation.

Agency and Responsibility

When listening with an attuned ear to clients, it is often easy to discern whether they see themselves as the agent of their lives and therefore take responsibility for their actions as well as the situations. Early in the growth process, clients tend to blame others or their circumstances or report feeling like a victim. They describe events happening *to them*, with others serving as the agents in the story. In contrast, as they begin to become more self-actualized, the same circumstances are described with the client as the agent or protagonist of the story, and they take responsibility for the situation and their response.

Recognition and Expression of Feelings

Humanistic counselors carefully observe a person's ability to recognize, own, express, and experience their emotions. As people become more self-actualized, they more readily access and manage emotions. When some clients begin counseling, they have extreme difficulty identifying their emotions: when asked what they are feeling they can only describe what they are thinking. Through the counseling process, they learn to identify and more fully experience their emotions. Finally, the counselor helps them to "own" them (take responsibility) and respectfully express them in appropriate contexts with appropriate people.

Here-and-Now Experiencing

Once a counselor has helped a client to more readily identify emotions, the next step is to be able to experience and express emotions as they arise in the present moment. Typically, clients are first able to do this in a safe environment in session with their counselor and then in less controlled, real-life situations. Clients who learn how to experience emotions in the here-and-now can feel emotions as they arise, are consciously aware of feeling those emotions, and can do so without overreacting to them. For example, if a client gets disappointing news about not getting a job or promotion, he can feel the disappointment, is aware that he is feeling the disappointment, yet does not overreact by getting angry, depressed, or self-harming (drinking, etc.).

Personal Constructs and Facades

Carl Rogers paid careful attention to the social roles and facades his clients played. His counseling approach aimed to get people to move beyond these limiting personal constructs—rigid definitions of self—to move toward a more fluid form of identity that was constantly evolving and expanding. The more rigid one holds to a personal construct—"I am a hard worker" or "I am beautiful"—the more limited one's life becomes because so much energy must go toward maintaining the particular identity. Thus, humanistic counselors look for more tentatively held ideas of self and personhood as a sign of living more authentically.

Complexity and Contradictions

News flash: You are a hypocrite. I am a hypocrite. We are all riddled with contradictions, complexities, and confusions. As a person becomes more self-aware, the better able one is to see these contradictions and accept them as part of what it means to be human.

Shoulds

Also targeted by Gestalt and cognitive counselors, "shoulds" and "oughts" are socially imposed rules about how one should think, feel, and behave. Every culture has these shoulds; in fact, in essence each culture is a list of shoulds. Thus, it is impossible to live with other humans and not have a list of socially defined shoulds. The key is how one relates to them. If a person swallows them whole and contorts themselves to fit into these shoulds, the authentic self has little room for expression. Instead, the ideal is to thoughtfully balance one's need for authentic self-expression with the socially imposed shoulds, sometimes having to forgo social acceptance to maintain one's integrity. That said, someone who flaunts going against cultural norms is not expressing the authentic self but rather finding identity by being a reactive rebel, who is still defined by socially imposed shoulds—just in negative relief.

Acceptance of Others

Relating to other humans is challenging. Even in the best of relationships, at a certain point a fundamental difference or failure occurs that leaves one or both feeling betrayed, hurt, or angry. Accepting imperfection in others tends to occur when one begins to accept it in oneself. Thus, humanistic counselors carefully assess clients' abilities to accept others and to modify their expectations of others to be more realistic. In theory, it would be great if everyone spoke with kind words in a kind tone to everyone. In theory, it would be great if everyone could follow through on their promises and act with integrity in difficult situations. The more you are in relationship with others, the more you realize that such perfection is not possible. That said, it is important to keep striving for these ideals and to balance this realism with realistic expectations for thoughtful and kind behavior.

Trust of Self

Finally, humanistic counselors assess the extent to which clients are able to experience their identity as a *process* rather than as a stable object. People who experience their identity as a stable "thing" are attached to labels, routines, status, objects, and anything else that symbolizes their identities. As a person becomes more self-actualized, these things matter less and less, and a person becomes more comfortable with the idea that identity is fluid and evolving. Important identity factors today—grades, degree, job, relationship, child—will likely be less important at some point in the future. Self-actualization involves trusting the ongoing unfolding of the self with less and less need to label it, pin it down, or claim it.

Existential Analysis

Existential Analysis

*Sources of Life Meaning (as described or demonstrated by client):*________________

____

____

General Themes of Life Meaning: ❑ Personal achievement/work ❑ Significant other ❑ Children ❑ Family of origin ❑ Social cause/contributing to others ❑ Religion/spirituality ❑ Other: ________________

Satisfaction with and clarity on life direction: ❑ Clear sense of meaning that creates resilience in difficult times ❑ Current problems require making choices related to life direction ❑ Minimally satisfied with current life direction; wants more from life ❑ Has reflected little on life direction up to this point; living according to life plan defined by someone/something else ❑ Other: ________________

Based on existential logotherapy (Frankl, 1963), existential analysis of a client's life situation involves looking at their life from the highest possible vantage point. It's such a "big picture" view that it is easy to forget when one is focused on so many other details, such as frequency of symptoms, childhood history, and current relationships. However, this wide-angle view often provides invaluable information about how to expedite the counseling process. Two initial areas for assessment are:

- Sources of life meaning: What inspires the client and makes them feel whole and fulfilled?
- Satisfaction with and clarity of life direction: Does the client have a clear sense of purpose and direction for his/her life? Is life on or off track?

The importance of these perennial existential questions has had a boost from science in recent years. In studying happiness and life satisfaction, positive psychologists report a strong correlation between having a sense of meaning and purpose and being happy (Seligman, 2002). Thus, counselors need to understand where clients find meaning and purpose at the outset of counseling in order to effectively guide treatment to help the client achieve greater levels of happiness.

An existential analysis of meaning and purpose is particularly useful when working with certain types of clients. For example, when working with clients who have suicidal feelings, counselors can assess for sources of life meaning and life satisfaction to determine how serious the threat is and how best to motivate a client to value life again.

Similarly, clients who struggle with depression have often lost their sense of direction in life and need to have their life dreams reinvigorated. As is developmentally expected, most teens I work with struggle with issues of life meaning and direction and appreciate being able to discuss these personal issues with an open-minded and patient adult. In all cases, knowing where clients draw their inspiration reveals what will ultimately motivate them toward change, no matter what the initial presenting concern.

Gestalt Contact Boundary Disturbances

Gestalt Contact Boundary Disturbances

- ❑ *Desensitization:* Failing to notice problems
- ❑ *Introjection*: Take in others' views whole and unedited
- ❑ *Projection*: Assign undesired parts of self to others
- ❑ *Retroflection*: Direct action to self rather than other
- ❑ *Deflection*: Avoid direct contact with another or self
- ❑ *Egotism:* Not allowing outside to influence self
- ❑ *Confluence*: Agree with another to extent that boundary blurred

Describe: ______________________________

____

As described in Chapter 10, Gestalt counselors view each moment of lived experience primarily in terms of a form of *contact* between the self (organism) and outside world (others and environment; Perls, Hefferline, & Goodman, 1951; Yontef, 1993). If a person is able to make direct contact and authentically *encounter* the outside world, the person is living a fully authentic life. However, for a variety of reasons—early life lessons, fears, social dictates—people avoid genuine contact to protect themselves. These *contact boundary disturbances* refer to distortions in perceptions of self or others.

An encounter involves a continuum of seven phases, beginning with initial perception, moving toward direct encounter, and ending in withdrawal. The human experience involves an endless ebb and flow of making contact with one person/object/idea and then withdrawing; then making contact and withdrawing from another; in an endless series of connections and disconnections. A person can avoid contact at any of the seven phases using specific resistance processes at each stage (Woldt & Toman, 2005):

Continuum Phase	Resistance Process	Example of Resistance
1. *Sensation/Perception:* Organism perceives input from environment.	*Desensitization:* Failing to notice problems	Ignoring increasing violence by partner in fights
2. *Awareness:* One's lived experience becomes focused on the environmental sensation.	*Introjection:* Take in others' views whole and unedited	Becoming what your parents wanted you to be
3. *Excitement/Mobilization:* The organism mobilizes to prepare for contact.	*Projection:* Assign undesired parts of self to others	Rejecting sexual aspects of self and then perceiving others as "oversexed"
4. *Encounter/Action:* The organism takes action to engage the other.	*Retroflection:* Direct action to self rather than other	Rather than creating conflict with others, focus criticism on self
5. *Interaction/Full Contact:* A back-and-forth exchange happens; the self becomes part of "we."	*Deflection:* Avoid direct contact with another or self	Working long hours to avoid spouse or avoiding own emotions

(continued)

6. *Assimilation/Integration:* The organism takes in and integrates new information, behavior, etc.	*Egotism:* Not allowing outside to influence self	Claiming to be "in love," but not being open to changing self to meet needs of relationship
7. *Differentiation/Withdrawal:* The organism withdraws from contact and returns to its individual state.	*Confluence:* Agree with another to extent that boundary blurred	Agreeing with spouse to extent that one no longer allows self to have a divergent opinion

Digital Download Download from CengageBrain.com

When assessing clients, Gestalt counselors look for where their clients are "stuck" in the cycle of making contact and direct their interventions to encourage clients to make contact and complete the encounter cycle.

Cognitive-Behavioral Conceptualization

Baseline of Symptomatic Behavior

Baseline of Symptomatic Behavior

Symptom #1 (behavioral description): ____________________

Frequency: ____________________

Duration: ____________________

Context(s): ____________________

Events Before: ____________________

Events After: ____________________

Symptom #2 (behavioral description): ____________________

Frequency: ____________________

Duration: ____________________

Context(s): ____________________

Events Before: ____________________

Events After: ____________________

Baseline Assessment of Symptomatic Behavior originated in behavioral counseling (Spiegler & Guevremont, 2003), but now it is commonly required by insurance companies and other third-party payers whose preferred model is the *medical model*, which focuses on observable symptoms. Therefore, if you like to get paid, it's a good idea to perfect the art of baseline assessment. Thankfully, compared to everything else in this assessment, it's a snap.

Steps to Baseline Assessment

Step 1. Define the problem behavior in specific, observable behaviors that are easily counted.

Examples: To measure depression, you could measure any of the following: (a) hours per day with depressed mood; (b) days per week with mild, moderate, or severe depressed mood; (c) days per week avoiding social contact and/or normal activities.

Step 2: Get a Baseline
Create a chart for the client that collects the following data:

- *Frequency of problem behavior:* Measured in minutes, hours, days, weeks.
- *Duration and/or severity of each episode:* Duration can be in minutes or hours; severity is typically measured as mild, moderate, or severe.
- *Context in which the behavior happened:* Could be place, relationship, timing, or some other potentially contextual trigger for the behavior.
- *Events before each episode:* Used to identify potential triggers (e.g., rain, an argument).
- *Events after each episode:* Used to identify potential reinforcement and/or clarify trigger of the behavior (e.g., when her husband comes home the wife's anxiety diminishes).

Sample of Baseline Assessment Chart

	Frequency	Duration/ Severity	Context	Events Before	Events After
Monday					
Tuesday					
Wednesday					
Thursday					
Friday					
Saturday					
Sunday					

The client then completes the chart for a period of one to four weeks to get a baseline assessment of the problem behavior. This becomes the measuring point for progress once treatment commences, and progress can thus be closely measured. Relying on the most objective data available in mental health, baseline assessment is considered one of the best measures of progress. However, for those who have spent some time collecting such data, it becomes quickly apparent that because these data rely heavily on client recall and description, they are less consistent and reliable as one might hope. In fact, often a spouse or parent may be a more reliable source of behavioral information than the client trying to remember his or her internal states.

A-B-C Analysis of Irrational Beliefs

A-B-C Analysis of Irrational Beliefs

Activating Event ("Problem"): ____________________

Consequence (Mood, behavior, etc.): ____________________

Mediating Beliefs (Unhelpful beliefs about event that result in C): ____________________

1. ____________________

2. ____________________

3. ____________________

One of the more common assessment techniques in cognitive-behavior approaches, Albert Ellis's (1999) A-B-C framework is used to identify problematic beliefs that result in undesirable emotions and behaviors. The A-B-C framework works as follows:

A = Activating Event ➔ B = Belief ➔ C = Consequence

In this case, A, the activating event, triggers B, a belief, that results in C, a consequence. In theory, this happens with all events all the time. However, when a person has what Ellis terms an irrational, or what I prefer to call a problematic, belief, the consequences are essentially the presenting problem for which the client is seeking help.

Here are some examples:

- A = Fight with boyfriend ➔ B = Our relationship is in trouble; no one will ever love me ➔ C = Feeling depressed; acting desperate; text messaging every two minutes; eating a pint of ice cream.
- A = Trip to shopping mall ➔ B = People judge me by the way I look; I am not as good as everyone else; something is wrong with me ➔ C = Feelings of inadequacy; feeling anxious and panicked; afraid to make eye contact; avoiding people; leaving the mall early; overspending online at home.

The role of the counselor is to help identify **B**, the unhelpful belief, because most clients *experience* the chain of events as A ➔ C and describe it as "I am depressed *because* my boyfriend and I had a fight" not "I am depressed because I believe no one will ever love me." To identify these underlying beliefs, counselors can ask questions such as the ones below.

Questions for Identifying Unhelpful Beliefs

- When you think about the Activating Event (helps to name it), why does it make sense to then feel ________________ (C) or do ________________ (C)?

Example: When you think about going to the mall (A), why does it make sense to feel anxious (C) and leave as soon as possible (C)?

- What beliefs do you have about yourself and/or ________________ (A) that may lead you to feel ________________ (C) or do ________________ (C)?

Example: What beliefs do you have about you or your relationship that may lead you to feel depressed or act impulsively after a fight?

Digital Download Download from CengageBrain.com

Beck's Schema Analysis

Beck's Schema Analysis

Identify frequently used cognitive schemas:

❑ *Arbitrary inference:*________________

❑ *Selective abstraction:*________________

❑ *Overgeneralization:*________________

❑ *Magnification/Minimization:*________________

❑ *Personalization:*________________

❑ *Absolutist/Dichotomous thinking:*________________

❑ *Mislabeling:*________________

❑ *Mindreading:*________________

Another common cognitive assessment technique is *schema analysis*, pioneered by Aaron Beck (1976). Schema is a technical psychological term that refers to a structured set of beliefs about some aspect of the world, such as one's worth, others' motives, or luck. To connect back up with Ellis's A-B-C framework, Beck's schema analysis can be viewed as a categorization of specific unhelpful beliefs. Assessing unhelpful beliefs using Beck's categorization of schemas can be very helpful in the counseling process by naming the beliefs more concretely and by identifying habitual patterns of thought. Categories of schema include, but are not limited to, the following:

- *Arbitrary Inference:* Drawing conclusions without sufficient or relevant evidence, including pessimism and catastrophizing (e.g., assuming someone is angry with you just because they do not return a phone call when expected).
- *Selective Abstraction:* Making assumptions based on certain facts while ignoring other—usually more positive—facts (e.g., assuming that you will lose a long-term friend due to a minor miscommunication).
- *Overgeneralization:* Holding extreme beliefs based on relatively little data (e.g., because I was not a good soccer player in elementary school, I am terrible at all sports).
- *Magnification and Minimization:* Overemphasizing or underemphasizing a particular fact and drawing inaccurate conclusions; in statistical terms, making assumptions based on an unrepresentative data set (e.g., believing that no one thinks you are beautiful because of a comment that one person made).
- *Personalization:* Assuming that an external event or someone else's action somehow says something about you (e.g., believing something is wrong with you because a partner cheats on you—hint, hint, *you* didn't make the choice to be unfaithful).
- *Absolutist or Dichotomous Thinking:* Categorizing things as all-good or all-bad or in either-or extremes (e.g., either she loves me or she doesn't).
- *Mislabeling:* Unfairly characterizing one's entire identity based on limited events (e.g., I am a terrible counselor because one client did not return for a second session).
- *Mindreading:* Believing you know what another person is thinking without sufficient supporting evidence (e.g., I know he does not like me because of the look on his face when I am at the meetings).

Family Systemic Conceptualization

Stage of Family Life Cycle

Family Life Cycle Stage

❑ Single Adult ❑ Marriage ❑ Family with Young Children ❑ Family with Adolescent Children ❑ Launching Children ❑ Later Life

Describe struggles with mastering developmental tasks in one of these stages: ______

Boundaries with

Parents: ❑ Enmeshed ❑ Clear ❑ Disengaged ❑ NA: *Describe:* ______

Significant Other: ❑ Enmeshed ❑ Clear ❑ Disengaged ❑ NA:*Describe:* ______

Children: ❑ Enmeshed ❑ Clear ❑ Disengaged ❑ NA: *Describe:* ______

Extended Family: ❑ Enmeshed ❑ Clear ❑ Disengaged ❑ NA: *Describe:* ______

Other: Name ❑ Enmeshed ❑ Clear ❑ Disengaged ❑ NA: *Describe:* ______

Typical style for regulating closeness and distance with others: ______

(continued)

Triangles/Coalitions

❑ Coalition in family of origin: *Describe:* ____________________

❑ Coalitions related to significant other: *Describe:* ____________________

❑ Other coalitions: ____________________

Hierarchy between Self and Parent/Child ❑ NA

With own children: ❑ Effective ❑ Rigid ❑ Permissive

With parents (for child/young adult): ❑ Effective ❑ Rigid ❑ Permissive

Complementary Patterns with Name:

❑ Pursuer/distancer: ❑ Over-/underfunctioner ❑ Emotional/logical ❑ Good/bad parent ❑ Other: *Describe*

Example of complementary pattern: ____________________

Intergenerational Patterns

Substance/Alcohol Abuse: ❑ NA ❑ History: ____________________

Sexual/Physical/Emotional Abuse: ❑ NA ❑ History: ____________________

Parent/Child Relations: ❑ NA ❑ History: ____________________

Physical/Mental Disorders: ❑ NA ❑ History: ____________________

Family Strengths: *Describe:* ____________________

Stage of Family Life Cycle Development

When assessing families, it is helpful to identify their stage in the life cycle (Carter & McGoldrick, 1999). Each stage is associated with specific developmental tasks; symptoms arise when families are having difficulty mastering these tasks:

- *Leaving Home: Single Adult:* Accepting emotional and financial responsibility for self.
- *Marriage:* Commit to new system; realigning boundaries with family and friends.
- *Families with Young Children:* Adjust marriage to make space for children; join in child-rearing tasks; realign boundaries with parents/grandparents.
- *Families with Adolescent Children:* Adjusting parental boundaries to increase freedom and responsibility for adolescents; refocus on marriage and career life.
- *Launching Children:* Renegotiating marital subsystem; developing adult-to-adult relationships with children; coping with aging parents.
- *Family in Later Life:* Accepting the shift of generational roles; coping with loss of abilities; middle generation takes more central role; creating space for wisdom of the elderly.

Interpersonal Boundaries

A family counseling term that has found its way into many self-help books, *boundaries* are the rules for negotiating interpersonal closeness and distance (Minuchin, 1974). These rules are generally unspoken and unfold as two people interact over time, each defining when, where, and how he/she prefers to relate to the other. Structural counselors characterize boundaries in one of three ways: clear, diffuse, or rigid, all of which are strongly influenced by culture.

Clear Boundaries and Cultural Variance: Clear boundaries refer to a range of possible ways couples can negotiate a healthy balance between closeness (we-ness) and separation (individuality). Cultural factors shape how much closeness versus separation is preferred. Collectivist cultures tend toward greater degrees of closeness whereas individualistic cultures tend to value greater independence. The best way to determine if a couple's boundaries are clear or not is to determine whether or not symptoms have developed in the individual, couple, or family. If they have, it is likely that there are problems with the boundaries being too *diffuse* or too *rigid*. Most people who come in for counseling have reached a point where previous boundaries and rules for relating that may have worked in one context are no longer working. For relationships to weather the test of time, couples, families, and even friends must constantly renegotiate their boundaries (rules for relating) to adjust to each person's evolving needs. The more flexible people are in negotiating these rules, the more successful they will be in adjusting to life's transitions and setbacks.

Enmeshed/Diffuse Boundaries: When a couple or family begins to overvalue togetherness at the expense of respecting the individuality of each, their boundaries become *diffuse* and relationship becomes *enmeshed* (note: technically, boundaries are not enmeshed; they are diffuse). In these relationships, individuals may feel that they are being suffocated, that they lack freedom, or that they are not cared for enough. Often, in these relationships, people feel threatened whenever the other disagrees or does not affirm them, resulting in an intense tug-of-war to convince the other to agree with them. Couples with diffuse boundaries may also have diffuse boundaries with their children, families of origin, and/or friends, which results in these outside others becoming overly involved in one or both of the partners' lives (e.g., involving parents, friends, or children in a couple's arguments).

Disengaged/Rigid Boundaries: When relationships emphasize independence over togetherness, boundaries can become *rigid* and the relationship *disengaged*. In these relationships, people may not allow others to influence them, often choosing careers over relationship priorities, and frequently may have minimal emotional connection. In couple partnerships that are disengaged, one or the other may compensate for distance in the couple relationship by having diffuse boundaries with children, friends, family, or an outside love interest (e.g., an emotional or physical affair). Often difficult to accurately assess, the key indicator of rigid boundaries is whether or not they are creating problems individually or for the partnership.

Questions for Assessing Boundaries

Here are some sample questions to think about while working with an individual, couple, or family to assess boundaries:

- Does the couple have clear couple boundaries that are distinct from their parenting and family-of-origin relationships?
- Does the couple spend time alone not talking about the children?
- Do family members experience anxiety or frustration when there is a difference of opinion?
- Is one hurt or angry if another has a different opinion or perspective on a problem?
- Do they use "we" or "I" more often when speaking? Is there a balance?
- Does each have a set of personal friends and activities separate from the family and partnership?
- How much energy goes into the family versus career and outside interests?
- What gets priority in their schedules? Children? Work? Personal activities? Couple time?

Digital Download Download from CengageBrain.com

Triangles/Coalitions: Problem Subsystems and Triangles

Problem systems are identified in most systemic family counseling approaches. Triangles (Kerr & Bowen, 1988), covert coalitions (Minuchin & Fishman, 1981), or cross-generational coalitions (Minuchin & Fishman, 1981) all refer to a similar systemic process: tension between two people is resolved by drawing in a third (or fourth, "*tetrad*"; Whitaker & Keith, 1981) person to stabilize the original dyad. Many counselors include inanimate objects or other processes as potential "thirds" in the triangulation process, such as drinking, drug use, work, hobbies, and such, which are used to help one or both partners soothe their internal stress at the expense of the relationship.

Counselors assess for triangles and problematic subsystems in several ways:

- Clients overtly describe another party as playing a role in their tension; in these cases the clients are aware at some level of the process going on.
- When clients describe the problem or conflict situation, another person plays the role of confidant or takes the side of one of the partners (e.g., one person has a friend or another family member who takes his/her side against the other).
- After being unable to get a need met in the primary dyad, a person finds what they are not getting in another person (e.g., a mother seeks emotional closeness from a child rather than from her partner).
- When counseling is inexplicably "stuck," there is often a triangle at work that distracts one or both parties from resolving critical issues (e.g., an affair, substance abuse, a friend who undermines agreements made in counseling, and so on).

Identifying triangles early in the assessment process enables counselors to intervene more successfully and quickly in a complex set of family dynamics.

Hierarchy between Child and Parents

A key area in assessing parent and child relationships is the parent-child hierarchy. When assessing parental hierarchy, counselors must ask themselves: Is the parent-child hierarchy developmentally and culturally appropriate? If the hierarchy is appropriate, there are generally minimal problems with the child's behavior. Generally, if the child is exhibiting symptoms or there are problems in the parent-child relationship, there is some problem in the hierarchical structure: either an excessive (authoritarian) or insufficient (permissive) parental hierarchy given the family's current sociocultural context(s). Immigrant families most always have two different sets of cultural norms for parental hierarchy (the traditional and the current cultural context), resulting in a difficult task of finding a balance between the two.

Assessing hierarchy is critical because it tells the counselor where and how to intervene. Often, inappropriate interventions are used if the counselor assesses only the symptoms. For example, although children with ADHD have similar symptoms—hyperactivity, defiance, failing to follow through on parents' requests, etc.—these same symptoms can occur in two dramatically different family structures: either too much or too little parental hierarchy. In the cases where the parental hierarchy is too rigid, the counselor works with the parents to soften this, develop a stronger personal relationship with the child, and set developmentally and culturally appropriate expectations. On the other hand, if there is not enough parental hierarchy, the counselor works with the parents to increase their consistency with consequences and to increase their attention to setting limits and rules. Thus, the same set of symptoms can require very different interventions.

Complementary Patterns

Complementary patterns characterize most couple relationships to a certain degree and can also characterize sibling relationships, friendships, and other relationships. *Complementary* in this case refers to each person taking on opposite or complementary roles, which exist on a range from functional to problematic. For example, a complementary relationship of introvert/extrovert can exist in a balanced and well-functioning relationship as well as in an out-of-balance, problematic relationship; the difference is in the rigidity of the pattern. Classic examples of complementary roles that often become problematic include pursuer/distancer, emotional/logical, overfunctioner/underfunctioner, friendly parent/strict parent, and the like. In fact, Gottman (1999) indicates that the female-pursue (demand) and male-withdraw pattern exists to some extent in the majority of marriages he studied. However, in distressed marriages, this becomes exaggerated and begins to be viewed as innate personality traits. Assessing for these patterns can help counselors intervene around these interactional dynamics. In most cases, people readily identify their complementary roles in their complaints about a relationship: "he's too strict with the kids"; "she always emotionally overreacts"; "I have to do it all the time"; "she never wants sex." These broad, sweeping descriptions of the other denote a likely problematic complementary pattern.

Intergenerational Patterns

Assessing for intergenerational patterns is easiest when using a genogram (McGoldrick, Gerson, & Petry, 2008), which provides a visual map of intergenerational patterns. Counselors can create comprehensive genograms, which map numerous intergenerational patterns, or problem-specific genograms, which focus on patterns related to the presenting problem and how family members have dealt with similar problems across generations (e.g., how other couples have dealt with marital tension). Patterns that frequently included in genograms are:

- Substance and alcohol abuse and dependence
- Sexual, physical, and emotional abuse
- Personal qualities and/or family roles; complementary roles (e.g., black sheep, rebellious one, overachiever/underachiever, etc.)
- Physical and mental health issues (e.g., diabetes, cancer, depression, psychosis, etc.)
- Historical incidents of the presenting problem, either with the same people or how other generations and family members have managed a similar problem.

Postmodern-Feminist Conceptualization

Solutions and Unique Outcomes

Solutions and Unique Outcomes

Attempted Solutions that DIDN'T or DON'T work:

1. ______________________________

2. ______________________________

3. ______________________________

Exceptions and Unique Outcomes: Times, places, relationships, contexts, etc., when problem is less of a problem; behaviors that seem to make things even slightly better:

1. ______________________________

2. ______________________________

3. ______________________________

Miracle Question Answer: If the problem were to be resolved overnight, what would client be doing differently the next day? (Describe in terms of doing X rather than not doing Y).

1. ______________________________

2. ______________________________

3. ______________________________

Attempted Solutions that DID NOT Work

When assessing solutions, counselors need to assess two kinds: those that have worked and those that have not. The MRI group (Watzlawick et al., 1974) and CBT counselors (Baucom & Epstein, 1990) are best known for assessing what has not worked, although they use these in different ways when they intervene. With most clients, it is generally easy to assess failed previous solutions.

Questions for Assessing Solutions That Did Not Work

- *What have you tried to solve this problem?*

Most clients respond with a list of things that have not worked. If they need more prompting, counselors may ask:

I am guessing you have tried to solve this problem (address this issue) on your own and that some things were not as successful as you had hoped. What have you tried that did not *work?*

Previous Solutions That DID Work/Unique Outcomes

Assessing previous solutions that helped is much harder, because most clients are less aware of when the problem is not a problem and of how they have kept things from getting worse. Solution-focused (de Shazer, 1988; O'Hanlon & Weiner-Davis, 1989) and narrative counselors (Freedman & Combs, 1996; White & Epston, 1990) have developed most of the assessment strategies for assessing what has worked.

Questions for Assessing Solutions and Unique Outcomes

- *What keeps this problem from being worse than it is right now?*
- *Is there any solution you have tried that worked for a while? Or made things slightly better?*
- *Are there times or places when the problem is less of a problem or when the problem is not a problem?*
- *Have you ever been able to respond to the problem so that it is less of a problem or less severe?*
- *Does this problem occur in all places with all people or is it better in certain contexts?*

These questions generally require more thought and reflection on the part of the client and often require more follow-up questions on the part of the counselor. The answers to these questions often provide invaluable clues about how best to proceed and intervene in counseling.

Miracle Question

The original solution-generating question, the *miracle question* serves to both (a) conceptualize and assess, and (b) set goals in solution-based counseling. The question goes as follows:

Miracle Question: Imagine that you go home tonight and during the middle of the night a miracle happens: ***all the problems you came here to resolve*** are miraculously resolved. However, when you wake up, you have no idea a miracle has occurred. What are some of the first things you would notice that would be different? How would you know that the problems that brought you here were resolved?

The key to successfully using this question to conceptualize the case involves (a) emphasizing that the miracle isn't just any ol' miracle but that it specifically resolves *problems that brought you here* today, and (b) getting specific, behavioral descriptions of what is different (not what the client wouldn't be doing or feeling). When delivered well, this single intervention can generate just about all of your client goals for treatment. For example, when working with a client who reports feeling depressed, a properly delivered miracle question would uncover goal-informing information, such as the client would (a) wake up excited about the day, (b) go for a run, (c) hug and kiss his wife, (d) read a passage from his favorite Rumi book, and (e) arrive at work on time and warmly greet coworkers.

Narrative, Dominant Discourses, and Diversity

Narrative, Dominant Discourses, and Diversity

- *Ethnic, Class, and Religious Discourses: How do key cultural discourses inform what is perceived as a problem and the possible solutions?*______________________

____

- *Gender and Sexuality Discourses: How do the gender/sexual discourses inform what is perceived as a problem and the possible solutions?*______________________

____

- *Community, School, and Extended Family Discourses: How do other important community discourses inform what is perceived as a problem and the possible solutions?*____

____

*Identity Narratives: How has the problem shaped each client's identity?*__________

____

*Local or Preferred Discourses: What is the client's preferred identity narrative and/or narrative about the problem? Are there local (alternative) discourses about the problem that are preferred?*____

Assessing dominant social discourses in which a client's problems are embedded often creates a broader and new perspective on a client's situation (Freedman & Combs, 1996; White & Epston, 1990). I frequently find that this broader perspective helps me feel more freedom and possibility, increasing my emotional attunement to clients and allowing me to be more creative in my work. For example, when I view a client's reported "anxiety" as part of a larger discourse in which the client feels powerless, such as being a sexual minority, I begin to see the anxiety as part of this larger social dance. I also see how it is possible for this person to put less "faith," weight, or credence to the dominant discourse and generate new stories about what is "normal" sexual behavior and what is not. By discussing the difficulty in concretely defining what is "normal" sexual behavior and what is not, the client and I can begin to explore the truths that this person has experienced. We join in an exploratory process that offers new ways for the client to understand the anxiety as well as his/her identity.

Common dominant discourses or broader narratives that inform clients' lives include:

- Culture, race, ethnicity, immigration
- Gender, sexual orientation, sexual preferences
- Family of origin experiences, such as alcoholism, sexual abuse, adoption, etc.
- Stories of divorce, death, and loss of significant relationships
- Wealth, poverty, power, fame
- Small town, urban, regional discourses
- Health, illness, body image, etc.

Identity Narratives

When a client comes for counseling, the problem discourse has almost always become a significant part of one or more person's *identity narrative*, the story people tell themselves as to who they are. For example, a child having problems in school may begin to think, "I am stupid," while his mother may also be feeling like, "I have failed as a mother" because of her child's academic performance. Obviously, these negative sweeping judgments of a person's value or ability need to be addressed in counseling. Assessing these early in the process is useful to understand how to engage and motivate each person.

Local and Preferred Discourses

Local discourses are the stories that occur at the "local" (as opposed to dominant societal) level (Andersen, 1997). These narratives often are built upon personal beliefs and unique interpretations and often contradict or significantly modify dominant discourses. Although it is theoretically possible for local discourses to contribute to the problem (e.g., having more oppressive versions of dominant discourses), they are most often a significant source of motivation, energy, and hope for addressing problems. Most often, local discourses are a person's "personal truth" that they have been hiding or are ashamed of because of anticipated disapproval from others. Local discourses can address common subculture values, such as valuing certain religious or sexual practices, or highly unique to an individual, such as wanting to sell everything and travel the world. Local discourses are often the source of *preferred discourses* in narrative counseling (Freedman & Combs, 1996), which are the preferred version of one's life and identity that serve as the goal in narrative counseling.

Case Conceptualization, Diversity, and Sameness

Just in case you were beginning to feel like you finally understood something about case conceptualization, let me throw a wrench or two into the mix: diversity and sameness. The problem with case conceptualization and assessments in general (this applies to the next several chapters as well) is that there are no objective standards against which a person can be measured for "healthy boundaries," "logical thinking," or "clear communication." Healthy, emotionally engaged boundaries look quite different in a Mexican American family and an Asian American family. In fact, problematic boundaries in a Mexican American family (e.g., cool, disengaged) may look *more like* healthy (e.g., quietly respectful) than problem boundaries (e.g., overly involved) in an Asian American families. Thus, counselors cannot rely simply on objective descriptions of behavior in assessment. Instead, counselors must consider the broader culture norms, which may include *more than one* set of ethnic norms as well as local neighborhood culture, school contexts, sexual orientation subculture, religious communities, and so forth. Although you will undoubtedly take a course on cultural issues that will go into more depth on this topic and will read that professional codes of ethics requires respecting diversity, it takes working with a diverse range of individuals and families and a willingness to learn from them to cultivate a meaningful sense of cultural sensitivity. I believe this to be a lifelong journey.

Ironically, I have found that new counselors in training today sometimes have the most difficulty accepting diversity in clients from *within* their culture of origin or who are in some ways similar to the counselor. The more similar clients are to us, the more we expect them to share our values and behavioral norms, making us more likely to have a low threshold for differentness. For example, middle-class Caucasian counselors often expect middle-class Caucasian clients to have particular values toward emotional expression, marital arrangements, extended family, and parent-child relationships, and may be quick to encourage particular systems of values, namely their own. Thus, whether working with someone very similar to or very different from yourself, counselors need to *slowly* assess and evaluate, always considering clients' broader sociocultural context and norms. Counselors who excel in conceptualization and assessment approach these tasks with profound humility and a continual willingness to learn.

Questions for Personal Reflection and Class Discussion

1. What areas of the case conceptualization do you find most interesting and intriguing? Which seem least useful?
2. Which area of the conceptualization fits with how you typically think of human problems and struggles? Which area seems most foreign to your typical way of thinking?
3. Which areas of the conceptualization do you think will be most useful when working with:
    - Someone who is depressed? Why?
    - Someone who has anxiety? Why?
    - Someone who has relationship difficulties? Why?
    - Someone who is grieving? Why?
    - A child with ADHD? Why?
    - Someone with a substance use disorder? Why?
4. What specific areas might be most useful when working with a Latina client who was sexually abused as a child? Why?
5. Which areas of the conceptualization seem most useful for:
    - Understanding why the client has a problem?
    - Setting useful treatment goals?
    - Intervening the best with the problem?
    - Helping a client grow and develop new coping skills?

Online Resource

Family History Maker: U.S. Department of Health and Human Services
www.hhs.gov/familyhistory/

References

Anderson, H. (1997). *Conversations, language, and possibilities.* New York: Basic.

Anderson, H., & Gehart, D. R. (Eds.). (2007). *Collaborative therapy: Relationships and conversations that make a difference.* New York: Brunner-Routledge.

Bateson, G. (1972). *Steps to an ecology of mind.* New York: Ballentine.

Bateson, G. (1979/2002). *Mind and nature: A necessary unity.* Cresskill, NJ: Hampton.

Baucom, D. H., & Epstein, N. (1990). *Cognitive-behavioral marital therapy.* New York: Brunner/Mazel.

Beck, A. (176). *Cognitive therapy and emotional disorders.* New York: International University Press.

Bowlby, J. (1988). *A secure base: Parent-child attachment and healthy human development.* London: Routledge.

Carter, B., & McGoldrick, M. (1999). *The expanded family life cycle: Individuals, families, and social perspectives* (3rd ed.). New York: Allyn & Bacon.

Chapman, A. (2006). Erickson's psychosocial development theory. Retrieved from http://www.businessballs.com/erik_erikson_psychosocial_theory.htm.

de Shazer, S. (1988). *Clues: Investigating solutions in brief therapy.* New York: Norton.

Eckstein, D. (2009). An understanding of each person's personal prefernces. Retrieved from http://www.santafecoach.com/DRC/drcpp-test%20theory.htm#comfortpar.

Ellis, A. (1999). *Reason and emotion in psychotherapy* (revised). New York: Kensington.

Frankl, V. (1963). *Man's search for meaning.* Boston: Beacon.

Freedman, J., & Combs, G. (1996). *Narrative therapy: The social contruction of preferred realities.* New York: Norton.

Gergen, K. J. (1999). *An invitation to social construction.* Thousand Oaks, CA: Sage.

Gottman, J. M. (1999). *The marriage clinic: A scientifically based marital therapy.* New York: Norton.

Johnson, S. M. (2004). *The practice of emotionally focused marital therapy: Creating connection* (2nd ed.). New York: Brunner-Routledge.

Kerr, M., & Bowen, M. (1988). *Family evaluation.* New York: Norton.

Lambert, M. J., & Ogles, B. M. (2004). The efficacy and effectiveness of psychotherapy. In M. J. Lambert (Ed.), *Bergin and Garfield's handbook of psychotherapy and behavior change* (5th ed., pp. 139–193). New York: Wiley.

McGoldrick, M., Gerson, R., & Petry, S. (2008). *Genograms: Assessment and intervention* (3rd ed.). New York: Norton.

Miller, S. D., Duncan, B. L., & Hubble, M. (1997). *Escape from Babel: Toward a unifying language for psychotherapy practice*. New York: Norton.
Minuchin, S. (1974). *Families and family therapy*. Cambridge, MA: Harvard University Press.
Minuchin, S., & Fishman, H. C. (1981). *Family therapy techniques*. Cambridge, MA: Harvard University Press.
Morgan, O. (2006). *Counseling and spirituality: Views from the profession*. Pacific Grove, CA: Wadsworth.
O'Hanlon, W. H., & Weiner-Davis, M. (1989). *In search of solutions: A new direction in psychotherapy*. New York: Norton.
Perls, F., Hefferline, R. F., & Goodman, P. (1951). *Gestalt therapy: Excitement and growth in the human personality*. New York: Julian Press.
Rogers, C. (1961). *On becoming a person: A counselor's view of psychocounseling*. London: Constable.
Seligman, M. (2002). *Authentic happiness: Using the new positive psychology to realize your potential for lasting fulfillment*. New York: Free Press.
Sperry, L. (2001). *Spirituality in clinical practice: Incorporating the spiritual dimension in psychotherapy and counseling*. New York: Routledge.
Spiegler, M. D., & Guevremont, D. C. (2003). *Contemporary behavior therapy* (4th ed.). Pacific Grove, CA: Brooks/Cole.
St. Clair, M. (2000). *Object relations and self psychology: An introduction*. Belmont, CA: Brooks/Cole.
Walsh, F. (Ed.) (2003). *Spiritual resources in family therapy*. New York: Guilford.
Watzlawick, P., Weakland, J., & Fisch, R. (1974). *Change: Principles of problem formation and problem resolution*. New York: Norton.
Whitaker, C. A., & Keith, D. V. (1981). Symbolic-experiential family therapy. In A. S. Gurman & D. P. Kniskern (Eds.), *Handbook of family therapy* (pp. 187–224). New York: Brunner/Mazel.
White, M., & Epston, D. (1990). *Narrative means to therapeutic ends*. New York: Norton.
Woldt, A. L., & Toman, S. M. (Eds.) (2005). *Gestalt therapy: History, theory, and practice*. Thousand Oaks, CA: Sage.
Yontef, G. (1993). *Awareness dialogue and process: Essays on Gestalt therapy*. Highland, NY: Gestalt Journal Press.

Case Conceptualization Form

COPIES OF THIS FORM ARE AVAILABLE ON THE CENGAGE WEBSITE AND THE BOOK'S WEBSITE: WWW.MASTERINGCOMPETENCIES.COM

COUNSELING CASE CONCEPTUALIZATION

Date: __________ **Clinician:** __________ **Client/Case #:** __________

I. Introduction to Client

Identify primary client and significant others

Client

Select Client Type Age: ___ Select Ethnicity Select Relational Status Occupation/Grade: __________

Other: __________

Significant Others

Select Person Age: ___ Select Ethnicity Select Relational Status Occupation/Grade: __________

Other: __________

Select Person Age: ___ Select Ethnicity Select Relational Status Occupation/Grade: __________

Other: __________

Select Person Age: ___ Select Ethnicity Select Relational Status Occupation/Grade: __________

Other: __________

Select Person Age: ___ Select Ethnicity Select Relational Status Occupation/Grade: __________

Other: __________

II. Presenting Concern(s)

Client Description of Problem(s): __________

Significant Other/Family Description(s) of Problems: __________

Broader System Problem Descriptions: Description of problem from referring party, teachers, relatives, legal system, etc.:

Name: __________

Name: __________

III. Background Information

Trauma/Abuse History (recent and past): __________

(*continued*)

Substance Use/Abuse (current and past; self, family of origin, significant others): ___

Precipitating Events (recent life changes, first symptoms, stressors, etc.): ___

Related Historical Background (family history, related issues, previous counseling, etc.): ___

IV. Client Strengths and Diversity

Client Strengths

Personal: ___

Relational/Social: ___

Spiritual: ___

Diversity: Resources and Limitations

Identify potential resources and limitations available to clients based on their age, gender, sexual orientation, cultural background, socioeconomic status, religion, regional community, language, family background, family configuration, abilities, etc.

Unique Resources: ___

Potential Limitations: ___

Complete All of the Following Sections for a Complete Case Conceptualization or Specific Sections for Theory-Specific Conceptualization.

V. Psychodynamic Conceptualization

Psychodynamic Defense Mechanisms

Check 2–4 most commonly used defense mechanisms

❑ Acting Out: *Describe:* ___

❑ Denial: *Describe:* ___

❑ Displacement: *Describe:* ___

❑ Help-rejecting Complaining: *Describe:* ___

❑ Humor: *Describe:* ___

❑ Passive Aggression: *Describe:* ___

❑ Projection: *Describe:* ___

❑ Projective Identification: *Describe:* ___

(continued)

❑ Rationalization: *Describe:* ______

❑ Reaction Formation: *Describe:* ______

❑ Repression: *Describe:* ______

❑ Splitting: *Describe:* ______

❑ Sublimation: *Describe:* ______

❑ Suppression: *Describe:* ______

❑ Other: ______

Object Relational Patterns

Describe relationship with early caregivers in past: ______

______

______

Was the attachment with the mother (or equivalent) primarily: ❑ Generally Secure

❑ Anxious and Clingy ❑ Avoidant and Emotionally ❑ Distant Other: ______

Was the attachment with the father (or equivalent) primarily: ❑ Generally Secure

❑ Anxious and Clingy ❑ Avoidant and Emotionally ❑ Distant Other: ______

Describe present relationship with these caregivers: ______

______

______

*Describe relational patterns with partner and other current relationships:*______

______

______

Erickson's Psychosocial Developmental Stage

Describe development at each stage up to current stage

Trust vs. Mistrust (Infant stage): ______

Autonomy vs. Shame and Doubt (Toddler stage): ______

Initiative vs. Guilt (Preschool age): ______

Industry vs. Inferiority (School age): ______

Identity vs. Role Confusion (Adolescence): ______

Intimacy vs. Isolation (Young adulthood): ______

Generativity vs. Stagnation (Adulthood): ______

Ego Integrity vs. Despair (Late Adulthood): ______

Adlerian Style of Life Theme

❑ Control: ______

❑ Superiority: ______

❑ Pleasing: ______

❑ Comfort: ______

Basic Mistake Misperceptions: ______

(*continued*)

VI. Humanistic-Existential Conceptualization

Expression of Authentic Self

Problems: Are problems perceived as internal or external (caused by others, circumstance, etc.)?
❑ Predominantly internal ❑ Mixed ❑ Predominantly external

Agency and Responsibility: Is self or other discussed as agent of story? Does client take clear responsibility for situation? ❑ Strong sense of agency and responsibility ❑ Agency in some areas
❑ Little agency; frequently blames others/situation ❑ Often feels victimized

Recognition and Expression of Feelings: Are feelings readily recognized, owned, and experienced?
❑ Easily expresses feelings ❑ Identifies feelings with prompting ❑ Difficulty recognizing feelings

Here-and-Now Experiencing: Is the client able to experience full range of feelings as they are happening in the present moment? ❑ Easily experiences emotions in present moment ❑ Experiences some present emotions with assistance ❑ Difficulty with experiencing the present moment

Personal Constructs and Facades: Is the client able to recognize and go beyond roles? Is identity rigid or tentatively held? ❑ Tentatively held; able to critique and question ❑ Some awareness of facades and construction of identity ❑ Identity rigidly defined; seems like "fact"

Complexity and Contradictions: Are internal contradictions owned and explored? Is client able to fully engage the complexity of identity and life? ❑ Aware of and resolves contradictions ❑ Some recognition of contradictions
❑ Unaware of internal contradictions

Shoulds: Is client able to question socially imposed shoulds and oughts? Can client balance desire to please others and desire to be authentic? ❑ Able to balance authenticity with social obligation
❑ Identifies tension between social expectations and personal desires ❑ Primarily focuses on external shoulds
List shoulds: ______________________________

Acceptance of Others: Is client able to accept others and modify expectations of others to be more realistic?
❑ Readily accepts others as they are ❑ Recognizes expectations of others are unrealistic but still strong emotional reaction to expectations not being met ❑ Difficulty accepting others as they are; always wanting others to change to meet expectations

Trust of Self: Is client able to trust self as process (rather than as stable object)? ❑ Able to trust and express authentic self ❑ Trust of self in certain contexts ❑ Difficulty trusting self in most contexts

Existential Analysis

Sources of Life Meaning (as described or demonstrated by client): ______________________________

____

____

General Themes of Life Meaning: ❑ Personal achievement/work ❑ Significant other ❑ Children ❑ Family of origin ❑ Social cause/contributing to others ❑ Religion/spirituality ❑ Other: ______________
Satisfaction with and clarity on life direction:

(continued)

❑ Clear sense of meaning that creates resilience in difficult times

❑ Current problems require making choices related to life direction

❑ Minimally satisfied with current life direction; wants more from life

❑ Has reflected little on life direction up to this point; living according to life plan defined by someone/something else

❑ Other: ______________________________

Gestalt Contact Boundary Disturbances

❑ *Desensitization:* Failing to notice problems

❑ *Introjection*: Take in others' views whole and unedited

❑ *Projection*: Assign undesired parts of self to others

❑ *Retroflection*: Direct action to self rather than other

❑ *Deflection*: Avoid direct contact with another or self

❑ *Egotism:* Not allowing outside to influence self

❑ *Confluence*: Agree with another to extent that boundary blurred

*Describe:*______________________________

____

VII. Cognitive-Behavioral Conceptualization

Baseline of Symptomatic Behavior

Symptom #1 (behavioral description): ______________________________

Frequency: ______________________________

Duration: ______________________________

Context(s): ______________________________

Events Before: ______________________________

Events After: ______________________________

Symptom #2 (behavioral description): ______________________________

Frequency: ______________________________

Duration: ______________________________

Context(s): ______________________________

Events Before: ______________________________

Events After: ______________________________

A-B-C Analysis of Irrational Beliefs

Activating Event ("Problem"):

Consequence (Mood, behavior, etc.):

Mediating Beliefs (Unhelpful beliefs about event(s) that result(s) in C):

1. ______________________________
2. ______________________________
3. ______________________________

(continued)

Beck's Schema Analysis

Identify frequently used cognitive schemas:

❑ *Arbitrary inference:* ______________________________

❑ *Selective abstraction:* ______________________________

❑ *Overgeneralization:* ______________________________

❑ *Magnification/Minimization:* ______________________________

❑ *Personalization:* ______________________________

❑ *Absolutist/Dichotomous thinking:* ______________________________

❑ *Mislabeling:* ______________________________

❑ *Mindreading:* ______________________________

VIII. Family Systems Conceptualization

Family Life Cycle Stage

❑ Single Adult ❑ Marriage ❑ Family with Young Children ❑ Family with Adolescent Children ❑ Launching Children ❑ Later Life

❑ Describe struggles with mastering developmental tasks in one of these stages: ______________________________

____

Boundaries with

Parents: ❑ Enmeshed ❑ Clear ❑ Disengaged ❑ NA: *Describe:* ______________________________

Significant Other: ❑ Enmeshed ❑ Clear ❑ Disengaged ❑ NA: *Describe:* ______________________________

Children: ❑ Enmeshed ❑ Clear ❑ Disengaged ❑ NA: *Describe:* ______________________________

Extended Family: ❑ Enmeshed ❑ Clear ❑ Disengaged ❑ NA: *Describe:* ______________________________

Other: Name ❑ Enmeshed ❑ Clear ❑ Disengaged ❑ NA: *Describe:* ______________________________

Typical style for regulating closeness and distance with others: ______________________________

Triangles/Coalitions

❑ Coalition in family of origin: *Describe:* ______________________________

❑ Coalitions related to significant other: *Describe:* ______________________________

❑ Other coalitions: ______________________________

Hierarchy between Self and Parent/Child ❑ NA

With own children ❑ Effective ❑ Rigid ❑ Permissive

With parents (for child/young adult): ❑ Effective ❑ Rigid ❑ Permissive

Complementary Patterns with Name: ______________________________

❑ Pursuer/distancer ❑ Over-/underfunctioner ❑ Emotional/logical ❑ Good/bad parent ❑ Other: *Describe*

Example of complementary pattern: ______________________________

Intergenerational Patterns ______________________________

Substance/Alcohol Abuse: ❑ NA ❑ History: ______________________________

Sexual/Physical/Emotional Abuse: ❑ NA ❑ History: ______________________________

(*continued*)

Parent/Child Relations: ❑ NA ❑ History: ____________________

Physical/Mental Disorders: ❑ NA ❑ History: ____________________

Family Strengths: *Describe:* ____________________

IX. Solution-Based and Cultural Discourse Conceptualization (Postmodern)

Solutions and Unique Outcomes

Attempted Solutions that DIDN'T or DON'T work:

1. ____________________
2. ____________________
3. ____________________

Exceptions and Unique Outcomes: Times, places, relationships, contexts, etc. when problem is less of a problem; behaviors that seem to make things even slightly better:

1. ____________________
2. ____________________
3. ____________________

Miracle Question Answer: If the problem were to be resolved overnight, what would client be doing differently the next day? (Describe in terms of doing X rather than not doing Y).

1. ____________________
2. ____________________
3. ____________________

Dominant Discourses informing definition of problem:

- *Ethnic, Class, and Religious Discourses: How do key cultural discourses inform what is perceived as a problem and the possible solutions?* ____________________
- *Gender and Sexuality Discourses: How do the gender/sexual discourses inform what is perceived as a problem and the possible solutions?* ____________________
- *Community, School, and Extended Family Discourses: How do other important community discourses inform what is perceived as a problem and the possible solutions?* ____________________

Identity Narratives: How has the problem shaped each client's identity? ____________________

Local or Preferred Discourses: What is the client's preferred identity narrative and/or narrative about the problem? Are there local (alternative) discourses about the problem that are preferred? ____________________

CHAPTER

3

Introduction to Clinical Assessment and Diagnosis

Step 2: Identify Oases and Obstacles

Aside from feeling like you had a full workout after completing a case conceptualization, you have a comprehensive understanding of your client and the key issues: limiting core beliefs, ineffective interpersonal dynamics, level of self-actualization, and so on. You should feel confident with clear direction, ready to put on your walking shoes and start the counseling journey. But before you go rushing off, you need to get a more detailed map that will help you avoid obstacles and identify potential rest stops, which, in more technical terms, is a clinical assessment: the complement to case conceptualization.

Clinical assessment focuses on the psychiatric and medical symptoms of clients, allowing you to have a better sense of how to more effectively partner with them as you start your journey. Although most of the time what you learn from a clinical assessment will not reveal information that causes you to radically shift direction from your case conceptualization, sometimes it does—and when it does, you will be very glad you spent the time assessing.

Lay of the Land

Given the complexity of clinical assessment, the next two chapters will introduce you to this intricate art. In this chapter, you will learn about:

- Definition and purpose of clinical assessment and diagnosis
- Diversity and cultural issues related to clinical assessment and diagnosis
- Counseling models relationship to clinical assessment and diagnosis
- Contemporary issues in diagnosis: recovery model and parity diagnosis
- The newly revised DSM-5, its organization, new diagnosis format, and assessments
- Counseling and the mental status exam

In Chapter 4, you will learn how to complete a clinical assessment form.

Clinical Assessment and Diagnosis

Mental health professionals from all disciplines—counseling, psychology, family therapy, psychiatry, psychiatric nursing, and social work—share a common set of competencies related to clinical assessment, which includes the following:

- Performing a mental status exam to identify psychological symptoms
- Making mental health diagnoses using the DSM-5 (*Diagnostic and Statistical Manual*, 5th Edition)
- Monitoring for client safety
- Identifying medical and psychiatric conditions that warrant medical attention outside the counselor's scope of practice
- Case management, including referrals to necessary social services

Although these basic skills are required of all, practitioners have a surprising degree of freedom in terms of *how* they perform these tasks. Counselors are free to use structured or unstructured interview methods; written or verbal assessments; standardized or original instruments. The "best" method depends on the clinical setting and client characteristics. Although considered standard practice, counselors should be mindful that clinical assessment and diagnosis have both benefits and potential liabilities.

Purpose of Clinical Assessment and Diagnosis

Clinical assessment and mental health diagnosis serve several practical purposes. They can help counselors (a) coordinate care with other professions, (b) decide how best to keep clients and the public safe, (c) determine the need for referrals and additional services, and (d) help identify potential courses of treatment. Diagnostic language provides a relatively simple way for a wide range of medical and mental health professionals to serve the same client—if we all had different systems of identifying problems, coordinating care would be far more challenging. In addition, certain diagnoses are known to be correlated with particular crisis issues, such as depression and suicide and self-harm; thus, diagnosis can help clinicians remember to screen for potential crisis and enable them to more effectively assist clients seeking additional resources. Furthermore, certain diagnoses have a well-established research base that helps the clinician identify a preferred treatment method, such as behavioral interventions for phobias.

Moreover, some clients find that having a diagnosis is helpful, even liberating. For example, many survivors of sexual abuse are relieved to hear that the symptoms they are experiencing—hypervigilance, nightmares, and flashbacks—are part of a larger syndrome, Post-Traumatic Stress Disorder, and that this condition has a good prognosis. Similarly, depending on their view of mental health diagnosis, some clients with whom I have worked report feeling relief when they learn that they (or their partner) meet the criteria for Major Depressive Disorder, a condition that is less severe or humiliating than they feared (such as "lazy," "uncaring," "out of love," or "really crazy").

In addition to potential clinical benefits, there are some practical benefits for researchers and third-party payers. An inspiring example: Because researchers around the globe have had the diagnoses of "autism" and "Asperger's syndrome" to collectively study, they have been able to move forward a focused research agenda that has dramatically changed our understanding of and the prognosis for these disorders (APA, 2013). Without an agreed-upon set of diagnostic definitions and criteria, researchers would have had no way to coordinate their efforts in order to better the lives of children and families struggling with these issues. In a similar fashion, having agreed-upon descriptions and criteria for mental health concerns makes it possible for third-party payers to reimburse persons diagnosed with a particular condition, enabling mental health services to be paid through health insurance and similar mechanisms. Although not everyone may agree that having insurance involved in mental health treatment is ultimately desirable, it is a reality for many needing services, and most clients of average or lower financial means would have much greater difficulty using services without the help of insurance.

Clinical Assessment and Diagnosis: Limitations and Cautions with Diversity

With several clear benefits, how could mental health diagnosis possibly be a problem or even dangerous? Like most things in life, clinical assessment and diagnosis are a double-edged sword. Many advocates have concerns about diagnosis with diverse populations, particularly marginalized ethnic groups, gay/lesbian/bisexual/transgendered individuals, and women. In addition, several theoretical schools of counseling and psychotherapy have concerns about the effects of clinical assessment and diagnosis on the client as well as the counseling relationship. The most notable critiques come from humanistic, family systems, and postmodern counselors and therapists.

Diagnosis and Our Inescapable Cultural Lenses

Each counselor views a client through a unique lens. As a counselor, your lens is your personal culture, values, history, beliefs, and norms. These are generally things that make us who we are, and they cannot be cast aside by simply telling yourself to be "neutral." In addition, systemic counselors remind us that we are part of the system we are trying to observe, thus significantly influencing the behavior of the observed (Keeney, 1983). Think about it: the last time you were in a doctor's office describing your medical problem, were you your "normal self"? Most of us significantly alter how we speak and act when working with a professional, making it more difficult for the professional to get an accurate read of what is happening. Additionally, any words the counselor uses to describe the client comes from the *counselor's* worldview, not the client's. Counselor's descriptions of clients reveal more about the *counselor* than the client: clinical assessment reveals what the counselor and the broader mental health culture values as "good," "healthy," and "valuable" enough to focus on.

Postmodern philosophers are keenly aware of the intersubjectivity that occurs in counseling relationships. Two "horizons of meaning" or worldviews meet when counselor and client talk (Gadamer, 1975). Because counselors cannot step out of their cultures, beliefs, personalities, histories, or theoretical training in order to be neutral and unbiased, counselors must always interpret the client from where they are standing, their particular horizon of meaning. For example, a Latina counselor who grew up in a well-to-do suburb will have a different interpretation of an urban teen's story than a Latina whose parents were migrant farm labors, with neither being necessarily more "accurate" than the other. The "nearness" of the suburban counselor does not ensure greater accuracy because the counselor may have *more* biases from repeat encounters with this type of client; the rural counselor may be more "objective" or more biased, depending on how aware the counselor is of his/her "horizon of meaning" and its effects on viewing the client. Thus, counselors' ability to become aware of their lenses (horizon for making meaning and interpreting others) increases their ability to see the other person more clearly and with less unreflected bias. When beginning the journey of becoming a counselor, everyone is very limited in the awareness of the lenses through which they view others. Part of the goal of training is to help awaken counselors to see the lenses through which they view their clients.

At the same time, however, professional training provides counselors with an entirely new set of lenses that take the form of theories of health and normalcy. These can also be problematic, especially when working with people who are inherently different from the norm, such as cultural, sexual, or other minority clients. The *DSM* is the *Diagnostic and Statistical Manual.* Statistics are based on *norms*, making it difficult to accurately apply DSM criteria with those whose demographics vary significantly from the norm. Clinical assessment is one of the most dangerous places for counselors to practice if they are not clearly aware of their personal biases, because there is little feedback if one gets off course.

For example, when you try using a counseling technique that is not appropriate for a client, it is often immediately obvious because the client will refuse to participate or in some way signal that he/she does not like the idea—the major exception to this is a client who wants to please the counselor. Similarly, if one's case conceptualization is incorrect, the client will not progress and/or new information comes to light that helps the counselor refine the conceptualization as part of the hypothesizing process itself; case conceptualization is by nature a process of hypothesizing, gathering feedback from the family through interactions, then refining the hypothesis based on this information. However, when doing clinical assessment, it is easier to get off course.

The medical model that informs DSM diagnosis is based on the concept that the professional has access to a more precise truth, and thus the counselor is less likely to continually question and refine diagnoses and mental status reports (Anderson, 1997). The model is predicated on the assumption that it is easy to distinguish between normal and abnormal behaviors, which is more difficult in the psychological than physical realm. For example, behaviors such as drinking, talking, emoting, eating, worrying, or seeing ghosts have different meanings and norms depending on one's family, culture, social class, and so on. Thus, although it *appears* that we begin with a clear set of norms of mental health, when a counselor begins to fully attend to the broader social context of the client, it becomes much less clear where normal ends and abnormal begins. In fact, some argue that because the concept of "mental illness" lacks any reliable corollary measurement of health, it is more of a socially constructed myth than factual science (Hansen, 2003). Furthermore, just because medications can ameliorate psychiatric symptoms, this does not validate particular diagnostic categories, just the drugs' effectiveness. Thus, counselors must cautiously and thoughtfully approach diagnosis, especially with diverse clients.

Diagnosis and Gender

Although in the development of the most recent version of the DSM its authors tried to reduce gender bias (APA, 2013), historically the enterprise of psychiatric diagnosis is frequently critiqued for pathologizing feminine traits and behaviors while failing to develop diagnoses for issues more likely to affect men (Eriksen & Kress, 2008). Feminists argue that diagnoses such as nymphomania, hysteria, neurasthenia, erotomania, kleptomania, and masochism have served to unnecessarily pathologize and subordinate women (Eriksen & Kress, 2008). In particular, personality diagnoses, such as borderline, dependent, and histrionic, can be understood as an exaggeration of otherwise socially promoted female qualities. Furthermore, several studies have shown that women who enter treatment are more likely to be characterized as "unhealthy" by professionals simply because they exhibit typical female qualities, such as greater emotional expression, less independence, and less goal-directed activity, and are more easily influenced by others (Eriksen & Kress, 2008). Thus, counselors need to carefully attend to gender bias when making diagnoses, carefully considering whether female clients are being overpathologized. Conversely, some argue that men may be underdiagnosed, especially if they are reticent to talk about emotions, and are therefore are potentially undertreated.

DSM-5, Social Justice, and the Cultural Case Formulation

As part of their attempt to address the cultural bias of the DSM, the most recent edition of the DSM includes a cultural formulation and cultural interview protocol to assist clinicians in considering cultural and diversity issues when conducting a clinical assessment and making a diagnosis (APA, 2013). In particular, counselors committed to social justice may find this interview useful in their work. Similar to case conceptualization in Chapter 2, *cultural formulation* invites clinicians to take a step back and learn from clients about how their problems (or apparent problems) are understood within their cultural context and also consider relevant sociopolitical and social justice issues. When living in situations where they are ostracized, marginalized, or abused, most people act and behave in ways that may appear odd or pathological due to the inherent trauma, stigma, and social pressures. For example, in some cases, people *are* out to get your client—the client isn't paranoid and actually needs assistance with ensuring personal safety. In other cases, what may look like paranoia, depression, or anxiety may actually be best understood as Post-Traumatic Stress Disorder due to abuse or maltreatment related to cultural and social differences. Thus, counselors need to perform a broad, socially aware assessment of their clients to ensure accurate and appropriate diagnoses. Building on the cultural formulation in the DSM-IV, the DSM-5 includes a revised outline for cultural formulation as well as an interview guide, complete with sample prompts and questions to be used in session to gather cultural information (see Cultural Formulation and Assessment below; APA, 2000, 2013, pp. 752–775).

Counseling Models and Diagnosis: Philosophical and Practical Concerns

Although counselors will be required to diagnose their clients in most treatment environments, this does not mean that diagnosis should necessarily *drive* treatment. In fact, several approaches to counseling are based on the assumption that *diagnosis may not be the most useful means for conceptualizing treatment or how counselors and therapists best position themselves in relation to clients to promote change.* Most notably, humanistic, family, and postmodern counselors do not conceptualize treatment around a diagnosis, and in fact, many of their proponents caution *against* using any diagnosis at all.

Humanistic Concerns with Diagnosis

One of the leading humanistic counselors, Carl Rogers did not organize his approach using diagnostic labeling. He announced his concerns in some of his earliest writings: diagnosis "is unnecessary for psychotherapy, and may actually be a detriment to the therapeutic process" (1951, p. 220). His concerns included that the diagnostic process limits the counselor's ability to authentically relate to clients. In addition, it puts the counselor in an expert position, with the responsibility to "treat" the client, and thereby failing to support and foster self-actualization in the client, which Rogers defined as the ultimate goal of therapy.

Diagnostic labeling is antithetical not only to the general spirit but also to the underlying theoretical premises of Rogers's person-centered counseling (Freeth, 2007; Schmid, 2004; Sugarman, 1978). Grounding their work in a phenomenological view of humans, person-centered counselors are "interested in a person's subjective experience, as it is for that person, without trying to define or explain it" (Freeth, 2006, p. 55). Since the focus of this approach is on the client's inner, subjective experience, external diagnostic labels *distract* counselor and client alike from the primary realm of focus. Furthermore, rather than the counselor informing the client of a diagnosis, "it is the client who defines the meaning of his/her experiencing and thus 'informs' the counselor" [about classifying his/her experience] (p. 36).

In a classic review of the humanistic literature, Sugarman (1978) identified five primary points of critique of diagnosis by humanists:

Humanistic Critique of Diagnosis

1. *Reductionistic:* The first concern is that clinical assessment and diagnosis is reductionist: it loses sight of the whole person and instead breaks the person down into discrete parts that malfunction. The individuality of client is lost as the person is lumped into categories of similar others.
2. *Artificial:* The assessment and diagnosis system is artificial, not arising from the client's natural environment or inner process but instead derived from the professional's worldview. Furthermore, when conducted in a clinical environment, the assessor is unable to accurately assess the person in context.
3. *Ignores the Relationship:* The diagnostic process frequently does not take into account the counselor-client relationship and how it might affect client behaviors in session and reports of behavior out of session.

(*continued*)

4. *Judgment:* The diagnostic process puts the counselor in the position of making a type of judgment about the client, which in many cases makes it hard to embody the humanistic principle of unconditional positive regard.
5. *Intellectualism:* Humanists also argue that the assessment and diagnostic process intellectualizes problems of the human condition, instead of engaging such problems from a position of spontaneity and authenticity and recognizing their existential nature of suffering.

Given that diagnosis does not inform humanistic *treatment*, does that mean that person-centered counselors are exempt from the general practice of clinical assessment and diagnosis? There may have been a time when the answer to this question could be a more confident "yes." But increasingly, counselors are expected to conduct a clinical assessment and diagnosis regardless of their theoretical orientation, especially if they want to avoid lawsuits or ethical violations, because most professionals, insurance companies, and ethics codes would consider diagnosis part of "standard care." In fact, a recent review of the literature traces the ongoing debate between humanistic counseling psychologists, who insist on staying true to their philosophical position against labeling, and those advocating the more pragmatic need to collaborate with other professionals and work within contemporary environments (Larsson, Brooks, & Loewenthal, 2012). Toward this end, it may be helpful to clearly distinguish between the process of diagnosis and treatment because—at least for humanistic counselors and therapists—clinical assessment and diagnosis may *not* be the most useful means of *conceptualizing the actual treatment*.

Family Systems Concerns with Diagnosis

Systemic counselors have similar concerns about the effects of diagnostic labels on clients, yet they identify a different set of potential problems. Systemic counselors base their work on the foundational assumption that "all behavior makes sense in context" (Ray & Watzlawick, 2005/2009, p. 186). A seminal systemic practitioner, Don Jackson (1967/2009) describes the "myth of normality" in his classic essay of that title, arguing that the practice of diagnosis promotes a dangerous perception that "normal" behavior can be readily identified and separated from pathological behavior. Instead, systemic clinicians argue that all behavior has a meaning and purpose in its given context.

By only focusing on a person's behavior—rather than the entire interactional sequence between people—systemic counselors argue that a single person is unfairly characterized as somehow possessing a pathology that serves a role within a complex relational web (Selvini-Palazzoli, Boscolo, Cecchin, & Prata, 1978; Watzlawick, Weakland, & Fisch, 1974). This artificial distinction can lead to blaming or pathologizing a single person for an inherently relational dynamic. A classic example is diagnosing one partner as depressed when the depression serves a role within the couple system. Similarly, often diagnosable behavior in children, such as opposition and defiance, labels the child's behavior as problematic; yet this behavior serves a meaningful systemic function, such as a focus of attention that unites an otherwise distressed couple. Similar to humanistic counselors, systemic family counselors and therapists rarely use clinical diagnosis to conceptualize treatment and intervention even when they work in contexts that require it.

Postmodern Concerns with Diagnosis

Postmodern practitioners, such as narrative and collaborative counselors, are skeptical of diagnoses because these become labels that clients use to inform their identity, often silencing a person's strengths, resiliencies, and capabilities (Anderson, 1997; Gergen, Anderson, & Hoffman, 1996). The danger is that once a person is given a diagnostic label, it is easy to interpret future behaviors and events through this lens, becoming a self-fulfilling prophecy. For example, when a child is diagnosed with ADHD, parents, teachers, and the child tend to develop telescopic vision, focusing their attention on the child's hyperactivity and attention, but missing exceptions to the label and other elements of the child's identity, such as mentoring a younger sibling, a musical talent, or a pro-family attitude.

When working in contexts where diagnoses are regularly used, postmodern counselors conceptualize the diagnosis as one of several voices in the counseling conversation. In the case of narrative counselors, they often literally give the diagnosis a name and voice by externalizing the diagnosis (see Chapter 14) as Depression or Anorexia and talk about it as if it were a person or external force so that clients separate themselves linguistically from their problems (White & Epston, 1990): So what does Anorexia tell you to convince you that you're fat? Does Anorexia have certain tactics that it uses to stop you from eating? Are there times when you have not fallen prey to Anorexia's tactics? This linguistic separation enables clients to relate to their symptoms in new and more proactive ways. Again, similar to humanists and systemic counselors, postmodernists are challenged with balancing their philosophical position with the demands of current practice standards.

So, What Is a Competent Counselor to Do?

Included in professional standards, counselors are expected to be competent in clinical assessment and diagnosis. Few argue this point. The question then becomes *what role* should diagnosis play in counseling. Hansen (2003) argues that, although a necessary skill, diagnosis plays a minor role in the daily practice of counseling. He argues that diagnosis addresses overt psychiatric symptoms, which is the focus of psychiatry. But counseling, on the other hand, is focused on the client as a whole and the internal psychology of clients, which are less directly related to the overt symptoms that define mental health diagnosis. He contends that counselors learn diagnosis primarily for its economic utility (i.e., getting paid) rather than for its clinical utility (i.e., providing competent counseling). He recommends that it is important to learn about the inherent limitations of diagnosis, especially for women, the impoverished, and minorities (Eriksen & Kress, 2008; Zalaquett, Fuerth, Stein, Ivey, & Ivey, 2008), and to balance diagnosis with thoughtful case conceptualization (see Chapter 2).

Contemporary Issues in Diagnosis

DSM-5 and Dimensional Assessment

In 2013, the American Psychiatric Association released the DSM-5, which represents the most significant change to mental health diagnosis in over 30 years. Some of the more noteworthy changes in this manual include the removal of the five-axis diagnosis system, reorganization of the chapters, and inclusion of new assessment measures (APA, 2013). However, the most significant changes associated with this version of the manual are arguably at a more fundamental and philosophical level: the DSM-5 represents the initial efforts at a shift away from identifying discrete categories of mental disorders, for which there is less supportive evidence, and a move toward a dimensional approach to diagnosis that recognizes the heterogeneity of symptoms within and across disorders (APA, 2013). For example, the new DSM conceptualizes substance use problems along a spectrum of mild to severe rather than in two discrete categories of abuse and dependence, for which only arbitrary distinctions could be made. Although there is insufficient science to propose alternative definitions for most disorders at this time, the new structure of the manual is designed to serve as a bridge between the historic, categorical approach to diagnosis to the more likely future version with a dimensional approach, which will better account for the wide variation and forms that mental health disorders can take.

Toward this end, the National Institute of Mental Health will focus future research on Research Domain Criteria (RDoC), a project designed to "transform [mental health] diagnosis by incorporating genetics, imaging, cognitive science, and other levels of information to lay the foundation for a new classification system" (Insel, 2013, para. 3). Future federally funded research will focus more on general domains of symptoms and functioning than on specific diagnoses, as it has done in the past. Thus, future research may include all clients in a mood disorder clinic rather than exclude participants who don't meet strict diagnosis criteria. The overarching goal will be to develop a system of mental health diagnosis that more accurately captures the complexity of human psychological functioning. These potential changes would begin to address some of the concerns raised by humanistic, systemic, and postmodern critics about the effects of labeling on a person's identity and the counseling process.

Mental Health Recovery and Diagnosis

At the same time psychiatrists and researchers are reconceptualizing the future direction of mental health diagnosis, consumer movements related to mental health treatment have become formally recognized and mainstreamed. An international movement, the mental health recovery is quickly reshaping how government-funded agencies view diagnosis and mental illness (Davidson, Tondora, Lawless, O'Connell, & Rowe, 2008; Fisher & Chamberlin, 2004; Onken, Craig, Ridgway, Ralph, & Cook, 2007; Repper & Perkins, 2006). With its origins in consumer self-help in the 1930s, the *recovery movement* captured the attention of rehabilitation and substance abuse professionals in the 1990s and mental health policy makers since 2000, having been formally adopted by most first-world countries. In the United States, the 2002 New Freedom Commission on Mental Health proposed transforming the national mental health system using a paradigm of recovery, and in 2004 the U.S. Department of Health and Human Services launched a nationwide recovery campaign (Fisher & Chamberlin, 2004; U.S. Department of Health and Human Services, 2004).

The recovery movement has been widely adopted due to emerging research findings. In the 1990s, the World Health Organization released research findings from a cross-national study on recovery from severe mental illness, which revealed surprising results: 28% of patients diagnosed with severe mental illness (e.g., schizophrenia, bipolar, etc.) make a *full recovery* and 52% reported a *social recovery* (e.g., able to return to work, satisfying family relationships, etc.; Ralph, 2000). Similarly, Jaakko Seikkula's (2002) and his colleagues' (Haarakangas, Seikkula, Alakare, & Aaltonen, 2007) Open Dialogue approach to treating clients with psychotic symptoms, a collaborative counseling approach that shares similar principles to the Recovery Model, has even more impressive outcomes: 83% of first-episode psychosis patients return to work and 77% have no remaining psychotic symptoms after two years of treatment. These findings do not fit with medical model assumptions about severe mental illness—assumptions that the genetic and biological predispositions precluded meaningful recovery (Ramon, Healy, & Renouf, 2007). Thus, the Recovery Model is about helping clients lead rich, meaningful lives rather than simply reducing symptoms related to a mental health diagnosis, a perspective that resonates with the field of counseling and its historically uneasy relationship with the medical model and its emphasis on pathology.

The U.S. Department of Health and Human Services (2004) defines mental health recovery as "... a journey of healing and transformation enabling a person with a mental health problem to live a meaningful life in a community of his or her choice while striving to achieve his or her full potential" (p. 2). The recovery model uses a *social* model of disability rather than a medical model; thus, it deemphasizes diagnostic labeling and emphasizes *psychosocial functioning*, an emphasis that is the hallmark of family counseling approaches. The "National Consensus Statement on Mental Health Recovery" includes *10 Fundamental Components of Recovery* (U.S. Department of Health and Human Services, 2004):

Components of Mental Health Recovery-Oriented Care

- **Self-Direction:** Consumers (clients) exercise choice over their path to recovery/treatment.
- **Individualized/Person-Centered:** Paths to recovery are individualized based on a person's unique strengths, resiliencies, preferences, experiences, and cultural backgrounds.

(*continued*)

- **Empowerment:** Consumers have the authority to choose from a range of options and participate in decision making; professional relationships that encourage decision making and assertiveness.
- **Holistic:** Recovery encompasses all aspects of life: mind, body, spirit, and community.
- **Nonlinear:** Recovery is not a step-by-step process but an ongoing process that includes growth and setbacks.
- **Strengths-Based:** Recovery focuses on valuing and building upon strengths, resiliencies, and abilities.
- **Peer Support:** Consumers are encouraged to engage with other consumers in pursuing recovery.
- **Respect:** For recovery to occur, consumers need to experience respect from professionals, their communities, and other systems.
- **Responsibility:** Consumers are personally responsible for their recovery and self-care.
- **Hope:** Recovery requires a belief in the self and a willingness to persevere through difficulty.

These elements play leading roles in many counseling theories, most notably approaches such as humanism (e.g., responsibility and self-directed; Chapter 10), solution-based counseling (e.g., emphasis on client strengths, empowerment, and hope; Chapter 13), and postmodern (e.g., views "client as the expert"; people as separate from problems; dealing with social stigma, peer support, etc.; Chapter 14). The Recovery Movement's approach to harnessing client strengths to help them fashion meaningful lives while reducing the expert role of the counselor fits with many counseling approaches to working with clients diagnosed with severe mental illness. Although diagnosis still has its place, both counseling models and the Recovery Model share the premise that diagnosis is not the most beneficial driving force of treatment—as it is in the medical model—instead, the client's motivation for a quality life directs the course of treatment.

Counselors can draw from numerous approaches to facilitate mental health recovery (Gehart, 2012a). For example, using principles from narrative therapy (Chapter 14), a counselor could help clients restore their identity narratives related to their diagnoses:

- How has being diagnosed with mental illness changed how you see yourself, your role in relationships, and/or your role in society? Where did you get these ideas? Do you think they are fair and accurate?
- Do you think being diagnosed with XXX changes your value as a person? Why or why not? How? Where did these ideas come from?
- How did you define yourself before the [diagnosis or symptoms] began? How did you develop these ideas about who you were? Did others see you this way? Do you think this depiction is still true today in some ways?
- Do you believe that you can still lead a meaningful life with the symptoms you are experiencing? If not, where did you get this idea? If so, how can you make this happen? (Gehart, 2012b, p. 451).

Parity and Non-Parity Diagnoses

A seemingly minor development in mental health that will significantly shape the future of the field, certain mental health disorders have recently been deemed "equal" to physical health conditions in laws regulating insurance reimbursement. The Paul Wellstone and Pete Domenici Mental Health Parity and Addiction Equity Act was passed as part of the Economic Stabilization Act of 2008. This act requires that insurance companies reimburse for mental health and substance abuse disorders the same as any other physiological disorders, thereby requiring insurance companies to cover mental issues as part of their health plans. Prior to the bill's passage, only approximately 30 states had mental health parity laws.

State mental health parity laws, which tend to be more comprehensive than the federal act passed in 2008, often distinguish between "parity" diagnoses and "non-parity" diagnoses. When a client is diagnosed with a *parity* mental health diagnosis, insurance plans must reimburse the same as they would for physiological disorders, which most critically implies that the number of sessions cannot be artificially limited, as was the prior practice with HMO-type plans, and co-pays must be the same as those for physiological disorders. Parity diagnoses typically include severe mental health disorders and must be the *primary diagnosis* (first one listed) in order for insurance co-pays and reimbursement policies to apply. Parity diagnoses typically include:

- Anorexia and bulimia
- Bipolar disorder
- Major depressive disorder
- Obsessive-compulsive disorder
- Panic disorder
- Pervasive-developmental disorder
- Schizoaffective disorder
- Schizophrenia
- Any mental health disorder in children (including Adjustment Disorders)

Introduction to Changes in the DSM-5

Even if you are of the generation that was never trained using the DSM-IV (APA, 2000), you are guaranteed to encounter client files, supervisors, billing systems, and other texts that refer to it. So, this following section is designed to help both Generation-IV and Generation-5 counselors successfully engage with the core features of the DSM-5 and its most critical cross-diagnosis changes.

Title

One of the first changes a seasoned clinician may notice is the shortened title: ***DSM-5*** (note that using a hyphen is the correct format). The APA decided to stop using the Roman numeral system (DSM-V is considered incorrect) and switch to Arabic numerals to more easily allow for multiple text revisions in the years ahead. Digital technologies will enable updated publication of a DSM-5.1 and DSM-5.2, etc. Given expected changes, such as new diagnosis codes with the ICD-11 due out in 2015 (see ICD section below), more frequent text revisions may be particularly important in the future.

Manual Structure

Unlike the DSM-IV, there are three major sections of the DSM-5 (in addition to the appendices):

- Section I: DSM-5 Basics
  - History of the manual
  - Use of the manual and cautionary statements
  - Definition of a mental disorder
- Section II: Diagnostic Criteria and Codes
  - 20 chapters that describe recognized disorders
- Section III: Emerging measures and models
  - Emerging assessment measures
  - Cultural formulation
  - Alternative DSM-5 model for personality disorders
  - Conditions for further study

- Appendices
  - Highlights of changes
  - Glossaries of technical terms and cultural concepts of distress
  - Various listings of the disorders and codes

Reorganization of Diagnostic Chapters

For those familiar with the DSM-IV, one of the most notable changes in the DSM-5 is the reorganization of chapters in the new Section II. The chapters have been reorganized to more closely group disorders by known etiologies, underlying vulnerabilities, symptom characteristics, and shared environmental factors. The intention behind this reorganization is to facilitate more comprehensive diagnostic and treatment approaches and facilitate research across related disorders (APA, 2013).

Of particular note, the DSM-IV chapter "Disorders Usually Diagnosed in Infancy, Childhood, and Adolescents" was removed, and these disorders have been placed into other chapters based on common causes. Each DSM-5 chapter is organized developmentally, with those occurring in childhood toward the front of the chapter and those associated with later life toward the end.

DSM-5 Chapters Describing Mental Health Disorders (Section II)

1. Neurodevelopmental Disorders
2. Schizophrenia Spectrum and Other Psychotic Disorders
3. Bipolar and Related Disorders
4. Depressive Disorders
5. Anxiety Disorders
6. Obsessive-Compulsive and Related Disorders
7. Trauma- and Stressor-Related Disorders
8. Dissociative Disorders
9. Somatic Symptom Disorders
10. Feeding and Eating Disorders
11. Elimination Disorders
12. Sleep-Wake Disorders
13. Sexual Dysfunctions
14. Gender Dysphoria
15. Disruptive, Impulse Control, and Conduct Disorders
16. Substance Use and Addictive Disorders
17. Neurocognitive Disorders
18. Personality Disorders
19. Paraphilic Disorders
20. Other Conditions that May Be the Focus of Clinical Attention (V/Z codes)

Note: Similar to the DSM-IV, the DSM-5 does not include chapter numbers; the above numbers are added to facilitate learning and answer the burning question: how many chapters is that?

Diagnostic Code Changes and the ICD

The five-digit coding system most mental health practitioners are familiar with from the DSM-IV is derived from another set of diagnostic codes, those published in the *International Statistical Classification of Diseases and Related Health Problems* (ICD). Published by the WHO, the ICD is the most widely used set of diagnostic codes, and like the DSM, it attempts to statistically classify health disorders. It is used internationally by virtually all physical health practitioners and is used in most other countries for mental health diagnosis as well. The codes in the DSM-IV correlated to the ICD-9 (the ninth edition). These same codes are included in the DSM-5.

However, in October 2014, the United States finally adopted ICD-10 codes, which have been used in other countries since 1994 (the ICD-10 was released by WHO in 1990). The United States delayed implementation of ICD-10 codes due to the bureaucratic complexity and expense of the task in such a large health care system. The

ICD-10 codes are alphanumeric codes that are included in the DSM-5 in parentheses and gray text next to the old ICD-9 codes. Of particular note, the former "V-codes" have become Z and T codes in the ICD-10 system (see example below).

To complicate matters further, during the revision of the DSM-5, the WHO worked with the APA to correlate DSM-5 and ICD-11 codes and criteria for mental illness. The ICD-11 is due out in 2015; however, it may be a while until the ICD-11 codes are implemented in the United States. The ICD-11 codes are expected to be longer alphanumeric codes than those in the ICD-10 to allow for a greater number of diagnostic codes, which is a significant issue for the medical health professions.

	ICD-9	ICD-10
Diagnostic Code Format	###.##	A##.#
Sample Diagnosis: Major Depression, Recurrent, Severe	296.33	F33.2
Sample Diagnosis: Disruption of Family by Separation or Divorce	V61.03	Z63.5

New Diagnosis Format

The five-axis system used in the DSM-IV was removed from the DSM-5, and a nonaxial (i.e., single-line) system is used instead (APA, 2013). The nonaxial diagnosis approach was identified as an option in the DSM-IV-TR; however, most clinicians and third-party payers used the five-axis approach. In the nonaxial system, diagnoses from the former Axis I (mental health diagnosis), Axis II (personality disorders and mental retardation), and Axis III (physical health issues affecting mental health) are simply listed out, generally on a single line or set of lines. In addition, former Axis IV issues (psychosocial and environmental problems that may affect the diagnosis, treatment, and prognosis) are recorded similar to other diagnoses using ICD-9 "V codes" or ICD-10 "Z codes." The former Axis V (global assessment of functioning or GAF score) has been removed. Although no required replacement for the GAF was identified, the WHODAS (WHO Disability Assessment Schedule) is included in Section III of the DSM-5 as an optional global measure of disability (APA, 2013). As in the former diagnosis system, the principal diagnosis or reason for visit should be listed first.

Quick Review: DSM-IV Five-Axis Diagnosis Format

For those unfamiliar with the five-axis system, it is reviewed here because you will find it referred to both in professional literature and in client files for years to come.

DSM-IV Five-Axis Diagnosis Format

- **Axis I:** Clinical disorders that are the focus of treatment, including developmental and learning disorders; primary reason for visit listed first.
- **Axis II:** Underlying or pervasive conditions, including personality disorders, defensive mechanisms, and mental retardation.
- **Axis III:** Medical conditions and disorders
- **Axis IV:** Psychosocial stressors and environmental conditions that may be contributing to condition and/or its treatment, such as:
    - problems with the primary support system (family, partner, etc.)
    - economic or housing problems
    - problems accessing health care

(*continued*)

- legal situations
- social, school, and/or occupational issues

- **Axis V:** Global Assessment of Function (GAF) score: a score from 0 to 100 indicating level of functioning.
  - **70 and above:** Indicates adaptive coping, with higher scores indicating greater mental health
  - **60–69:** Mild symptoms; *most third-party payers require a client's level of functioning be 69 or below to be a reimbursable medical expense.*
  - **50–59:** Moderate symptoms
  - **40–49:** Severe symptoms
  - **39 and below:** Significant impairment that generally requires hospitalization and intensive treatment

Digital Download Download from CengageBrain.com

DSM-5 Equivalents to DSM-IV Format

DSM-IV Five-Axis System	DSM-5 Equivalent
Axis I: Mental Health Disorders	Record on diagnosis line (primary reason for visit listed first)
Axis II: Personality Disorders and Mental Retardation	Record on diagnosis line (primary reason for visit listed first)
Axis III: General Medical Conditions	Record on diagnosis line (especially those important to understanding mental disorder)
Axis IV: Psychosocial and Environmental Problems	Record on diagnosis line using V, Z, or T codes from chapter on "Other Conditions that May Be the Focus of Clinical Attention"
Axis V: Global Assessment of Functioning	Optional use of WHODAS scale

Digital Download Download from CengageBrain.com

The formatting of a DSM-5 diagnosis is simpler than the former five-axis diagnosis. In most cases, third-party payers, such as insurance companies, will provide several numbered lines; these do not correlate to axes but rather are a prompt to write one diagnosis per line. The diagnostic code generally goes first and then the name of the diagnosis followed by any specifiers (see Specifiers below).

Insurance Company/Third Party Prompt:

Diagnosis(es)

1. ______________________________

2. ______________________________

3. ______________________________

4. ______________________________

The diagnosis is written as follows:

DSM-5 Diagnosis Format Sample (ICD-9 Codes)

1. 296.32 Major depressive disorder, recurrent, moderate, with mild anxious distress
2. 309.81 Post-traumatic stress disorder, with delayed onset
3. V60.1 Inadequate housing
4. V60.2 Extreme poverty

As of October 2015, the above diagnosis reads as follows:

DSM-5 Diagnosis Format Sample (ICD-10 Codes)

1. F33.1 Major depressive disorder, recurrent, moderate, with mild anxious distress
2. F43.10 Post-traumatic stress disorder, with delayed onset
3. Z59.1 Inadequate housing
4. Z59.5 Extreme poverty

Subtypes and Specifiers

The DSM-5 includes several new subtypes and specifiers. Subtypes identify mutually exclusive subgroups within the diagnostic category, whereas specifiers are more general. All subtypes are diagnosis-specific and many are described below with individual diagnoses. Similarly, many specifiers are used with only specific diagnoses; however, several new specifiers are used across several or all diagnoses in the manual. These specifiers are used to note information about a person's condition that may be useful for treatment decisions, often alerting clinicians to additional symptoms or qualities of symptoms that need specific attention in treatment planning. When adding a specifier, the diagnostic code does not change; however, the specifier is written *after* the name of the diagnosis on the diagnosis line (see diagnosis examples above).

Cross-Diagnostic Specifiers

- With catatonia (for neurodevelopmental, psychotic, mood, etc.)
- With anxious distress (depression and bipolar disorders; see example above)
- With panic attacks (all disorders)
- With poor insight (OCD and certain anxiety disorders)
- With mixed features (bipolar and mood disorders)
- In remission or partial remission

In addition, many of the specific diagnoses have new specifiers, such as "with limited prosocial emotions" for conduct disorder (APA, 2013). The new manual clearly lists these condition-specific specifiers after diagnostic criterion in bold text, making it easy to identify and include the specifiers.

Dimensional Assessment

As mentioned above, emerging research supports a more dimensional approach (variation of intensity on a given symptom or dimension) to mental health diagnosis, in contrast to its historical categorical approach (APA, 2013). Current research is not sufficiently developed to warrant a radical reorganizing of the manual using a dimensional approach; however, in the years ahead, the DSM is likely to move in this direction. Nonetheless, the current DSM takes steps in this direction by organizing chapters by etiology and by separating internalizing from externalizing disorders (APA, 2013). In addition, for certain diagnoses where there was sufficient evidence to support the change, dimensional assessments—such as mild, moderate, and severe—were introduced rather than retaining separate and discrete categories to indicate levels of severity. Among the diagnoses that use dimensional assessment in the DSM-5 are:

- Schizophrenia (pen-and-paper assessment available for free download)
- Depression (pen-and-paper assessment available for free download)
- Separation anxiety disorder (pen-and-paper assessment available for free download)
- Specific phobia (pen-and-paper assessment available for free download)
- Social anxiety disorder (pen-and-paper assessment available for free download)
- Panic disorder (pen-and-paper assessment available for free download)
- Agoraphobia (pen-and-paper assessment available for free download)
- Generalized anxiety disorder (pen-and-paper assessment available for free download)
- Post-traumatic stress disorder (pen-and-paper assessment available for free download)
- Acute stress disorder (pen-and-paper assessment available for free download)
- Dissociative symptoms (pen-and-paper assessment available for free download)
- Intellectual disability
- Sexual disorders
- Substance abuse
- Anxious distress specifier

These dimensional assessments are intended to help clinicians assess severity and simplify tracking progress during treatment.

NOS versus NEC Diagnosis

Due to their overuse and lack of clinical utility, the NOS (not otherwise specified) diagnoses of the DSM-IV have been replaced in the DSM-5 with Not-Elsewhere-Classified (NEC) diagnoses, which may be an "other specified disorder" or an "unspecified disorder."

Other Specified Disorder

The other specified disorder allows the clinician to document the specific reason a particular client does not meet the criteria for a specific diagnosis (APA, 2013). This is done by recording the name of the diagnostic category followed by the specific reason the person does not meet the criteria. The text lists common examples of how to write the "other specified" diagnosis for a given diagnosis. For example, in the chapter on depression, three examples of "other specified" are given:

- Recurrent brief depression
- Short-duration depressive episode (4–13 days)
- Depressive episode with insufficient symptoms (APA, 2013, p. 183)

Thus, if a client has depressive symptoms for several weeks but does not meet the diagnostic threshold, the diagnosis would read:

"311. Other specified depressive disorder, depressive episode with insufficient symptoms"

Unspecified Disorders

When the clinician cannot specify or chooses not to specify the characteristics of the disorder, then the "unspecified disorder" can be used. This is used when a client experiences significant clinical distress but does not meet the criteria for the disorder. This can be used when there is insufficient information, such as in emergency rooms, to make a full diagnosis.

Example: "311. Unspecified depressive disorder"

Counseling Approach to Clinical Assessment

Mental Status Exam

In most clinical environments, counselors are asked to conduct some form of semi-structured diagnostic interview with clients, most frequently called a *mental status exam* (aka, MSE). Numerous models for conducting a mental status exam exist (Burgess, 2013; Morrison, 2006; Nussbaum, 2013), and most clinicians develop a custom approach that best fits their approach and practice context. Mental status exams are used to gather information necessary to make a diagnosis. Most exams cover the following areas of functioning:

Common Elements of a Mental Status Exam (MSE)

- **Appearance:** Observations of client's overall appearance: age, weight, height, grooming, and manner of dress.
- **Attitude:** Observations of client's attitude toward the interviewer: cooperative, uncooperative, hostile, guarded, suspicious, or regressed.
- **Behavior:** Observations of client behavior, such as eye contact, gait, tics, tremors, repetitive movements, hyperactivity, or other qualities of movement.
- **Mood:** The client's *reported* emotional state, such as euthymic, dysphoric, euphoric, angry, anxious.
- **Affect:** Observations of the client's outer expression of emotion: congruent, incongruent, flat, labile, etc.
- **Speech:** Observations of the client's manner of speech: speed, volume, rate, spontaneity, etc.
- **Thought Process and Content:** Client descriptions of thought processes and/or inferences based on client comments; may include delusions, obsessions, phobias, etc.
- **Perceptions:** Client reports of unusual sensory experiences, such as hallucinations, illusions, or depersonalization.
- **Cognition:** Assessed using structured questions, cognition refers to basic executive functions, such as orientation to time/person/place, alertness, memory, etc.
- **Insight:** Assessment of the client's overall ability to recognize any pathology, possible causes, and implications.
- **Judgment:** Assessment of the client's overall ability to make sound, reasoned decisions. If impaired, additional safety precautions may be necessary.

Digital Download Download from CengageBrain.com

Counseling Relationship and the MSE

Mental status exams are based on the medical model, requiring a more hierarchical, detached counseling relationship than most counselors prefer. This shift in the counseling relationship is often confusing for clients and practitioners alike and can interfere with the effectiveness of later interventions that require a more empathetic and/or egalitarian counseling relationship. Ideally, counselors develop strategies for conducting a mental status exam that preserves the type of counseling alliance they intend to use throughout treatment. One of the easiest ways to do this is to clearly flag the mental status exam as a more formal set of questions you will ask the client as part of the assessment process and that "regular" counseling sessions will be more conversational and/or less structured. Otherwise, clients may develop the expectation that the counselor will be structuring sessions in a more formal way and may have trouble shifting gears when the counselor then expects the client to speak freely.

Preparing Client for a Structured Mental Status Exam: Example Introduction

Counselors wanting to establish a more collaborative, nonhierarchical relationship with clients can introduce the mental status questions as follows:

"As part of getting to know you, I want to ask you about how you are doing in several areas of functioning to make sure I have a good sense of how I can best help you. So, I am going to go down a list and ask you some standard questions. Normally, I won't necessarily be so structured or ask so many questions about things that may not be your primary area of concern."

Cross-Cutting Assessments

One of the most significant practical changes in the DSM-5 is the introduction of cross-cutting symptom assessments, pen-and-paper measures that can be used as part of the mental status exam process (APA, 2013). *Cross-cutting symptoms* are those symptoms that are seen across diagnoses; these are broad and general areas of functioning, such as mood, anxiety, and insomnia. Based on general medicine's review of symptoms, these measures are used to help clinicians systematically review key domains of psychological functioning, to assist with making a diagnosis and determining overall functioning. These measures are *not* intended for systematically determining a diagnosis but rather for broad overall assessment and to help guide the clinician in the correct direction for making a diagnosis. Based on well-established measures, the cross-cutting symptom measures involve two levels of assessment: level 1 and level 2.

Level 1 Cross-Cutting Symptom Measure

A single, short assessment measure, the Level 1 Cross-Cutting Symptom Measure is initially given to clients at the beginning of treatment to determine if further assessment is needed in a given area. The adult version has 23 items and measures 13 domains of functioning, and the child version has 25 items and measures 12 domains of functioning. The assessment asks clients if "during the past two (2) weeks, how much (or how often) have you [or your child, on the child measure] been bothered by the following problems?" (APA, 2013, p. 738). Each of the 23–25 questions addresses basic areas of functioning, such as "little interest or pleasure in doing things," "feeling down, depressed, or hopeless," or "thoughts of actually hurting yourself" (APA, 2013, p. 738).

Level 1 Domains for Adults

- Somatic symptoms
- Sleep problems
- Inattention (not on adult)
- Depression
- Anger
- Irritability (not on adult)
- Mania
- Anxiety
- Psychosis
- Repetitive thoughts and behaviors
- Substance use
- Suicidal ideation/attempts

Level 1 Domains for Children

- Somatic symptoms
- Sleep problems
- Inattention (not on adult)
- Depression

- Anger
- Irritability (not on adult)
- Mania
- Anxiety
- Psychosis
- Repetitive thoughts and behaviors
- Substance use
- Suicidal ideation/attempts

Level 2 Assessments

If a client scores at or above the specific cutoff score in a given domain, then a Level 2 Cross-Cutting Symptom Measure is given (except for suicidal ideation, psychosis, memory, dissociation, or personality functioning, which do not have level 2 measures). A child-specific cross-cutting symptom measure is available for children 6–17; these measures are completed by a parent or guardian. These measures are available for free download from the APA-hosted websites (www.psychiatry.org/dsm5 and www.dsm5.org).

WHODAS 2.0

Another assessment measure that may be used as part of the clinical assessment is the WHODAS 2.0: World Health Organization Disability Assessment Schedule 2.0 (APA, 2013). The most likely replacement for the former Axis V, this measure is a 36-item, self-administered test for adults to assess disability across six domains of functioning: communication, getting around, self-care, getting along with people, life activities, and participation in society. The instrument can be scored in two ways:

- *Simple scoring* involves simply adding up points without weighting individual items; this type of scoring can be done by hand.
- *Complex scoring* involves weighting scores based on multiple levels of difficulty for each item. This method requires a computer program from the WHO website, which can convert the score to a 100-point scale, with 100 being full disability.

The instrument is available in the APA resources for the DSM-5, and the adult version is published in the text.

Cultural Formulation and Assessment

As mentioned above, when working with diverse clients, best practices include conducting a cultural formulation interview to identify specific cultural issues that may be affecting the presentation and significance of symptoms (APA, 2013). Building on the cultural formulation in the DSM-IV, the DSM-5 includes a revised outline for cultural formulation as well as an interview guide, complete with sample prompts and questions to be used in session to gather cultural information (APA, 2013, pp. 752–775).

The elements of the cultural formulation include:

- *Cultural identity of the individual:* Involves identifying important racial, ethnic, and cultural reference groups as well as other clinically relevant aspects of identity, such as religious affiliation, socioeconomic status, sexual orientation, and migrant status.
- *Cultural conceptualization of distress:* Requires outlining the cultural constructs and significance of presenting symptoms.
- *Psychosocial stressors and cultural features of vulnerability and resilience:* Entails identifying specific stressors and supports related to cultural factors, including the role of religion, family, and social networks.
- *Cultural features of the relationship between the individual and the clinician:* Requires identifying the cultural, linguistic, and social status issues that may impede communication, therapeutic relationship, diagnosis, and treatment.
- *Overall cultural assessment:* Involves a summary of the key findings and implications of salient issues for diagnosis and treatment.

Diagnostic Reflections

As you may have surmised by now, diagnosis and clinical assessment are topics that elicit strong emotions in many: some in favor, some against, and some in between. In fact, your response to reading this chapter is likely to be diagnostic in itself. Are you excited? Concerned? Frightened? Confused? It is important to know where you stand on diagnosis and why. For some, experiences in their personal life have left an indelible impression that puts them on one side or the other. Whatever your position, I encourage you to be open to learning from your clients and colleagues in the years ahead. I have found that the issues are far more complex and nuanced than they initially appear and that the "truth" and pros and cons can vary significantly from one person to another. Like many things in life, when it comes to diagnosis, any simple answers are probably not the whole story.

Questions for Personal Reflection and Class Discussion

1. Describe the benefits and risks to diagnosis that you believe to be most critical?
2. What ethical guidelines would you propose for ensuring that clients benefit most and are exposed to the least risk in the process of diagnosis?
3. What potential improvements and limitations do you see with dimensional assessment?
4. Describe the benefits and risks of the recovery in mental health movement.
5. Describe what you might do to preserve a strong counseling relationship with clients when conducting a mental status exam.
6. Describe your concerns about how culture, social class, immigration status, and sexual orientation/identity might impact the diagnosis process? What suggestions do you have for addressing these issues?

Online Resources

Official DSM-5 website with access to Cross-Cutting Measures, WHODAS 2.0, and cultural assessment, as well as fact sheets for specific disorders and videos on the changes.
www.psychiatry.org/dsm5

Originally serving as the site to solicit public feedback on the DSM-5, this site documents the development of the DSM-5, including monographs, conference proceedings, and related reference lists, and also includes many of resources on the sister site: psychiatry.org/dsm5, including the online measures for download.
www.dsm5.org

References

American Psychiatric Association. (2000). *Diagnostic and statistical manual for mental disorders* (4th ed., Text Revision). Washington, DC: Author.

American Psychiatric Association (APA). (2013). *Diagnostic and statistical manual for mental disorders* (5th ed.). Washington, DC: Author.

Anderson, H. (1997). *Conversations, language, and possibilities*. New York: Basic.

Burgess, W. (2013). *Mental status examination* (2nd ed.). Seattle, WA: CreateSpace Independent Publishing Platform.

Davidson, L., Tondora, J., Lawless, M. S., O'Connell, M. J., & Rowe, M. (2008). *A practical guide to recovery-oriented practice: Tools for transforming mental health care*. New York: Oxford University Press.

Eriksen, K., & Kress, V. E. (2008). Gender and diagnosis: Struggles and suggestions for counselors. *Journal of Counseling and Development*, *86*, 152–161.

Fisher, D. B., & Chamberlin, J. (2004, March). Consumer-directed transformation to a recovery-based mental health system. Retrieved from http://mentalhealth.samhsa.gov/publications/allpubs/NMH05-0193/default.asp. Accessed on August 16, 2008.

Freeth, R. (2006). Focusing on relationship—is there room for another paradigm in psychiatric intensive care? *Journal of*

Psychiatric Intensive Care, 2(2), 55–58. doi:10.1017/S1742646407000295

Freeth, R. (2007). *Humanising psychiatry and mental health care: The challenge of the person-centered approach*. London: Blackwell.

Gadamer, H. (1975). *Truth and method*. New York: Seabury.

Gehart, D. R. (2012a). The mental health recovery movement and family therapy, part I: Consumer-led reform of services to persons diagnosed with severe mental illness. *Journal of Marital and Family Therapy, 38*(3), 429–442. doi:10.1111/j.1752-0606.2011.00230.x

Gehart, D. R. (2012b). The mental health recovery movement and family therapy, part II: A collaborative, appreciative approach for supporting mental health recovery. *Journal of Marital and Family Therapy, 38*(3), 443–457. doi:10.1111/j.1752-0606.2011.00229.x

Gergen, K., Anderson, H., & Hoffman, L. (1996). Is diagnosis a disaster?: A constructionist trialogue. In F. Kaslow (Ed.), *Relational diagnosis*. New York: Wiley.

Haarakangas, K., Seikkula, J., Alakare, B., & Aaltonen, J. (2007). Open dialogue: An approach to psychotherapeutic treatment of psychosis in Northern Finland. In H. Anderson & D. Gehart (Eds.), *Collaborative therapy: Relationships and conversations that make a difference* (pp. 221–233). New York: Brunner-Routledge.

Hansen, J. T. (2003). Including diagnostic training counseling curricula: Implications for professional identity development. *Counselor Education and Supervision, 43*, 96–107.

Insel, T. (2013, April). *Director's blog: Transforming diagnosis*. Retrieved from http://www.nimh.nih.gov/about/director/2013/transforming-diagnosis.shtml

Jackson, D. D. (1967/2009). The myth of normality. In W. Ray (Ed.), *Don D. Jackson: Interactional theory in the practice of therapy: Selected papers, Vol. 2* (pp. 217–224). Phoenix, AZ: Zeig, Tucker & Tucker. (Originally published in *Medical Opinion & Review*, 3(5), 28–33).

Keeney, B. P. (1983). *Aesthetics of change*. New York: Guilford.

Larsson, P., Brooks, O., & Loewenthal, D. (2012). Counselling psychology and diagnostic categories: A critical literature review. *Counselling Psychology Review, 27*(3), 55–67.

Morrison, J. (2006). *Diagnosis made easier*. New York: Guilford.

Nussbaum, A. (2013). *The pocket guide to the DSM-5 diagnostic exam*. Washington, DC: American Psychiatric Association.

Onken, S. J., Craig, C., Ridgway, P., Ralph, R. O., & Cook, J.A. (2007). An analysis of the definitions and elements of recovery: A review of the literature. *Psychiatric Rehabilitation Journal, 31*, 9–22.

Ralph, R. (2000). *Review of the recovery literature: Synthesis of a sample recovery literature 2000*. National Association for State Mental Health Program Directors. Retrieved from www.bbs.ca.gov/pdf/mhsa/resource/recovery/recovery_oriented_resources.pdf. Accessed on September 2, 2008.

Ramon, S., Healy, B., & Renouf, N. (2007). Recovery from mental illness as an emergent concept and practice. *Australia and the UK International Journal of Social Psychiatry, 53*(2), 108–122.

Ray, W., & Watzlawick, P. (2005/2009). The interactional approach: Enduring conceptions from the Mental Research Institute. In W. Ray & G. Nardone (Eds.), *Paul Watzlawick: Insight may cause blindness and other essays* (pp. 171–198). Phoenix, AZ: Zeig, Tucker, & Tucker. (Orignally published in the *Journal of Brief Therapy*, 6(1), 1–20).

Repper, J., & Perkins, R. (2006). *Social inclusion and recovery: A model for mental health practice*. UK: Baillière Tindall.

Rogers, C. (1951). *Client-centered therapy*. Boston, MA: Houghton Mifflin Company.

Schmid, P. (2004). Back to the client: A phenomenological approach to the process of understanding and diagnosis. *Person-Centered and Experiential Psychotherapies, 3*(1), 36–51.

Seikkula, J. (2002). Open dialogues with good and poor outcomes for psychotic crises: Examples from families with violence. *Journal of Marital and Family Therapy, 28*(3), 263–274.

Selvini-Palazzoli, M., Boscolo, L., Cecchin, G., & Prata, G. (1978). *Paradox and counterparadox*. New York: Jason Aronson.

Sugarman, A. (1978). Is psychodiagnostic assessment humanistic? *Journal of Personality Assessment, 42*(1), 11–21.

U.S. Department of Health and Human Services. (2004). National consensus statement on mental health recovery. Retrieved from http://mentalhealth.samhsa.gov/publications/allpubs/sma05-4129. Accessed on August 26, 2008.

Watzlawick, P., Weakland, J., & Fisch, R. (1974). *Change: Principles of problem formation and problem resolution*. New York: Norton.

White, M., & Epston, D. (1990). *Narrative means to therapeutic ends*. New York: Norton.

Zalaquett, C. P., Fuerth, K. M., Stein, C., Ivey, A. E., & Ivey, M. B. (2008). Reframing the DSM-IV-TR from a multicultural/social justic perspectivve. *Journal of Counseling and Development, 86*, 364–371.

CHAPTER

4

Completing a Clinical Assessment

Clinical Assessment Form

Chances are you will fill out many clinical assessment forms, and they will likely vary wildly in their appearance. However, if you take a moment to look carefully, you will find they have virtually the same information on all of them. The clinical assessment in this chapter includes elements common to most outpatient clinical assessments: client demographics, presenting problem, mental status, diagnosis, medication information, risk assessment, case management, prognosis, and overview of plan. So, although you are likely to complete forms that appear quite different from this, chances are the content is about the same.

CLINICAL ASSESSMENT			
Clinician:______	Client ID #: ______	Primary configuration: ❑ Individual ❑ Couple ❑ Family	Primary Language: ❑ English ❑ Spanish ❑ Other: ______

List client and significant others

Adult(s)

Select Gender Age: ______ Select Ethnicity Select Relational Status Occupation: ______ Other identifier: ______

Select Gender Age: ______ Select Ethnicity Select Relational Status Occupation: ______ Other identifier: ______

Child(ren)

Select Gender Age:______ Select Ethnicity Grade: Select Grade School: ______ Other identifier: ______

Select Gender Age:______ Select Ethnicity Grade: Select Grade School: ______ Other identifier: ______

Others: ______

(continued)

Presenting Problems

		Complete for children:
❑ Depression/hopelessness	❑ Couple concerns	❑ School failure/decline in performance
❑ Anxiety/worry	❑ Parent/child conflict	❑ Truancy/runaway
❑ Anger issues	❑ Partner violence/abuse	❑ Fighting w/peers
❑ Loss/grief	❑ Divorce adjustment	❑ Hyperactivity
❑ Suicidal thoughts/attempts	❑ Remarriage adjustment	❑ Wetting/soiling clothing
❑ Sexual abuse/rape	❑ Sexuality/intimacy concerns	❑ Child abuse/neglect
❑ Alcohol/drug use	❑ Major life changes	❑ Isolation/withdrawal
❑ Eating problems/disorders	❑ Legal issues/probation	❑ Other: ____________
❑ Job problems/unemployed	❑ Other: ____________	

Mental Status Assessment for Identified Patient

Interpersonal	❑ NA	❑ Conflict ❑ Enmeshment ❑ Isolation/Avoidance ❑ Harassment ❑ Other: ____________
Mood	❑ NA	❑ Depressed/Sad ❑ Anxious ❑ Dysphoric ❑ Angry ❑ Irritable ❑ Manic ❑ Other: ____________
Affect	❑ NA	❑ Constricted ❑ Blunt ❑ Flat ❑ Labile ❑ Incongruent ❑ Other: ____________
Sleep	❑ NA	❑ Hypersomnia ❑ Insomnia ❑ Disrupted ❑ Nightmares ❑ Other: ____________
Eating	❑ NA	❑ Increase ❑ Decrease ❑ Anorectic restriction ❑ Binging ❑ Purging ❑ Other: ____________
Anxiety	❑ NA	❑ Chronic worry ❑ Panic ❑ Phobias ❑ Obsessions ❑ Compulsions ❑ Other: ____________
Trauma Symptoms	❑ NA	❑ Hypervigilance ❑ Flashbacks/Intrusive memories ❑ Dissociation ❑ Numbing ❑ Avoidance efforts ❑ Other: ____________
Psychotic Symptoms	❑ NA	❑ Hallucinations ❑ Delusions ❑ Paranoia ❑ Loose associations ❑ Other: ____________
Motor Activity/ Speech	❑ NA	❑ Low energy ❑ Hyperactive ❑ Agitated ❑ Inattentive ❑ Impulsive ❑ Pressured speech ❑ Slow speech ❑ Other: ____________
Thought	❑ NA	❑ Poor concentration ❑ Denial ❑ Self-blame ❑ Other-blame ❑ Ruminative ❑ Tangential ❑ Concrete ❑ Poor insight ❑ Impaired decision making ❑ Disoriented ❑ Other: ____________

(continued)

Socio-Legal	❑ NA	❑ Disregards rules ❑ Defiant ❑ Stealing ❑ Lying ❑ Tantrums ❑ Arrest/Incarceration ❑ Initiates fights ❑ Other: ______
Other Symptoms	❑ NA	______

Diagnosis for Identified Patient

Contextual Factors considered in making diagnosis: ❑ Age ❑ Gender ❑ Family dynamics ❑ Culture ❑ Language ❑ Religion ❑ Economic ❑ Immigration ❑ Sexual/Gender orientation ❑ Trauma ❑ Dual diagnosis/Comorbid ❑ Addiction ❑ Cognitive ability ❑ Other: ______

Describe impact of identified factors on diagnosis and assessment process: ______

DSM-5 Code	Diagnosis with Specifier *Include V/Z/T-Codes for Psychosocial Stressors/Issues*
1. ______	1. ______
2. ______	2. ______
3. ______	3. ______
4. ______	4. ______
5. ______	5. ______

Medical Considerations

Has patient been referred for psychiatric evaluation? ❑ Yes ❑ No

Has patient agreed with referral? ❑ Yes ❑ No ❑ NA

Psychometric instruments used for assessment: ❑ None ❑ Cross-cutting symptom inventories

❑ Other: ______

Client response to diagnosis: ❑ Agree ❑ Somewhat agree ❑ Disagree ❑ Not informed for following reason: ______

Current Medications (psychiatric & medical) ❑ NA

1. ______; dose ______ mg; start date: ______
2. ______; dose ______ mg; start date: ______
3. ______; dose ______ mg; start date: ______
4. ______; dose ______ mg; start date: ______

Medical Necessity: *Check all that apply*

❑ Significant impairment ❑ Probability of significant impairment ❑ Probable developmental arrest

Areas of impairment: ❑ Daily activities ❑ Social relationships ❑ Health ❑ Work/School ❑ Living arrangement

❑ Other: ______

(*continued*)

Risk and Safety Assessment for Identified Patient

Suicidality	Homicidality	Alcohol Abuse
❑ No indication/Denies	❑ No indication/Denies	❑ No indication/Denies
❑ Active ideation	❑ Active ideation	❑ Past abuse
❑ Passive ideation	❑ Passive ideation	❑ Current; Freq/Amt: ______
❑ Intent without plan	❑ Intent without means	**Drug Use/Abuse**
❑ Intent with means	❑ Intent with means	❑ No indication/Denies
❑ Ideation in past year	❑ Ideation in past year	❑ Past use
❑ Attempt in past year	❑ Violence past year	❑ Current drugs: ______
❑ Family or peer history of completed suicide	❑ History of assaulting others	Freq/Amt: ______
	❑ Cruelty to animals	❑ Family/Sig. other use

Sexual & Physical Abuse and Other Risk Factors

❑ Childhood abuse history: ❑ Sexual ❑ Physical ❑ Emotional ❑ Neglect

❑ Adult with abuse/assault in adulthood: ❑ Sexual ❑ Physical ❑ Current

❑ History of perpetrating abuse: ❑ Sexual ❑ Physical ❑ Emotional

❑ Elder/Dependent adult abuse/neglect

❑ History of or current issues with restrictive eating, binging, and/or purging

❑ Cutting or other self harm: ❑ Current ❑ Past: Method: ______

❑ Criminal/Legal history: ______

❑ Other trauma history: ______

❑ None reported

Indicators of Safety

❑ NA

❑ At least one outside support person

❑ Able to cite specific reasons to live or not harm

❑ Hopeful

❑ Willing to dispose of dangerous items

❑ Has future goals

❑ Willingness to reduce contact with people who make situation worse

❑ Willing to implement safety plan, safety interventions

❑ Developing set of alternatives to self/other harm

❑ Sustained period of safety: ______

❑ Other: ______

Elements of Safety Plan

❑ NA

❑ Verbal no harm contract

❑ Written no harm contract

❑ Emergency contact card

❑ Emergency therapist/agency number

❑ Medication management

❑ Plan for contacting friends/support persons during crisis

❑ Specific plan of where to go during crisis

❑ Specific self-calming tasks to reduce risk before reach crisis level (e.g., journaling, exercising, etc.)

❑ Specific daily/weekly activities to reduce stressors

❑ Other: ______

Legal/Ethical Action Taken: ❑ NA ❑ Action: ______

(continued)

Case Management

Collateral Contacts

- Has contact been made with treating *physicians or other professionals*: ❑ NA ❑ Yes ❑ In process. Name/Notes: ______
- If client is involved in mental health *treatment elsewhere*, has contact been made? ❑ NA ❑ Yes ❑ In process. Name/Notes: ______
- Has contact been made with *social worker*: ❑ NA ❑ Yes ❑ In process. Name/Notes: ______

Referrals

- Has client been referred for *medical assessment*: ❑ Yes ❑ No evidence for need
- Has client been referred for *social services*: ❑ NA ❑ Job/Training ❑ Welfare/Food/Housing ❑ Victim services ❑ Legal aid ❑ Medical ❑ Other: ______
- Has client been referred for *group* or other support services: ❑ Yes: ______ ❑ In process ❑ None recommended
- Are there anticipated *forensic/legal processes* related to treatment: ❑ No ❑ Yes; describe: ______

Support Network

- Client social support network includes: ❑ Supportive family ❑ Supportive partner ❑ Friends ❑ Religious/ Spiritual organization ❑ Supportive work/social group ❑ Other: ______
- Describe anticipated effects treatment will have on others in support system (children, partner, etc.): ______
- Is there anything else client will need to be successful? ______

Expected Outcome and Prognosis

❑ Return to normal functioning ❑ Anticipate less than normal functioning ❑ Prevent deterioration

Client Sense of Hope: Select

Evaluation of Assessment/Client Perspective

How were assessment methods adapted to client needs, including age, culture, and other diversity issues? ______

Describe actual or potential areas of client-clinician agreement/disagreement related to the above assessment: ______

______, ______ ______

Clinician Signature License/Intern Status Date

______, ______ ______

Supervisor Signature License Date

How to Complete a Clinical Assessment

Identifying Client Information

Clinical assessments typically start out with some form of identifying salient client demographics, such as gender, age, ethnicity, sexual orientation, relational status, occupation, language, or other important information, such as immigration status or significant physical disorders or conditions. It is also important to identify significant others, especially if crisis issues are identified or if relational issues are a concern.

Presenting Problems

The presenting problems include what clients identify as the initial problems when they enter counseling, including the primary reason they are seeking treatment (e.g., a child's behavior problem) as well as secondary issues they may more casually mention (e.g., marital tension). The list of presenting problems provides a quick overview of the client's and/or family's current difficulties as *they* define them: the mental status exam and diagnosis is where clinicians get to document their perspectives.

Mental Status Exam and Diagnosis

Mental Status Exam

A mental status exam is used to develop a comprehensive overview of clients' mental health functioning to support diagnoses (Burgess, 2013). As described above, counselors may use interviews or standardized instruments, such as the Cross-Cutting Measures from the DSM-5, to help gather the information necessary to complete the written mental status section (APA, 2013). Thus, completing this section takes far less time than gathering the information. For those new to diagnosis, the end of this chapter includes a definition of the common terms used in a mental status exam. Typical areas of functioning assessed are:

- Interpersonal: Conflict, enmeshment, isolation, harassment, etc.
- Mood (subjective experience): Depressed, anxious, dysphoric, angry, irritable, manic, etc.
- Affect (expression of emotion): Constructed, blunt, flat, labile, incongruent.
- Sleeping patterns: Hypersomnia, insomnia, disrupted, nightmares, etc.
- Eating patterns: Increased, decreased, anorectic restriction, binging, purging, etc.
- Trauma symptoms: Hypervigilance, flashbacks, dissociation, numbing, avoidance, etc.
- Psychotic symptoms: Hallucinations, delusions, paranoia, loose associations, etc.
- Motor activity: Low energy, hyperactive, agitated, inattentive, impulsive, pressured speech, slow speech, etc.
- Thought: Poor concentration, denial, self-blame, other-blame, ruminative, tangential, concrete, poor insight, impaired decision making, disoriented, etc.
- Socio-legal issues: Disregards rules, defiant, stealing, lying, tantrums, arrest, initiates fights, etc.

DSM-5 Diagnosis

Contextual Factors Before making a diagnosis, counselors should take a moment to consider contextual factors, such as age, ethnicity, family dynamics, language, religion, economic issues, sexual orientation, trauma history, addictions, and cognitive ability, and how these might affect the diagnosis process. For example, often a woman from a culture that values emotional expression who has a history of trauma will present with histrionic features that are more a function of cultural communication than an actual personality disorder; thus, symptoms generally dissipate as trauma is treated. Taking such issues into consideration improves the accuracy of diagnosis. The cultural formulation interview can help clinicians effectively address diversity issues when making a diagnosis.

Making a Diagnosis When making a diagnosis, clinicians consult the *DSM (Diagnosis and Statistical Manual)*; each diagnosis requires that a certain number of criteria be met to make the diagnosis; *these criteria should be clearly reflected in the mental status exam*. For example, if you identify depression, hallucinations, and trauma symptoms in the mental status section, the diagnosis should clearly account for all of these symptoms. Additionally, before making a diagnosis, medical causes, trauma, and substance abuse should be considered and ruled out. When writing the diagnosis, it is important to include the proper code as well as the diagnosis with all specifiers written out, because the codes do not include the specifiers.

Medical Considerations Depending on the client's symptoms and level of functioning, counselors may want to refer out for an evaluation for medication; diagnoses with symptoms that typically warrant referral include depression, anxiety, mania, psychosis, trauma, disordered eating, alcohol/substance abuse, sleep disorders, and so forth. If medication is prescribed, counselors are expected to keep a written record of the medication, dose, and start date. Increasingly, counselors are also asked to document whether clients have been told about and/or agree with the diagnosis; this is common in recovery-oriented contexts (see above).

Medical Necessity In order to qualify for reimbursement, third-party payers require that counselors document that the condition meets the criteria for *medical necessity*, which means there is presently significant impairment in functioning, a high probability of significant impairment, and/or probable developmental arrest in children. Areas of impairment may include:

- Daily activities (e.g., getting out of bed, feeding self, chores, etc.)
- Social relationships (e.g., maintaining satisfying marriage, friendships, etc.)
- Health (e.g., maintaining physical health)
- Work/School (e.g., able to maintain employment, complete school tasks, etc.)
- Living arrangement (e.g., having a place to live, etc.)

Risk Management

Clinicians must also assess for crisis and danger during clinical assessments, including the potential for suicide, homicide, substance abuse (past, present, or by others), and sexual/physical abuse history. If a client has any indicators of potential problems in these areas, counselors should assess for indicators of safety, generate a safety plan, and document legal actions taken.

Assessing Suicidality and Homicidality

Clients who present with depression and hostility for others should be assessed for suicidal and/or homicidal intentions. Each state has different laws governing precisely when and how a counselor can take action to protect clients, the public, and property from danger. In most states, counselors must take some form of action to protect clients who have a clear plan and intent for killing themselves or others; when there is no clear plan or intent, then counselors are still ethically bound to create safety plans in case the situation escalates. Documentation should include salient risk factors to support a clinician's subsequent actions.

- *No indication:* No verbal, nonverbal, or situational indications of danger.
- *Denial:* Client was directly asked and denies suicidal and/or homicidal intent.
- *Passive Ideation:* Client "would like to be dead" or "have the other person gone" but denies any plan or willingness to kill self or another.
- *Active Ideation:* Client thinks about killing themselves or others.
- *Attempt:* Client has attempted to kill themselves or another at any point; a significant risk factor.
- *Family History:* A family history of suicide is another significant risk factor.

Assessing Substance Abuse

Substance and alcohol abuse is generally considered one of the most difficult areas of functioning to assess, because clients often underreport or deny their use, especially if problematic (Saha, Harford, Goldstein, Kerridge, & Hasin, 2012). Often, these issues are not fully revealed early in treatment; thus, counselors should routinely and frequently inquire about substance and alcohol use throughout treatment, especially in cases where progress is not readily being made.

Sexual Abuse, Physical Abuse, and Other Risk Factors

Research over the past decade has highlighted the importance of identifying past and current trauma in order to improve treatment outcomes (Grasso, Ford, & Briggs-Gowan, 2013). Counselors should assess both with written and verbal self-report, bearing in mind that some clients will wait until later in treatment to reveal their experiences of trauma. Common forms of trauma include child abuse, abuse to an adult, or elder abuse.

Child Abuse

Four types of child abuse are generally outlined in state laws:

- *Sexual abuse:* Inappropriate sexual contact with a minor by adult or another minor; may or may not be consensual (defined by state laws).
- *Physical abuse:* Hitting, beating, kicking, or otherwise inflicting bodily harm by hand, with an object, and/or other means (e.g., locking child in enclosed space); includes most forms of spanking.
- *Emotional abuse:* Inflicting severe psychological harm, such as fear of death, physical intimidation, intense rejection and disapproval, and such.
- *Neglect:* Failing to provide for basic physical needs of child, such as sufficient food, clothing, shelter, health needs, and so on.

In most states, all forms of child abuse except emotional abuse legally require a child abuse report to authorities (e.g., child protective services, sheriff, police, and the like) of that state.

Elder and Dependent Adult Abuse

In addition to childhood abuse, it is important to assess for partner abuse (physical, sexual, and/or emotional) and as well as other forms of assault in adulthood. As most states do not have mandated reporting for such abuse, counselors have a greater ethical imperative to help these clients take steps toward ensuring their own safety by creating safety plans (see below: Davies, Lyon, & Monti-Catania, 1998). Most significantly, most states have laws for reporting elder and dependent adult abuse and neglect, which include the categories above in addition to *financial abuse*, illegal or unauthorized use of a person's property, money, pension, etc.

Other Risk Factors

- *Anorexia, Bulimia, and Other Eating Disorders:* Eating disorders are one of the most dangerous mental health disorders, anorexia frequently cited as having one of the highest fatality rates of any mental health diagnosis, with a significant number committing suicide (Arcelus, Mitchell, Wales, & Nielsen, 2011). These disorders most always require coordinated care with a medical professional.
- *Cutting and Self-Harm:* Cutting, burning, and other forms of self-harm are used to cope with emotional pain; counselors need to interview clients to determine if there is suicidal intent or if the self-harm is intended for another purpose, such as relieving emotional pain. Even when a client self-harms without suicidal intent, counselors should consider this a safety issue that needs to be carefully monitored and addressed (Selekman, 2006).
- *Criminal or Legal History:* Criminal or legal history is helpful in assessing potential for harm and danger.
- *Other Traumas:* In addition to abuse, other common forms of trauma include war, loss, and natural disasters.

Indicators of Safety

In addition to assessing for danger, counselors should assess for the potential for safety: what factors are in place to keep the client safe? The balance of these two potentials helps counselors determine the overall level of crisis (Davies et al., 1998; Dolan, 1991; Selekman, 2006).

Indicators of Safety

- At least one outside support person.
- Able to cite reasons to live and/or not harm others (e.g., "I couldn't do it because of my kids").
- Hope; goals for future.
- Willing to dispose of dangerous items (e.g., gun).
- Agrees to reduce contact with people who make the situation worse.
- Agrees to safety plan and develops an alternative to harming self/other.

Safety Plans

Safety plans should be developed for any situation in which potential risk is identified, such as passive suicidal ideation, history of cutting, history of abuse, and such. Safety plans should be tailored to each client's individual needs using combinations of the below components as well as unique elements for each client.

Safety Plan Components

- Verbal or written agreement or contract to not harm themselves or others.
- A card with emergency contact numbers for local hotlines, supportive friends, counselor's emergency contact number, and such.
- Working with medical professionals prescribing medication to reduce crisis potential.
- Specific action plan regarding who to call and what to do if a crisis begins to arise.
- Identifying tasks to calm self, such as journaling, exercising, etc., at low levels of pre-crisis stress.
- Specific daily or weekly activities to reduce overall level of stress and triggers for crisis.

Scaling for Safety

A variation of solution-oriented scaling questions (O'Hanlon & Weiner-Davis, 1989), I have found scaling for safety one of the most useful techniques for stabilizing crisis situations with clients willing to make change, including severe depression, suicide, cutting, eating disorders, substance abuse, and violence. Using a white board, I have clients define both emotionally and behaviorally a "1" when things are good, "5" when things are neutral or okay, and a "10," the crisis point when a dangerous activity occurs. I then have them describe a 6–9 in terms of emotions and behaviors, looking for the point at which the client has the ability to relatively easily take action, generally a 7. Then, we develop a realistic safety plan at this point, what the client will do, whom they will call, etc., when they begin to "feel" and "act" at a level 7. If the client engages in the behavior after the plan is in place, it should be revised to take action at a lower level on the scale. For most clients, this is specific and realistic enough to avoid getting close to the crisis behavior.

	Behaviors and Actions	Thoughts/Feelings
10: Crisis/Dangerous Act Occurs		
9		
8		

(*continued*)

7		
6		
5: Doing/Feeling Okay		
4		
3		
2		
1: Feeling Great		

- Number at which I feel I still have enough control to easily enact safety plan: ______________________
- Top 5 warning signs that I have hit #______________________.
- 5 Things I can do when I hit #______________________.

Digital Download Download from CengageBrain.com

Commitment to Treatment

In cases involving suicide, Rudd, Mandrusiak, and Joiner (2006) recommend obtaining a "Commitment to Treatment" agreement rather than a no-harm contract, which, although standard practice, has no empirical support. A commitment to treatment is an agreement between the client and counselor in which the client agrees to commit to the treatment process, and it has three elements:

1. Identifying the roles, obligations, and expectations of both the counselor and client in treatment,
2. Communicating openly about all aspects of treatment, including suicidal thoughts and plans, and
3. Accessing agreed-upon emergency resources during a crisis that might threaten the client's ability to fulfill his/her commitment to treatment (e.g., a crisis during which the client contemplates suicide).

Rudd et al. (2006) believe that obtaining a commitment to treatment provides a more useful clinical intervention than a no-harm contract in which clients sign a contract agreeing not to harm themselves and to contact emergency services. In contrast, the commitment to treatment provides a more hopeful and useful framework for both client and counselor by clearly outlining each person's responsibilities and encouraging open communication. Rather than emphasizing *not* committing suicide, the focus is on *committing* to meaningfully participate in psychotherapy treatment.

Case Management

Case management refers to a collaborative process of working with clients to develop a comprehensive plan of care that takes into account resources and services necessary to ensure a successful treatment outcome. Counselors rendering mental health services must develop *treatment plans* (see Chapter 5) that detail how they plan to address the client's presenting problems as part of standard practice. In addition, counselors need to "think outside of the counseling room" to coordinate care with other professionals, advocate for clients, and help clients identify and access the resources necessary for counseling to be effective. Common case management activities include:

Making Collateral Contacts

- Contacting and coordinating care with
  - Client's physician, psychiatrist, and/or other health professionals
  - Other mental health professionals (e.g., group therapists, family therapist, etc.)
  - Involved social workers or probation officers

Referrals to Resources to Support Need to Achieve Clinical Goals

- Referring client for a medical/psychiatric assessment to rule out medical causes and/or exacerbating conditions.
- Referring client for social services such as job training, welfare, housing, victim services, legal assistance, etc.
- Referral for group counseling and/or psychoeducational classes (e.g., parenting classes).
- Referral for legal and/or forensic services (e.g., custody evaluations).

Creating a Support Network

- Helping client connect with new or existing social supports, such as religious groups, friends, family, etc.
- Considering the effects of treatment on significant others in the system (e.g., effect of treating substance dependence on family).
- Identifying any unique needs the client has in order to be successful (e.g., transportation, safe place to exercise, a computer, etc.).

Prognosis

Finally, a clinical assessment often includes a general *prognosis*, or expected outcome, which is typically framed in terms of "return to normal functioning." In some cases, based on the diagnosis, symptoms, history, and evidence base, a counselor can confidently state that return to normal functioning is not anticipated. As part of this, hope can also be assessed, as it is a significant common factor that affects treatment outcomes; the more hope a client has, the greater the chance of a positive outcome (Miller, Duncan, & Hubble, 1997).

Evaluation of Assessment

The final section of the Clinical Assessment encourages counselors to reflect on how they have adapted the assessment to fit the client's unique needs, including diversity factors, effects of treatment on the client, and areas of client-counselor agreement/disagreement. Considering these factors helps counselors develop a plan that is more likely to be successful and helps identify potential pitfalls.

Communicating with Other Professionals

When speaking to medical doctors and psychiatrists involved in a patient's care, counselors need to speak their "medical" language, even if this is not the language they use to conceptualize the case. Much like learning to speak a foreign language, counselors learn to translate from one language to another in their heads. With time and practice, counselors learn to actually "think" in the foreign language and speak more fluidly and eloquently, expressing more and more complex ideas. As with any foreign language, it often helps to "go abroad" and spend time living in an environment where the language is spoken as the primary language. In the mental health world, such environments take the form of inpatient, intensive outpatient, county mental health, and similar settings.

Medical terminology is a technical language with preferred vocabulary found in its dictionary, the DSM-5. The essence of this language is summarized in the following four principles:

- **Use DSM Symptom Language**
  Rather than use vernacular descriptions of client symptoms, medical terminology requires the use of symptoms that are the foundation for making diagnoses.

- Panic attack (rather than "nervous breakdown")
- Depressed mood (rather than "feeling down")
- Irritability (rather than "feeling upset")

- **Use Behavioral Descriptions**
  When symptoms can be described in more detail using behavioral description, the behavioral description should be added.
  - Yells at partner (rather than "gets angry")
  - Loss of interest in hobbies (rather than "doesn't care anymore")
  - Loses focus on homework after 15 minutes (rather than "doesn't pay attention")
- **Include Duration of Symptoms**
  - Depressed mood for 3 months
  - Hypomanic episode for 3 days
  - Auditory hallucinations reported since age 14
- **Include Frequency of Symptoms**
  - Tantrums 3–4 times per week for past year
  - Violence outburst every 1–2 months for past 3 years
  - Binging and vomiting 2 times per week for past 6 months

By simply using symptom and behavioral descriptors with frequency and duration, you will quickly be on your way to fluency in medical terminology and improving your communication with other professionals. Thus, to end the chapter, I leave you with a comprehensive list of the symptoms and mental status terms to get you started on learning the language of clinical assessment—a good time for a cup of tea and a highlighter.

Mental Status Terms

Interpersonal Issues

- *Conflict:* Frequent arguments and conflict with one or more persons.
- *Enmeshment:* Boundaries with one or more persons are diffuse, not allowing for significant sense of independence (e.g., needing the other to always agree to feel okay; unable to tolerate differences with significant others; feelings easily hurt and/or easily feels rejected).
- *Isolation/Avoidance:* Avoids social contact to manage difficult feelings; reports actively isolating self or feeling isolated; reports few social contacts.
- *Emotional Disengagement:* Clients are in a relationship but lack meaningful emotional connection with one or more significant persons in their life.

Common Mood Descriptors

- *Mood versus Affect:* Mood is how a person reports feeling inside; affect is the outer expression of emotion.
- *Depressed:* Feeling of sadness and unhappiness; "blue," "down."
- *Anxious:* Generalized worry about unspecified or vague negative events happening.
- *Dysphoric:* General state of unease or dissatisfaction with life.
- *Angry:* Feeling indignant or wronged about a specific happening.
- *Irritability*: Generalized feelings of anger or upset without a specific object of anger; angry reactions are easily triggered.
- *Manic*: Unusually energetic feelings of elation, euphoria, or irritability.

Common Affect Descriptors

- *Constricted or Restricted:* Emotional expression is restrained but emotions are evident.
- *Blunt or Blunted:* Emotional expression is severely restrained; little emotional reactivity.

- *Flat:* Associated with psychosis and severe pathology; emotional expression is virtually nonexistent.
- *Labile:* Mood vacillates frequently, rapidly, and abruptly.
- *Incongruent:* Expressed affect distinctly incongruent with described mood (e.g., appears angry but reports no negative moods).

Common Sleep Descriptors

- *Hypersomnia:* Sleeping more than usual.
- *Insomnia:* Unable to get usual amounts of sleep, due to difficulties falling or staying asleep.
- *Disrupted Sleep:* Sleep disturbed by nightmares, night terrors, or other issues.
- *Nightmares:* Dreams that frighten the dreamer; occur during REM sleep.
- *Night Terrors:* A general sense of panic or terror is experienced while sleeping without dream content; the sleeper generally cannot be roused during night terrors, although he/she may scream or act panicked; occur in slow-wave sleep, not REM.

Common Eating Descriptors

- *Anorectic Restriction:* Restrictive eating that characterizes anorexia.
- *Binging:* Episodes of uncontrolled overeating.
- *Purging:* Following a binge episode, an attempt to rid body of food by vomiting, overexercising, fasting, or laxative abuse.
- *Body Image Distortion:* Image of body, particularly related to weight, is grossly inconsistent with others' perception and medical weight norms.

Common Anxiety Descriptors

- *Anxiety:* Anticipation of danger, problems, or misfortune that creates uneasiness, tension, and/or somatic symptoms.
- *Chronic Worry:* A specific form of anxiety that involves dwelling on anticipated problems.
- *Panic Attacks:* Discrete periods of intense anxiety or terror that may be characterized by shortness of breath, pounding heart, sense of losing control, or sense of doom; may be unexpected or situationally bound.
- *Phobias:* Persistent, irrational fears of specific objects or situations.
- *Obsessions:* Intrusive and recurrent thoughts, impulses, or images that cause marked distress.
- *Compulsions:* Repetitive behaviors or mental acts (counting, praying, etc.) that one is driven to perform to reduce some form of distress; generally the act is not realistically related to the distress.

Common Trauma Symptoms

- *Hypervigilance:* On constant alert for potential danger; out of proportion for actual situation.
- *Flashbacks/Intrusive Memories:* Sudden and disturbing memory or visceral sensations; may be cued or uncued.
- *Dissociation:* Disruption in integration of consciousness, memory, identity, and/or perception; may come on suddenly or gradually.
- *Emotional Numbing:* Inability to access emotional experiences; may be general or related to specific events.
- *Avoidance efforts:* Avoiding triggers and associations to past trauma.

Common Psychotic Descriptors

- *Hallucinations:* Sensory perceptions (sight, sound, touch, smell, or taste) that have no external stimuli; perceptions are experienced as real.
- *Delusions:* False beliefs based on an incorrect inference about external reality that is rigidly maintained despite substantial evidence to the contrary. May be bizarre (considered culturally implausible) or nonbizarre.

- *Paranoia:* Suspicion that one is being harassed or persecuted with little corroborating evidence; less severe than delusion.
- *Loose Associations:* Thought disorder characterized by frequent derailment from topic of conversation, jumping from thought to thought often triggered by a "loose" connection to a word or phrase.

Common Motor Activity Descriptors

- *Low Energy:* Little movement or energy behind movement.
- *Hyperactive:* Excessive motor activity, such as fidgeting or moving about; not necessarily associated with tension or discomfort.
- *Agitated:* Excessive activity associated with inner tension or frustration.
- *Inattentive:* Unable/Unwilling to pay attention.
- *Impulsive:* Acts on urges without reflecting on potential or likely consequences.
- *Pressured speech:* Speech is rapid, frenetic, and urgent beyond what seems appropriate for context or content.
- *Slow speech:* Speech is unusually slow and/or deliberate for context or content.

Common Thought Descriptors

- *Poor Concentration or Attention:* Inability to sustain the attention expected for the developmental level.
- *Denial:* Inability or refusal to acknowledge clearly evident problems that most others in the situation identify as problems.
- *Self-Blame:* Tendency to blame self for things that are outside of personal control and/or that others hold greater responsibility for.
- *Other-Blame:* Tendency to blame others for things that are primarily a personal responsibility.
- *Ruminative:* Compulsively focused attention on particular topic or problem.
- *Tangential:* Tendency to make comments that move conversation away from original topic to a tangentially or loosely related topic; typically done when discussing a difficult subject.
- *Concrete:* Thinking focused on actual objects and events with little use of concepts or higher-order thinking.
- *Poor Insight:* Unusually great difficulty identifying one's own thoughts, feelings, and motivations.
- *Impaired Decision Making:* Pattern of making decisions that result in negative consequences for self and others.
- *Disoriented:* Not well oriented to time, place, and/or person.

Questions for Personal Reflection and Class Discussion

1. Which part of the mental status exam seems easiest to you? Most difficult?
2. What type of questions might you ask to assess for suicide risk? Which clients would you ask these questions?
3. What type of questions might you ask to assess for childhood abuse? Which clients would you ask these questions?
4. How would you go about creating a safety plan with a client?
5. What elements of case management will likely be most challenging for you? Why?

Online Resources

Official DSM-5 website with access to Cross-Cutting Measures, WHODAS 2.0, and cultural assessment as well as fact sheets for specific disorders, and videos on the changes.
www.psychiatry.org/dsm5

Originally serving as the site to solicit public feedback on the DSM-5; this site documents the development of the DSM-5, including monographs, conference proceedings, and related reference lists, and also includes many of resources on the sister site: psychiatry.org/dsm5, including the online measures for download.
www.dsm5.org

References

American Psychiatric Association. (2013). *Diagnostic and statistical manual for mental disorders* (5th ed.). Washington, DC: Author.

Burgess, W. (2013). *Mental status examination* (2nd ed.). Seattle, WA: CreateSpace Independent Publishing Platform.

Davies, J. M., Lyon, E., & Monti-Catania, D. (1998). *Safety planning with battered women: Complex lives/difficult choices*. Thousand Oaks, CA: Sage.

Dolan, Y. (1991). *Resolving sexual abuse: Solution-focused therapy and Ericksonian hypnosis for survivors*. New York: Norton.

Grasso, D. J., Ford, J. D., & Briggs-Gowan, M. J. (2013). Early life trauma exposure and stress sensitivity in young children. *Journal of Pediatric Psychology*, *38*(1), 94–103. doi:10.1093/jpepsy/jss101

Miller, S. D., Duncan, B. L., & Hubble, M. A. (1997). *Escape from Babel: Towards a unifying language for psychotherapy practice*. New York: Norton.

O'Hanlon, W. H., & Weiner-Davis, M. (1989). *In search of solutions: A new direction in psychotherapy*. New York: Norton.

Rudd, M. D., Mandrusiak, M., & Joiner, T. E. Jr. (2006). The case against no-suicide contracts: Commitment to treatment statement as a practice alternative. *Journal of Clinical Psychology in Session*, *62*, 243–251.

Saha, T. D., Harford, T., Goldstein, R. B., Kerridge, B. T., & Hasin, D. (2012). Relationship of substance abuse to dependence in the U.S. general population. *Journal of Studies on Alcohol and Drugs*, *73*(3), 368–378.

Selekman, M. (2006). *Working with self-harming adolescents: A collaborative, strength-oriented therapy approach*. New York: Norton.

CHAPTER

5

Treatment Planning

More Than a Number

Shanna was 12 when I met her. She was alone in witnessing her mother die of a stroke three years before. Her aunt tried to take care of her the first year, but had to give her up to social services because she did not want the trouble. To be fair, Shanna was trouble. She frequently ran away, talked back, and didn't do her homework. Her foster parents—there were several in the past two years—had similar experiences. So, when I submitted my treatment plan to county mental health, I included the following in my goals.

1. Reduce episodes of running away to none; sustain for three months.
2. Reduce arguing with foster parents to no more than one mild episode per week.
3. Increase completion of homework to 90% every week; sustain for three months.
4. Work through grief related to loss of mother.

My treatment plan was rejected. So, I called the county mental health department to ask how best to revise the plan. The assessor on the other end of the phone said, "You just need to make the last goal measurable." In trying to get her to lighten up, I jokingly said, "Something like count how many tears she cries each week?" To my great surprise, she said, "Something along those lines would be perfect. Perhaps measure how long she cries each day." That's when I realized I was dealing with a bureaucracy's need for a line to be filled rather than discussing therapeutic process or client needs. First of all, reality check: I doubt I will get an accurate report of such a statistic from her or her mother. Secondly, since healthy grieving often involves quite a few tears, how meaningful would that goal really be in terms of measuring progress from week to week with a child grieving her mother? Finally, aren't we losing our sense of humanity and compassion? This is a child who traumatically lost her mother. I actually felt sad for not only my client but also for the woman on the end of the phone who must spend her days quibbling about such matters that she too must know are not getting to the heart of the matter (pun intended).

All of this flashed through my head along with a note to myself to not joke about HMO treatment plans, and I suggested we strike the fourth goal from the plan and approve it with the first three. She agreed. I then documented in my notes how I worked on grief to help her let go of the guilt that held her back from building a relationship with her foster parents and kept her from investing herself in school so she could make a life for herself.

However, the outrage I felt over the dehumanizing practice of reducing a child's grief to a simple matter of counting tears did not dissipate. So, in an act of rebellion and classic sublimation (see Chapter 8 for definition), I did all that an academic could do to make a difference in the world: I wrote a book (yeah, we are a wimpy lot when it comes to revolution). It's been almost 15 years since then, and my treatment plan approach has had to evolve to keep up with new demands from third-party payers. In this chapter, you are going to learn a more comprehensive model for treatment planning that should enable you to get yours approved for payment the first time you submit—without counting tears.

Step 3: Select a Path

After you complete your case conceptualization and clinical assessment, the next step is to develop a treatment plan that addresses the problems you worked so diligently to identify. Treatment plans are fun and perhaps one of the most creative acts of a counselor. However, they also come with the burden of professional responsibility. Since numerous good plans can be developed for any one client, counselors are free to choose—and are responsible for choosing—a theory and techniques that are the best fit for *this client*, the specific *problem*, and the particular counselor-client relationship. In developing a treatment plan, counselors need to consider the evidence base related to the client issue, client demographics, and theory chosen. Ultimately, a counselor's job is to promote an effective intervention process that addresses the client's concerns, and coherent, thoughtful treatment plans are a primary vehicle for demonstrating the ability to do so.

The Brief History of Mental Health Treatment Planning

This section is brief because the history of mental health treatment planning is quite short. The original theorists did not talk or write about treatment planning, and, in fact, if you search the literature you will not find any published in a form that a managed care company would approve for payment. If the approved approach to treatment planning isn't found in mental health literature, where did it come from? The short answer: the medical field.

Symptom-Based Treatment Plans

The type of treatment planning that the vast majority of counselors must complete in order to receive third-party payment and, arguably, to maintain standard practice of care in the 21st century is derived from the medical model: it's what medical doctors use for medical treatment. Within the field of mental health, Jongsma and his colleagues (Dattilio & Jongsma, 2000; Jongsma, Peterson, & Bruce, 2006; Jongsma, Peterson, McInnis, & Bruce, 2006; O'Leary, Heyman, & Jongsma, 1998) have developed the most extensive models for this form of treatment planning, which is focused solely on clients' medical symptoms and referred to as *symptom-based treatment plans*. Most publications on mental health treatment planning use a similar symptom-based model (Johnson, 2004; Wiger, 2005). The strength of these plans is that they are relevant to those in the medical community; the weakness is that they do not sufficiently help counselors to conceptualize their treatment in useful ways.

For example, if a parent brings a child to counseling who is having tantrums and the counselor develops a plan around the presenting problem (e.g., "reduce child's tantrums to less than once per week"), and follows that plan without thoroughly conceptualizing the case from a theoretical perspective, treatment is less likely to be successful. In this particular situation, a systemic assessment will typically reveal that there are marital and/or parenting issues that contribute to the presenting problem. In a surprising number of cases, I find doing couples counseling that targets tension in the marriage is required to effectively reduce the child's tantrums. The danger of symptom-based treatment planning is that the counselor will *under*utilize counseling theories to conceptualize and *over*focus on symptoms. Or to borrow from the cliché, they are likely to miss the forest because they are focusing on the trees. Arguably, a "good" counselor would not do this; however, today's workplace realities include (a) heavy caseloads, (b) pressure to complete diagnosis and treatment plans by the end of the first session, and (c) highly structured paperwork and payment systems, all of which make it hard for a "good" counselor to do a good job. Thus, symptom-based treatment planning, although convenient, may not be the best choice for today's practice environments.

Theory-Based Treatment Plans

In Gehart and Tuttle (2003), I promoted theory-based treatment planning, which involved using theory to generate more clinically relevant treatment plans than the symptom model offers. Berman (1997) developed a similar approach for traditional psychotherapies. The strength of these models was that they include goals that are informed by clinical theories. However, after using theory-based plans with new trainees, I discovered theory-based goals and interventions are easily confused because they use the same theory-based language. Furthermore, it was difficult for most students to address diagnostic issues and clinical symptoms in these theory-based plans because the language of these two systems is radically different. So I have developed a new, "both/and" model that draws from the best of theory-based and symptom-based treatment plans and adds more recent elements of measurability.

Clinical Treatment Plans

Clinical treatment plans provide a straightforward yet comprehensive overview of treatment. They are the "Hummers" of the treatment plan world: luxury meets invincibility. If you can do these, you can go anywhere and do just about any other treatment plan out there.

Clinical treatment plans include the following elements:

- **Introduction:** The treatment plan starts with a brief introduction to the planned modalities (individual, couple, family, and/or group), frequency, and expected length of treatment.
- **Treatment Tasks:** Treatment tasks are "standard practice" tasks that the counselor should perform at each stage of counseling, namely the initial, working, and closing phases of counseling. These tasks are informed by theory as well as ethical and legal requirements. These are rarely included in other plans, but spell out standards of practice that are important to consider and document.
- **Diversity:** For each treatment task, the counselor identifies how specifically the counseling process will be adjusted to address diversity issues, such as age, gender, ethnicity, ability, sexual identity, and so on. This part rarely goes into a formal plan for reimbursement; however, it is a profound step for becoming a counselor who is competent with cultural and diversity issues. Because, although you may technically use the same intervention to develop a counseling relationship with all clients when using a particular theory, you should be altering its implementation when working with a 6-year-old girl, 14-year-old young man, or an 80-year-old army veteran.
- **Client Goals:** The key element of all treatment plans, client goals are unique to each client and describe what behaviors, thoughts, feelings, or interactions will be either increased or decreased as a result of treatment. Client goals are derived from the assessment of the presenting problem and are in theory-specific language. These goals are included in virtually all forms of treatment plans in one way or another.
- **Interventions:** Each goal includes two to three interventions that describe how the counselor plans to achieve these goals using the counselor's chosen theory. Interventions may or may not be included in other types of treatment plans.
- **Client Perspective:** The final section describes areas of client agreement and concern with the outlined plan. Increasingly, public mental health agencies include some indication that the client agrees with the plan, often a signature or statement that the plan was shared with the consumer.

Treatment Plan Format

TREATMENT PLAN

Date: __________ Case/Client #: __________

Clinician Name: __________ Theory: __________

Modalities planned: ❑ Individual Adult ❑ Individual Child ❑ Couple ❑ Family ❑ Group: __________

Recommended session frequency: ❑ Weekly ❑ Every two weeks ❑ Other: __________

Expected length of treatment: ______ months

Initial Phase of Treatment

Initial Phase Treatment Tasks

1. Develop working relationship. *Diversity considerations: [Describe how you will adjust to respect cultured, gendered, and other styles of relationship building and emotional expression.]*
   Relationship-building approach/intervention:
   a. __________

2. Assess individual, systemic, and broader cultural dynamics. *Diversity considerations: [Describe how you will adjust assessment based on cultural, socioeconomic, sexual orientation, gender, and other relevant norms.]*
   Assessment strategies:
   a. __________
   b. __________

3. Define and obtain client agreement on treatment goals. *Diversity considerations: [Describe how you will modify goals to correspond with values from the client's cultural, religious, and other value systems.]*
   Goal-setting intervention:
   a. __________

4. Identify needed referrals, crisis issues, collateral contacts, and other client needs.
   a. *Crisis assessment intervention(s):* __________
   b. *Referral(s):* __________

Initial Phase Client Goals: Manage crisis; reduce distressing symptoms

1. ❑ Increase ❑ Decrease __________ (personal/relational dynamic using terms from theory) to reduce __________ (symptom).

(continued)

Interventions:

a. ____________________

____

b. ____________________

____

Working Phase of Treatment

Working Phase Treatment Task

1. Monitor quality of the working alliance. *Diversity considerations: [Describe how you will attend to client response to interventions that indicate clinician using emotional or relational norms that are not consistent with client's cultural background.]*

   a. *Assessment Intervention:* ____________________

   ____

2. Monitor client progress. *Diversity considerations: [Describe how you will attend to cultural, gender, social class, and other diversity elements when assessing progress.]*

   a. *Assessment Intervention:* ____________________

   ____

Working Phase Client Goals (2–3 Goals). Target individual and relational dynamics using theoretical language (e.g., decrease avoidance of intimacy, increase awareness of emotion, increase agency, etc.)

1. ❑ Increase ❑ Decrease____________________ (personal/relational dynamic using terms from theory) to reduce____________________ (symptom).

   Interventions:

   a. ____________________

   ____

   b. ____________________

   ____

2. ❑ Increase ❑ Decrease ____________________ (personal/relational dynamic using terms from theory) to reduce ____________________ (symptom).

   Interventions:

   a. ____________________

   ____

   b. ____________________

   ____

3. ❑ Increase ❑ Decrease ____________________ (personal/relational dynamic using terms from theory) to reduce ____________________ (symptom).

   Interventions:

   a. ____________________

   ____

(continued)

b. ____

____

Closing Phase of Treatment

Closing Phase Treatment Task

1. Develop aftercare plan and maintain gains. *Diversity considerations: [Describe how you will access resources in the communities of which they are a part to support them after treatment ends.]*
   Intervention:
   a. ____
   ____

Closing Phase Client Goals (1–2 Goals): Determined by theory's definition of health and normalcy

1. ❑ Increase ❑ Decrease ____________________(personal/relational dynamic using terms from theory) to reduce ____________________(symptom).
   Interventions:
   a. ____
   ____
   b. ____
   ____
2. ❑ Increase ❑ Decrease ____________________(personal/relational dynamic using terms from theory) to reduce ____________________(symptom).
   Interventions:
   a. ____
   ____
   b. ____
   ____

Client Perspective

Has treatment plan been reviewed with client: ❑ Yes ❑ No; If no, explain: ____________________

*Describe areas of Client Agreement and Concern:*____________________

____________, ________ ______ ____________, ________ ______

Clinician's Signature, Intern Status Date Supervisor's Signature, License Date

You will find examples of completed treatment plans at the end of each chapter in Part II of the book.

Writing Useful Treatment Tasks

Treatment tasks are generally the easiest part of the treatment plan to develop because they are the most formulaic. Each theory has its own language and interventions for describing how to create a counseling relationship, and a good plan should reflect these differences. For example, a humanistic counselor focuses on the affective quality of the relationship, while a counselor using a cognitive counseling would have a more pragmatic and problem-focused approach.

Initial Phase Treatment Tasks

Perhaps not surprisingly, counselors have the most tasks in the initial phase of treatment. This is when the counselor establishes the foundation for counseling. Virtually all theories include in some form these four initial counselor tasks early in counseling:

- Establish a counseling relationship
- Assess individual, family, and social dynamics
- Develop treatment goals
- Case management: refer for medical/psychiatric evaluation; connect with needed community resources; rule out substance abuse, violence, and medical issues.

Although each theoretical approach has different ways to do these four tasks, the cross-theory similarities make it easy for counselors to conceptualize this early phase of treatment. If ever problems arise in treatment, counselors can be sure that one of these four initial tasks needs to be readdressed.

Working Phase Treatment Tasks

In the working phase, the primary task is to keep the ball rolling. As counseling progresses, counselors need to assess whether treatment is effective. Is the client making progress on the identified goals? Standardized measures, such as those in Chapter 7, can be used to more reliably measure progress. If treatment does not seem effective, what might be the reason and how can counseling be adjusted to accomplish those goals?

Similarly, counselors need to monitor to ensure that they maintain a strong rapport with clients. As counseling progresses, the counseling relationship can be weakened by numerous obvious and not-so-obvious factors, including lack of progress, a necessary confrontation, a counselor's ill-timed self-disclosure, a misinterpreted comment, a random remark by a stranger, or the outcome of a Google search. Thus, counselors must continue to monitor the relationship to ensure that there is a solid working foundation for the treatment plan. Monitoring of the relationship should always be done by observation and verbally "checking in" every few weeks. In addition, counselors can use instruments such as the Session Rating Scale described in Chapter 7.

Closing Phase Treatment Tasks

Simply put, the primary task of the closing phase is for counselors to make themselves unnecessary in clients' lives. During this phase of counseling, counselors work with clients to develop aftercare plans that include identifying (a) what they did to make the changes they have made, (b) how they will maintain their success, and (c) how they will handle the next set of challenges in their lives. Each counseling model has different ways of doing this, but there is a cross-theoretical consistency as well as a consistent logic to this task that is useful in most counseling situations. When done well, clients leave counseling feeling better able to handle the inevitable problems that will continue to arise in their lives. As systemic practitioner John Weakland reportedly stated, "Clients come in experiencing the same damn problem over and over. Therapy is successful when life is one damn problem after another" (Gehart & McCollum, 2007, p. 214).

Diversity and Treatment Tasks

For each treatment task, you should also note how you will address diversity issues, such as culture, ethnicity, race, sexual orientation, gender orientation, religion, language, ability, age, gender, and such. For example, with almost every client, you will need to adjust your relationship style, slightly to significantly, for some form of diversity, such as age, ethnicity, or gender. Similarly, any assessment of functioning should always take into consideration diversity variables.

In virtually all cases, a diversity note can address gender, age, ethnicity, and socioeconomic status. You don't need to address all of these every time, but you should specifically identify at least one significant one for each treatment task. Additionally, counselors can also note here how to address *counselor-client differences* in terms of these diversity factors.

Examples of how diversity may be addressed in treatment tasks:

- Use of humor with teens and men
- More formal, respectful relational style with immigrants or clients from ethnic backgrounds that prefer such relations with professionals (*respecto* with Latino clients)
- Use of *personalismo* with Hispanic/Latino clients
- Including spirituality and religious beliefs and resources
- Including more extended family or tribe members with clients who come from backgrounds where the extended family/tribal system is the primary system
- Use of present-focused, problem-focused approaches with clients who do not value exploring the past
- Using interventions, assessments, and questions that enable Asian clients to avoid shameful discussions
- Including culturally appropriate resources and persons in therapy
- Assessing family of choice with gay, lesbian, bisexual, or transgendered clients
- Accounting for the stress of marginalization and discrimination in assessment

If this seems like a daunting task, it is. I believe it is impossible to "master" diversity issues as a counselor. Instead, it is an ever-unfolding journey of developing new competencies in this area; each client, friend, family member, and stranger in your life offers you an opportunity to learn more. I hope you take them up on the offer each time. However, I realize you may want something more concrete to help you get started. One place to start learning about how to address diversity in counseling is this book. Each theory chapter (Chapters 8–14) includes a section that describes some of the ways the theory can be used with select ethnic, racial, and sexually diverse groups. The case studies in this book also have examples for you to use. Additionally, for ethnicity and religion, McGoldrick, Giordano, and Garcia-Preto (2005) describe the cultural norms for emotional expression and communication, typical family dynamics, and common clinical issues for 53 different ethnicities. In addition, counselors should also be familiar with the basics of working with children (Adler-Tapia, 2012), men (Good & Brooks, 2005), and older adults (Knight, Nordhus, & Satre, 2003). As you meet clients with more specific diversity issues—such as an unfamiliar religion, disability, or chronic medical condition—it is an ethical responsibility for counselors to educate themselves about the client's circumstances to better understand how to engage and support them best.

Writing Useful Client Goals

Whereas writing symptom-based goals such as "reduce depressed mood" is ridiculously simple, writing truly useful clinical goals is a significant challenge because it requires using counseling theory to describe the complex interplay between your client's presenting problem, personal dynamics, relational dynamics, and manifest psychiatric symptoms. In most cases, meaningful client goals strategically target two to three key threads that link these seemingly unrelated dynamics and issues. If you ever tried to open a large bag of flour (sugar, cat litter, bird seed, etc.) sealed with a braided thread, you know how this works. When you find the right thread to pull on, you achieve your goal effortlessly and quickly. If you can't find the right thread, nothing moves, and you get wildly frustrated. Similarly in counseling, when you know which threads to pull on, things go surprisingly smoothly. When you don't, things don't move and frustration ensues. To help you find the right thread from the beginning, I am going to walk you slowly through the details of the process.

The Goal-Writing Process

There are no clear rules for goal writing that work for every situation because each client is unique. However, there are some general guidelines that can be useful.

Guidelines for Writing Useful Goals

- **Start with a Key Concept/Assessment Area from Theory of Choice:** Start with "increase" or "decrease" (or similar verb that indicates change) followed by a description using language from your chosen theory as to what is going to change.
- **Link to Symptoms:** Describe what symptoms will be addressed by changing the personal/relational dynamic.
- **Use Client's Name:** When you use the client's name (or equivalent confidential notation), you ensure that it is a unique goal rather than a formulaic one.

Anatomy of a Client Goal

"Increase/Decrease" + [theoretical concept/assessment area] + "to reduce" + [symptom]

Part A (covers "Increase/Decrease" + [theoretical concept/assessment area]) — Part B (covers "to reduce" + [symptom])

Each part of the goal has a different function:

Function of Part A and Part B of Goal Statement

Part A: Gives the counselor a clear focus of treatment that fits with the theory of choice, and

Part B: Provides third-party payers with a clear description of how psychiatric symptoms will be affected.

Part A is most useful to counselors for conceptualizing treatment; Part B is most useful to third-party payers who require a medical model assessment. When counselors write goals that address both A and B, they allow themselves maximum freedom and flexibility to work in their preferred way, while translating their work so that third-party payers get their needs met as well.

Sample Goals:

- *Increase* positive self-talk about body *to reduce* binging and body image distortion. (Cognitive-behavioral)
- *Reduce* compliance to socially imposed "shoulds" related to making others happy *to reduce* AF sense of hopelessness and depressed mood. (Humanistic)
- *Increase* frequency of social interaction and reengagement in music, sports, hobbies *to reduce* severity of depressed mood. (Solution-focused)

Initial Phase Client Goals

During the initial phase of counseling, in most cases the first one to three sessions, client goals generally involve stabilizing crisis symptoms, such as suicidal and homicidal thinking, severe depressive or panic episodes, stabilizing eating and sleeping patterns, managing child, dependent adult, and elder abuse issues, addressing substance and alcohol abuse issues, and stopping self-harming behaviors such as cutting. In addition to stabilizing crisis issues, some theories have specific clinical goals that should be addressed in the initial phases. For example, solution-based counselors begin working on clinical symptoms in the first session by setting small, measurable goals toward desired behaviors as well as increasing clients' level of hope (O'Hanlon & Weiner-Davis, 1989).

Working Phase Client Goals

Working phase client goals address the dynamics that create and/or sustain the symptoms and problems for which clients came to counseling. These are the goals that most interest third-party payers. The secret to writing great working phase client goals is framing the goal *in the theoretical language* used for conceptualization; then link this language to the psychiatric symptoms. When counselors state the goal using theoretical language, this enables them to document a coherent treatment using their preferred language of conceptualization, rather than language that is geared for those prescribing medication.

For example, when a client is diagnosed with depression, many counselors include a goal such as "reducing depressed mood." Let's not kid ourselves: a person does not need a Master's degree and 2,000–4,000 hours of training to come up with such a goal. This medical model, symptom-based goal does not provide clues as to what the counselor will actually do. Furthermore, all documentation for the case will need to monitor the client's level of depression each week. In contrast, a clinical client goal should address the theoretical conceptualization that will guide the reduction of depression. Some examples include:

- *Psychodynamic:* Reduce rationalization to increase ability to directly experience emotions and reduce depressed mood and improve ability to emotionally connect in marriage.
- *Humanistic:* Increase ability to experience authentic emotions in the present moment to reduce depressed mood and increase sense of agency.
- *Cognitive-behavioral:* Reduce placating behaviors in marriage and at work to increase congruent communication and positive mood.
- *Narrative counseling:* Reduce influence of family's and societal evaluations of self-worth to increase sense of autonomy and reduce depressed mood.

Each of these goals addresses a client's depressed mood and provides a clear clinical conceptualization and sense of direction, thereby being much more useful to counselors than the medical goal of "reduced depressed mood."

Closing Phase Client Goals

Closing phase client goals address (a) larger, more global issues that clients bring to counseling, and/or (b) moving the client toward greater "health" as defined by the counselor's theoretical perspective. The former type of goals often takes the form of clients presenting with one issue, perhaps marital discord, and then later wanting to also address their parenting issues in the later stages of counseling. Similarly, often a client may present with depression or anxiety and in the later phase want to address relationship issues or an unresolved issue with their family of origin. Also, a couple may present with several pressing issues, such as conflict and sexual concerns to be treated in the working phase, and in the later phase they want to examine more global issues, such as redefining their identities and relational agreements.

The second type of client goal in the later phases is driven by the counselor's agenda. Some theories, such as humanistic and psychodynamic, have very clearly defined theories of health that counselors work toward. Other theories, such as systemic and solution-focused therapies, have less clearly defined long-term goals and theories of health for people. Thus, closing phase goals often include an agenda item that clients may not have verbalized. For example, in humanistic counseling, increased authenticity is a long-term goal that is embedded in the theory that should be included in long-term goals for clients. With such a general goal, it helps to add more detail, such as "increase sense of authenticity *in the marriage OR in career OR in social interactions"*; the more specific the goal, the more likely it is to be achieved.

Writing Measurable Goals

Many third party payers require goals be "measurable," meaning that somehow the client and therapist will know when the goal is achieved. Starting the goal with "increase/decrease" helps in this effort. In addition, some third parties want therapists to specify exactly what the criterion will be to determine if the goal has been met. To meet this requirement, you may use the following:

Measure: Able to sustain __________ for period of ______ ❑ weeks ❑ months.

Examples:

- Able to sustain positive mood for period of 2 ❑ weeks ☒ months.
- Able to sustain positive relational interactions for period of 2 ❑ weeks ☒ months.
- Able to sustain sobriety for period of 6 ❑ weeks ☒ months.
- Able to sustain C grade point average for period of 4 ❑ weeks ☒ months.

Writing Your First Set of Goals

When it comes time to write your first few treatment plans, you may find it helpful to take the time to do some preparatory work following these five steps.

Preparatory Steps to Writing Useful Client Goals

Step 1: Complete a thorough case conceptualization (Chapter 2) and clinical assessment (Chapters 3–4).

Step 2: Identify any crises or pressing issues that need to be managed early in treatment (Chapters 3–4).

Step 3: Identify two to three themes from the case conceptualization and clinical assessment.

Step 4: Identify the long-term theoretical goals from theory of choice.

Step 5: Complete a Goal Writing Worksheet.

The Basic Steps

Step 1: Case Conceptualization and Clinical Assessment

You can use the forms in Chapters 2 and 3 to conduct a thorough assessment. The case conceptualization is the most important and difficult step, and the one most new counselors would prefer to skip. Why? It requires significant reflective and critical thinking; it is *not* formulaic. It will take some time to apply theoretical concepts to your client's actual situation. You will struggle. It is most often *not* as clear as in the textbook (as is true of most things in life). But in that struggle, you will actually learn how to use theory. You will become a competent counselor. The clinical assessment is generally a bit more straightforward. So set aside time to do these, and know that it is well worth the effort—you have officially begun your license exam preparation. Whatever you master now, you will not need to pay to learn once you are out of school.

Step 2: Crises or Pressing Issues

In the clinical assessment, the counselor identified crisis issues such as the following:

- Suicidal or homicidal threats
- Potential, current, or past child, dependent adult, or elder abuse
- Current or past domestic or social violence
- Alcohol or substance abuse issues
- Need for an evaluation for medication or other medical issues that could impact treatment
- Eating disorders, self-mutilation, or other danger symptoms that need immediate attention
- Severe depressive, psychotic, or panic episodes or other serious symptoms that need to be stabilized for outpatient treatment

If any of these issues has been identified, it should be addressed in the Initial Client Goals section; if not, the counselor can include an early-stage goal that relates to the presenting problem.

Step 3: Themes from the Case Conceptualization and Clinical Assessment

After completing these two assessments, sit back and ask the following questions:

- What two to three key patterns emerged in the case conceptualization?
- How do these fit with the clinical assessment?
- What theory do I want to use, and how would it describe these key themes?

Step 4: Long-Term Goals

Some theories, including psychodynamic (Chapter 8), Adlerian (Chapter 9), experiential-humanistic (Chapter 10), and cognitive-behavioral (Chapter 11), have theoretically defined long-term goals, such as clear interpersonal boundaries, differentiation, or self-actualization. When using such therapeutic models, counselors begin with larger goals in mind and design the middle phase goals to prepare clients for the closing phase goals.

Step 5: Complete Goal Writing Worksheet

Finally, the following Goal Writing Worksheet will help you put all of this together in a neat package to ensure you have your bases covered:

- Client's reported problem
- Problematic relational dynamic identified in the case conceptualization
- Clinical and/or relational symptoms
- Evidence-based practice (optional)

Goal Writing Worksheet

Presenting Problem: These are used to help identify problem dynamics.

What does the client say is the problem(s)? Use the client's words and phrases as much as possible.

1. ______________________________

2. ______________________________

3. ______________________________

Case Conceptualization: Theory-Based Description of Problem Dynamics: These are used to write your goals.

Develop a case conceptualization based on "The Viewing: Case Conceptualization" section of each theory chapter. Identify two to four of the most salient problematic relational dynamics or discourse from the case conceptualization; these are the dynamics that are most likely to be contributing to the client's presenting problem. In some cases, you will see that certain dynamics overlap or are related; in these situations, try to summarize these overlapping dynamics into one point below.

1. ______________________________

2. ______________________________

3. ______________________________

(*continued*)

Clinical Symptoms

Identify two to four of the most salient psychological symptoms or issues from the clinical assessment (e.g., depression, anxiety, substance use, conflict with loved ones, isolation, loss of interest, hallucinations, and such). List these below.

1. ______________________________

2. ______________________________

3. ______________________________

Put It All Together

This keeps you honest: Do all the pieces fit together?

Presenting Problem	*Dynamic*	*Symptom*
1.		
2.		
3.		

Note: If for any reason you have symptoms that don't seem to be related to the dynamics you chose, review your case conceptualization again. The pieces should fit together.

Evidence-Based Practice (Optional): This helps you determine theory and technique.

Use PsychInfo or a similar search engine to do a review of the research literature related to (a) the client's presenting problem, (b) diagnosis, (c) personal demographics/diversity factors, and/or (e) your intended therapy approach. Describe the key interventions, techniques, or guidelines below.

1. ______________________________

2. ______________________________

3. ______________________________

Based on the most salient dynamics and evidence base, as well as your client's needs, which theory and/or techniques do you plan to use with this case?

____

Digital Download Download from CengageBrain.com

Writing Useful Interventions

The final element of treatment plans is including interventions to support each treatment task or client goal. Once you have conceptualized treatment and identified treatment tasks and client goals, identifying useful interventions is generally quite easy. The interventions should come from the counselor's chosen theory and be specific to the client.

Guidelines for Writing Interventions

- **Use Specific Interventions from Chosen Theory:** Interventions should be clearly derived from the theory used to conceptualize treatment tasks and client goals. If an intervention from another theory is integrated, the modifications should be clearly spelled out.
- **Make Specific to Client:** Use confidential notation (e.g., AF for adult female and AM for adult male) to make the goal as specific and clear as possible. For example, "Increase insight regarding AF's pattern of pursuing and AM's tendency to withdraw."
- **Include Exact Language When Possible:** Whenever possible, counselors should use the exact question or language a counselor would use to deliver the intervention (e.g., "On a scale from 1 to 10, how would you rate your current level of satisfaction in the marriage?").

Client Perspectives

Finally, counselors need to ask themselves—or better yet, their clients—what do my clients think of this plan?

- Are these the things the clients want to change?
- Are these interventions and activities my clients would be willing to try?
- Do the goals and interventions "fit" with my client's personality, cultural background, gender style, values, educational level, cognitive level, lifestyle, and so on?
- Are there areas where the clients and I have different ideas about what might be the source of the problem?
- Will we be starting where my client wants to start making changes or where there is the most immediate distress?
- Does the plan make sense to my client?

Considering the client's perspective is crucial to designing a plan that is likely to be effective. Counselors should discuss the plan directly with clients and ensure that there is a shared understanding about the goals, strategies for change, and outcomes. Many agencies have moved to having clients sign the treatment plan to ensure agreement. If you choose to do this, I recommend you include only the Client Goals from the treatment plan in this chapter to avoid overwhelming the client with too much jargon.

Do Plans Make a Difference?

Now that you know how to create a detailed treatment plan, I want to also let you in on a little secret: like most things in life, counseling rarely goes according to plan. Life happens; new problems arise; original ones lose their importance; new stressors change the playing field. Does that make them useless? Absolutely not. Treatment plans help counselors in numerous ways, just not the way it appears at first:

- Treatment plans help counselors think through which dynamics need to be changed and how.
- Treatment plans provide counselors with a clear understanding of the client situation so that they can more quickly and skillfully address new crisis issues or stressors that arise.

- Treatment plans give counselors a sense of confidence and increase clarity of thought that makes it easier to respond on the spot to new issues.
- Treatment plans ground counselors in their theory and increase understanding of how their theory relates to clinical symptoms.

All this is to say: do not be surprised when counseling does not go according to plan; instead, expect it. And know that the time you took to create a treatment plan makes you much better able to respond to the unplanned.

Questions for Personal Reflection and Class Discussion

1. Do you think treatment plans are a good idea? Why or why not?
2. For which type of presenting problems do you think treatment plans will be most useful or accurate? For which type the least? Why?
3. Do you think having predefined long-term goals based on a theory of health is helpful? Why or why not?
4. What particular issues do you think are most important to consider when working with diverse clients?
5. Who benefits more from treatment plans: the counselor or client?

Online Resource

Symptom-Based Treatment Planners
www.jongsma.com

References

Adler-Tapia, R. (2012). *Child psychotherapy: Integrating developmental theory into clinical practice*. New York: Springer.

Berman, P. S. (1997). *Case conceptualization and treatment planning*. Thousand Oaks, CA: Sage.

Dattilio, F. M., & Jongsma, A. E. (2000). *The family therapy treatment planner*. New York: Wiley.

Gehart, D., & McCollum, E. (2007). Engaging suffering: Towards a mindful re-visioning of marriage and family therapy practice. *Journal of Marital and Family Therapy*, *33*, 214–226.

Gehart, D. R., & Tuttle, A. R. (2003). *Theory-based treatment planning for marriage and family counselors: Integrating theory and practice*. Pacific Grove, CA: Brooks/Cole.

Good, G. E., & Brooks, G. R. (2005). *The new handbook of psychotherapy and counseling with men: A comprehensive guide to settings, problems, and treatment approaches* (Rev. & abridged ed.). San Francisco, CA: Jossey-Bass.

Johnson, S. L. (2004). *Counselor's guide to clinical intervention: The 1-2-3's of treatment planning* (2nd ed.). San Diego, CA: Academic Press.

Jongsma, A. E., Peterson, L. M., & Bruce, T. J. (2006). *The complete adult psychotherapy treatment planner* (4th ed.). New York: Wiley.

Jongsma, A. E., Peterson, L. M., McInnis, W. P., & Bruce, T. J. (2006). *The child psychotherapy treatment planner* (4th ed.). New York: Wiley.

Knight, B. G., Nordhus, I., & Satre, D. D. (2003). Psychotherapy with older adults. In G. Stricker, T. A. Widiger, & I. B. Weiner (Eds.), *Handbook of psychology: Clinical psychology, Vol. 8* (pp. 453–468). Hoboken, NJ: John Wiley & Sons Inc.

McGoldrick, M., Giordano, J., & Garcia-Preto, N. (2005). *Ethnicity in family therapy* (3rd ed.). New York: Guilford.

O'Leary, K. D., Heyman, R. E., & Jongsma, A. E. (1998). *The couples psychotherapy treatment planner*. New York: Wiley.

O'Hanlon, W. H., & Weiner-Davis, M. (1989). *In search of solutions: A new direction in psychotherapy*. New York: Norton.

Wiger, D. E. (2005). *The psychotherapy documentation primer* (2nd ed.). New York: Wiley.

CHAPTER 6

Progress Notes

Step 4: Document It

The fourth step of the competent counseling journey involves a breadcrumb trail: documenting where you've been and what you have done. Most human activities leave some sort of trace: footprints, a new creation, or debris of some sort. But counseling leaves little if anything behind: zero emissions. This undetectable nature of counseling is largely driven by legal and ethical guidelines to maintain confidentiality and client privacy. The problem with this setup is that third parties who have a vested interest in the counseling process—most often insurance companies and other third-party payers—demand some evidence that (a) it is actually happening, and (b) they are getting what they are paying for. In lieu of recording sessions or sending teams of observers to our offices, counselors leave evidence of their competence by documenting their work in *progress notes*, an official record of what happens in each meeting with the client.

Progress notes are counselors' primary means of showing that they are rendering professional care that conforms to legal and ethical standards. Unless in black and white, the counselor's professional opinion, supervisor's assessment, and even the client's enthusiastic exclamation that "the counselor is great" do not mean much to third-party payers. Instead, the default means of determining whether the counseling rendered conforms to standard practice is by reviewing progress notes. Thus, this documentation provides the primary line of defense in lawsuits and claims against the counselor. Additionally, counselors themselves use progress notes to remind themselves of what they did and said last week, last month, or last year.

Ideally, progress notes can and should be used to help counselors reflect upon and improve their services.

In years past, multiple and dramatically varied models and advice were given to new counselors about how to write progress notes; in my early days of training I was told such things as: don't make it legible, keep it brief, document as much as possible. Thankfully, relatively recent federal legislation provides counselors with increased clarity as to what should and should not be in progress notes, taking the guesswork out of the most frequently used clinical document in mental health.

On a Different Note: Progress versus Psychotherapy Notes

In 2003, the U.S. Department of Health and Human Services began enforcing a new set of medical documentation guidelines outlined in HIPAA (Health Insurance Portability and Accountability Act; USDHHS, 2003). Along with solving other health-care-related issues such as portability of health care insurance coverage, HIPAA regulations include new privacy standards for medical documentation. Most significant for counselors—actually, startling to those who had been practicing for years—was the new distinction between two sets of clinical documentation: *progress and psychotherapy notes* (Halloway, 2003). Formerly, keeping two sets of notes was somewhere between unethical and illegal, depending on how you handled requests for information. However, this new legislation allowed just that, in order to increase patient privacy.

Progress Notes: The "Official" Medical File

- Records that are shared with other medical professionals, clients (upon written request), and/or in response to subpoenas.
- Third-party payers generally have detailed requirements for the content of these notes.
- Under normal circumstances, clients in most states have rights to access these records.

Psychotherapy Notes: Counselor's Case Conceptualization File

- *Psychotherapy notes must be kept separate from the formal medical file* (i.e., separate physical file); if they are not kept separate, they are considered part of the medical file and do not have special protections.
- If kept separately, psychotherapy notes have a much higher level of protection under HIPAA legislation and are rarely, if ever, disclosed to an outside third party.
- There are no requirements to keep such records (e.g., you *don't* have to keep these, but you *may*).
- These are the distinct property of the counselor; clients do not have rights to these records.
- Contents typically include case conceptualizations, personal impressions, analysis of the client, hypotheses, and such.
- There are no standards for what information should be placed in these records, if kept, because their purpose is to help counselors think through, plan out, and/or reflect on client progress.

Since *psychotherapy* notes are kept separate and private with few guidelines, I am not going to get into your private affairs. You (and your supervisor until you are licensed) determine what goes in these notes. *Progress* notes are another matter—they have lots of form rules that we will focus on for the rest of the chapter.

Progress Notes

Ethical Mandates of HIPAA Progress Note

1. *Maximize client privacy*
   while simultaneously
2. *Documenting competent treatment that conforms to professional standards of care.*

When writing progress notes, you are balancing two ethical mandates: (a) maximize client privacy and confidentiality, while at the same time (b) documenting that you are providing competent treatment. Balancing these two equally important mandates is a bit tricky at first, but, like riding a bicycle, the balancing act gets easier with practice.

With regard to protecting client privacy, I like to quip that your progress notes should be written as if they were going to be printed on the front page of the *New York Times*. What do I mean by this? That any and all potential and unintentional stakeholders, including the client, would read the article in the *Times* and say, "Yea. That is what happened. No arguing the facts." Thus, progress notes document the basic facts and medical information that relate to a particular session. Most critically, counselors document (a) progress and setbacks related to psychiatric symptoms, (b) interventions used to treat those symptoms, and (c) the client response to those treatments. By focusing on these elements, counselors simultaneously maximize client privacy while documenting prudent care, thereby meeting both ethical mandates.

When writing progress notes, counselors should avoid including any highly subjective observations ("Client is unaware of how upset she really is with mother") as well as avoid putting in details of events, names of third parties, specific places, negative statements about others, for example ("She compares herself with Betty Jones, who left her husband for another man"). Rather than a dramatic *Harlequin romance* filled with intrigue and emotional turmoil, counseling progress notes should read like cold, dry medical records, lacking soul and anything "juicy." Such notes increase client privacy by not including potentially damaging information, such as fantasies of an affair, details about family interactions, and names of colleagues and friends. Thus, even if printed on the front page of the *Times*, progress notes detailing "five days of moderate depression" that the counselor treated by using "scaling questions to identify small tasks for the week" would hardly raise an eyebrow—and in any case would certainly be cut by the editor before going to press.

Crisis situations are the most notable exception to this general principle of minimal private information. When stabilizing a suicidal, self-harming, abused, or homicidal client, counselors must include detailed information about the assessment of safety, the safety plan (including names/roles of people who are part of the plan), and specific actions taken to ensure safety and follow legal requirements. Detailed notes when stabilizing a crisis situation provide the counselor with additional "insurance" by documenting prudent, professional care in high-risk legal situations and also provide other health care professionals involved in treating the client with the information they need.

Progress Note Ingredients

HIPAA guidelines and third-party payers provide guidance about what to include in a progress note, increasing the uniformity of progress notes in the field. These common ingredients include:

- **Client Identification:** Client case number (generally no name on weekly notes to further protect client confidentiality)
- **Time:** Date, time, and length of session; location if appropriate
- **Who:** Who attended session
- **Progress and Symptoms:** Client progress, including improvement/worsening of symptoms as well as *frequency*, *severity*, and/or *duration* of the psychiatric symptoms/conditions for which they are seeking help
- **Assessment and Crisis:** Assessment for crisis issues and description of how they are managed
- **Interventions:** Interventions used and client response to the intervention
- **Plan:** Plan for future sessions; modification to treatment plan
- **Signature:** Provider's original signature (not initials) with professional license/degree

Variations on a Theme: Types of Progress Notes

The necessary elements for progress notes are generally agreed upon. However, just like any list of ingredients, there are many ways to combine them to serve up different dishes. Translated into the world of progress notes, this means that there is more than one right way to do a progress note. Many counselors choose to conform to HIPAA by adapting pre-HIPAA forms of progress notes, SOAP, DAP, and such, to the new standards; others use formats they create or that an agency has developed. Although it seems logical to assume that HIPAA regulations have unified progress note formats, my annual trips to agencies around town indicate that there are more flavors of progress notes than ice cream flavors stocked at your local Baskin-Robbins™. The most common are SOAP, DAP, and BIRP notes.

SOAP Notes

Perhaps the original format for progress notes, SOAP notes are widely used in all medical contexts: SOAP stands for Subjective, Objective, Assessment, Plan (Wiger, 2005). Many medical professionals, including general practice doctors, chiropractors, and occupational counselors, use SOAP notes because they are designed for documenting the treatment of physical conditions, SOAP notes can be somewhat awkward when applied to mental health, especially with the new HIPAA regulations. Thus, the interpretation of each section can vary significantly across practitioners and agencies.

- *Subjective Observations:* Description of client's narrative and/or reported symptoms.
- *Objective Observations:* Counselor's observations, test results, findings from physical examination, vital signs. Note: counselor's observations need to be stated in purely behavioral terms, describing the behaviors, grooming, and such, observed in the room.
- *Assessment:* Summary of symptoms, assessment, and diagnosis; differential diagnosis considerations.
- *Plan:* Plan to treat listed symptoms, including instructions and medications given to client.

One of the key components not clearly identified in SOAP is where to put the interventions used in session. In most cases, this should go under "plan," which broadly refers to what the counselor *plans* to do about the assessed problems. This "plan" can refer to what the counselor did in session, homework, as well as next week's session.

DAP Notes

Developed in response to early managed care requirements, DAP (Data, Assessment, Plan) notes are one of the more common formats for progress notes (Wiger, 2005).

- *Data:* What happened or what was said in session, interventions, clinical observations, test results, symptoms, stressors, etc.
- *Assessment:* Assessment of symptoms, outcome of current session, and overall course of counseling, treatment plan goals/objectives being met, areas needing more work, areas of progress, etc.
- *Plan:* Homework, interventions for next session, timing of next sessions, changes to treatment plan. Some counselors use "P" for progress and describe improvements that the client has made related to the presenting problems and symptoms.

Although there is a general outline, DAP notes can be interpreted in numerous ways, thus each practitioner or agency often develops its unique style, emphasizing different information in each section.

BIRP Notes

A newer format that is increasingly popular is BIRP: Behavior, Intervention, Response, Plan. This format is closest to the one used in this text:

- *Behavior:* A behavioral description of symptoms that typically includes duration, severity, and frequency.
- *Intervention:* A description of interventions used in session.
- *Response:* Description of client response to the interventions.
- *Plan:* Plan for next session and/or changes to the treatment plan.

The All-Purpose HIPAA Progress Note

Harkening back to the pre-HIPAA era, neither DAP or SOAP are ideally laid out for mental health practitioners. Therefore, to facilitate trainee learning and simplify file audits by third-party payers, I developed the following Progress Note to address HIPAA requirements and the most common requirements of third-party payers, both private insurance and public agencies, in a format that is easier to follow.

PROGRESS NOTE FOR CLIENT #_______

Date: _______ **Time:** _____:_____ ❑ am/❑ pm **Session Length:** ❑ 45 min. ❑ 60 min. ❑ Other: _______ minutes

Present: ❑ Adult Male ❑ Adult Female ❑ Child Male ❑ Child Female ❑ Other: _______

Billing Code: ❑ 90791 (eval) ❑ 90834 (45 min. therapy) ❑ 90837 (60 min. therapy) ❑ 90847 (family)

❑ Other: _______

Symptom(s)	Duration and Frequency Since Last Visit	Progress
1: _______	_______	❑ Improved ❑ Progressing ❑ Maintained ❑ Regressed ❑ None ❑ Variable ❑ Not addressed
2: _______	_______	❑ Improved ❑ Progressing ❑ Maintained ❑ Regressed ❑ None ❑ Variable ❑ Not addressed
3: _______	_______	❑ Improved ❑ Progressing ❑ Maintained ❑ Regressed ❑ None ❑ Variable ❑ Not addressed

Explanatory Notes on Symptoms: ____________________

In-Session Interventions and Assigned Homework

____

Client Response/Feedback

____

Plan

❑ Continue with treatment plan: plan for next session: ____________________

❑ Modify plan: ____________________

Next session: Date: __________ Time: __________:__________ ❑ am/❑ pm

Crisis Issues: ❑ No indication of crisis/client denies ❑ Crisis assessed/addressed: describe below

____

____________________, ____________________ ____________________

Clinician's Signature License/Intern Status Date

(continued)

Case Consultation/Supervision ❑ Not Applicable

Notes: ____

____

Collateral Contact ❑ Not Applicable

Name: __________ Date of Contact: __________ Time: __________:__________ ❑ am/❑ pm

❑ Written release on file: ❑ Sent/❑ Received ❑ In court docs ❑ Other: _______

Notes: ____

____

______________________, ______________________ ______________________

Clinician's Signature License/Intern Status Date

______________________, ______________________ ______________________

Supervisor's Signature License Date

Examples of completed progress notes are located at the end of each of the chapters in Part II of the book.

How to Complete a Progress Note

Here are simple instructions on how to complete a progress note:

Client #

To protect client confidentiality, client names should never be put on file labels or progress notes. Ideally, if a progress note slipped out of a file, it would be impossible to identify the client if the note accidentally slipped out of a binder at Starbucks (yeah, it's happened—which is why the notes should never leave your agency's building, and why you should never leave the building after seeing clients until your progress notes are completed).

Date/Time/Session Length

Start each note with the date of the session; time session started; and length of session. Typically, individual, couple, and family sessions are limited to 25 or 50 minutes, while group sessions may be an hour to an hour-and-a-half.

Persons Present

Most clinicians use some form of abbreviation instead of the client name or word "client" to refer to the client and significant others. Some simply use "cl" to abbreviate for client. However, when working with couples and families, that does not suffice. Similarly, most individual clients refer to their significant others frequently, thus it helps to have an abbreviation for them, too, especially if a supervisor will be reading the note. Thus, after years of writing my own and reading others', I recommend the following notation system that works well for individuals, couples, and families as well as supervisors trying to track scores of clients they have never met:

AF: Adult Female: If more than one, add age (AF34; AF62) or simply AF1 and AF2
AM: Adult Male: If more than one, add age (AM24; AM58) or AM1 and AM2
CF#: Child Female plus age (e.g. CF8 = eight-year-old girl)
CM#: Child Male plus age (e.g. CM8 = eight-year-old boy)

CPT Billing Codes

Insurance companies use CPT (Current Procedural Terminology) codes established and updated by the American Medical Association to identify what type of service was provided. As of January 1, 2013, new CPT codes for mental health practitioners were issued:

Psychotherapy CPT Billing Codes

- **90791:** Psychiatric diagnostic evaluation (generally used for the first session)
- **90832:** Psychotherapy, 30 minutes with patient and/or family member
- **90834:** Psychotherapy, 45 minutes with patient and/or family member (used for standard 45–50 minute session)
- **90837:** Psychotherapy, 60 minutes with patient and/or family member
- **90845:** Psychoanalysis
- **90846:** Family psychotherapy, 45–50 minutes
- **90847:** Family psychotherapy, conjoint psychotherapy with patient present, 45–50 minutes
- **90849:** Multiple-family group psychotherapy
- **90853:** Group therapy (other than multiple-family group)
- **90839:** Psychotherapy for crisis, first 60 minutes; use **90840** for each additional 30 minutes
- **90785:** Interactive complexity code used with evaluation and psychotherapy codes: 90791, 90832, 90834, 90837, and 90839

Most county mental health agencies have their own set of billing codes, which are often not standardized within the same state, but they generally use billing categories similar to the CPT codes.

Symptom Progress

The defining element of a progress note, counselors document changes in (e.g., hopefully progress related to) the *duration, frequency, and severity* of symptoms from session to session. These symptoms should clearly match the diagnosis or other documented focus of clinical attention. Additionally, symptom progress should be stated in behavioral, psychiatric, and measurable terms.

- *Behavioral:* Describe symptoms in behavioral terms when possible
  - Conflict (number of conflicts rather than general descriptor of argumentative)
  - Panic attack (number of attacks)
  - Ran away (number of times)
- *Psychiatric:* Use psychiatric terms as much as possible
  - Depressed mood (preferred to sad)
  - Irritable (rather than moody)
  - Hypervigilance (rather than fearful)
  - Anxious (rather than stressed)
- *Measurable:* Include duration, frequency, and severity whenever possible.
  - *Duration:* How long did the symptoms last? Can be measured in minutes, hours, or days.
  - *Frequency:* How many times did it occur over a stated period? Ideally reported in numbers, but can be "most" or "rarely."
  - *Severity:* How severe were symptoms? Generally stated in terms of mild, moderate, or severe.

Examples of clear symptom progress statements include:

  - *Client reports mild [severity] depressed mood [symptom] 5/7 days [frequency]*
  - *Client reports one panic attack [symptom] past week [frequency], moderate severity.*
  - *Client reports decrease conflict with parents [symptom]; 2 short [severity] arguments past week [frequency].*

Examples of vaguely written symptom documentation includes:
Too vague: Client reports "doing better" this week.
Too vague: Overall improvement in symptoms.

Interventions

Once the symptoms are identified, progress notes clearly identify which interventions the counselor used to help the client address problems. The interventions should be theory- and client/symptom-specific. The "intervention" sections of each of the theory chapters in this book (Chapters 8–14) provide a wealth of options to make this task easy.

- *Used solution-focused scaling to identify steps to reduce depression over next week.*
- *Used empty-chair technique to practice sharing feelings with spouse.*
- *Offered attachment hypothesis to provide insight into relational pattern.*

Avoid general and vague statements that don't clearly convey professional psychotherapy intervention, such as:

- "Discussed work stress": not necessarily a counseling intervention that warrants insurance reimbursement.
- "Talked about fears": how does this distinguish you from a bartender or hairstylist?

Client Response

Increasingly, counselors document how clients respond to treatment: whether or not they responded well to interventions and what did and did not work. Over the years, I have found this section particularly helpful in prompting me to reflect on what types of interventions work with a particular client, thus, quite frankly, it's the most useful section for me to improve my work as a clinician.

- *Client receptive to reframe related to work issues; less receptive to reframe of pattern related to relationship.*
- *Client actively engaged in empty-chair technique; optimistic could employ at home.*
- *Client expressed enthusiasm about mindfulness exercises.*

Plan

Describe plan for next session and/or plans to modify treatment plan.

- *Will bring in partner to next session.*
- *Follow up on journal assignment: letter to future self.*
- *Continue to assess for suicidal ideation.*

Crisis Issues

Counselors document any crisis issues that arose in session and/or any issues that were followed up on from prior sessions. If there had been crisis issues, such as cutting or suicidal ideation, it is good to continue noting *in writing* that the counselor checked in during session. If a crisis issue was detected, counselors must clearly detail (a) the assessment process and data used to support conclusions and (b) the specific actions taken to ensure safety of client and/or public. Documenting crisis situations requires much more detailed and specific information compared to documenting general progress and intervention.

- *Client reported suspected abuse to child in family; reported child hit with belt on more than one occasion; report called in to CPS at 7:15 pm; taken by Christine K.; full report placed in file.*
- *Client reported passive suicidal ideation "wish I were dead"; denied plan or intent; "I would never do it because of my kids"; developed safety plan of 3 names to call; went over emergency contact for counselor.*
- *Client reported cutting twice this week; developed safety plan that client agreed to use scaling for safety to develop alternative action at level 7; client readily agreed to plan.*
- *Client denies cutting this week; no new cuts on wrists evident.*

Consultation and Supervision

When obtaining supervision, peer consultation, or legal consultation (from a lawyer), counselors should document recommendations and/or information, especially regarding ethical and legal issues.

Collateral Contacts

Whenever you contact another professional or family member regarding a client, such as a teacher, physician, psychiatrist, social worker, parent, or others, the contact needs to be documented, noting that a release is on file.

- *Consulted with psychiatrist; reports increasing Celexa to 60 mg; believes marital issues and child care duties fueling client depression; I shared solution-focused treatment plan with goals targeting mood, marital conflict, and parenting.*
- *School counselor reports that Math/Science teacher (Mr. Thomas) reports CM12 does not complete class work, interrupts lecture, and has conflict with peers; earning C in class. PE teacher reports similar problems; C in class. English and Social Studies teachers have not reported problems; B, C, respectively.*

Signature

Finally, counselors must (a) sign the progress note by hand (no initials) and (b) indicate license status. If unlicensed, the supervisor typically also signs the progress note.

A Time and Place for Progress Notes

The proper timing of writing progress notes is simple: immediately following the session. Counselors conduct 45–50 minute sessions so that the progress notes can be written in the 10–15 minutes in between. If not between sessions, counselors must complete progress notes before leaving at the end of the day. Anything else gets you into gray ethical areas because memory is not as detailed a day or two (especially a week or more) later—no matter how good your memory is. Trust me, I've tried it once or twice, and it does not work; therefore, I recommend you put daily progress notes in your "religious practice" category: they get done *every time, on time*, motivated by the fear of eternal damnation or worse—the wrath of an ethics review board.

Additionally, there is only one place for progress notes when they are not in your hands: a locked file cabinet. Like all medical professionals, counselors are required to keep client files and progress notes securely locked when not in immediate use; in some cases, under two sets of locks (e.g., locked file cabinet in a locked room). Computers, emails, and digital files containing client information require high levels of computer security outlined in the HIPAA policy (USDHH, 2003), including passwords, spyware, anti-virus software, secure file transfers, anti-spam software, secure socket layer (SSL) protocols, encryption, individual firewalls, and so on. Additionally, *any piece of paper that has identifying client information*, such as phone message pads or calendars, must also be locked when not in use. In most states, counselors must keep records for seven years past the age of majority (adulthood), after which time they may be destroyed (e.g., shredded). The upside of these security requirements is that they keep your desk clean, and, for many, the ritual act of shredding has the benefit of releasing pent-up stress and frustration.

Final Note on Notes

Progress notes are the heart of clinical documentation, and in many ways the most important documents we produce, because they provide the clearest record of what happens behind closed doors. Progress notes are the only place where we can document that we conducted ourselves as professionals, rendering appropriate and necessary medical services. They are the documents most likely to be viewed by outsiders should documents be released or subpoenaed. So we must take care to ensure that they protect us as well as our clients' privacy. The art of writing progress notes is one of the most important clinical skills to master. Thankfully, we get ample opportunity to practice!

Questions for Personal Reflection and Class Discussion

1. Do you think the increased standardization of progress notes is helpful or unhelpful? Constraining or reassuring?
2. What surprises you most about the common ingredients in a progress note? Do you think something is missing?
3. How might documenting mental health symptoms from week to week help the counseling process? How might it limit the process?
4. What challenges do you see with managing client documents in the digital age?

Online Resources

American Psychiatric Association Page for 2013 Psychiatric CPT Codes
www.psych.org/cptcodingchanges

CPT Codes from the AMA
www.ama-assn.org

HIPAA Guidelines
www.hhs.gov/ocr/hipaa

References

Halloway, J. D. (2003). More protections for patients and psychologists under HIPAA. *Monitor on Psychology, 34*(2), 22.

United States Department of Health and Human Services (USDHHS) (2003). *Summary of HIPAA privacy rule.* Washington, DC: Author. Retrieved December 2, 2007 from www.hhs.gov/ocr/hipaa.

Wiger, D. E. (2005). *The psychotherapy documentation primer* (2nd ed.). New York: Wiley.

CHAPTER

7

Evaluating Progress in Counseling

Step 5: Evaluating Progress

Have you ever noticed that often the drive to a new place seems to take longer than the drive home? This common perception—or misperception—results from anticipation and the additional attention required when traveling in a new area: what's around the next bend? Where do I need to turn? And where can I refuel? Similarly, relying on perception to determine where you are and how far you've gone on the counseling journey can be misleading. Just like on a road trip, it helps to have milestones to know how far you've come and how far you have left to go. However, unlike milestones on the open highway, measures of progress are less obvious in the field of counseling.

Increasingly, insurance companies, state legislators, and other third-party payers are asking counselors to measure and evaluate progress (Lambert & Hawkins, 2004). This is a daunting task, especially when compared to other medical professions. It is relatively easy to determine if a surgery is successful, physical therapy made a difference, or a medication is working. These are physical things that can be measured with a fair degree of reliability. But when counselors are asked to measure whether depression is getting better, anxiety is less, or a person is worrying less, measurement becomes trickier. If we could x-ray a person's mind or psyche and get an objective measure of levels of mood, that might help. If we could control for all the factors that contribute to a person's moods and behaviors—including relationship ups and downs, work stress, news headlines, physical illness, and weather—that would also give us a clearer sense of whether we are helping. If we could factor out the biases of our own personalities, histories, and moods, that might also give us a clearer picture. Instead, counselors need to be more creative and thoughtful when measuring progress. One approach to doing so is gathering multiple sources of data, often referred to as *triangulation*, to get a sense of whether clients are improving (Lambert & Hawkins, 2004). Toward this end, counselors have two general options for measuring progress, the fourth step of competent counseling:

- **Nonstandardized:** Client's and counselor's subjective reports of progress
- **Standardized:** Measures that have been standardized to measure specific psychological variables

Nonstandardized Evaluation of Progress

Nonstandardized evaluation of progress involves either the client or counselor descriptions, gathered verbally or in writing. In either case, the evaluation needs to be included in the written documentation for the client (e.g., their "file"). Increasingly, third-party payers require client evaluations of their progress in addition to counselor descriptions. Many insurance companies have shifted from having counselors complete treatment plans and assessments to the client completing progress checklists to assess if counseling is warranted and/or effective. Although there is some research to support the idea that client assessment of their level of functioning is useful, it is nonetheless a "self-report" that is generally considered less reliable than standardized and often even a neutral third party's evaluation (e.g., the counselor, who cannot be neutral as a participant).

Pros of Nonstandardized Evaluation

Basically, there is no reason not to use nonstandardized evaluations of client progress; the more challenging question is whether to add standardized measures of progress.

The Pros:

- Financial costs are minimal
- Can be done every session
- Including client and counselor perspectives creates greater validity
- More easily adapted for diverse clients
- When used weekly, helps to provide feedback on what is not working so counselor can adjust treatment plan

Cons of Nonstandardized Evaluation

- Not as reliable or valid as standardized measures
- Difficult to do with children if parents are not there to help provide information (although this is an even bigger problem with standardized instruments)
- More difficult to do with persons with severe pathology and/or who are unable to accurately recall events between sessions
- With certain couples or families, data should be collected on paper to get assessments that are not influenced by the comments of other members

Strategies

The easiest way to gather this information is to ask:

- For clients to assess their progress since the last meeting
- About changes in specific symptoms and/or progress toward goals (e.g., how often were you depressed/have a panic attack/binge, etc.?)
- For clients to rate change by using solution-focused scaling questions (Chapter 13; Berg & de Shazer, 1993)

Counselors can document both the clients' and their own assessment of progress, either (a) in a narrative (using phrases or sentences) or (b) using a scale.

Examples of Narrative Descriptions of Progress

- Client reports an increase in depressive episodes over the week (5/7 days)
- Client reports a decrease in conflict over the week; only 1 major argument
- Client reports no change in difficulty sleeping in past week (1–2 hours to fall asleep)

Examples of Documenting Using a Scale

Client Report: Improve ______ No Change ______ Worsening of following symptoms: ______

Counselor Observation: Improve ______ No Change ______ Worsening of following symptoms: ______

Scaling: Worst things have been 1 ______ 5 ______ 10 Goal achievement

Standardized Evaluation of Progress

Introduced in Chapter 3 as part of clinical assessment, standardized measures of progress are generally considered more accurate and reliable. These evaluations involve pen-and-paper or electronic questionnaires that are completed by clients and/or significant others. These measures have been tested for reliability and validity and allow counselors to more carefully track changes and compare a single client with a norm group, which is most meaningful when the client is similar to the comparative group (e.g., level of functioning, culture, age, etc.).

The common critique of these evaluations is that each person completing them has unique frames of reference and situations that make it difficult to meaningfully interpret the scores. Generally, the more diverse your clientele, the more difficult it is to accurately interpret these scores. For example, I once had a student who worked with a Chinese immigrant (sessions were in Mandarin), and she used a standardized instrument to collect initial symptoms and symptoms at the end of the semester three months later. Although the client appeared to have made significant progress, the instrument indicated that she had gotten *worse*. When the student followed up with the client about whether things were significantly worse, the client stated that she had minimized the reporting of symptoms initially because she did not trust the counselor and was uncomfortable admitting to certain problems. After she had developed a good rapport with the counselor, she felt free to more accurately answer the questions, which is consistent with her cultural values of saving face. The moral of the story is that standardized forms only work if the client is able to "play by the rules" and answer questions the way the authors intended. Clearly, counselors need to proceed with caution when trying to interpret standardized forms, and it is critical that counselors talk with clients when the results are unexpected.

Pros

- Considered more reliable and valid
- Better able to make cross-client comparisons
- Better able to make comparisons across time

Cons

- Almost all standardized forms must be purchased; some require a fee for each administration of the instrument, which can quickly become expensive
- May require more counselor time and/or equipment and resources (e.g., computers, copies)
- Requires more client time, and many clients are reluctant to give this time due to their busy lives and must be "sold" on the idea
- Not all are standardized for diverse populations and/or available in client's primary language

Effects on Counseling Relationship

Using questionnaires *always* impacts the counseling relationship; counselors need to be thoughtful about how they communicate about formal assessments and help clients make sense of the counseling relationship, especially if the counselor approaches the counseling relationship from a more egalitarian position (e.g., a postmodern, feminist, or humanistic approach).

Assessment in a Diverse Society

Meaningful and accurate assessment is especially difficult with diverse clients, requiring that counselors use clinical judgment and multiple forms of assessment to approach the endeavor (Hui & Triandis, 1985). Numerous issues need to be considered when assessing persons from diverse backgrounds.

Standards and Norms

Standardized assessment instruments are designed to compare the individual test taker's results to that of a norm group. For this comparison to be meaningful, the norm group must be similar to the person taking the test, especially similar in terms of culture. The majority of tests have been normed on middle-class Caucasians (sometimes limited to males) and thus should only be applied to the norm group (Brems, 1998). Increasingly, test developers are providing population-specific norms, but again, these have limits due to the dramatic variability in a given population based on differences in acculturation, language, immigration status, and social class. Although there is significant diversity within norm groups, the spectrum of diversity is much broader and more problematic with cultural subgroups. For example, although socioeconomic status creates significant diversity in any cultural group, most people growing up in the United States are familiar with questions from a medical or other professional, regardless of class. In contrast, this may not be the case with an immigrant subpopulation, and for those from oppressive governments, there may be notable fear, distrust, or reasonable paranoia of such a process. Ultimately, counselors need to use clinical judgment to determine the appropriateness of a standardized test for a given client.

Acculturation and Test Taking

Clients' levels of acculturation significantly impact how they experience and respond in assessment situations, particularly formal verbal or written assessments (Hui & Triandis, 1985). For some, most notably immigrants, the process of formal assessment—such as written multiple-choice questions or a formalized verbal questionnaire—may be a truly foreign experience compared to those who grew up in countries where standardized testing is common from the first years in school (Cofresí & Gorman, 2004). For example, a rural immigrant unfamiliar with standardized tests may spend most of the time baffled by a professional asking him to fill in childlike bubbles to seemingly random questions, when all he wants is visitation with his child. It is almost inevitable that a person unaccustomed to standardized tests would be more anxious and confused in such circumstances, and that's before language is factored into the equation. Similarly, a person with a learning disability, or who had difficulty or minor trauma related to test taking as a child, may also respond to such standardized tests with more anxiety than those who feel comfortable or even confident with such test-taking situations.

Expectations of Interpersonal Interactions

Furthermore, persons from cultural backgrounds that value community and strong affective connection, such as women and Latino cultures (Cofresí & Gorman, 2004), may have difficulty interpreting the detached and impersonal interpersonal interactions that typify the proper administration of standardized tests. Counselors are then in a difficult situation trying to balance assessment protocols that call for detachment and objectivity while interacting in a culturally appropriate manner. As the daughter of southern European immigrants, I have always found myself anxious and uncomfortable in formalized assessment situations when the test administrators are "all business," refusing to smile or respond to a friendly hello. Even though I now know intellectually that their behavior is appropriate for the context, it is virtually impossible to "be myself" in response to a person who from my perspective seems to be responding in an exceptionally bizarre fashion. When you begin to imagine someone who is unaware of the reasons that a test administrator might be acting so oddly, it becomes clear that the test-taking situation can elicit highly atypical behavior, thus generating misleading results.

Language and Bilingualism

Counselors should make every effort to conduct assessments in the client's language of preference and greatest fluency. However, the issue of language is more complicated than one might initially expect. If the person being assessed is not fluent—both *linguistically* and *culturally*—in the language of the test, then the assessment process will have little meaning. Therefore, although it is tempting to give "bilingual" clients an assessment in English, it is only appropriate if the client is sufficiently fluent both in the language and cultural references. To further complicate matters, those who are bilingual and bicultural may express themselves differently in one language versus another (Cofresí & Gorman, 2004), and the language itself may bring out different aspects of self and correspond to different memories. For example, many people find that they are more emotional in their native language than in their second language. Alternatively, others report that the language itself brings out different elements of their personality, with Latin languages such as Spanish or Italian resulting in more emotional expression and a technical language like German or English conveying a more logical side of themselves.

When a standardized test is professionally translated into the client's language, counselors should be aware that some languages have such variability that they cannot be entirely confident that the assessment questions have been correctly understood. For example, both Spanish and Chinese are spoken by numerous subpopulations, each with unique idiomatic expressions and word use that vary by region, socioeconomic class, and political affiliations. In all fairness, the same problem can happen with subpopulation in a majority culture too. As a young girl growing up in Southern California, I was given an intelligence test that included a "what's wrong with this picture" question that had the shadow from a pile of snow going in the wrong direction. At that point in my life I had only seen cartoon renderings of snow, and I remember being confused at first with the drawing until I realized that this was supposed to be a picture of something *real*—not a cartoon—and thus the laws of physics should be applied. Had they used a palm tree, I would not have had to pause to translate the scene from a drawing to reality. To this day, when I see snow, I always check out the shadows to make sure they are going in the same direction. Thus, even within the same cultural group, test questions can be easily misunderstood.

Real-World Options for Standardized Evaluations of Progress

In an ideal world (or obsession-compulsive fantasy, depending on your perspective) advocated by academics, theoreticians, and researchers, counselors would measure client progress by having them complete a series of the *most* reliable and valid assessment instruments at regular intervals over the course of counseling. This is great in theory—that is, until you factor in the fact that reliability and validity generally are correlated with the *length* of the instrument (Lambert & Hawkins, 2004; Miller, Duncan, Brown, Sparks, & Claud, 2003). For those working in typical clinical settings—community agencies and private practices—the reality is that neither clients nor clinicians are enthusiastic about completing lengthy questionnaires, whether used for initial diagnosis (see tests described in Chapter 3) or client progress. Short and sweet is the reality with most clients and counselors. Thankfully, counselors have an increasing number of options that fit these requirements.

General Guidelines

- **First Session:** Because there is evidence that most change occurs early in counseling, the initial measures of symptoms and functioning should occur in the first session (Lambert & Hawkins, 2004).
- **Five Minutes or Less:** Lambert and Hawkins (2004) recommend instruments that take no longer than five minutes to complete.
- **Regular (Weekly/Monthly) Intervals:** Pre- and post-test measures often work for research studies, but defining "post" in real-world practice is much more difficult because clients may drop out rather than announce their intention to end treatment. Therefore, counselors should develop a regular interval for measuring client progress. Depending on the instrument and session setting, weekly, monthly, or quarterly may be appropriate.
- **Before the Session:** It does not take much time to learn that asking clients to complete a questionnaire *before* the session is generally much more successful than afterwards, when clients are often in a rush to leave. When used before, questionnaires are useful for developing an agenda for the session.

- **Framing the Measurement:** If the counselor conveys the message that the measurement is helpful in treatment, most clients will be willing to spend five minutes to improve their treatment outcomes. Lambert and Hawkins (2004) recommend using a metaphor such as a medical doctor getting blood pressure or "vital signs" at the beginning of each visit: this information helps the doctor or counselor to be more useful to the client.

Ultra-Brief Measures

Counselors have several options for measuring both client symptoms and general functioning with instruments that are *ultra-brief*, requiring as little as one minute to complete, or *brief* assessments, requiring less than ten minutes to complete.

Outcome Rating Scale (ORS)

Miller et al. (2003) developed the Outcome Rating Scale as an ultra-brief version of the Outcome Questionnaire (see below) in response to client and counselor complaints that even 45 questions were too many. It was designed by clinicians for clinicians and is the most clinician-friendly of the outcome measures. The ORS is composed of only four visual analog scales and takes less than a minute to complete, making it ideal for weekly use and highly economical: the ORS is free via the Internet, with photocopying the only remaining cost. The scale measures four areas of functioning:

- **Overall** (general sense of well-being)
- **Individually** (personal well-being)
- **Interpersonally** (family and close relationships)
- **Socially** (work, school, friendship)

Outcome Rating Scale (ORS)

Name ____________ Age (Yrs): _____
ID# ____________ Sex: M/F
Session# ____ Date: __________

Looking back over the last week, including today, help us understand how you have been feeling by rating how well you have been doing in the following areas of your life, where marks to the left represent low levels and marks to the right indicate high levels.

Individually:
(Personal well-being)

I----Examination Copy Only----I

Interpersonally:
(Family, close relationships)

I----Examination Copy Only----I

Socially:
(Work, School, Friendships)

I----Examination Copy Only----I

Overall:
(General sense of well-being)

I----Examination Copy Only----I

Institute for the Study of Therapeutic Change

www.talkingcure.com

Two versions for children are also available: the Child Outcome Rating Scale, which includes a similar scale to the adult version, and the Young Child Outcome Rating Scale, which uses happy, neutral, and unhappy faces to measure how the child is feeling (Duncan et al., 2003). Scoring is simple: A ruler is used to measure how far on the 10 cm scale the client scored, and cutoff scores are used to address potential problems.

The ORS has high internal consistency (.93), test-retest reliability (.84), and moderate concurrent validity with the OQ-45.2 (.59; Miller et al., 2003). Given its ultra-brief format, it is not as sensitive as other outcome measures, such as the OQ-45.2; nonetheless, it has been demonstrated to be sensitive enough to measure change in clinical settings, which is the primary aim of the everyday practitioner. The ORS's greatest strength is its feasibility for regular and consistent use in real-world practice settings (Miller, Duncan, & Hubble, 2004). When counselors were trained in using either the ORS or OQ-45.2 for outcome measures, 86% of counselors were still using the ORS after one year, compared to only 25% of counselors who were using the 45-item OQ-45.2 (Miller et al., 2003), a dramatic difference.

Session Rating Scale (SRS)

Also developed by Duncan et al. (2003), the Session Rating Scale, Version 3 (SRS V3.0) is typically used with the ORS. Whereas the ORS is given at the *beginning* of the session, the SRS is used at the *end* of the session to measure counseling alliance, and it was consistently found to be one of the best predictors of positive outcome (Orlinsky, Rønnestad, & Willutzki, 2004). Specifically, *client* ratings of alliance rather than counselor ratings of alliance are the better predictor of outcome (Bachelor & Horvath, 1999). In a study conducted by Whipple et al. (2003), counselors who had access to both alliance and outcome information were twice as likely to achieve clinically significant change.

Session Rating Scale (SRS V.3.0)

Name ______________ Age (Yrs):______
ID#______________ Sex: M/F
Session#_____ Date: ______________

Please rate today's session by placing a hash mark on the line nearest to the description that best fits your experience.

Relationship:

I did not feel heard, understood, and respected	I----Examination Copy Only----I	I felt heard, understood, and respected

Goals and Topics:

We did *not* work on or talk about what I wanted to work on and talk about	I----Examination Copy Only----I	We worked on and talked about what I wanted to work on and talk about

Approach or Method:

The therapist's approach is not a good fit for me.	I----Examination Copy Only----I	The therapist's approach is a good fit for me.

Overall:

There was something missing in the session today	I----Examination Copy Only----I	Overall, today's session was right for me

Institute for the Study of Therapeutic Change

www.talkingcure.com

Like the ORS, the SRS consists of only four analog scales:

- **Relationship:** Does the client feel heard, understood, and respected?
- **Goals/Topics:** Does the client feel that the session focused on what he/she wanted to work on?
- **Approach/Method:** Was the counselor's approach a good fit?
- **Overall:** Was the session helpful ("right") for the client?

Similar to the ORS, two versions for children are also available: the Child Session Rating Scale (CSRS), which includes a similar scale to the adult version, and the Young Child Session Rating Scale (YCSRS), which uses happy, neutral, and unhappy faces to measure how the child is feeling (Duncan et al., 2003). Scoring is simple: A ruler is used to measure how far on the 10 cm scale the client scored, and cutoff scores are used to address potential problems. Research has identified a very high cutoff score for this instrument, meaning that when clients start indicating there are minor problems with alliance, counselors need to swiftly address these issues to ensure a positive outcome. This scale can be particularly helpful for newer counselors wanting to ensure a strong alliance.

The SRS has good internal consistency (.88) with a test-retest reliability of .64, which is comparable to other alliance measures (Duncan et al., 2003). The concurrent validity of the measure, when compared to a similar measure, is .48, providing evidence that a similar construct is being measured. Similar to the ORS, the greatest strength of the SRS is its feasibility and user-friendliness, with the SRS being used by 96% of clinicians introduced to it, compared to only 29% of clinicians using the 12-item Working Alliance Inventory.

Brief Measures

Brief measures refer to assessment instruments that require less than ten minutes to complete. Two of the more common ones are the Outcome Questionnaire (OQ) and the Symptom Checklist (SCL).

Outcome Questionnaire (OQ-45.2)

The Outcome Questionnaire (OQ-45) was designed to measure outcome in clinical settings (Lambert et al., 1996). The questionnaire has a total of 45 items, takes less than five minutes to complete, and includes three subscales:

- Symptom Distress (clinical, mental health symptoms)
- Interpersonal Relationships
- Social Role Performance

There is also a youth version, the Youth Outcome Questionnaire (YOQ), which can be completed by parents, and a Youth Outcome Questionnaire Self Report (YOQ-SR) for youth from 12 to 18. Briefer, single-scale (only a global score), 30-item versions are available for the OQ and YOQ, and a 10-item version is also available for the OQ. These measures are affordable and easy to administer, score, and interpret, with the briefer versions more practical for frequent measurement.

The OQ-45.2 has good test-retest reliability (.66–.86) and internal consistency (.7–.9; Lambert & Hawkins, 2003). Its minor weakness is that the subscales are highly correlated with one another, meaning that they may not be measuring unique constructs. Most of the research on the validity and reliability has been conducted on the *summary* score, and clinicians are encouraged to use this as the primary measure of progress (Lambert & Hawkins, 2004).

Sample Questions from the Outcome Questionnaire

	Never	Rarely	Sometimes	Frequently	Always Almost
1. I get along well with others	❑	❑	❑	❑	❑
2. I tire quickly	❑	❑	❑	❑	❑
3. I feel no interest in things	❑	❑	❑	❑	❑
4. I feel stressed at work/school	❑	❑	❑	❑	❑
5. I blame myself for things	❑	❑	❑	❑	❑
6. I feel irritated	❑	❑	❑	❑	❑
18. I feel lonely	❑	❑	❑	❑	❑
19. I have frequent arguments	❑	❑	❑	❑	❑
20. I feel loved and wanted	❑	❑	❑	❑	❑
21. I enjoy my spare time	❑	❑	❑	❑	❑
22. I have difficulty concentrating	❑	❑	❑	❑	❑
23. I feel hopeless about the future	❑	❑	❑	❑	❑
24. I like myself	❑	❑	❑	❑	❑

Developed by Michael J. Lambert, Ph.D. and Gary M. Burlingame, Ph.D. For more information contact: OQ Measures LLC. © Copyright, 2005. Printed with permission.

Symptom Checklist (SCL-90-R) and Brief Symptom Inventory (BSI)

The Symptom Checklist is a 90-item test that assesses for mental health symptoms and their intensity (mild, moderate, severe). It is designed for individuals 13 and older and requires 12–15 minutes to complete. The Brief Symptom Inventory (BSI) is based on the SCL but is, as the name indicates, briefer. The BSI has 53 items, is designed for individuals 13 and older, and takes 8–10 minutes to complete. Both measures have nine symptom subscales and three global indices:

Subscales:

- Somatization
- Obsessive-Compulsive
- Interpersonal Sensitivity
- Depression
- Anxiety
- Hostility
- Phobic Anxiety
- Paranoid Ideation
- Psychoticism

Global Indices:

- Global Severity Index: overall psychological distress
- Positive Symptom Distress Index (PSDI): Intensity of symptoms
- Positive Symptom Total (PST): Number of self-reported symptoms

Ultra-brief six- and ten-item versions that correlate to the overall distress scores have also been developed (Rosen et al., 2000), a more feasible option for everyday practice. The SLQ-90-R has good test-retest validity, ranging from .63 to .86 for online versions and .68 to .84 for pen-and-paper versions (Derogatis & Fitzpatrick, 2004; Vallejo, Jordán, Díaz, Comeche, & Ortega, 2007). The internal consistency coefficients are also good, ranging from .70 to .90.

Behavior and Symptom Identification Scales (BASIS)

Available as a 24- or 32-item pen-and-paper measure of client outcome, the Behavior and Symptom Identification Scales (BASIS-24 and BASIS-32) ask clients to rate from 0 to 4 their level of difficulty in various areas of functioning, including work, relationships, mood, and such. Requiring computer scoring, the more comprehensive BASIS-24 provides counselors with scores in each of the following areas:

- Overall Score: General Measure of Functioning
- Depression and Functioning
- Relationships
- Self-Harm
- Emotional Lability
- Psychosis
- Substance Abuse

The BASIS-32, which can be scored by hand, includes the following scores:

- Overall Functioning
- Relation to Self and Others
- Depression and Anxiety
- Daily Living and Role Functioning
- Impulsive and Addictive Behavior
- Psychosis

Normed in Britain, the BASIS-24 demonstrates good reliability (coefficient α values for combined clinical sample across subscales ranging from .75 to .91) and good validity (effect size for change of the BASIS-24 was 0.56; Cameron et al., 2007), and it is considered an effective measure of client progress.

Specific Measures of Progress

The above measures are some of the more common measures of client progress and outcome. In some cases, more specific measures can be used, such as the Beck Depression Inventory or the Beck Anxiety Inventory, which could be used with clients diagnosed with depression or anxiety, respectively. Such measures are good options when these, often less expensive measures, are already used as part of the initial assessment.

Final Thoughts on Assessing Client Progress

Increasingly, counselors are assessing client progress more closely and precisely than before. Although assessment involves additional paperwork and time, numerous quick and effective options are available that integrate easily in today's practice environment. Counselor attitude is critical to the success and usefulness of an assessment system: if counselors believe in it, they communicate this to clients, and the assessments become a helpful resource for helping clients achieve their goals. When counselors see assessment as a burden or unnecessary, it becomes a lifeless bureaucratic task of little use to anyone.

Questions for Personal Reflection and Class Discussion

1. Overall, do you think formal evaluation is more helpful or problematic? When do the benefits outweigh possible limitations?
2. What benefits or risks do you see in using formal evaluation with diverse clients? How might you address any concerns?
3. When you fill out evaluation forms at a doctor's office, how accurate do you think you are in remembering and/or truthfully reporting symptoms? When, or about what, are you least likely to be accurate?

4. Which of these assessments do you see as most promising or useful? Which are you most skeptical about using?
5. In which contexts or with what type of client do you think you are most likely to use formal evaluation? Which ones least likely?

Online Resources

American Psychological Association Assessment Resources
www.apa.org/science/programs/testing/find-tests.aspx

Behavior and Symptom Identification Scale (BASIS)
www.basissurvey.org/

Outcome Rating Scale (ORS) and Session Rating Scale (SRS)
Free download at http://heartandsoulofchange.com/measures/

Outcome Questionnaire 45 (OQ-45):
For purchase at www.oqmeasures.com

Symptom Checklist 90 (SC-90)
Purchase from www.pearsonassessments.com/tests/scl90r.htm

Other Resources

Health and Psychosocial Instruments (HaPI) Database

www.ovid.com/site/catalog/DataBase/866.jsp

Your university may subscribe to the HaPI database that references over 15,000 psychological assessment instruments. The database does not provide full-text versions of the instruments, but instead provides a comprehensive list of what exists, including questionnaires, interview schedules, coding schemes, and the like.

References

Bachelor, A., & Horvath, A. (1999). The therapeutic relationship. In M. A. Hubble, B. L. Duncan, & S. D. Miller (Eds.), *The heart and soul of change* (pp. 133–178). Washington, DC: APA Press.

Berg, I., & de Shazer, S. (1993). Making numbers talk: Language in therapy. In S. Friedman (Ed.), *The new language of change: Constructive collaboration in psychotherapy.* New York: Guilford.

Brems, C. (1998). Cultural issues in psychological assessment: Problems and possible solutions. *Journal of Psychological Practice, 4*, 88–117.

Cameron, I. M., Cunningham, L., Crawford, J. R., Eagles, J. M., Eisen, S. V., Lawton, K., Naji, S. A., & Hamilton, R. J. (2007). Psychometric properties of the BASIS-24© (Behaviour and Symptom Identification Scale–Revised). *Mental Health Outcome Measure. International Journal of Psychiatry in Clinical Practice, 11*, 36–43.

Cofresí, N., & Gorman, A. A. (2004). Testing and assessment issues with Spanish-English bilingual Latinos. *Journal of Counseling & Development, 82*, 99–106.

Derogatis, L. R., & Fitzpatrick, M. (2004). The SCL-90-R, the Brief Symptom Inventory, and the BSI-81. In M. E. Murish (Ed.), *The use of psychological testing for treatment planning and outcome.* New York: Routledge.

Duncan, B. L., Miller, S. D., Sparks, J. A., Claud, D. A., Reynolds, L. R., Brown, J., & Johnson, L. D. (2003). The Session Rating Scale: Preliminary psychometric properties of a "working" alliance measure. *Journal of Brief Therapy, 3*, 3–12.

Hui, C. H., & Triandis, H. C. (1985). Measurement in cross-cultural psychology: A review and comparison of strategies. *Journal of Cross-Cultural Psychology, 16*, 131–152.

Lambert, M. J., Hansen, N. B., Umphress, V. J., Lunnen, K., Okiishi, J., Burlingame, G. M., Huefner, J. C., & Reisinger, C. W. (1996). *Administration and scoring manual for the Outcome Questionnaire (OQ-45.2).* Wilmington, DE: American Professional Credentialing Services.

Lambert, M. J., & Hawkins, E. J. (2004). Measuring outcome in professional practice: Considerations in selecting and using brief outcome instruments. *Professional Psychology: Research and Practice, 35*, 492–499.

Miller, S. D., Duncan, B. L., & Hubble, M. A. (2004). Beyond integration: The triumph of outcome over process in clinical practice. *Psychotherapy in Australia, 10*(2), 2–19.

Miller, S. D., Duncan, B. L., Brown, J., Sparks, J. A., & Claud, D. A. (2003). The Outcome Rating Scale: A preliminary study of the reliability, validity, and feasibility of a brief visual analog measure. *Journal of Brief Therapy*, 2, 91–100.

Orlinsky, D. E., Rønnestad, M. H., & Willutzki, U. (2003). Fifty years of process-outcome research: Continuity and change. In M. J. Lambert (Ed.), *Bergin and Garfield's handbook of psychotherapy and behavior change* (5th ed., 307–390). New York: Wiley.

Rosen, C. S., Drescher, K. D., Moos, R. H., Finney, J. W. Murphy, R. T., & Gusman, F. (2000). Six- and Ten-Item Indexes of Psychological Distress Based on the Symptom Checklist-90. *Assessment*, 7, 103–111.

Vallejo, M. A., Jordán, C. M., Díaz, M. I., Comeche, M. I., & Ortega, J. (2007). Psychological assessment via the internet: A reliability and validity study of online (vs Paper-and-Pencil) versions of the General Health Questionnaire-28 (GHQ-28) and the Symptoms Check-List-90-Revised (SCL-90-R). *Journal of Medical Internet Research*, 10.

Whipple, J. L., Lambert, M. J., Vermeersch, D. A., Smart, D. W., Nielsen, S. L., & Hawkins, E. J. (2003). Improving the effects of psychotherapy: The use of early identification of treatment and problem strategies in routine practice. *Journal of Counseling Psychology*, *50*(1), 59–68.

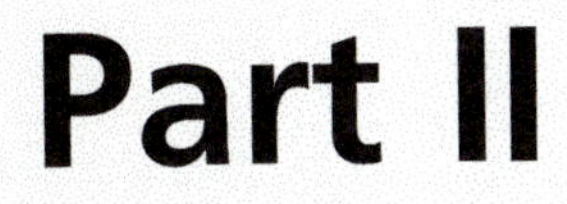

Part II

Theory-Informed Case Documentation

CHAPTER

8

Psychodynamic Counseling and Psychotherapy

Lay of the Land

Over a century in development, psychoanalytic and psychodynamic theories include a wide range of practices, including "blank slate" analysts whose clients free-associate on a couch; empathically engaged counselors who address early childhood relationships; relationally oriented therapists who co-construct interpretations with clients; and brief psychodynamic practitioners who use manualized treatment with substance abuse. These—along with Adler's Individual Psychology (Chapter 9)—are all considered *depth psychologies,* because they explore the *unconscious* mind.

The original psychotherapy, Freudian psycho*analysis*, is the root of all psychodynamic approaches, with ego psychology, object relations, self psychology, relational, and intersubjectivity theories being the most direct descendants. Although there is some debate over the terms, everyone agrees *psychoanalysis* always refers to Freud's original approach, and most agree that it describes long-term counseling with multiple weekly sessions in which an analyst analyzes a person's personality using ego psychology, object relations, self psychology, or a relational approach. In psychoanalysis, the analyst is more likely to use more of a "blank slate" approach, often uses a couch, and typically does not engage clients with warmth—an oft-mocked approach in Woody Allen movies and other Hollywood films. For better or worse, this form of treatment in contemporary contexts is increasingly rare.

In contrast, psycho*dynamic* therapy refers to a more standard, shorter-term (but typically still long), one-session-per-week outpatient counseling approach that addresses a specific presenting problem, such as depression or anxiety, rather than the general project of personality analysis. To keep you thoroughly confused, ego psychology, object relationship, self psychology, and relational psychoanalysis can be used for either psychoanalytic or psychodynamic approaches. And if that wasn't complex enough, "analytic" and "psychodynamic" are sometimes also used to refer to the work of Carl Jung, who split from Freud to develop his own theory early in their careers.

Although there are many ways to categorize the various threads of psychodynamic approaches, the most highly recognized threads include:

- *Psychoanalysis or Drive Theory:* Based on Freud's original theories, classic psychoanalysis is a relatively rare but still practiced approach that focuses on analysis of innate drives and transference issues.

- *Ego Psychology:* Similar to Freudian theory in terms of the working relationship, ego psychology focuses on analysis of how the ego uses defense mechanisms to manage innate drives.
- *Object Relations Theories:* Using a more empathic and warmer counseling relationship, object relations theorists focus on repairing the client's early "object" and relational patterns, often through corrective experiences during the counseling relationship. There are several schools of object relations theory, each using a unique system of analysis; however, they can generally be divided into schools that (a) integrate drive theory or (b) are purely relational.
- *Interpersonal Analysis:* Related to object relations, Sullivan's (1953, 1954) interpersonal analysis is unique in that the analysis process relies heavily on observable data and focuses almost exclusively on interpersonal interactions rather than unconscious processes.
- *Self Psychology:* Based on the work of Kohut, self psychology involves empathic immersion in the client's inner world, analysis of selfobjects, and a focus on building self-esteem.
- *Relational and Intersubjectivity Theories:* Recent approaches that emphasize the intersubjective nature of reality and employ a more collaborative counseling relationship, including the co-construction of interpretations with clients.
- *Brief Psychodynamic Theories:* Time-limited, evidence-based approaches that have been demonstrated effective with depression and substance abuse.

Basic Psychodynamic Assumptions

The vast majority of psychodynamic theorists share the following basic assumptions (Greenberg & Mitchell, 1983; Mitchell & Black, 1995; St. Clair, 2000):

- A person's history affects present behaviors and relationships.
- There is an unconscious mind that exerts significant influence over present behavior.
- The personality is structured into various substructures, such as ego, id, and superego.
- A person's personality is significantly impacted by early relationships in life, especially with one's mother.
- Insight into one's personality and internal dynamics can help resolve various psychopathologies.
- Clients *project* onto the counselor interrelational patterns from earlier unresolved issues, most often with the clients' parents; the *transference* of these patterns can be analyzed and used to promote change in the counseling relationship.

Psychodynamic Theory

In a Nutshell: The Least You Need to Know

At its most basic level, psychodynamic theory is about analyzing an individual's personality—characteristic habits of mind—to better understand how these dynamics affect the presenting problem and general quality of life. Psychoanalytic and psychodynamic approaches share the basic practice of:

a) analyzing or conceptualizing personality structures and functioning,
b) fostering client insight into their personality dynamics, and then
c) working through these insights toward action. The different schools vary in the quality of the counseling relationship (e.g., neutral versus empathic) and the preferred concepts for case conceptualization (e.g., defense mechanisms, ego/id/superego, universal unconscious, etc.).

For example, Freudian drive theorists and ego psychologists use a more dispassionate counseling relationship to encourage and use projection to promote change, whereas object relations, self psychologists, and intersubjectivity theorists use more empathy and warmth to create a relationship that can foster corrective experiences. The broad (oversimplified but useful for those new to these approaches) differences between major schools are summarized below.

	Schools					
	Drive Theory	Ego Psychology	Object Relations	Self Psychology	Interpersonal	Relational/ Intersubjectivity
Theorist	S. Freud	A. Freud Erickson Horney	Kernberg Klein Fairbairn Mahler Winnicott	Kohut	Sullivan	Mitchell Greenberg Stolorow
Focus of analysis	Drive theory; id; instincts	Ego; defense mechanisms	Intrapsychic representations of caregivers	Relationship with self and selfobjects	Observable interactions; self system	Interpersonal world; relational matrix
Root cause of problems	Conflicts between id and superego	Defense mechanisms used to manage infantile drives	Pathological internal object relations	Distorted images of self	Keeping elements of interpersonal interactions out of awareness	Distorted expectations of interpersonal world
Mechanism of change	Making unconscious conscious	Developing more mature defense mechanisms; increasing ego strength	Integration of good and bad in objects; release bad objects from subconscious; realistic view of others	Developing a more realistic self-image and sense of self-worth	Developing the ability to maintain health interpersonal relations	Developing more realistic expectations and interpretations of relationships
Client–counselor relationship	Detached expert; blank slate for client	Detached expert; blank slate for client	Empathic; uses relationship to reflect on object relation patterns	Empathic; uses mirroring to help restore self-image	Uses relationship to explore interpersonal dynamics	Uses relationship to explore interpersonal relationship patterns
Commonly used techniques	Free association; dream analysis	Analysis of defense; free association; dream analysis	Analysis of early relationships, present relationship with counselor and others	Analysis of self-object relations; mirroring; empathy	Analysis of behaviors in interpersonal relationships	Exploring client's experience of the relationship with counselor

The Juice: Significant Contributions to the Field

If you remember one thing from this chapter, it should be …

Transference and Countertransference

Transference A classic psychoanalytic concept that has remained central to virtually all schools, *transference* refers to when a client projects onto the counselor attributes that stem from unresolved issues with primary caregivers; counselors use the immediacy of these interactions to promote client insight and work through these conflicts (Kernberg, 1997; Luborsky, O'Reilly-Landry, & Arlow, 2008). The process of transference reveals unconscious templates that clients bring to relationships over and over again. For example, if a client had a critical parent, the client is likely to interpret silence, neutrality, and vague comments as critical. In extreme cases, without repeated, enthusiastic, over-the-top expressions of verbal confirmation (i.e., "you're amazing, fantastic—the *best* client I *ever* had"—and, no, such statements are not appropriate in counseling), these clients will always feel criticized and/or looked down upon and will often desperately seek approval from the analyst.

Drive theorists and ego psychologists encourage transference by maintaining a strict neutral stance that encourages clients to project unresolved issues onto the counselor; the analyst can then interpret these for the client. For example, the analyst may analyze transference by stating, "When I sit here quietly listening, you seem to think that I am judging you to be inadequate, much the same way your father used to do when you were little." In object relations, self psychology, and relational approaches, counselors use transference slightly differently because they use a more empathic relationship rather than neutrality to build their relationships with clients. When transference happens in these relationships, the counselor discusses the transference patterns with the client and explains how it emerged in the current relationship: "You seem to think that my quietly listening implies that I am somehow judging you. Would it surprise you to know that I am not? I am simply listening intently." Psychoanalysts also vary on their opinion about whether a "real" nontransference relationship is possible in treatment or whether all interactions are inherently a form of transference, with some arguing that even a positive therapeutic alliance "reflect(s) transference dispositions stemming from a normally achieved trusting relationship between the infant and the mother" (Kernberg, 1997, p. 10).

Recent scholars have added an important caveat to analyzing transference: the client might just be right! In most cases, there is usually a grain of truth in any perception (Gill, 1982). Thus, analysts should not consider all client perceptions and reactions as simply transference; in most cases, the client's perspective has a trace to significant amounts of truth. In addition, relational theorists maintain that the analyst's personality unavoidably influences the client's transference: the analyst *cannot not* affect how the client behaves (Greenberg & Mitchell, 1983). Furthermore, analysts recognize "the concept of 'resistance' as potentially fostering an adversarial relation between patient and analyst, and imposing the analyst's views on the patient" (Kernberg, 1997, p. 9). The process of sorting transference out from accurate description becomes particularly confusing when gender, age, culture, economic, educational, and other diversity issues are taken into consideration. What is accurately perceived as respectful in one culture (e.g., looking someone in the eye when you speak) is considered exceptionally rude in another; such minor differences quickly cascade into a series of misinterpretations on the part of both parties. Thus, it is imperative that counselors be cautious when examining transference, considering the contrasting of their gender, sexual orientation, culture, economic status, education level, and that of the client's.

Countertransference As if matters were not complex enough, counselors also need to consider the issue of *countertransference*. Countertransference refers to when counselors project back onto clients, losing their therapeutic neutrality and having strong emotional reactions to the client. The understanding of countertransference has broadened over the years to include not only the analyst's problematic unconscious projections but also the total emotional reaction (Kernberg, 1997). Thus, countertransference can be used in two basic ways, with different schools of psychoanalysis emphasizing one over the other.

- *Countertransference as Unconscious Projection:* Especially early in training or around a personal issue for the counselor, the countertransference reaction represents an unconscious projection on the part of the analyst that needs to be explored in supervision, and it is often inappropriate to discuss with clients.
- *Countertransference as Conscious Experiencing of the Other:* If the counselor has self-awareness and can accurately sort out the sources of countertransference, it can be used to help the counselor and client better understand how others experience the client and the reactions the client may trigger in others (Luborsky et al., 2008). In this case, countertransference is used with the client to promote insight.

More traditional approaches, such as ego psychology and drive-theory–based object relations, focus primarily on the client's transference, with less focused attention on the analyst's countertransference. In marked contrast, "interpersonal psychoanalysis gives almost symmetrical [equal] attention to transference and countertransference," giving it a more central role in the process of assessment and treatment (Kernberg, 1997, p. 7).

Corrective Emotional Experience Once transference and countertransference patterns have been carefully considered and assessed, relationally focused analysts use this information to provide clients with a *corrective emotional experience*, in which the analyst responds differently than what the client experienced in childhood to facilitate resolution of an inner conflict. For example, if a client interprets the analyst's refusal to vociferously agree as an aggressive stance, the analyst can use the opportunity to help the client understand that her neutral stance is not an attack, but simply another means of showing support and interest.

Self-Assessment Questions to Manage Transference and Countertransference

- What does the client perceive in me *specifically*: an attitude, emotion, behavior, thought?
- What behaviors, comments, and nonverbals is the client responding to?
- Which elements of the client's experience are accurate descriptions of what is happening?
- Which elements of the client's experience seem to be related to one of their prior relationships or relationship with a caregiver?
- Are there differences between us that might explain the client's perception of me, such as age, gender, culture, sexual orientation, education, and so on?
- Did I have any inner emotional reaction to the client's transference? Do I feel angry, insulted, self-righteous? Or am I able to maintain a calm, nonreactive empathy?
- Do I have any countertransference issues that I am aware of? May there be some that I am not aware of?
- Who does this client remind me of most? How do I react to that person? Is that repeating here?
- Is there anyone in the client's life who might also have the similar response I am having? How does that person respond to the client? How can I use my response to provide a more effective response?

Try It Yourself

Answer these questions based on a session with a client or a role-play you have done.

Big Picture: Overview of Counseling Process

Listening, Interpretation, and Working Through

In general, current psychodynamic counseling involves three generic phases:

1. Listening with empathy to reduce defensiveness and increase willingness to hear interpretations
2. Interpretation to promote insight
3. Working through insight to promote new action

- *Listening and Empathy:* The primary tool of psychoanalytic counselors is listening objectively to the client's story without offering advice, reassurance, validation, or confrontation. Empathy may be used to help the client open to nondefensively hearing the counselor's interpretation of unconscious dynamics.
- *Interpretation and Promoting Insight:* In the next phase, the focus is to encourage insights into personal and interpersonal dynamics, which the counselor promotes by offering interpretations to the client using various case conceptualization approaches; the form of case conceptualization is the most distinguishing feature between the various schools.
- *Working Through:* Finally, *working through* refers to the process of repeatedly getting in touch with repressed strivings and defense responses, so that the unconscious can be made conscious (St. Clair, 2000). The counselor facilitates this process by providing a realistic ego to help the client tolerate delay and anxiety as the client revisits, explores, and struggles to accept and understand drives, urges, and patterns that have been unrecognized. However, this is just the first step of the working through process. Working through ultimately involves translating these insights into action. Insight into your tendency to project childhood patterns onto your partner is relatively easy; changing how you respond to your partner on a daily basis is more challenging.

Basic Psychodynamic Process

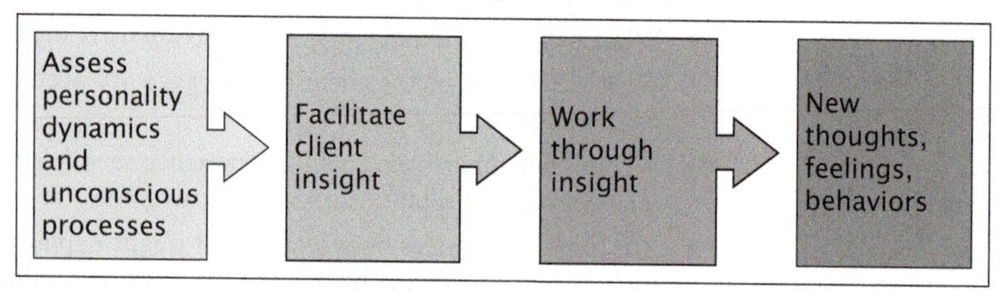

Psychoanalysis

Psychoanalysis refers to an intensive approach designed to create significant and sustainable *personality change* (Abend, 2001; St. Clair, 2000). Analysts typically meet with patients (preferred term) 3–5 days per week for several years. Thus, a person doesn't casually stumble into analysis, nor should an analyst slyly lure someone into long-term analysis. It should be a process that is entered upon with full knowledge and consent (McWilliams, 1999). The counseling process in psychoanalysis follows the above process, with the basic process of analysis–insight–working through–action process frequently repeating at deeper and more profound levels. As analysis progresses, the process should—if all is going well—accelerate, with the client relying less and less on the analyst for insight and becoming more adept at working through new insights and translating them to real-world change. Psychoanalysis is typically an expensive endeavor for patients, and therefore it tends to attract wealthier and psychologically minded people who highly value insight.

Psychodynamic Counseling and Psychotherapy

In contrast to analysis, psychodynamic counseling and psychotherapy target specific symptoms or problems, such as depression or recovering from a divorce, with sessions typically occurring once per week and lasting several months to a couple of years depending on client needs (Altman, 2008). More recently, brief forms of psychodynamic counseling have been developed to last 12–16 sessions. Again, the same basic process is employed but the goals are narrower, creating clearer criteria for termination (i.e., when the client is able to maintain prior level of work and social activity, then counseling is done). As you can imagine, psychodynamic counseling is more common than psychoanalysis. Any of the schools in this chapter—drive theory, ego psychology, object relations, self psychology, and relational approaches—can be used in either psychoanalysis or psychodynamic counseling.

Making Connection: Counseling Relationship

Introduction to Psychoanalytic Relationships: One- and Two-Person Relationships

Each school of psychodynamic counseling has a different approach to relationships, ranging from a highly distant "blank-slate" role of the drive theory analyst to a highly engaged, deeply human intersubjective approach. Mitchell (1988) differentiates these into two general types: *one-person* versus *two-person* psychology. In approaches that emphasize *one-person psychology*, the entire focus and process of analysis is on—you guessed it—one person, the client. Although historically the primary form of relationship in psychodynamic approaches, the one-person psychology relationship is increasingly rare and is typically only used in formal analysis that emphasizes drive theory and ego psychology (Marmor, 1995).

In *two-person psychology*, analysis includes—bet you can guess this—two people: counselor and client. In these approaches, counselors are keenly aware of their impact on clients. First articulated by object relations and self psychology practitioners and developed most fully by relationally oriented practitioners, two-person psychology is increasingly used by the majority of psychodynamic practitioners. That said, it is perhaps best to think of these existing on a continuum with newer forms of psychodynamic practice emphasizing the more relational two-person psychology and more traditionally oriented and analytically focused counselors emphasizing one-person psychology.

Transference and Countertransference (See "The Juice" above) Neutrality and the Blank Slate (Drive Theory and Ego Psychology)

Freudian and ego psychology analysis typically maintains *neutrality* in relation to clients to provide a "blank slate" upon which clients can project unconscious material that the analyst can then use to promote insight. This stance, sometimes referred to as the *rule of abstinence*, requires that the analyst not gratify the client's instinctual demands, such as wanting more connection with the counselor or for the counselor to agree with the client on various topics. Kernberg explains, "The psychoanalyst, I believe, should behave as naturally as possible, without any self-revelation and without gratifying the patient's curiosity and transference demands, and acting, outside his specific technical function, within ordinary norms of social interaction" (1997, p. 12).

This neutral stance is *not* used simply to frustrate clients but is considered essential to better helping them. Especially in formal analysis, the analyst keeps responses short, offers little new information to the conversation, is slow to reveal personal information or opinions (either verbally or nonverbally), and avoids discussing topics unrelated to the process at hand. By being more of a recipient, the analyst can carefully observe clients to study their internal and unconscious processes, and, most importantly, *allow for transference*. For example, if a client harbors fears of not being smart enough, the client is likely to project these fears onto the analyst's cool interactions and assume that the analyst thinks she is dumb or her fears silly. The less-than-chatty approach is, when done well, done from a place of empathy (albeit unexpressed) and desire to help clients more quickly gain insight into relational patterns and use these insights to make meaningful life change.

Holding Environment (Object Relations)

Winnicott (1965) originally discussed *holding environment* as it relates to good enough mothering (see below) and refers to the nurturing environment provided by the mother that enables the child to move from an unintegrated state to having a structured, integrated self. A successful holding environment reduces overwhelming stimuli that the child cannot yet manage—thus requiring skillful empathy on the part of the mother/caregiver. By protecting the child against overwhelming events, the child avoids ego fragmentation and develops positive feelings about the self and sense of being real.

The concept of a holding environment is also used to refer to the counselor-client relationship in which the counselor provides a supportive, nurturing environment that enables the client to develop a structured, integrated self and a positive sense of self, which in the case of many clients does not happen as successfully as it could have (Brown, 1981). When applied to the counseling process, holding environment refers to providing structure, consistency, and routine to filter out overwhelming stimuli and enable the client to develop the ego strength to do the work of psychoanalysis. In this process, the structure of the counseling process takes care of ego maintenance functions so that the client has freed energy to work through and resolve conflicts and developmental crises.

Empathy (Object Relations, Self Psychology, Relational Theory)

Empathy—the ability to grasp another's internal reality—is required of all good counselors. However, the counselor's use and demonstration of empathy vary dramatically based on the counselor's theory. For example, traditional Freudian analysis relies heavily on empathy, but empathy is not expressed as a warm, "I-feel-your-pain" manner but rather through highly logical interpretive insight that requires empathy to ascertain. Within the psychodynamic circles, Kohut was the first strong advocate for supportive expressions of empathy in psychoanalysis and used it primarily when there was tension between the client and analyst to allow for corrective emotional experiences (Kohut, 1984). However, he was not the first to use it: "Although self psychology must not claim that it has provided psychoanalysis with a new kind of empathy, it can claim that I have supplied analysis with new theories which broaden and deepen the field of empathic perception" (p. 175). Kohut described the practice of empathy as the analyst verbalizing to the client that he grasped what the client is feeling, demonstrating that the client has been understood. Thus, empathic expression involves first grasping and then sharing aloud this understanding. The concept of empathy has been broadened to include empathizing with that which the client cannot tolerate in himself, projections, and other forms of dissociations from self (Kernberg, 1997).

Mirroring (Self Psychology)

A term from self psychology, *mirroring* refers to the counselor confirming the client's sense of self. Kohut believed that healthy adults "continue to need the mirroring of the self by selfobjects [persons experienced as part of self functioning and identity] throughout life" (St. Clair, 2000, p. 146). When met with indifference by someone with whom one is trying to connect, a person is left feeling helpless and empty and with a lowered sense of self-esteem. Thus, counselors provide mirroring for clients by confirming their worth, both verbally and nonverbally. This differs from empathy, which involves identifying and reflecting back the client's subjective reality, particularly an emotional state. In the case study at the end of this chapter, the counselor uses mirroring with Ken, who is struggling with suicidal thoughts and basing his self-worth on his professional achievements.

Relational Psychoanalysis and Intersubjectivity

Based on social constructionist theory (see Chapter 14), relational and intersubjective psychoanalysis approaches maintain that the analyst cannot be neutral but is an active agent in the dynamic interactions that occur in session. Greenberg (2001) identifies four assumptions that relational psychoanalysts use in understanding the counseling relationship; these are views that are not shared with any other psychodynamic school:

1. The analyst has a deep, personal influence on the client and has more influence than is typically acknowledged.
2. The impact of the analyst's behavior can never be understood while it is happening, if ever.
3. The analyst cannot adopt any posture, including neutrality or empathy, that guarantees a predictable atmosphere and relationship; instead, each relationship must be uniquely negotiated to suit both client and counselor.
4. The analyst is a subjective participant in the analysis process; objective neutrality is impossible.

In the relational psychoanalysis, the analyst's role is to provide useful ideas and explore their relational interactions to help clients reach their goals. Unlike other schools of psychoanalysis, they do not presume that they have a more accurate truth, understanding, or interpretation of the client's life than the client does. Relational psychoanalysts strive to create an intersubjective relationship with clients in which both the analyst and client mutually influence each other, co-creating interpretations and better understandings of self and other.

Personal Analysis

From its inception and perhaps more than any other approach, psychoanalysis has required that analysts go through analysis themselves in order to be helpful to clients. In fact, a person's credibility as an analyst is often established by whom one sought for analysis. If a counselor has not deeply explored unconscious patterns, they will inevitably project these onto clients, act out based on these unconscious patterns, and/or misinterpret elements from clients' lives. Thus, in order to "train" to be a psychodynamic counselor, one must first go through what is typically several years of analysis oneself. In fact, many would consider it *unethical* to practice analysis and psychodynamic counseling without experiencing the process oneself.

The Viewing: Case Conceptualization

Introduction to Psychodynamic Case Conceptualization

You will quickly note that "The Viewing" section is far, far longer and more complex than "The Doing" section in this chapter. Should you want to curse me halfway through, just remember that would be a form of "projection" (see Defenses below): I am just the messenger here. What is important to note is that most of the work for the clinician in psychodynamic counseling is in the *viewing*, the case conceptualization—not flashy interventions. Admittedly, case conceptualization doesn't get more intricate than this; the upside is that it is one of the most comprehensive approaches available. Increasingly, when conceptualizing, psychodynamic practitioners borrow freely from one school or another—drive theory, ego psychology, object relations, self psychology, relational theory, and even brief approaches, rather than stay rigidly wedded to one theory or another (McWilliams, 1999). This enables counselors to custom-tailor case conceptualizations for a single client. Psychodynamic case conceptualization may include an assessment of numerous areas of personality functioning and related dynamics, including:

- Levels of consciousness
- Structures of the self
- Drive theory
- Psychosexual stages
- Defense mechanisms
- Psychosocial stages of development
- Object relations patterns
- Good enough mothering
- Stages of separation
- Selfobjects
- Relational matrix
- Unconscious organizing principles related to culture

Levels of Consciousness: Conscious, Preconscious, and Unconscious (Drive Theory)

One of his earliest and most enduring contributions, Freud described three levels of consciousness: the conscious, preconscious, and unconscious. The *conscious* mind includes sensations and experiences that the person is aware of, such as awareness that you are tired, hungry, and/or currently reading a long (hopefully not too boring) chapter on psychoanalysis. Freud believed the conscious mind comprised a small part of mental life. The *preconscious* holds memories and experiences that a person can easily retrieve at will, such as what you ate for dinner last night, lines from your favorite song, or elements of this chapter for your final exam. The *unconscious* holds memories, thoughts, and desires that the conscious mind cannot tolerate and is the source of innate drives; Freud believed this to be the largest level of consciousness and focused his work on making conscious material conscious. Thus, most Freudian techniques are methods for making the unconscious conscious, such as dream analysis and free association. More recent practitioners distinguish the "present" unconscious from a person's childhood or "past" unconscious, and often begin treatment by analyzing here-and-now unconscious meanings that are more experience-near and easier for clients to relate to (Kernberg, 1997). Let's just hope that the contents of this chapter do not remain deeply hidden in your unconscious when it comes time to take the test.

Structures of the Self: Id, Ego, and Superego (Drive Theory)

The psychodynamic term *self* refers to the organization and integration of all psychic structures that comprise the individual (St. Clair, 2000). An object relationship always takes place between the entire self and an object; not between elements of the self—such as ego or id—and an object. Freud conceptualized the self as having three structures, which are used to conceptually understand and discuss psychodynamics, and are not thought of as actual "things":

- *Das Es* ("The It"): Latinized for English speakers as *Id* (the Latin term makes it sound more technical and mysterious than simply saying "the it"): Unorganized part of the personality that is motivated by instinctual drives; it inspires us to act according to the "pleasure principle." This part of the personality is almost if not exclusively unconscious. Infants are born with only id impulses and develop other personality structures in the first few years of life.
- *Das Ich* ("The I"): Latinized for English speakers as *Ego*: The ego operates according to the "reality principle," striving to meet the needs of the id in socially appropriate ways. More a part of a person's conscious mind, the ego is the part of the personality that involves intellect, cognition, defense mechanisms, and other executive functions, and serves as a mediator between the id and superego.
- *Das Über-Ich* (The Over/Above-I): Latinized for English speakers as *Superego*: Always striving for perfection, the superego represents ego and social ideals and generally prohibits the id's drives and fantasies that are not socially acceptable.

Freudian analysts conceptualize client problems by examining how the ego manages the ongoing conflicts between the id's drives and the superego's prohibitions. In many cases, the ego "manages" these tensions using a defense mechanism.

Drive Theory (Drive Theory and Ego Psychology)

Freud conceptualized the human psyche as a type of machine: "he built his theory on a vision of man [*sic*] emphasizing the internal workings of a psychic apparatus fueled by the energy of instinctual drive" (Greenberg & Mitchell, 1983, p. viii). When energy within this system arises that cannot be "discharged," it must be managed and/or channeled in some fashion, such as denying or redirecting it. Freud identified the energy of the system as *libido*, a sexual energy, and after World War I added the *death drive*, the source of aggressive energy, as another form of energy that must be similarly managed. These energies are *instinctual drives* that are an inherent part of being human, experiences shared by all; however, when these drives are not properly acknowledged and managed, symptoms can develop. Freud's *psychosexual developmental model* (see below) described the development and maturation of libido energy. Although Freud did not develop a parallel model for the death drive, Melanie Klein, an object relations theorist, developed her ideas around the concept of the aggressive death drive (Altman, 2008; Klein, 1932/1975). Other object relations theorists developed alternative drive theories that posited the drive for relationship; however, these relational drive theories primarily are used to describe the human need to seek relationship and generally do not include the mechanistic elements of Freud's drive theory.

Psychosexual Stages of Development and the Oedipal Complex (Drive Theory)

Based on drive theory and regarded as some of his most controversial ideas, Freud's *psychosexual stages of development* describe how the personality—id, ego, superego—developed during the first five years of life. Freud believed that children experience general sexual/sensual gratification through various parts of the body until they reach adolescence when sexuality pleasure becomes localized in the genitals. He acknowledged that this theory "may indeed sound strange enough ... [but] we shall indeed be ... richer by a motive for directing our attention to these most significant after-effects of infantile impressions which have hitherto been so grossly neglected" (Freud, 1963a, p. 13).

Contemporary practitioners are frequently divided into two general "camps": those who use drive theory and the psychosexual stages (Freudian drive theory analysts, ego psychologists, and some object relations practitioners) and those who believe drive theory and the psychosexual stages to be incompatible with object relations theory (self psychologists, interpersonal theorists, and the remaining object relations practitioners; Greenberg & Mitchell, 1983; Kernberg, 1997). There is also debate as to how literally versus metaphorically to interpret the psychosexual stages, with Americans tending to be more literal than their continental counterparts. Feminists have long critiqued Freud's psychosocial stages on numerous fronts, including the unabashed male bias that assigns a higher value to masculinity and uses masculinity as the standard by which females are understood (Friedan, 1963; Messer & Warren, 1995). Nonetheless, Freud's psychosexual stages provide a template for understanding how sexuality and aggressive drives may shape the personality and, more importantly, shape the development of the superego and morality.

Oral Stage: Dependency and Security (Birth–18 months) During this period, infants are dependent upon their mothers to gratify their needs, which they do orally: sucking, biting, and spitting. If infants rely too heavily on the mother during this stage, they become *dependent* in adulthood. On the other hand, infants who too infrequently have their needs met may become *insecure* as an adult. In case formulation, psychodynamic counselors may refer to "orally dependent" personalities that have an exaggerated need to be nurtured.

Anal Stage: Control (18 months–3 years) During the anal stage, toddlers learn to control their sphincters, thus learning to manage the polarities of relaxation and rigidity. Children who become fixated in this stage may be *anal retentive,* developing an overly strong need to control urges and maintain control, or *anally explosive,* unable to maintain control over instinctual urges.

Phallic Stage: Morality and Superego (3–6 years) The most controversial of Freud's theories and a sure-fire way to add zest to any conversation that lacks enthusiasm, the phallic stage is marked by the Oedipus/Electra complexes, castration anxiety, and penis envy. Named after Sophocles's famous Greek tragedy, the *Oedipal complex* refers to what Freud believed to be a universal pattern in which boys directed their sensual impulses toward their mothers and had aggressive impulses toward their fathers; similarly, the *Electra complex* refers to girls who desire their fathers and want to eliminate their mothers. Children successfully resolve these libidinal instincts by developing a *superego* that enables them to identify with the same-sex parent and change from erotic to nonsexual love for the opposite-sex parent. *Castration anxiety* refers to a boy's fear that he may be castrated as punishment for masturbating, Oedipal urges, or other expressions of libidinal energy, all of which were strictly prohibited in Freud's era when boys were frequently warned that their penises would fall off if they play with them. On the other hand, girls may develop *penis envy,* wondering if they had done something wrong and already lost theirs. These theories developed from his early female patients reporting sexual advances by older men. Initially, Freud believed the reports to be what we now call sexual abuse; but later he believed that they must have been fantasies. As you might imagine, modern feminists as well as gay/lesbian advocates vociferously object to these theories, as they imply that homosexuality is a failure in development, that young children sexually desire their parents, and that sexual abuse can be blamed on children who "seduce" their parents.

Perhaps best understood in a more metaphoric sense, the important outcome of the phallic stage is the development of the superego and a sense of morality: "The superego embodies a successful identification with the parents' superego and gives permanent expression to their influence" (St. Clair, 2000, p. 26). Freud similarly emphasized the importance of the ultimate outcome as developing a conscious or superego so that one can successfully participate in society: "Whether one has killed one's father or has abstained from doing so is not really the decisive thing. One is bound to feel guilty in either case" (Freud, 1931/1961, p. 89).

Latency Stage: Sexuality Latent (6–12 years) In the latency period, libidinal energy is channeled to normal childhood activities, such as school, friendship, and hobbies; this is a period in which libidinal sexual conflicts are not typically present.

Genital Stage: Adult Sexuality (12+years) In this stage, sexual energy is focused on members of the opposite sex. If issues were not appropriately resolved in earlier stages, they are likely to create difficulties and symptoms in adulthood.

Symptoms as Intrapsychic Conflict: Primary and Secondary Gains

Presenting symptoms, such as a phobia, depression, or psychosomatic complaint, are viewed as expressions of inner or *intrapsychic conflict*, often a metaphor for emotions that cannot otherwise be consciously acknowledged and/or expressed (Luborsky et al., 2008). The analyst views these symptoms as clues to the client's underlying inner conflicts. The goal of therapy in such cases is to gain awareness and enable safe expression of these emotions. For example, a client who complains of chronic back pain may be feeling burdened in a relationship or at work, or a client who has a fear of heights may be afraid of realizing his full potential.

Primary gains and *secondary gains* of a particular symptom are also considered in assessment (McWilliams, 1999). Primary gains refer to the primary benefit of the symptom. For example, the primary gain of a teen's depression may be that the loss of energy and interest enables him to avoid an activity that causes distress in some way (e.g., he may feel that he is not good at sports and being too depressed to go to practice allows him to get out of this). In addition, there are often *secondary gains*, which are benefits that are not immediately related but a natural consequence nonetheless. For example, the depression may get him attention from girls at school, released from normal chores, out of visits to extended family, or—whoops!—whatever he wants because a counselor takes his side against his parents. Thus, professionals need to be careful that they don't inadvertently create secondary gains in the name of being helpful, which requires careful thought because what might be therapeutic for one client is a secondary gain for another.

Defense Mechanisms (Drive Theory, Ego Psychology, Object Relations, and Self Psychology)

Defense mechanisms are automatic responses to perceived psychological threats and are often activated on an unconscious level (Luborsky et al., 2008). When the ego is unable to reconcile tensions between the id and superego and/or manage unacceptable drives, it may use one or more defense mechanisms to manage the seemingly irreconcilable conflict. When used periodically, defense mechanisms can be adaptive ways of coping with stress; when used regularly they become quite problematic. Freud began identifying these early in his work and later theorists have continued adding to the list. Here are some of the more common forms of defense mechanisms (also see Chapter 2 for additional discussion of defense mechanisms). In the case study at the end of this chapter, the client's long-term reliance on several defense mechanisms to suppress emotions eventually resulted in depression, suicidal thinking, and misuse of pain medication; the counselor helps him bring these emotions into his consciousness so he can more effectively deal with them.

Denial One of the first defenses identified by Freud, denial is the refusal to accept an external reality or fact because it is too threatening and may involve the reversal of facts (Luborsky et al., 2008). Denial is commonly seen in families with substance and alcohol abuse as well as people in dead-end jobs and relationships.

Introjection The earliest form of identification used by infants, introjection describes when one "takes in whole" behaviors, beliefs, and attitudes of another. In the case of infants, their earliest object relations are formed by introjections of their caregivers. Introjections can have positive or negative emotional valence. Initially infants "split" these into two sets of memories, and in healthy development these become integrated (Kernberg, 1976). Adults who use the defense of introjection "swallow whole" the opinions, style, and characteristics of others in order to identify with them or gain their approval.

Splitting (Object Relations and Self Psychology) A defense that is of particular interest to object relations and self psychologists, splitting refers to the inability to see an individual as an integrated whole that has both positive and negative qualities (St. Clair, 2000). Splitting is normal for infants, but as they mature, infants are better able to understand that the mother who feeds them when they are hungry ("good" mother) is the same as the one who straps them into an uncomfortable car seat ("bad" mother). When an adult uses splitting as a defense mechanism, the person switches from seeing people as all-good or all-bad: idealizing and then villainizing. In some cases, they can rapidly alternate between an all-good or all-bad view of the same person, creating significant chaos in relationships. As you can imagine, this results in very difficult interpersonal relationships; my teen clients refer to them as the "drama queens and kings." Splitting is a defense that is commonly seen in borderline personality disorders.

Projection Projection refers to falsely attributing one's own unacceptable feelings, impulses, or wishes onto another, typically without being aware of what one is doing (e.g., seeing others as greedy but not recognizing this characteristic in oneself; Mitchell & Black, 1995). In clinical practice, this is often seen in the case where one partner has cheated and then projects these intentions onto the faithful partner; this can happen whether or not the infidelity has been discovered.

Projective Identification Similar to simple projection, projective identification involves falsely attributing to another one's own unacceptable feelings. However, in this case, "what is projected is not simply discrete impulses, but a part of the self—not just aggressive impulses, for example, but a bad self, now located in another" (Mitchell, & Black, 1995, p. 101). Since what is projected is part of the self, there is a continued unconscious identification that maintains a typically strong and animated connection and control. Furthermore, in many cases the person's controlling behaviors often result in the other person acting in such a way as to confirm the projection, making it difficult to clarify who did what to whom first. The classic example of this is jealousy: a person is jealous of his partner's relationship with other men, but claims that is because of her behavior. His jealousy causes her to be more secretive to avoid conflict, which further confirms his hypothesis about her, quickly creating a negative, downward spiral. Projective identification can also take the form of a radical activist against violence (pick one: animal, child, embryo, women, etc.) who projects aggressive impulses on others and then puts obsessive effort into promoting nonviolence, often using violent metaphors and sometimes violent means. Even when advocating noble causes, such a person tends to recklessly pursue the perceived evil in others to the point where their personal relationships, career, and well-being are harmed.

Repression A central concept in Freud's approach and considered one of the two basic defenses by Kernberg (along with splitting; 1976), repression describes the *unconscious process* that occurs when the superego seeks to *repress* the id's innate impulses and drives (St. Clair, 2000). In drive theory, repression is the cause of a wide range of neurotic symptoms, such as obsessions, compulsions, hallucinations, psychosomatic complaints, anxiety, and depression. Because it happens outside of awareness, repression is considered more pathological than *suppression*, in which the person consciously pushes the impulse out of mind.

Suppression Unlike repression, suppression is the *intentional* avoidance of difficult inner thoughts, feelings, and desires. When thoughtfully chosen, this defense can be very useful when facing difficult emotions over extended periods of time, such as grief, complicated loss, and so forth.

Erickson's Psychosocial Stages of Development (Ego Psychology)

One of the most widely used developmental models, Erickson's (1994; Erickson & Erickson, 1998) eight-stage psychosocial model of development describes developmental crises that must be negotiated at eight significant points in life (also see Chapter 2). If these crises are not mastered, difficulties are encountered in subsequent stages. His stages closely parallel Freud's psychosexual stages initially but then extend across the life span.

Trust versus Mistrust: Infant Stage Applicable to the first year or two of life, infants in this stage develop a healthy balance of trust and mistrust based on their experiences with early caregivers. A healthy balance of trust translates to a general sense of hope and safety in the world while simultaneously knowing when caution is warranted. Persons who have had traumatic childhoods or whose parents overly protected them often have confusion over when, where, and who to trust, resulting in either a sense of being unrealistically entitled or needlessly afraid.

Autonomy versus Shame and Doubt: Toddler Stage During toddlerhood, children develop a sense of autonomy and influence in their lives while also learning the limits of their abilities. If caretakers are either neglectful or overly protective, children become overburdened with a sense of shame and may grow up to have lingering issues that manifest as extreme self-doubt or debilitating shame and/or shyness. Alternatively, if parents do not allow their children to experience shame and self-doubt, these children tend to become impulsive and inconsiderate of others.

Initiative versus Guilt: Preschool and Kindergarten Age During preschool and kindergarten, children transition through a developmental stage in which they develop a sense of initiative and purpose tempered by guilt when their actions hurt others. Children who have either overly protective or neglectful parents may develop a strong sense of guilt and insecurity about making their own choices leading to risk avoidance and inhibition. Alternatively, children who have an underdeveloped awareness of guilt and how their actions affect others become overly aggressive.

Industry versus Inferiority: School Age In the early years in school, children learn new skills, developing a sense of competence from which they build their sense of self-worth; thus, the task at this stage is to engage in industrious activities to build confidence in their abilities. Children who are frequently criticized or compared to others and found to be lacking develop a pervasive sense of inferiority. Recent research also shows that overly praised children who are protected from experiencing failure and obstacles also develop a sense of inferiority because they are thwarted from developing a genuine sense of mastery (Seligman, 2002). Thus, contrary to their parents' intentions, children who are constantly sheltered from the feelings of losing a game, getting bad grades, being left out, and similar feelings of inferiority are actually likely to develop a lingering sense of inadequacy as they get older that can manifest as "underachieving" down the road. Alternatively, overly identifying with one's industriousness can result in obsessiveness in their activities.

Identity versus Identity Confusion: Adolescence Few developmental stages are more infamous—or as well researched—as adolescence. Erickson saw this as a time of identity development when a person first begins to answer questions, such as who am I and how do I fit in? Developmentally, this is a time of exploring possible identities and social roles, which often takes the form of wild outfits, colorful hair, rebellious music, rotating social groups, and other ways to magnificently annoy one's parents. Teens who are not allowed to explore their identity or are made to feel guilty for not pursuing certain life paths may experience role confusion, failing to identify a clear or viable sense of identity. Alternatively, role confusion can also take the form of failing to adopt a viable social role and instead developing a reactive identity that is based on a rebellious need to "not be" what someone wants, often taking the form of drug use, a radical social group, gang membership, or high school dropout. In such cases, teens are not able to conceive of themselves as productive members of one's family or society.

Intimacy versus Isolation: Young Adulthood In recent generations, young adulthood has become much longer than in years prior, due to more people seeking higher education and changing views of marriage and "settling down." During this time, a person establishes intimate relationships in their personal, social, and work life, developing their own families and social network. People who struggle at this stage can become either overly focused on their relationships, possibly becoming sexually promiscuous or overly identified with being in a relationship, or becoming increasingly socially isolated.

Generativity versus Stagnation: Adulthood The developmental tasks of adulthood focus on feeling as though one meaningfully contributes to society and the succeeding generations and is often measured by whether one is satisfied with life accomplishments. A midlife crisis refers to feeling as though one's life is stagnant, off course, and/or in need of fixing, which some pursue by trying to make radical life changes—sometimes these help and at other times get a person even more off course. Often, the consequences of developmental deficiencies from prior stages come to a head during this time and can now be worked through and more readily addressed. Additionally, developmental issues at this stage can take the form of being overly involved and extended in one's social or work world, or alternatively, becoming cynical and disconnected.

Integrity versus Despair: Late Adulthood The final developmental stage is an increasingly important one for counselors to understand as more elderly are receiving professional services. During this stage, people balance a sense of integrity with a sense of despair as they look back over their life and face the inevitability of death. Those who are able to face the end of life with a greater sense of integrity and wisdom are able to integrate the experiences of their life to make meaning and accept what and who they have been. In contrast, others struggle to make peace with their lives and with life more generally and experience inconsolable sadness and loss, or alternatively, develop a false sense of self-importance that is conveyed as arrogance and self-righteousness.

Object Relations Theory

A term first coined by Freud and objectionable (no pun intended) to modern ears, *object* in psychodynamic theory is used to refer to the "object" of a person's desire, attention, or "drive" (think "object of my affection"; St. Clair, 2000). So, yes, it often refers to a person, most often one's mother. It derives from subject/object distinction in classic grammar: the subject (of the sentence) does something (verb) to an object. Objects can be *internal* (operating in one's internal world) or *external* (existing in the "real" world). Freudian drive theory analyzes how a person relates to the "objects" of their psychosexual and life/death drives. In contrast, object relations theory explores how a person relates to external and internal objects to understand personality dynamics. Object relations theorists believe that the personality results from the *internalization* and *introjection* of external interaction patterns with objects, namely primary caregivers (Fiarbairn, 1954; Kernberg, 1976; St. Clair, 2000). *The relationships with caregivers become the templates for all future relationships*, and, hence, are carefully assessed and analyzed to understand problems later in life.

Object relations theorists are most concerned with how the infant internalizes relationships in the first three years of life and analyze how this affects adult personality development. Initially, "introjections [of caregivers] with positive valence and those with negative valence are thus kept completely apart .... simply because they happen separately and because of the ego's incapacity to integrate introjections not activated by similar valences" (Kernberg, 1976, p. 35). The most critical task in the first three years then becomes to integrate "good" and "bad" objects into a coherent, realistic understanding of another and avoid the defense mechanism of *splitting* and *repression* (see above). When a young child is abused or frustrated and lacks any control over the situation, a common coping strategy is to "split" the object into "good" and "bad" aspects and then internalize the "bad" aspect, making the external and uncontrollable object "good" and the self "bad." Thus, to emotionally survive, abused children may hate themselves and love their abusive caregivers, resulting in a pattern of continued victimization in adulthood. The focus of treatment in such cases is to identify, make conscious, and integrate these good and bad parts to create a more coherent identity, realistic expectations of others, and new relationship patterns.

Good Enough Mothering and the True Self (Object Relations)

Good news for perfectionists, Winnicott's observations revealed that mothers who were generally (but not perfectly) able to respond to their infant's communication and needs while allowing them to move toward independence provided "good enough" mothering, allowing the child to develop a *true self*. When relating from the true self, a person can spontaneously express needs and desires while maintaining a clear distinction between self and other. In contrast, if the mother is too cold and distant and/or too chaotic, good enough mothering does not occur and the child may develop a *false self* that is overly anxious to comply with others, feel "unreal," and struggle in relationships. Winnicott's goal in therapy was to help clients repair parenting damage and restore a sense of true self. Modern research on brain development provides support for Winnicott's theory by linking healthy brain development with the quality of parental interaction with infants (Siegel, 1999).

Stages of Separation and Individuation (Mahler's Object Relations)

Margaret Mahler described a *separation-individuation* process during the first three years of life during which time the infant develops an intrapsychic sense of self, which gives the child a sense of being an independent entity. Thus, her theory describes how a person is "psychologically born." She described a three-phase developmental process (Mahler, Pine, & Bergman, 1975; St. Clair, 2000):

Stage 1: Normal Infant Autism During the first month, newborns are unable to differentiate their actions and that of their caretakers; the primary task is to maintain a homeostatic equilibrium outside the womb.

Stage 2: Normal Symbiosis During the second month of life, a psychological shell begins to form for the infant that encloses the symbiotic relationship of mother and child as a dual entity. From this point on, infants begin to be aware of the need-satisfying object (i.e., mother). Mahler believed that severely disturbed children regressed to this mental state of fusion. Good mothering encourages the child toward sensory awareness of the environment.

Stage 3: Separation and Individuation In the final phase that begins at five months and continues until three years of age, the child both (a) individuates, developing intrapsychic autonomy, and (b) separates, creating psychological differentiation from the mother. This third stage has four subphases:

Subphase 1: Differentiation and Body Image: The child begins to physically distance slightly from the mother when practicing motor skills, often "checking back" to make sure the mother is still there.

Subphase 2: Practicing: Once infants begin to walk, they increasingly venture away with periodic returns for emotional connection. This is a period in which the child feels omnipotence and a peak in an idealized state of self.

Subphase 3: Rapprochement: During the second half of the second year, toddlers become more aware of physical separateness, their sense of omnipotence declines, and they reexperience separation anxiety. This phase is marked by inner conflicts resulting in demands for closeness alternating with demands for autonomy.

Subphase 4: Emotional Object Constancy and Individuality: Beginning in the third year of life, children begin to develop emotional object constancy using an integrated inner image of the good and bad aspects of mother that provides comfort in her physical absence. This whole object representation allows the children to develop a unified self-image.

Narcissism and Selfobjects (Self Psychology)

Kohut's self psychology is a unique form of object relations that Kohut developed from his work with persons diagnosed with narcissistic personality disorder (St. Clair, 2000). Freud implied that narcissistic people could not be treated because they could not form relationships with others. In contrast, Kohut (1977) conceptualized such persons as having narcissistic object relations, viewing objects (i.e., others) as if they were parts of the self and/or performing a crucial function for the self. Kohut reversed Freud's assumptions that drives preceded a sense of self: "In Kohut's theorizing it is the self that develops and is the motivational centre of the person. Evidence of the 'drives', 'drivenness', rage, or perversions are the manifestations of structural vulnerabilities, experiences of selfobject failures, a breakdown of the self. That was the direction in which Kohut led psychoanalytic exploration" (Lachmann, 1993, p. 227).

As conceptualized by Kohut, the selfobjects are those persons or objects that are experienced as part of the self or are used in service of the self to provide identity (Kohut, 1984; St. Clair, 2000). They are not whole objects but rather a series of unconscious patterns and themes. Young children develop selfobjects based on two things: (a) the *idealized image of the parents* ("my parents are perfect"), and (b) the *grandiose part of the self* ("I deserve to get what I want"). These two create a tension between what the child should do (what the parent would do; the idealized selfobject) and what the child wants to do (the grandiose self). The empathic relationship between the parents and child help the child develop a *cohesive self.* Nontraumatic failures of parental responsiveness—minor delays in responding to needs, such as a delay in getting a hot meal to a hungry child—actually serve to develop the nuclear self. In contrast, childhood traumas and deprivation prevent the healthy development of self; thus "the grandiose self and idealized objects continue in an unaltered form and strive for the fulfillment of their archaic needs" (St. Clair, 2000, p. 144). In these circumstances, the "selfobject experiences of all the preceding stages of his life reverberate unconsciously" (Kohut, 1984, p. 50), and these become the focus of self psychology treatment.

Relational Matrix

Abandoning drive theory, relational psychoanalysts use the *relational matrix* to organize, frame, and interpret clinical information (Mitchell, 1988). This matrix includes the self, the object, and transactional patterns, and redefines how "mind" is defined: "*Mind has been redefined from a set of predetermined structures emerging from inside an individual organism to transactional patterns and internal structures derived from an interactive, interpersonal field*" (p. 17; italics in original). According to relational theory, the "self" cannot be understood or even meaningfully experienced outside of interpersonal relationships. In fact, for relation theorists "*all* meaning is generated in relation, and therefore nothing is innate in quite the same way as it is in the drive model" (p. 61).

The relational approach conceptualizes the individual embedded within a web of relationships, called the *relational matrix* or *interactional field*, in which an individual connects with and differentiates from others. Rather than the individual, the basic unit of analysis is the interactional field, considering the *person-in-context* at all times, making it more applicable for diverse clients. Both intrapsychic and interpersonal dynamics are part of the field, and each affects the other. In the interactional field model, the self is experienced differently in each relationship, in each selfobject relation. Thus, the self is discontinuous, with different selves experienced in different relationships. For example, you may be confident with your best friend, insecure with a partner, and difficult to please with your parents.

Unconscious Organizing Principles and Culture

A particular form of relational theory, intersubjectivity theory draws on constructivist theory, self psychology, and relational analysis (Stolorow, Brandschaft, & Atwood, 1987). Based on postmodern constructivist philosophy, intersubjectivity theory posits that "people experience the world through the lens of their particular organizing frameworks—unique unconscious principles or templates—that formed based on early relational experiences" (Leone, 2008, p. 83). These unconscious principles are not a distortion or projection but rather an inescapable lens that each person develops in order to interpret his/her experiences. One *cannot not* have these principles or templates; without them a person cannot organize their experiences.

These unconscious organizing principles are shaped not only by early childhood relationships but also by culture. Culture by definition is a set of shared unconscious organizing principles (Rubalcava & Waldman, 2004; Waldman & Rubalcava, 2005). Each person within a given culture develops his/her own set of unconscious organizing principles based on early relationships as well as other diversity variables, such as gender, age, education, and so forth. During every moment of one's life, these unconscious organizing principles are used to inform one's sense of self, emotions, and behaviors. For example, whether a person interprets a friend's pat on the back as kind, rude, or inappropriate depends on these unconscious templates. Thus, intersubjectivity theorists radically redefine transference as a normal process that involves the client using unconscious organizing principles to interpret the counselor's behavior; the client cannot avoid doing this; nor can the counselor avoid countertransference. Intersubjectivity theorists use the immediacy of the counseling relationship to explore these principles and revise them as necessary to address current problems and relationships. In the case study at the end of this chapter, the counselor explores Ken's unconscious organizing principles about the importance of achievement in defining self that were shaped by his immigrant family and Japanese background.

Targeting Change: Goal Setting

General Goals of Psychoanalysis

Having specific theories of health, psychoanalysis approaches share similar long-term goals. These are general goals that define "mental health." They include:

- Decreased irrational impulses (early and middle phase)
- Increased ability to manage stress; decreased use of defense mechanisms (early and middle phase)
- Increased ego strength, self-esteem, and self-cohesion (middle and late phase)
- Increased insight followed by agency (middle and late phase)
- Increased emotional maturity and intelligence (middle and late phase)
- Decreased perfectionism (middle and late phase)
- Decreased internal conflict and personality integration (late phase)
- Increased ability to experience mature dependency and intimacy (late phase)

Irrational Impulses Often the earliest goals in treatment involve decreasing irrational impulses that result in compulsive or obsessive behaviors, self-destructive behaviors, substance abuse, depressive thinking, inappropriate, sexual impulses, and such (Messer & Warren, 1995). These impulsive behaviors and obsessive thoughts are typically what cause many clients to seek treatment, thus they are often highly motivated or at least somewhat eager to see a quick reduction in frequency. Goals can be written to target a simple decrease, especially initially (e.g., reduce binge eating to no more than once per week), or total elimination of the behavior (e.g., no episodes of binge eating to be sustained for two months).

Stress Management and Defenses Early goals also target decreasing a client's use of defense mechanisms and an increase in the client's ability to manage stress without them. When writing goals, the specific defense mechanisms being targeted should be specific, because most of us have a wide variety of favorites for use in different circumstances and relationships, each potentially requiring different interventions (e.g., denial, projection, introjection, passive aggression, and so on).

Ego Strength, Self-Esteem, and Self-Cohesion As the mediator between the id's pleasure-seeking impulses, superego's moral injunctions, and reality, the ego needs to be strong to keep a healthy balance. "Having ego strength" means that a person does not deny difficult realities but rather finds ways to cope that integrate the conflicting needs of the id, superego, and external world (McWilliams, 1999). By definition, the person does not blindly follow the id's pleasure-seeking drives, the superego's strict rules and dictates, or reality's most recent limits. Instead, the ego proactively engages the tension created by these opposing forces and seeks to find reasonable ways to mediate the differences and meet the various demands and needs without denying any. For example, when struggling with reading a difficult chapter, a person with ego strength may honor the needs of the id to find something better to do, the superego's demands to work harder, and reality's demands to prepare for a quiz by taking small breaks, asking for help, and/or setting aside extra time to study (so, go ahead, and enjoy your break; we'll be right here waiting for you).

Insight Followed by Agency "After the insight: agency." If agency, action, and change follow insight, then it is meaningful counseling. Therapeutic insight should strike like lightning, making it hard to return to one's old ways afterwards. If a client has frequent insight and nothing changes—then you need to work on the defense of intellectualization that is preventing the message from hitting home. Although Freud and many who came after him considered insight "curative," practitioners in more recent decades agree that if insight is not followed by change then it is not enough (McWilliams, 1999). Furthermore, relational and more modern practitioners believe insight is best arrived at collaboratively—counselor and client working together—rather than the traditional analyst *providing* the insight for the client.

Emotional Maturity and Intelligence Psychoanalytic practices help develop emotional maturity, which closely correlates to what Daniel Goleman (1995) recently called *emotional intelligence* (McWilliams, 1999). Emotional maturity or intelligence involves being aware of what one is feeling, understanding why one feels that way, and managing the emotions in a mature and intelligent way—rather than blindly reacting based on id-like impulses or rigid superego codes of morality. Recent neurological research supports the practice of finding words to expression emotion, because emotional memories stored in more primitive, nonlinguistic parts of the brain can be brought to the prefrontal cortex where it can be explored, understood, and transformed with language and greater understanding.

Perfectionism Another desired outcome of psychoanalytic counseling is to reduce the punitive nature of the superego, which typically takes the form of perfectionism (Messer & Warren, 1995). When a person's superego dominates the personality, the person becomes obsessed with following socially imposed rules and definitions of success without balancing the person's personal needs and drives. Although initially perfectionism often has many benefits in the form of worldly success, over time this strategy ultimately results in numerous potential neuroses, such as eating disorders, depression, and anxiety.

Personality Change Psychodynamic counseling approaches are designed to change personality and character structures; that is always the long-term goal, and arguably the most essential. Personality change is achieved by resolving internal and often unconscious conflicts, which involves a process of better understanding the self. Although initially Freud believed that insight was curative, most analysts today believe that insight is not enough: insight must be demonstrated by meaningful change in behaviors, thoughts, and feelings (Abend, 2001). Additionally, one of the most notable changes is in interpersonal relationships: clients should be able to have more meaningful and less conflictual relationships with significant people in their lives.

Mature Dependency and Intimacy By working through infant and childhood dependency issues, psychoanalysis enables adults to develop a mature and healthy dependency on others and the capacity for intimacy (McWilliams, 1999; Messer & Warren, 1995). Mature dependency involves acknowledging the human need for community, selecting supportive partners and friends, being emotionally vulnerable, and experiencing emotional and physical intimacy while still maintaining a clear identity. The other person is not expected to be all-nurturing or the panacea to life's problems, but instead is accepted as an integrated whole, both the good and bad parts. Furthermore, through psychoanalysis clients develop the capacity for adult intimacy, which involves psychological and sexual vulnerability.

The Doing: Interventions

Interpretation and Working Through Resistance

The most basic technique, all psychoanalytic approaches use interpretation of unconscious material to facilitate client insight. Numerous possibilities exist for interpretation:

- Dreams, fantasies, and daydreams
- Symptoms
- Transference and countertransference
- Favorite metaphors and word choice
- "Freudian" *slips of the tongue* (accidentally misspoken words that reveal unconscious motivations)
- Jokes and asides

Depending on the analyst's style of case conceptualization and analysis, the analyst may interpret sexually repressed material (drive theory), defense mechanisms (ego psychology), early childhood events (object relations), or selfobject conflicts (self psychology).

Like most things in life, the key to successful interpretation is timing! If the client is not ready, be prepared for *resistance*—in which case, the client is not ready to bring unconscious material to conscious awareness. In most cases, the closer the material is to preconsciousness, the more ready the client is for interpretation. For example, if the analyst has not felt the client was ready to hear an interpretation that she is angry at her partner but then she reports that she was "shaken" by a dream in which she was yelling at a character who represents her husband, the analyst may use this moment to present the interpretation.

Although interpretation was used initially to promote cognitive insight, analysts from all schools of psychoanalysis also increasingly attend to clients' affective experience in making and assessing the effectiveness of interpretation: "in the clinical situation the dominance of affective investment has come to be accepted almost universally as the most appropriate point for analytic intervention" (Kernberg, 1997, p. 8). The "affective investment" does not simply refer to the most readily visible emotions but rather to a holistic analysis of where emotional energy is invested across the entire range of conscious and unconscious processes, including transference, infantile material, countertransference, and so forth.

Steps to Providing Effective Interpretation

1. *Begin with case conceptualization:* Interpretation cannot be made willy-nilly, off-the-cuff, or as-the-spirit-moves. Instead, as a first step, the counselor needs to develop a well-crafted case conceptualization that thoughtfully reveals where the client invests most emotional energy (see the long Viewing section above for numerous options).
2. *Wait for the "Moment":* Once you have a clear sense of the client's dynamics and issues, don't rush into the next session ready to proclaim your insightful truth. In fact, it is hard to prepare a well-crafted interpretation because, to be effective, most need to be done when the client is ready to hear the interpretation, which is

(continued)

often after relating a new, often painful, difficult, or challenging event. In the struggle to understand what has just happened, most clients will then be more open to hearing an alternative perspective. The key is that when clients are still in the thralls of emotional upheaval, they are more likely to resist interpretation. So there is a sweet spot—somewhere between emotional turmoil and getting-over-it and getting the defenses back online, where clients pause to wonder, reflect, and ask why—that's the moment they are ready. Trust me, with time, you get better at finding this moment—it's generally obvious when you miss it.

3. *Work from the present to the past:* In most cases—and certainly no single set of steps will work for all forms of interpretation—begin by describing dynamics in the present issue (e.g., what just happened in session, what happened at work, between counselor and client, or whatever is most upsetting)—and then make links to the past (e.g., relationship with mother, father, past abuse, and so on; Kernberg, 1997).
4. *Assess client response:* Finally, you need to assess how clients respond to the interpretation. Do they resist: "I don't think that is what is happening at all"? Or do they agree: "Wow. I never thought of it before, but I think you are right"? Or do they fall somewhere in between: "I don't know. Some of that might be true"? Different schools and individual practitioners have different approaches to responding to each type of response. New counselors are probably safest using a more collaborative, relational approach, working with the client's reality, to reinterpret the interpretation in such a way that it not only "makes sense" in the client's subjective world but also translates to changes in action, feelings, and thoughts in their everyday life.

Empathy: Understanding-Explaining Sequence

Kohut (1984) describes an *understanding-explaining sequence* to both solidify the counseling relationship and provide meaningful interpretation. Most often, these two are presented together in a single utterance by the counselor. However, he emphasizes that in some cases, especially with people who have been severely traumatized, this phase may remain the only phase for a very long time.

Empathic Understanding-Explaining Sequence

This process involved two phases: the understanding and explaining phases.

1. *Understanding:* The understanding phase was an expression of empathy, "I can understand how my being late must have been upsetting for you."
2. *Explanation:* The second phase, the explaining phase, provides some form of interpretation that helps the client understand the source of the emotion, "We all care about how those around us see us and treat us, especially those who are important to us, much like our parents were to us years ago. Given your mother's unpredictability and your father's disinterest in you, my actions must have been especially upsetting."

Kohut used these two together to express a therapeutic expression of empathy that provides a corrective emotional experience and helps clients develop more cohesive sense of self.

Try It Yourself

Find a partner, share a recent life event, and role-play the empathic understanding-explaining sequence.

Kohut (1977) cautioned practitioners to look for evidence that a particular empathic interpretation was correct. He states, "We also know that there is one attitude that, after it has become an integral part of our clinical stance, provides us with an important safeguard against errors arising in consequence of our instinctive commitment to established patterns of thought: our resolve not to be swept away by the comfortable certainty of the 'Aha-experience' of intuited knowledge but to keep our mind open and to continue our *trial empathy* in order to collect as many alternatives as possible" (Kohut, 1977, p. 168). Kohut believed that only a gradual change in symptoms and behavior patterns provided evidence that one's empathic interpretations are correct. In the case study at the end of this chapter, the counselor uses the understanding-explaining sequence to help stabilize Ken by helping him understand the source of his suicidal thinking and hopelessness.

Free Association

Developed by Freud, free association involves asking a client to "just say what comes to mind" on a given topic, such as "your mother," allowing unconscious material to arise. The client may describe recent events, memories, feelings, fantasies, bodily sensations, or any other material. Analysts may have clients lay on a couch rather than sit in a chair to encourage a more relaxed and free-flowing thought process to encourage unconscious thoughts to emerge. The analyst listens carefully for unusual connections, idiosyncratic logic, slips of the tongue, and efforts to edit or hold back. After this process the analyst may provide interpretations to help promote insight into the client's process.

Dream Interpretation

"*... dreams in general can be interpreted, and that after the work of interpretation has been completed they can be replaced by perfectly correctly constructed thoughts which find a recognizable position in the texture of the mind*" (Freud, 1963b, p. 29).

Freud's approach to dream interpretation was revolutionary in his time, a period when scientists viewed dreams as a "somatic expression." In contradiction to the medical establishment, he proclaimed, "I must insist that the dream actually has significance, and that a scientific procedure in dream interpretation is possible" (Freud, 1900/1974, p. 83). Dubbed by Freud "the royal road to the unconscious," dream interpretation has been a key intervention since the beginning of psychoanalysis (Luborsky et al., 2008). In the tradition of Freud, the dreamer—not the analyst—is the key to symbolic meaning of the dreams; there are no predetermined meanings: "sometimes a cigar is just a cigar!" The dreamer's associations with symbols in the dream provide clues to underlying unconscious meaning of the dream. In dream analysis, dreams have two layers of meaning: the *manifest content* is the literal content of the dream and the *latent content* is the underlying, unconscious material that must be interpreted to be accessed.

Intersubjective Responding

Relational psychodynamic counselors rely on the counseling relationship itself to create opportunities for clients to gain insight and make change, referred to as *intersubjective responding*. Using a postmodern approach, they do not necessarily relate every experience in the counseling relationship to childhood experiences, but instead they stay focused on the present relationship and the client's interpretations of it, which may be related to culture, gender, economic status, or education, as well as childhood experiences. For example, if a client comments that she is frustrated because she does not feel like the counselor is telling her what he really thinks, the counselor will approach this comment from a nondefensive and nonassuming position, curiously exploring her perception, the expectations behind it, and their antecedents, which may be related to numerous factors, including childhood relationships.

Putting It All Together: Psychodynamic Case Conceptualization and Treatment Plan Templates

Theory-Specific Case Conceptualization: Psychodynamic

The prompts below can be used to develop a *theory-specific case conceptualization* using psychodynamic theory. The cross-theoretical case conceptualizations at the end of each theory chapter provide examples for writing a conceptualization that includes key elements of this theory-specific conceptualization. Comprehensive examples of theory-specific case conceptualizations are available in *Theory and Treatment Planning in Counseling and Psychotherapy* (Gehart, 2015).

- *Levels of Consciousness:* Describe salient dynamics of conscious versus unconscious processes.
- *Structures of the Self:* Describe the functioning and relationship between the client's ego, superego, and id.
- *Drive Theory:* Describe dynamics related to libidinal energy.
- *Secondary Gains:* Describe possible secondary gains related to client symptoms.
- *Defense Mechanisms:* Describe three to four of the client's most frequently used defense mechanisms, which may include:
    - Acting out
    - Denial
    - Displacement
    - Help-rejecting complaining
    - Humor
    - Passive aggression
    - Projection
    - Projective identification
    - Rationalization
    - Reaction formation
    - Repression
    - Splitting
    - Sublimation
    - Suppression
- *Erickson's Psychosocial Stages of Development:* Describe salient issues at development at each stage up to current stage:
    - Trust versus mistrust (infant stage)
    - Autonomy versus shame and doubt (toddler stage)
    - Initiative versus guilt (preschool age)
    - Industry versus inferiority (school age)
    - Identity versus identity confusion (adolescence)
    - Intimacy versus isolation (young adulthood)
    - Generativity versus stagnation (adulthood)
    - Integrity versus despair (late adulthood)
- *Object Relations Theory/True Self:* Describe attachment (secure, anxious, avoidant, or anxious-avoidant), general quality of relationship, and any attachment traumas with:
    - Early caregivers, in past and present
    - Current intimate relationships (partners, children, close friends)
- *Relational Matrix:* Describe the web of relationships and contexts through which the client understands self and world. Include intra- and interpersonal dynamics.
- *Unconscious Organizing Principles and Culture:* Describe unconscious organizing principles, highlighting those derived from racial, ethnic, gender, social class, sexual identity, ability, and other cultural dynamics.

Treatment Plan Template: Psychodynamic

Use this Treatment Plan template for developing a plan for clients with depressive, anxious, or compulsive types of presenting problems. Depending on the specific client, presenting problem, and clinical context, the goals and interventions in this template may need to be modified only slightly or significantly; you are encouraged to significantly revise the plan as needed. For the plan to be useful, goals and techniques should be written to target specific beliefs, behaviors, and emotions that the client is experiencing. The more specific, the more useful it will be to you.

Psychodynamic Treatment Plan

Initial Phase of Treatment

Initial Phase Counseling Tasks

1. Develop working counseling relationship. *Diversity considerations: Describe how you will specifically adjust to respect cultured, gendered, and other styles of relationship building and emotional expression.*
   a. *Relationship-building approach/intervention:* Use **empathy** and **mirroring** to provide a supportive, holding environment for client.
2. Assess individual, systemic, and broader cultural dynamics. *Diversity considerations: Describe how you will specifically adjust assessment based on cultural, socioeconomic, sexual orientation, gender, and other relevant norms.*
   Assessment strategies:
   a. Analyze **unconscious conflict** underlying symptoms and role of **defense mechanisms** in managing them.
   b. Analyze **object relations** and **selfobjects** patterns, including expressions in current relationships and historical development during infancy.
   c. Assess **relational matrix** and **culturally defined unconscious organizing principles** that shape the client's worldview.
3. Identify and obtain client agreement on treatment goals. *Diversity considerations: Describe how you will specifically modify goals to correspond with values from the client's cultural, religious, and other value systems.*
   Goal-making intervention:
   a. Discuss with client overarching goals, determining client's preference for brief psychodynamic symptom-reduction versus broader, long-term goals for restructuring client personality.
4. Identify needed referrals, crisis issues, and other client needs. *Diversity considerations: Describe diversity issues related to specific crisis issues and referral options.*
   a. *Crisis assessment intervention(s):* Assess for crisis potential by analyzing **defense mechanisms, transference, and object relations patterns**.
   b. *Referral(s):* Psychoanalytic process group as needed.

Initial Phase Client Goal

1. Decrease emotional reactivity to perceived **threats to self** to reduce [specific crisis symptoms].
   Interventions:
   a. Provide **empathy** using **understanding-explaining sequence** to reduce client's inaccurate perceptions of external threat to self.
   b. **Interpretation** to reduce need to use reactive **defense mechanisms** in response to incorrectly perceived threats.

(continued)

Working Phase of Treatment

Working Phase Counseling Tasks

1. Monitor quality of the working alliance. Diversity considerations: *Describe how you will specifically adapt expectations for age, gender, cultural, sexual orientation, socioeconomic, and other norms for relating.*
   a. *Assessment Intervention:* Monitor and work through **transference** and **countertransference.**
2. Monitor progress toward goals. *Diversity considerations: Describe how you will specifically adapt the monitoring of progress for age, ethnicity, educational level, language, and such.*
   a. *Assessment Intervention:* Monitor for changes in behavior and relationships outside of session; Outcome Questionnaire to measure client progress.

Working Phase Client Goals

1. Decrease [specify **defense mechanism**] to protect self from [specify perceived threat] to reduce [specific symptom: depression, anxiety, etc.].
   Interventions:
   a. **Interpretation** of role of **defense mechanism** and how it developed in early childhood experiences and is being inappropriately used currently.
   b. Analysis of **transference** in session when defenses are used in relationship to counselor.
2. Increase **ego strength** and **self-coherence** to reduce [specific symptom: depression, anxiety, etc.].
   Interventions:
   a. **Mirroring** to confirm client's sense of worth and value.
   b. **Empathy** using the **understanding-explaining sequence** to increase client's sense of coherence.
   c. **Dream interpretation** and **free association** to bring sources of inner conflict to conscious awareness.
3. Increase sense of personal agency informed by emotional intelligence to reduce [specific symptom: depression, anxiety, etc.].
   Interventions:
   a. **Intersubjective responding** to increase client's awareness of self in sessions versus various emotional-relational contexts.
   b. **Working through resistance** to translating insight into action.

Closing Phase of Treatment

Closing Phase Counseling Task

1. Develop aftercare plan and maintain gains. *Diversity considerations: Describe specific diversity considerations and unique resources for the ending treatment and sustaining gains posttreatment.*
   Intervention:
   a. Analyzing **transference** and abandonment issues as impending termination approaches.

Closing Phase Client Goals

1. Decrease internal conflict while increasing **personality integration** to reduce potential for relapse in [specific symptom: depression, anxiety, etc.].
   Interventions:
   a. **Dream analysis, free association**, and **analysis of transference** to identify internal conflicts generally and those related to ending treatment specifically.
   b. Enable client to identify, consciously contain, and successfully manage internal conflicts to allow for fuller personality integration.

(continued)

2. Increase ability to experience **mature dependency** and intimacy to reduce potential for relapse in [specific symptom: depression, anxiety, etc.].
   Interventions:
   a. Analyze **transference** and **work through resistance** to intimacy in in-session and out-of-session relationships.
   b. **Intersubjective responding** to critically examine the **unconscious organizing principles** the client uses to relate to others.

Tapestry Weaving: Working with Diverse Populations

Cultural and Ethnic Diversity

As traditionally practiced, psychoanalysis is generally considered not readily adaptable to other cultures (Greene, 2004; Luborsky et al., 2008) or sexual minorities (Glassgold & Iasenza, 2004) and has long been critiqued even from within the field as biased against women (Horney, 1939). Virtually all of the research on the approach has been exclusively with white clients (Watkins, 2012). However, more recently developed relational approaches enable psychodynamic practitioners to use a contextually sensitive approach that carefully incorporates the client's unique interpersonal context into the counseling process (Altman, 2008; Waldman & Rubalcava, 2005). Specifically, relational and intersubjectivity approaches recognize that both counselor and client "make sense of the other's affect, behavior, and expression in terms of their own unconscious cultural organizing principles"; these dynamics are considered when assessing the intersubjective field" (Rubalcava & Waldman, 2004, p. 138). Additionally, some practitioners such as Fred Pine (1990) have adapted psychoanalytic work to be more "supportive" when working with poor clients and clients with limited educational backgrounds. Pine uses "ego building" interventions, such as naming feelings and alerting clients before offering a potentially difficult-to-hear interpretation.

Latinos/Latinas Gelman (2004) conducted a grounded theory study to identify how Latino clinicians successfully adapted psychodynamic therapy with Latino clients. The counselors in his study reported that they modified the following elements to successfully work with Latinos using psychodynamic theory:

- *Counseling Relationship and Personalismo:* In Latino culture, warmth, respect, and cordiality are part of relating to others, a quality referred to as *personalismo*. This sense of personal connection was furthered by speaking the same language and sharing a common culture. Because of this change to the more typically reserved psychodynamic relationships, the clinicians noted that they felt there was a greater risk of overidentification with clients. Thus, greater self-awareness on the part of the counselor was required to attend to transference and countertransference dynamics.
- *Individuality and Individually Tailored:* The counseling process was individually tailored to each client, given the great heterogeneity of Latino cultures as well as the impact of socioeconomic status and acculturation.
- *Flexibility in Approach:* Similarly, clinicians reported using a more flexible psychodynamic approach, such as more allowable phone contact between sessions.
- *Address External Realities:* External realities, including psychosocial pressures, are included in the analytic process. Concrete problems are addressed within the psychodynamic process as part of the work.
- *Self-Disclosure:* Latino clinicians reported using more self-disclosure with Latino clients because it is culturally expected.
- *Gift Giving:* Because gift giving is an important part of their culture, counselors were more likely to accept culturally appropriate gifts when working with Latino clients.

- *Physical Contact:* Clinicians also reported a willingness to engage in reasonable and appropriate physical contact with Latino clients, including handshaking, back-patting, and reduced interpersonal space. They described carefully assessing the potential meaning of such contact with each individual client.
- *Activity and Direction:* Clinicians also reported being more active and directive, especially in terms of helping clients access resources.
- *Language as a Therapeutic Technique:* Clinicians report using language differently with Latino clients than non-Latino clients. When counseling was done in Spanish, the shift from a formal "you" (usted) to informal (tú) clearly signaled an increase in comfort and trust. Additionally, clinicians believed that speaking in one's native language accesses the psyche in a way that a second language cannot; thus, slipping into one's native language was seen as accessing more direct experience and emotions. Preference for using the second language was viewed as having several potential purposes and meanings: distancing from experience, distancing in the therapeutic relationship, demonstration of assimilation, or preference for an acculturated identity. Finally, language was used to modulate affect: with switching to the native language increasing affectivity and switching to the secondary language a means to reduce emotional charge.

East Asian Americans As many consider psychodynamic therapy ineffective with Asian clients, Yi (1995) proposes several modifications to traditional psychodynamic concepts using subjectivity theory (Stolorow et al., 1987).

- *Selfobject Relations:* As early mother-infant relations are believed to be the foundation of selfobject relations, it is important to recognize cultural differences that establish these patterns. In Asian cultures, mothers are more likely to positively mirror interdependence and respect for others rather than individuation, which is valued more in the West.
- *Confucian Self:* Given the profound influence of the highly structured and hierarchical Confucian value system, East Asians internalize similar hierarchical representations of self and other, with clearly defined roles. Unlike common Western conceptualizations of hierarchy, Confucian hierarchy implies mutual and reciprocal duties and responsibilities to the other—not unidirectional power.
- *Transference Considerations:* In Asian cultures, relating to authority involves a benign positive idealization of the authority figure's power and wisdom and an expectation of benevolent guidance and protection. This respect is often expressed by taking a receptive, listening stance. This traditional Asian approach to relating to authority figures, such as doctors and other professionals, must not be misinterpreted as some form of regression or passive dependency. Instead, psychodynamic counselors need to carefully consider the client's level of acculturation, assess the client within cultural norms, and co-create an appropriate counseling relationship.
- *Empathic-Introspective Approach:* Yi strongly supports using an empathic-introspective approach with Asian clients, empathically understanding the clients from within their subjective world and to use personal introspection on the part of the counselor to examine how his/her own personal subjective organizing principles are affecting the counseling process and interpretations of the clients. Counselors must continually examine their own assumptions and beliefs that are culturally bound, in order to more accurately make sense of the client's experiential world.

Sexual Identity Diversity

Freud is known for conflicting views and statements about homosexuality. He was a strong advocate for not criminalizing same-sex attraction and for proposing that everyone is capable of same-sex attraction but that most repress homo-erotic thoughts and feelings (Rubinstein, 2003). However, his theory of psychosexual development identifies heterosexuality as the "natural outcome" of healthy development, pathologizing of homosexuality as an "arrest in development" (Izzard, 2000, p. 107). Over the years, his views have had a significant impact on the field's views of homosexuality. In the 1940s, his followers took a more clearly pathologizing stance on same-sex attraction, citing his theories (Rubinstein, 2003). More recently, gay affirmative analysts also cite his work to support a nonpathologizing approach to working with same-sex attraction (Izzard, 2000; Rubinstein, 2003).

In recent decades, influenced by feminists and postmodernists, most psychodynamic counselors have assumed a more contemporary view of same-sex attraction that is nonpathologizing (Cornett, 1993; Izzard, 2000). Much of the literature has focused on changing the personal attitudes and practices of clinicians, with relatively little focusing on reconceptualizing theory (Izzard, 2000). That said, two of the more frequently discussed issues in psychodynamic literature related to conceptualizing psychoanalysis with gay and lesbian clients are internalized homophobia and the issue of the neutral therapeutic stance.

Internalized Homophobia: Shame and Self-Hatred

Psychodynamic analysis can help clinicians understand the process of internalized homophobia in gay, lesbian, and bisexual individuals (Izzard, 2000). Through the processes of identification and introjection, virtually all persons—gay or straight—in a heterosexist society develop homophobia. For those who are gay, this then becomes a source of self-hatred and shame. The lack of mirroring of their experience intensifies the sense of social stigma and isolation. The psychoanalytic process can be used to help clients work through the internalized homophobia and develop greater self-acceptance. As part of this acceptance process, clinicians also need to allow space for gay and lesbian clients to discuss the "shadow side" of same-sex attraction, which includes feelings of wishing for heterosexual attraction and/or being dissatisfied or disappointed in their orientation (Izzard, 2000). The emphasis for psychodynamic counselors theoretically, however, is the internalized homophobia and its remediation, rather than coping with the real experience of external homophobia in others. Thus, there is debate about how and whether to assume a more gay affirmative stance as a psychodynamic practitioner (Cornett, 1993).

Therapeutic Stance: Gay Affirmative versus Neutrality

The heart of psychodynamic approaches is clinician neutrality, which allows for the client's patterns of relating and intrapsychic material to clearly emerge and be seen (Izzard, 2000). In most forms of psychodynamic counseling, there is no affirmation or reassurance. This strict form of neutrality can be helpful for addressing internalized homophobia. However, it precludes an analyst from taking a "gay affirmative" stance (Cornett, 1993; Izzard, 2000). By definition, a gay affirmative stance is not a neutral position. In practice, gay affirmative counseling involves taking an advocate stance, offering affirmation of the client's sexual orientation, and may lead the counselor to preclude the exploration of the client's negative feelings about being gay. A gay affirmative stance includes greater attention to harassment and social realities. However, some worry that such a stance is an unhelpful overreaction to pathologizing same-sex attraction and does not allow the client to fully benefit from the psychoanalytic "working through" process (Shelley, 1998). Thus, Frommer (1995) recommends that analysts balance their commitment to neutrality that is critical to the analysis process while maintaining a realistic awareness of the daily impact of homophobia and marginalization.

Psychodynamics of Bisexuality Working with bisexual individuals requires sensitivity to their unique experiences (Friedman & Downey, 2010; Rubinstein, 2003). Bisexual individuals report attraction to both men and women, and each can vary in the homosexual/heterosexual balance over the course of a lifetime. Additionally, at different times in their lives, a person who experiences same-sex attraction may identify as heterosexual or homosexual depending on the sex of the partner. Like their gay counterparts, bisexual individuals must contend with internalized homophobia. However, in addition, many experience "biphobia," internalized self-oppression (Dworkin, 2001), as well as unrealistic expectations from self and others. Some assume that bisexuals "can't make up their minds" or "have a choice," which is often not the experience of bisexual attraction (Friedman & Downey, 2010). Instead, they typically report finding themselves "falling in love" with persons of either gender, creating confusion, complications, and significant life upheaval (Friedman & Downey, 2010). In addition, bisexual persons may struggle personally or interpersonally with negative assumptions, such as bisexuality involves a fear commitment, that they fear their true homosexual identity, or their inability to be faithful (Dworkin, 2001).

From a psychodynamic perspective, the unconscious conflict of bisexual individuals is different from those with heterosexual and same-sex attraction (Friedman & Downey, 2010). When a person is consistently attracted to one sex, the erotic image is stable and constant. In contrast, in bisexuality, the erotic image can change; this change is often highly influenced by external factors, including traumatic events and anxiety from unconscious conflicts about one's sexuality. Thus, the analyst needs to thoughtfully examine the underlying dynamics that affect the heterosexual/homosexual balance in bisexual individuals. One such factor is the sexual orientation of the counselor (if revealed) and any value judgments a counselor may make about sexual orientation (Friedman & Downey, 2010); thus, counselors need to carefully consider their potential impact on a given bisexual individual when discussing sexual orientation.

Research and the Evidence Base

Although often having a reputation for little research support, psychodynamic counseling has a respectable and growing evidence base (Leichsenring, 2009: Shedler, 2010). The best and most rigorously researched psychodynamic approaches are the brief psychodynamic methods, many of which are recognized as evidence-based approaches by the U.S. National Institutes of Health (Luborsky et al., 2008; Weissman, Markowitz, & Klerman, 2000, 2007). The strongest support for the effectiveness of general psychodynamic counseling comes from large-scale studies comparing psychodynamic to other approaches such as cognitive-behavioral and humanistic, as was recently done in the United Kingdom, indicating no significant difference in outcome between theories (Stiles, Barkham, Mellor-Clark, & Connell, 2008). More recent studies show a trend for sustained gains and even *increasing* gains after counseling has ended (Abbass, Hancock, Henderson, & Kisely, 2006; Leichsenring, 2009). In addition, there is support for specific psychodynamic concepts. For example, using the Core Conflictual Relationship Theme, Luborsky and associates (Luborsky et al., 2008; Luborsky & Crits-Christoph, 1998; Luborksy & Luborksy, 2006) have researched and found evidence that supports the psychoanalytic concept of transference. Additional research is needed to compare the different models or schools of psychodynamic theory to determine if they vary in effectiveness generally or for specific issues (Leichsenring, 2009). Finally, newer areas of research in psychodynamic counseling focus on the neurological and physiological correlates of psychodynamic processes and inform new ways of conceptualizing unconscious process and attachment (Marci & Riess, 2009; Roffman & Gerber, 2009).

Evidence-Based Treatment: Brief Psychodynamic Counseling

In a Nutshell: The Least You Need to Know

Several "brief, psychodynamic" approaches have been developed and validated through research (Book, 1998; Messer & Warren, 1995). These approaches use many of the same case conceptualization skills as traditional psychodynamic approaches; however, they differ in the quality of the counseling relationship, the specificity of the goals, and the directiveness of the interventions. These "brief" approaches may require 12–50 sessions, but typically end after 20. Similar to other psychodynamic approaches, they believe that early childhood relationships significantly affect problems later in life and that defense mechanisms should be targeted in treatment. Thus, most brief psychodynamic approaches aim to strengthen the ego so that it can better manage problem impulses and resolve inner conflicts. The counselor is more active in these approaches, quickly identifying core dynamics that are targeted for intervention; the counselor-client relationship is used as a learning forum for *corrective emotional experiences*, in which the counselor's response helps correct old traumas.

Big Picture: Overview of Counseling Process

Sifneos (1979) identifies five phases of brief psychodynamic counseling and psychotherapies:

1. *Client-counseling encounter:* The client and counselor develop a working rapport and mutually agree upon a focus of treatment. During this time, the counselor develops a case conceptualization of the client's dynamics, focusing on those that are related to the identified problem.
2. *Early treatment:* The counselor confronts idealistic, positive transference and helps the client to distinguish wishful thinking from realistic expectations of the counselor and counseling process.
3. *Height of treatment:* During this working phase, the past is explored to better understand current problems and transference issues that arise in session; clients are encouraged to use new ways of relating both in and out of session.
4. *Evidence of change:* Clients begin to apply what they learn in session to everyday life.
5. *Termination:* Once goals have been reached, counselors help them move toward termination rather than look for new goals. Careful attention is paid to issues of loss and separation as treatment ends.

Making Connection: Counseling Relationship

Corrective Emotional Experience

Rather than using transference and countertransference to promote insight into early childhood relationships, brief psychodynamic counselors use these immediate in-session interactions to promote *corrective emotional experiences*. Corrective emotional experiences involve using the counseling relationship to work through old childhood traumas and relational patterns (Mallinckrodt, 2010). For example, if a client perceives the counselor's professional mannerism as also implying disapproval, the counselor can use this opportunity to clarify that the professional boundaries are just that—professional boundaries—and do not imply any judgment or valuing of the client as a person, as may have been the case with the client's father or mother. When this is done with sincerity and without reactivity on the part of the counselor, this can be a profoundly healing experience for the client.

Specific Brief Psychodynamic Approaches

Interpersonal Psychotherapy

Originally developed for treating depression, *interpersonal psychotherapy* has been used with couples, older adults, bipolar disorder, eating disorders, anxiety disorders, and borderline personality disorder (Weissman et al., 2000, 2007). In one of the largest mental health studies conducted in the United States, interpersonal psychotherapy was compared with cognitive therapy and antidepressant medication and found to be as effective (Krupnick et al., 1994); thus, it has a well-respected evidence base. The approach is based on the assumption that stressful interpersonal experiences in adulthood trigger childhood attachment issues, resulting in depression or similar disorders. The approach focuses on building strong interpersonal relationships to reduce the likelihood of relapse.

Treatment is time-limited and focuses on the following four areas:

1. interpersonal deficits (i.e., lack of skills or knowledge),
2. role expectations and conflicts (i.e., creating realistic expectations),
3. role transitions (i.e., redefining relationships based on developmental and contextual needs), and
4. grief issues (i.e., dealing with past and current relational loss).

Interpersonal psychotherapy has three phases:

Phase 1: Initial Sessions: Focuses on identifying one or two concerns from the four areas listed above. The counseling process and diagnosis are explained so that the client fully understands the process and how it will help.

Phase 2: Intermediate Phase: During this working phase, the counselor actively helps the client address the targeted problems using a wide range of interventions that include psychoeducation, interpretation of patterns, advice giving, insight-stimulating questions, and behavior change techniques.

Phase 3: Termination: Termination requires 2–4 sessions to help the client develop confidence that they can handle future problems using the skills they have learned.

Core Conflict Relationship Theme Method

Luborsky and colleagues (Luborsky & Crits-Christoph, 1998; Luborsky & Luborsky, 2006; Luborsky et al., 2008) have developed the Core Conflictual Relationship Theme Method to operationalize transference in their brief, psychodynamic method. The method involves analyzing all accounts clients share about their interactions with others to identify core relationship themes that create conflict and problems. Counselors do this by analyzing three elements in each encounter reported by the client:

- W: The client's wish (W), either stated or implied (e.g., wanting to be loved, appreciated, acknowledged, etc.)
- RO: The response of others (RO), either real or imagined (e.g., rejection, disapproval, criticism, ignoring, etc.)
- RS: The response of self (RS) (e.g., anger, sadness, withdrawal, attacking other, blaming self, feeling trapped, etc.).

The counselor tracks these three elements in each problem encounter described by the client and helps the client to gain insight into these patterns and change their responses. Research shows that clients' wishes generally remain the same, but their responses and those of others change.

Time-Limited, Dynamic Psychotherapy

Designed for persons diagnosed with personality disorders, time-limited dynamic psychotherapy uses the counseling relationship to encourage corrective emotional experiences (Levenson, 2003). Clients interact with counselors the same way they do with others in their lives. Counselors using a time-limited, dynamic approach use their responses within the counseling relationship to provide new experiences for clients that enable them to change how they interact with others outside of session. The counselor has a positive, supportive approach that provides clients safety in exploring these long-standing relational patterns. Initially, counselors begin by identifying present relationship patterns but then move toward exploring early origins of these. Counselors help clients see how these patterns may have been adaptive earlier in life but no longer serve their purpose.

Questions for Personal Reflection and Class Discussion

1. Which ideas from this chapter do you find most personally relevant? Why?
2. Which ideas from this chapter do you think will be most helpful in working with clients?
3. What forms of countertransference are likely to be an issue for you?
4. What is your opinion about dream interpretation? What do you base this on?
5. What are the possibilities and limitations for using this approach with diverse clients? How might you address these limitations?
6. For which clients and/or presenting problems do you think this approach would be most appropriate? Least appropriate?

7. Which case conceptualization concept seems most useful for understanding a client's problem?
8. Which intervention do you think would be the most useful?
9. Do you think this approach is a good fit for you as a counselor or therapist? Why or why not?
10. In what ways would you need to grow, or what would you need to learn, to be able to use this approach well?

Online Resources

Associations

American Institute of Psychoanalysis
www.aipnyc.org

American Psychological Association, Division 39, Psychoanalysis
www.apa.org

American Psychoanalytic Association
www.apsa.org

Chicago Institute for Psychoanalysis
www.chicagoanalysis.org/

International Association for Relational Psychoanalysis and Psychotherapy
www.iarpp.org

International Psychoanalytic Association
www.ipa.org.uk

Los Angeles Institute and Society for Psychoanalytic Studies
www.laisps.org/

Psychoanalytic Institute of New York
www.psychoanalysis.org/

Journals

Contemporary Psychoanalysis
www.wawhite.org/

Journal of the American Psychoanalytic Association
www.apsa.org

Psychoanalytic Dialogues
www.theanalyticpress.com

References

*Asterisk indicates recommended introductory readings.

Abbass, A. A., Hancock, J. T., Henderson, J., & Kisely, S. (2006). Short-term psychodynamic psychotherapies for common mental disorders. *Cochrane Database of Systematic Reviews,* Issue 4, Article No. CD004687. doi:10.1002/14651858.CD004687.pub3

Abend, S. M. (2001). Expanding psychological possibilities. *The Psychoanalytic Quarterly, 70,* 3–14.

Altman, N. (2008). Origins and evolution of psychoanalytic theory. In J. Frew & M. D. Spiegler (Eds.), *Contemporary psychotherapies for a diverse world* (pp. 41–92). Boston, MA: Houghton Mifflin.

Book, H. E. (1998). *How to practice brief psychodynamic psychotherapy: The core conflictual relationship theme method.* Washington, DC: American Psychological Association.

Brown, L. J. (1981). The therapeutic milieu in the treatment of patients with borderline personality disorder. *Bulletin of the Menninger Clinic, 45,* 377–394.

Cornett, C. (1993). Dynamic psychotherapy of gay men: A view from self psychology. In C. Cornett (Ed.), *Affirmative dynamic psychotherapy with gay men* (pp. 45–76). Lanham, MD: Jason Aronson.

Dworkin, S. H. (2001). Treating the bisexual client. *Journal of Clinical Psychology, 57*(5), 671–680. doi:10.1002/jclp.1036.

Erickson, E. (1994). *Identity and the life cycle.* New York: Norton.

Erickson, E., & Erickson, J. (1998). *The life cycle completed: Extended version*. New York: Norton.

Friedan, B. (1963). *The feminine mystique*. New York: W. W. Norton.

Freud, S. (1900/1974). *The interpretation of dreams*. In J. Strachey (Ed.), *Standard edition of the complete psychological works of Sigmund Freud, Vol. 4*. London: Hogarth Press.

Freud, S. (1931/1961). *Civilization and its discontents (standard edition)*, (J. Strachey, trans.). New York: Norton.

Freud, S. (1963a). *Sexuality and the psychology of love*. (P. Rieff, Ed.). New York: Collier.

Freud, S. (1963b). *Dora: An analysis of a case of hysteria*. (P. Rieff, Ed.). New York: Collier.

Friedman, R. C., & Downey, J. I. (2010). Psychotherapy of bisexual men. *Journal of the American Academy of Psychoanalysis & Dynamic Psychiatry*, *38*(1), 181–197. doi: 10.1521/jaap.2010.38.1.181

Frommer, M. S. (1995). Countertransference obscurity in the psychoanalytic treatment of homosexual patients. In T. Domenici & R. Lesser (Eds.), *Disorienting sexuality: Psychoanalytic reappraisals of sexual identities* (pp. 65–82). London: Routledge.

Gehart, D. (2016). *Theory and treatment planning in counseling and psychotherapy* (2nd ed.). Pacific Grove, CA: Brooks Cole.

Gelman, C. (2004). Toward a better understanding of the use of psychodynamically informed treatment with Latinos: Findings from clinician experience. *Clinical Social Work Journal*, *32*(1), 61–77.

Gill, M. (1982). *The analysis of transference, Vol 1*. New York: International Universities Press.

Glassgold, J. M., & Iasenza, S. (Eds.) (2004). *Lesbians, feminism, and psychoanalysis: The second wave*. Binghamton, NY: Harrington Park Press.

Goleman, D. (1995). *Emotional intelligence*. New York: Bantam.

Greenberg, J. R. (2001). The analyst's participation: A new look. *Journal of the American Psychoanalytic Association*, *49*, 417–426.

*Greenberg, J. R., & Mitchell, S. A. (1983). *Object relations in psychoanalytic theory*. Cambridge: Harvard University Press.

Greene, B. (2004). African American lesbians and other culturally diverse people in psychodynamic psychotherapies: Useful paradigms or oxymoron? In J. M. Glassgold & S. Iasenza (Eds.), *Lesbians, feminism, and psychoanalysis: The second wave* (pp. 57–77). Binghamton, NY: Harrington Park Press.

Horney, K. (1939). *New ways in psychoanalysis*. New York: Norton.

Izzard, S. (2000). Psychoanalytic psychotherapy. In D. Davies & C. Neal (Eds.), *Therapeutic perspectives on working with lesbian, gay and bisexual clients* (pp. 106–121). Maidenhead BRK, England: Open University Press.

Kernberg, O. (1976). *Object relations theory and clinical psychoanalysis*. New York: Jason Aronson.

*Kernberg, O. (1997). Convergences and divergences in contemporary psychoanalytic technique and psychoanalytic psychotherapy. In J. K. Zeig (Ed.), *The evolution of psychotherapy: Third conference* (pp. 3–18). New York: Brunner/Mazel.

Klein, M. (1932/1975). *The psychoanalysis of children* (A. Strachey, trans.; Revised by H. A. Thorner). New York: Delacorte Press.

Kohut, H. (1977). *The restoration of the self*. New York: International Universities Press.

Kohut, H. (1984). *How does analysis cure?* Chicago, IL: University of Chicago Press.

Krupnick, J., Elkin, I., Collins, J., Simmens, S., Sotsky, S., Pilkonis, P., et al. (1994). Therapeutic alliance and clinical outcome in the NIMH Treatment of Depression Collaborative Research Program: Preliminary findings. *Psychotherapy: Theory, Research, Practice, Training*, *31*(1), 28–35. doi:10.1037/0033-3204.31.1.28.

Lachmann, F. (1993). Self psychology: Origins and overview. *British Journal of Psychotherapy*, *10*(2), 226–231. doi: 10.1111/j.1752-0118.1993.tb00651.x.

Leichsenring, F. (2009). Psychodynamic psychotherapy: A review of efficacy and effectiveness studies. In R. A. Levy & J. S. Ablon (Eds.), *Handbook of evidence-based psychodynamic psychotherapy: Bringing the gap between science and practice* (pp. 3–28). New York: Humana Press.

Leone, C. (2008). Couple therapy from the perspective of self psychology and intersubjectivity theory. *Psychoanalytic Psychology*, 25, 79–98. 10.1037/0736-9735.25.1.79.

Levenson, H. (2003). Time-limited dynamic psychotherapy: An integrationist perspective. *Journal of Psychotherapy Integration*, *13*(3–4), 300–333. doi:10.1037/1053-0479.13.3-4.300.

Luborsky, E. B., O'Reilly-Landry, M., & Arlow, J. A. (2008). Psychoanalysis. In R. J. Corsini & D. Wedding (Eds.), *Current psychotherapies* (8th ed.). Pacific Grove, CA: Thompson.

Luborsky, L., & Crits-Christoph, P. (1998). *Understanding transference: The core conflictual relationship theme method* (2nd ed.). Washington, DC: American Psychological Association.

Luborsky, L., & Luborsky, E. (2006). *Research and psychotherapy: The vital link*. Lanham, MD: Jason Aronson.

Mahler, M. Pine, F., & Bergman, A. (1975). *The psychological birth of the human infant*. New York: Basic Books.

Mallinckrodt, B. (2010). The psychotherapy relationship as attachment: Evidence and implications. *Journal of Social and Personal Relationships*, *27*(2), 262–270. doi:10.1177/0265407509360905.

Marci, C. D., & Riess, H. (2009). Physiologic monitoring in psychodynamic psychotherapy research. In R. A. Levy & J. S. Ablon (Eds.), *Handbook of evidence-based psychodynamic psychotherapy* (pp. 339–358). New York: Humana Press.

Marmor, J. (1995). The evolution of an analytic psychotherapist: A sixty-year search for conceptual clarity in the Tower of Babel. In J. K. Zeig (Ed.), *The evolution of psychotherapy: Third conference* (pp. 23–33). New York: Brunner/Mazel.

*McWilliams, N. (1999). *Psychoanalytic case formulation*. New York: Guilford.

Messer, S. B., & Warren, C. S. (1995). *Models of brief psychodynamic therapy: A comparative approach*. New York: Guilford.

*Mitchell, R. R., & Friedman, H. S. (1994). *Sandplay: Past, present, and future*. New York: Routledge.

*Mitchell, S. A. (1988). *Relational concepts in psychoanalysis: An integration*. Cambridge, MA: Harvard University Press.

*Mitchell, S. A., & Black, M. J. (1995). *Freud and beyond: A history of modern psychoanalytic thought*. New York: Basic.

Myers, I. B. (1998). *Introduction to type: A guide to understanding your results on the Myers-Briggs Type Indicator* (6th ed). Gainesville, FL: Center for Applications of Psychological Types.

Pine, F. (1990). *Drive, ego, object, and self*. New York: Basic Books.

Roffman, J. L., & Gerber, A. J. (2009). In R. A. Levy & J. S. Ablon (Eds.), *Handbook of evidence-based psychodynamic psychotherapy* (pp. 305–338). New York: Humana Press.

Rubalcava, L. A., & Waldman, K. M. (2004). Working with intercultural couples: An intersubjective-constructivist perspective. In W. J. Corbin (Ed.), *Transformations in self psychology: Progress in self psychology, Vol. 20* (pp. 127–149). Hillsdale, NJ: Analytic Press.

Rubinstein, G. (2003). Does psychoanalysis really mean oppression? Harnessing psychodynamic approaches to affirmative therapy with gay men. *American Journal of Psychotherapy*, *57*(2), 206–218.

Seligman, M. E. P. (2002). *Authentic happiness: Using the new positive psychology to realize your potential for lasting fulfillment*. New York: Free Press.

*Shedler, J. (2010). The efficacy of psychodynamic psychotherapy. *American Psychologist*, *65*(2), 98–109. doi:10.1037/a0018378.

Shelley, C. (Ed.). (1998). *Contemporary perspectives on psychotherapy and homosexualities*. London: Free Association Press.

Siegel, D. (1999). *The developing mind: How relationships and the brain interact to shape who we are*. New York: Guilford.

Sifneos, P. E. (1979). *Short-term dynamic psychotherapy: Evaluation and technique*. New York: Plenum.

St. Clair, M. (2000). *Object relations and self psychology: An introduction*. Belmont, CA: Brooks/Cole.

*Stiles, W., Barkham, M., Mellor-Clark, J., & Connell, J. (2008). Effectiveness of cognitive-behavioural, person-centred, and psychodynamic therapies in UK primary-care routine practice: Replication in a larger sample. *Psychological Medicine: A Journal of Research in Psychiatry and the Allied Sciences*, *38*(5), 677–688. doi:10.1017/S0033291707001511.

Stolorow, R. D., Brandschaft, B., & Atwood, G. E. (Eds.). (1987). *Psychoanalytic treatment: An intersubjective approach*. Hillsdale, NJ: Analytic Press.

Sullivan, H. S. (1953). *The interpersonal theory of psychiatry*. New York: Norton.

Sullivan, H. S. (1954). *The psychiatric interview*. New York: Norton.

Waldman, K., & Rubalcava, L. A. (2005). Psychotherapy with intercultural couples: A contemporary psychodynamic approach. *American Journal of Psychotherapy*, *59*, 227–245.

Watkins, C. R. (2012). Race/ethnicity in short-term and long-term psychodynamic psychotherapy treatment research: How "White" are the data? *Psychoanalytic Psychology*, *29*(3), 292–307. doi:10.1037/a0027449.

Weissman, M., Markowitz, J., & Klerman, G. (2000). *Comprehensive guide to interpersonal psychotherapy*. New York: Basic Books.

Weissman, M., Markowitz, J., & Klerman, G. (2007). *Clinician's quick guide to interpersonal psychotherapy*. New York: Oxford University Press.

Winnicott, D. W. (1965). *The maturational processes and the facilitating environment: Studies in the theory of emotional development*. New York: International University Press.

Yi, K. (1995). Psychoanalytic psychotherapy with Asian clients: Transference and therapeutic considerations. *Psychotherapy: Theory, Research, Practice, Training*, *32*(2), 308–316. doi:10.1037/0033-3204.32.2.308.

Psychodynamic Case Study: Suicidal Thoughts at Midlife

Ken, a 46-year-old Japanese American male, is referred because he is feeling hopeless and suicidal after being passed up again for a promotion at work. In his youth, his parents strictly enforced his study schedule and minimized time spent hanging out with friends, playing video games, and watching television. He graduated from high school and college at the top of his class and has since pursued a career in computer engineering. Although he is very good at what he does, he has never been able to move into upper management positions, and now fears he never will. He is unmarried mostly because he never made time for relationships in order to pursue his career. He admits he does not think he and his mother would ever agree on a suitable partner, although his mother continues to nag him about having a family. He lives close to his parents, and his mother is still very involved in caring for his apartment, cooking, and cleaning. He has been using pain medication for several years to manage severe back pain.

CASE CONCEPTUALIZATION

Date: August 1, 2013 **Clinician:** Kim **Client/Case #:** 80007

I. Introduction to Client

Identify primary client and significant others

Client

Adult Male Age: 46 Asian American Single heterosexual Occupation/Grade: Senior computer engineer

Other: Japanese (first generation); Lives close to parents

Significant Others

Client's Mother Age: 60 Asian American Married heterosexual Occupation/Grade: Homemaker

Other: Japanese (immigrant)

Client's Father Age: 62 Asian American Married heterosexual Occupation/Grade: Mechanical engineer

Other: Japanese (immigrant)

Select Person Age: ____ Select Ethnicity Select Relational Status Occupation/Grade: ______ Other: ______

Select Person Age: ____ Select Ethnicity Select Relational Status Occupation/Grade: ______ Other: ______

Others: ____________

II. Presenting Concern(s)

Client Description of Problem(s):

Client feels like he has "failed" in life. Although he makes good money, he has been turned down for a promotion into management three times. He feels as though he sacrificed having a family in order to have a successful career and now he has neither. He does not feel he has much to look forward to in the years ahead.

Significant Other/Family Description(s) of Problems: AM's parents believe he should be focusing on getting married and having a family. They are proud of his earning capacity, although they admit to being surprised and a bit ashamed that for the first time he has not been able to achieve the professional goals he has set for himself.

Broader System Problem Descriptions: Description of problem from referring party, teachers, relatives, legal system, etc.:

Boss: Describes AM as bright "one of the most talented system engineers" but not having the "people skills" needed for management.

______: ______

III. Background Information

Trauma/Abuse History (recent and past): AM does not report any physical or sexual abuse but does report his parents were very strict about grades and school "like most of my Asian friends' parents were."

(continued)

Substance Use/Abuse (current and past; self, family of origin, significant others): AM reports using pain medication daily to manage his back pain; he admits needing to take higher and higher doses to manage the pain.

Precipitating Events (recent life changes, first symptoms, stressors, etc.): AM has been passed over for 3 different promotions, the last one going to a colleague 10 years younger and newer to the company. The shame of this recent "passover" has resulted in thoughts of suicide and hopelessness. He reports symptoms of depression and thoughts of suicide on and off since high school, when he first remembers being depressed. However, he reports this most recent episode is the worst he has ever experienced.

Related Historical Background (family history, related issues, previous counseling, etc.): AM's parents immigrated from Japan in the 1960s to start their lives together in a country that would provide better opportunities for their children. They had two children, AM being the youngest; the eldest daughter became a physician and now has a family of her own. The father worked long hours and had a more formal relationship with the children. The mother was highly involved with the children, overseeing their homework, taking them to music lessons, and teaching them proper manners. As is typical of Japanese families, emotional restraint, respect for one's elders, and fulfilling obligations were emphasized. Although AM had a special place in the family as the eldest male, he has never felt that he fully lived up to his father's expectations of him. In contrast, he has always been his mother's favorite, with her protecting him and comforting him in any way she could. He and his sister were opposites, she being more outgoing and enjoying school, he tending to be shy and less willing to pursue rigorous academic study.

IV. Client Strengths and Diversity

Client Strengths

Personal: AM is hard-working, diligient, and respectful of others. He is able to support himself well and is excellent at his job.

Relational/Social: AM stays closely connected with his parents, sister, and relatives in the states. He has two close friends from college with whom he stays connected and has several colleagues with whom he enjoys working.

Spiritual: With no formal practice, AM finds great comfort in common Shinto and Zen Buddhist practices, such as creating sacred space, bonsai gardening, and mindfulness practices.

Diversity: Resources and Limitations

Identify potential resources and limitations available to clients based on their age, gender, sexual orientation, cultural background, socioeconomic status, religion, regional community, language, family background, family configuration, abilities, etc.

Unique Resources: AM has some connections with the Japanese American community; also has some interest in Shinto and Zen practices. He largely attributes his professional success to Japanese cultural values.

(continued)

Potential Limitations: Although in some ways a source of inspiration to pursue a career, AM also experiences his parents' immigrant value of excelling in his career as a form of pressure and at times a heavy burden. When he does live up to their standards and expectations, he feels like a failure because he knows they had to give up much to immigrate to the states, which they say was largely for the benefit of their children.

Complete All of the Following Sections for a Complete Case Conceptualization or Specific Sections for Theory-Specific Conceptualization.

V. Psychodynamic Conceptualization

Psychodynamic Defense Mechanisms

Check 2-4 most commonly used defense mechanisms

❑ Acting Out: *Describe:* ______

☒ Denial: *Describe:* AM uses denial in response to many of his inner conflicts and substance use.

❑ Displacement: *Describe:* ______

☒ Help-Rejecting Complaining: *Describe:* AM often complains (mostly to himself) about being single, but does little to change the situation.

❑ Humor: *Describe:* ______

❑ Passive Aggression: *Describe:* ______

❑ Projection: *Describe:* ______

❑ Projective Identification: *Describe:* ______

❑ Rationalization: *Describe:* ______

❑ Reaction Formation: *Describe:* ______

☒ Repression: *Describe:* AM uses repression to manage urges for greater freedom and expression of self.

❑ Splitting: *Describe:* ______

❑ Sublimation: *Describe:* ______

☒ Suppression: *Describe:* When strong emotions arise, AM suppresses them to avoid inappropriate displays of emotion, which is a common cultural practice.

❑ Other: ______

Object Relational Patterns

Describe relationship with early caregivers in past: AM's mother was highly involved in his life from childhood and extremely overprotective. His father worked often and their relationship was very formal with very few gestures of love or affection.

Was the attachment with the mother (or equivalent) primarily:

❑ Generally Secure ☒ Anxious and Clingy ❑ Avoidant and Emotionally Distant ❑ Other: ______

Was the attachment with the father (or equivalent) primarily:

❑ Generally Secure ❑ Anxious and Clingy ☒ Avoidant and Emotionally Distant ❑ Other: ______

(continued)

Describe present relationship with these caregivers: AM's mother continues to be overprotective of her "baby" and he overrelies on his mother to help him with household responsibilities.

Describe relational patterns with partner and other current relationships: AM at times will avoid his older sister because he feels she is much more successful than him and this makes him feel ashamed.

Erickson's Psychosocial Developmental Stage

Describe development at each stage up to current stage

Trust vs. Mistrust (Infant Stage): AM reports a normal infancy with a devoted mother and a general sense of trust.

Autonomy vs. Shame and Doubt (Toddler Stage): AM reports that shame more than guilt was used to motivate him and his sister to behave; autonomy was not strongly encouraged, especially by his mother at that age.

Initiative vs. Guilt (Preschool Age): Shame more than guilt was used to motivate initiative.

Industry vs. Inferiority (School Age): AM describes himself as "shamed" into industrious behavior and to view inferiority as the ultimate failure.

Identity vs. Role Confusion (Adolescence): AM's identity was increasingly tied to school performance in adolescence; he adhered closely to family roles.

Intimacy vs. Isolation (Young Adulthood): Choosing to excel in work rather than in his personal life, AM did not develop deep intimate connections in young adulthood.

Generativity vs. Stagnation (Adulthood): AM's current crisis is the feeling that he is beginning to stagnate professionally, having already failed to form a family.

Ego Integrity vs. Despair (Late Adulthood): ____________

Adlerian Style of Life Theme

❑ Control: ____________

☒ Superiority: AM's life has been organized around being superior to others in academic and professional contexts, neglecting personal and relational aspects of his life.

❑ Pleasing: ____________

❑ Comfort: ____________

Basic Mistake Misperceptions: AM believes his value and worth are predicated upon his professional accomplishments.

VI. Humanistic-Existential Conceptualization

Expression of Authentic Self

Problems: Are problems perceived as internal or external (caused by others, circumstance, etc.)?

❑ Predominantly internal
☒ Mixed
❑ Predominantly external

(continued)

Agency and Responsibility: Is self or other discussed as agent of story? Does client take clear responsibility for situation?

❑ Strong sense of agency and responsibility

☒ Agency in some areas

❑ Little agency; frequently blames others/situation

❑ Often feels victimized

Recognition and Expression of Feelings: Are feelings readily recognized, owned, and experienced?

❑ Easily expresses feelings

❑ Identifies feelings with prompting

☒ Difficulty recognizing feelings

Here-and-Now Experiencing: Is the client able to experience full range of feelings as they are happening in the present moment?

❑ Easily experiences emotions in present moment

❑ Experiences some present emotions with assistance

☒ Difficulty with present moment experiencing

Personal Constructs and Facades: Is the client able to recognize and go beyond roles? Is identity rigid or tentatively held?

❑ Tentatively held; able to critique and question

❑ Some awareness of facades and construction of identity

☒ Identity rigidly defined; seems like "fact"

Complexity and Contradictions: Are internal contradictions owned and explored? Is client able to fully engage the complexity of identity and life?

❑ Aware of and resolves contradictions

☒ Some recognition of contradictions

❑ Unaware of internal contradictions

Shoulds: Is client able to question socially imposed shoulds and oughts? Can client balance desire to please others and desire to be authentic?

❑ Able to balance authenticity with social obligation

❑ Identifies tension between social expectations and personal desires

☒ Primarily focuses on external shoulds

List shoulds: Client feels he "should" be more successful in his career and be married with children by this point in his life.

Acceptance of Others: Is client able to accept others and modify expectations of others to be more realistic?

❑ Readily accepts others as they are

☒ Recognizes expectations of others are unrealistic but still strong emotional reaction to expectations not being met

❑ Difficulty accepting others as is; always wanting others to change to meet expectations

Trust of Self: Is client able to trust self as process (rather than a stabile object)?

❑ Able to trust and express authentic self

❑ Trust of self in certain contexts

☒ Difficulty trusting self in most contexts

Existential Analysis

Sources of Life Meaning (as described or demonstrated by client): Client describes success in one's career and the ability to provide for a family as the primary purposes in life.

(continued)

General Themes of Life Meaning:

☒ Personal achievement/work
❑ Significant other
❑ Children
☒ Family of origin
❑ Social cause/contributing to others
❑ Religion/spirituality
❑ Other: ___

Satisfaction with and clarity on life direction:

❑ Clear sense of meaning that creates resilience in difficult times
❑ Current problems require making choices related to life direction
❑ Minimally satisfied with current life direction; wants more from life
☒ Has reflected little on life direction up to this point; living according to life plan defined by someone/something else
❑ Other: ___

Gestalt Contact Boundary Disturbances

☒ *Desensitization:* Failing to notice problems
❑ *Introjection*: Take in others' views whole and unedited
❑ *Projection*: Assign undesired parts of self to others
❑ *Retroflection*: Direct action to self rather than other
❑ *Deflection*: Avoid direct contact with another or self
❑ *Egotism:* Not allowing outside to influence self
❑ *Confluence*: Agree with another to extent that boundary blurred

Describe: AM will not acknowledge the impact that his back pain and increasing use of pain medication may be having on his life. He is additionally unaware of his social-skills problems possibly contributing to the reasons why he has been passed up for recent promotions.

VII. Cognitive-Behavioral Conceptualization

Baseline of Symptomatic Behavior

Symptom #1 (behavioral description): Suicidal thinking: mostly passive but increasingly considering plans.

Frequency: 1-3 times per week

Duration: 1-4 hours per episode

Context(s): Home alone; quiet; no tasks to do or people to visit.

Events Before: Long day at work; visiting "successful" sister; parents saying or implying something that suggests he should improve his situation.

Events After: Drinks; takes pain medication to help sleep; watches television or reads news on Internet.

Symptom #2 (behavioral description): Lack of initative or interest in pleasurable activities.

Frequency: Most days

Duration: 3-4 hours

Context(s): After comes home from work; weekends.

(continued)

Events Before: Less than enthusiastic about work in general but able to focus on specific tasks and projects at work; upon arriving home, immediately feels empty and uninterested in anything.

Events After: Watches television; surfs Internet; mother organizes precooked meals for him.

A-B-C Analysis of Irrational Beliefs

Activating Event ("Problem"): Passed up for promotion for third time.

Consequence (Mood, behavior, etc.): Depression; suicidal thinking; overuse of pain medication.

Mediating Beliefs (Unhelpful beliefs about event that result in C):

1. I am a failure.
2. I will never move beyond my current place in the company.
3. I missed my chance to have a family and there is nothing to look forward to.

Beck's Schema Analysis

Identify frequently used cognitive schemas:

❑ *Arbitrary inference:* ________

☒ *Selective abstraction:* Focuses on what he has not achieved rather than what he has achieved and other indicators of success

❑ *Overgeneralization:* ________

❑ *Magnification/Minimization:* ________

☒ *Personalization:* Personalizes neutral comments of others to imply that he is a failure.

☒ *Absolutist/dichotomous thinking:* I am a failure or success; I can have a great career or a family.

❑ *Mislabeling:* ________

☒ *Mindreading:* Assumes silence on the part of others indicates they are judging him.

VIII. Family Systems Conceptualization

Family Life Cycle Stage

☒ Single adult
❑ Marriage
❑ Family with Young Children
❑ Family with Adolescent Children
❑ Launching Children
❑ Later Life

Describe struggles with mastering developmental tasks in one of these stages: While AM would like to get married and have a family, he felt as though he needed to make a choice between that and having a successful career. Now he feels as though it is too late for him to marry and that he will be alone for the rest of his life.

Boundaries with

Parents ☒ Enmeshed ❑ Clear ❑ Disengaged ❑ NA: *Describe:* Mother is overprotective.

Significant Other ❑ Enmeshed ❑ Clear ❑ Disengaged ☒ NA: *Describe:* ________

(*continued*)

Children ❑ Enmeshed ❑ Clear ❑ Disengaged ☒ NA: *Describe:* ______

Extended Family ❑ Enmeshed ❑ Clear ☒ Disengaged ❑ NA: *Describe:* AM has always felt distant from more social and outgoing sister.

Other: Name ❑ Enmeshed ❑ Clear ❑ Disengaged ❑ NA: *Describe:* ______

Typical style for regulating closeness and distance with others: ______

Triangles/Coalitions

☒ Coalition in family of origin: *Describe:* Mother has always protected him from father's criticism and expectations.

❑ Coalitions related to significant other: *Describe:* ______

❑ Other coalitions: ______

Hierarchy between Self and Parent/Child ❑ NA

With own children ❑ Effective ❑ Rigid ❑ Permissive

With parents (for child/young adult) ☒ Effective ❑ Rigid ❑ Permissive

Complementary Patterns with Sister:

❑ Pursuer/distancer

❑ Over-/underfunctioner

❑ Emotional/logical

❑ Good/bad parent

☒ Other: *successful vs. unsuccessful*

Example of complementary pattern: AM feels he has lost competition with sister in terms of success because she has family.

Intergenerational Patterns

Substance/Alcohol Abuse: ❑ NA ☒ History: AM abusing pain medication; no other history of substance abuse in family.

Sexual/Physical/Emotional Abuse: ☒ NA ❑ History: ______

Parent/Child Relations: ❑ NA ☒ History: Hierarchical, structured families, with eldest male close to mothers.

Physical/Mental Disorders: ❑ NA ☒ History: Cancer history in family

Family strengths: Describe: Family supports one another; frequently gets together; want to see AM be happy.

IX. Solution-Based and Cultural Discourse Conceptualization (Postmodern)

Solutions and Unique Outcomes

Attempted Solutions that DIDN'T or DON'T work:

1. Working harder and harder;
2. Focusing all efforts in career and ignoring others;
3. Focusing all efforts in career and ignoring others.

(*continued*)

Exceptions and Unique Outcomes: Times, places, relationships, contexts, etc. when problem is less of a problem; behaviors that seem to make things even slightly better:

1. AM can cook when he wants to entertain friends;
2. AM has been promoted to senior status in division;
3. AM has two close friends from college.

Miracle Question Answer: If the problem were to be resolved overnight, what would client be doing differently the next day? (Describe in terms of doing X rather than not doing Y).

1. AF states he would be recognized by his superiors at work for his hard work and accomplishments.
2. AF would feel more confident in his abilities as a professional.
3. AF would participate in activities where he might potentially meet a romantic partner.

Dominant Discourses informing definition of problem:

- *Ethnic, Class and Religious Discourses: How do key cultural discourses inform what is perceived as a problem and the possible solutions?* AM has adopted cultural values of excelling academically and professionally. He also avoids bringing shame to himself and family. His thoughts of suicide fit within cultural traditions that ascribe honor to suicide as a means of responding to shame and failure. AM has not pursued intimate relationships or developed a family, having difficulty balancing the drive necessary to have a successful career with a relationship and family.
- *Gender and Sexuality Discourses: How do the gender/sexual discourses inform what is perceived as a problem and the possible solutions?* AM's emotional restraint is typical of first-generation Japanese American males, as is his focus on career. He has internalized his professional duties and duties to his family of origin but has not felt ready to also take on the role of being a husband and father, which is experienced as another source of failure and inadequacy.
- *Community, School, and Extended Family Discourses: How do other important community discourses inform what is perceived as a problem and the possible solutions?* As a computer engineer, AM is better relating to logical ideas and things than to people, possibily reinforcing his difficulty with intimate relationships.

Identity Narratives: How has the problem shaped each client's identity? AM is shifting from feeling like a successful person in most areas of life to feeling that he will end his life as a failure. His family is also experiencing signifcant shame for the first time regarding AM, which only compounds his sense of failure.

Local or Preferred Discourses: What is the client's preferred identity narrative and/or narrative about the problem? Are there local (alternative) discourses about the problem that are preferred? AM believes he is intelligent and good at what he does; he does not see how his lack of social skills may be affecting his promotion to a management position. He has also not allowed himself to fulfill his dream for a wife and family, but his desire for this is growing.

CLINICAL ASSESSMENT

Clinician: Kim	Client ID #: 80007	Primary configuration: ☒ Individual ❑ Couple ❑ Family	Primary Language: ☒ English ❑ Spanish ☒ Other: Japanese

List client and significant others

Adult(s)

Adult Male Age: 46 Asian American Single heterosexual Occupation: Senior computer engineer

Other identifier: Japanese, first generation

Select Gender Age: ____ Select Ethnicity Select Relational Status Occupation: ____ Other identifier: ____

Child(ren)

Select Gender Age: ____ Select Ethnicity Grade: Select Grade School: ____ Other identifier: ____

Select Gender Age: ____ Select Ethnicity Grade: Select Grade School: ____ Other identifier: ____

Others: ____

Presenting Problems

		Complete for children:
☒ Depression/hopelessness	❑ Couple concerns	❑ School failure/decline performance
❑ Anxiety/worry	❑ Parent/child conflict	❑ Truancy/runaway
❑ Anger issues	❑ Partner violence/abuse	❑ Fighting w/peers
❑ Loss/grief	❑ Divorce adjustment	❑ Hyperactivity
☒ Suicidal thoughts/attempts	❑ Remarriage adjustment	❑ Wetting/soiling clothing
❑ Sexual abuse/rape	❑ Sexuality/intimacy concerns	❑ Child abuse/neglect
❑ Alcohol/drug use	☒ Major life changes	❑ Isolation/withdrawal
❑ Eating problems/disorders	❑ Legal issues/probation	❑ Other: ____
☒ Job problems/unemployed	❑ Other: ____	

Mental Status Assessment for Identified Patient

Interpersonal	❑ NA	❑ Conflict ❑ Enmeshment ☒ Isolation/avoidance ❑ Harassment ☒ Other: Difficulty connecting with others
Mood	❑ NA	☒ Depressed/Sad ❑ Anxious ❑ Dysphoric ❑ Angry ❑ Irritable ❑ Manic ❑ Other: ____
Affect	❑ NA	☒ Constricted ❑ Blunt ❑ Flat ❑ Labile ❑ Incongruent ❑ Other: ____

(*continued*)

Sleep	❑ NA	☒ Hypersomnia ❑ Insomnia ❑ Disrupted ❑ Nightmares ❑ Other: ______
Eating	❑ NA	❑ Increase ☒ Decrease ❑ Anorectic restriction ❑ Binging ❑ Purging ❑ Other: ______
Anxiety	❑ NA	☒ Chronic worry ❑ Panic ❑ Phobias ❑ Obsessions ❑ Compulsions ❑ Other: ______
Trauma Symptoms	❑ NA	❑ Hypervigilance ❑ Flashbacks/Intrusive memories ❑ Dissociation ☒ Numbing ❑ Avoidance efforts ❑ Other: ______
Psychotic Symptoms	☒ NA	❑ Hallucinations ❑ Delusions ❑ Paranoia ❑ Loose associations ❑ Other: ______
Motor activity/ Speech	❑ NA	☒ Low energy ❑ Hyperactive ❑ Agitated ❑ Inattentive ❑ Impulsive ❑ Pressured speech ❑ Slow speech ❑ Other: ______
Thought	❑ NA	☒ Poor concentration ❑ Denial ☒ Self-blame ❑ Other-blame ☒ Ruminative ❑ Tangential ❑ Concrete ❑ Poor insight ❑ Impaired decision making ❑ Disoriented ❑ Other: ______
Socio-Legal	☒ NA	❑ Disregards rules ❑ Defiant ❑ Stealing ❑ Lying ❑ Tantrums ❑ Arrest/ incarceration ❑ Initiates fights ❑ Other: ______
Other Symptoms	☒ NA	______

Diagnosis for Identified Patient

Contextual Factors considered in making diagnosis: ☒ Age ☒ Gender ☒ Family dynamics ☒ Culture ❑ Language ❑ Religion ❑ Economic ☒ Immigration ❑ Sexual/gender orientation ❑ Trauma ❑ Dual diagnosis/comorbid ☒ Addiction ❑ Cognitive ability ❑ Other: ______

Describe impact of identified factors on diagnosis and assessment process: ______

DSM-5 Code	Diagnosis with Specifier *Include V/Z/T-Codes for Psychosocial Stressors/Issues*
1. F33.2	1. Major Depressive Disorder, Recurrent, Severe
2. r/o F11.20	2. Rule Out: Opioid Use Disorder, Mild
3. Z56.9	3. Other problem related to employment
4. ______	4. ______
5. ______	5. ______

Medical Considerations

Has patient been referred for psychiatric evaluation? ☒ Yes ❑ No

Has patient agreed with referral? ☒ Yes ❑ No ❑ NA

(*continued*)

Psychometric instruments used for assessment: ❑ None ☒ Cross-cutting symptom inventories

☒ Other: Will consult with MD to rule out potential abuse of Percocet

Client response to diagnosis: ❑ Agree ☒ Somewhat agree ❑ Disagree ❑ Not informed for following reason: ____

Current Medications (psychiatric & medical) ❑ NA

1. Percocet; dose 10/650 mg; start date: August 2010
2. Lexapro; dose 10 mg; start date: June 2013
3. ____; dose ____ mg; start date: ____
4. ____; dose ____ mg; start date: ____

Medical Necessity: *Check all that apply*

☒ Significant impairment ❑ Probability of significant impairment ❑ Probable developmental arrest

Areas of impairment: ☒ Daily activities ☒ Social relationships ☒ Health ☒ Work/School ❑ Living arrangement

❑ Other: ____

Risk and Safety Assessment for Identified Patient

Suicidality	Homicidality	Alcohol Abuse
❑ No indication/Denies	☒ No indication/Denies	☒ No indication/denies
☒ Active ideation	❑ Active ideation	❑ Past abuse
☒ Passive ideation	❑ Passive ideation	❑ Current; Freq/Amt: 1-2 drinks; 3-4 nights per week
☒ Intent without plan	❑ Intent without means	**Drug Use/Abuse**
❑ Intent with means	❑ Intent with means	❑ No indication/denies
❑ Ideation in past year	❑ Ideation in past year	❑ Past use
❑ Attempt in past year	❑ Violence past year	❑ Current drugs: Percocet Freq/Amt: 10/650mg or more
❑ Family or peer history of completed suicide	❑ History of assaulting others	❑ Family/sig.other use
	❑ Cruelty to animals	

Sexual & Physical Abuse and Other Risk Factors

❑ Childhood abuse history: ❑ Sexual ❑ Physical ❑ Emotional ❑ Neglect

❑ Adult with abuse/assault in adulthood: ❑ Sexual ❑ Physical ❑ Current

❑ History of perpetrating abuse: ❑ Sexual ❑ Physical ❑ Emotional

❑ Elder/dependent adult abuse/neglect

❑ History of or current issues with restrictive eating, binging, and/or purging

❑ Cutting or other self harm: ❑ Current ❑ Past: Method: ____

❑ Criminal/legal history: ____

❑ Other trauma history: ____

☒ None reported

(continued)

Indicators of Safety

❑ NA

❑ At least one outside support person

❑ Able to cite specific reasons to live or not harm

❑ Hopeful

☒ Willing to dispose of dangerous items

☒ Has future goals

❑ Willingness to reduce contact with people who make situation worse

☒ Willing to implement safety plan, safety interventions

☒ Developing set of alternatives to self/other harm

❑ Sustained period of safety: ____________

❑ Other: ____________

Elements of Safety Plan

❑ NA

☒ Verbal no harm contract

❑ Written no harm contract

☒ Emergency contact card

☒ Emergency therapist/agency number

☒ Medication management

❑ Plan for contacting friends/support persons during crisis

❑ Specific plan of where to go during crisis

☒ Specific self-calming tasks to reduce risk before reach crisis level (e.g., journaling, exercising, etc.)

☒ Specific daily/weekly activities to reduce stressors

❑ Other: ____________

Legal/Ethical Action Taken: ☒ NA ❑ Action: ____________

Case Management

Collateral Contacts

- Has contact been made with treating *physicians or other professionals*: ❑ NA ☒ Yes ❑ In process. Name/Notes: Dr. Rosetti; Aug 15, 2013; Consulted with MD on medication use and potential misuse; MD wants to continue with reduced Rx for Percocet before changing medications.
- If client is involved in mental health *treatment elsewhere*, has contact been made? ❑ NA ☒ Yes ☒ In process. Name/Notes: Pain Management Clinic
- Has contact been made with *social worker*: ☒ NA ❑ Yes ❑ In process. Name/Notes: ____________

Referrals

- Has client been referred for *medical assessment*: ☒ Yes ❑ No evidence for need
- Has client been referred for *social services*: ☒ NA ❑ Job/training ❑ Welfare/Food/Housing ❑ Victim services ❑ Legal aid ❑ Medical ❑ Other: ____________
- Has client been referred for *group* or other support services: ❑ Yes: _____ ❑ In process ☒ None recommended
- Are there anticipated *forensic/legal processes* related to treatment: ☒ No ❑ Yes; describe: ____________

Support Network

- Client social support network includes: ☒ Supportive family ❑ Supportive partner ❑ Friends ❑ Religious/spiritual organization ❑ Supportive work/social group ❑ Other: ____________
- Describe anticipated effects treatment will have on others in support system (children, partner, etc.): May create sense of loss and purposelessness for mother.
- Is there anything else client will need to be successful? ____________

(*continued*)

Expected Outcome and Prognosis

☒ Return to normal functioning ❑ Anticipate less than normal functioning ❑ Prevent deterioration

Client Sense of Hope: 3

Evaluation of Assessment/Client Perspective

How were assessment methods adapted to client needs, including age, culture, and other diversity issues?

Considered gender, age, and ethnic background when assessing for suicide risk and quality of emotional expression.

Describe actual or potential areas of client-clinician agreement/disagreement related to the above assessment:

Client less concerend about Percocet use; will consult with MD to consult on potential need to treat substance abuse.

____________________, __________ ________

Clinician Signature License/Intern Status Date

____________________, __________ ________

Supervisor Signature License Date

TREATMENT PLAN

Date: May 14, 2013 Case/Client #: 13009

Clinician Name: Kim Theory: Psychodynamic

Modalities planned: ☒ Individual Adult ❑ Individual Child ❑ Couple ❑ Family ❑ Group: ________

Recommended session frequency: ☒ Weekly ❑ Every two weeks ❑ Other: ________

Expected length of treatment: 12 months

Initial Phase of Treatment

Initial Phase Counseling Tasks

1. Develop working counseling relationship. *Diversity considerations:* Adapt expressions of emotion and empathy to resonate with client's cultural and gender norms; monitor interpretations to reduce potentially shaming client or his family.

   Relationship building approach/intervention:

   a. Empathy and mirroring to create a safe holding environment for the client; careful not to replicate patterns between client and his overly involved mother and detached father.

2. Assess individual, systemic, and broader cultural dynamics. *Diversity considerations:* Include assessment of client's family immigration history.

   Assessment strategies:

   a. Analyze object relations and selfobject patterns, including expressions in current relationship and family of origin in childhood.

   b. Analyze unconscious conflict underlying depression and role of defense mechanisms in managing depression.

3. Identify and obtain client agreement on treatment goals. *Diversity consideration:* Try to actively involve client in goal-making process and avoid his potential deference to authority figure.

   Goal-making intervention:

   a. Discuss with AM overarching goals, determining client's preference for brief psychodynamic symptom reduction vs. broader long-term goals for personality.

4. Identify needed referrals, crisis issues, and other client needs. *Diversity consideration:* Discuss with client's preferred and culturally appropriate role for his family for managing safety issues.

   a. *Crisis assessment intervention(s):* Assess for severity of suicide potential and substance abuse potential by analyzing defense mechanisms, relational support systems, and ability for AM to manage intense emotions.

   b. *Referral(s):* Referral to psychodynamic group in later phases of treatment to develop ability to create meaningful relations with others.

(continued)

Initial Phase Client Goal

1. Decrease emotional reactivity to perceived threats to self to reduce suicidal thinking and substance misuse.

   Interventions:

   a. Provide empathy using understanding-explaining sequence to reduce AM's perceptions of threats to self and sense of failure.

   b. Mirroring to increase sense of worth and valuing self.

Working Phase of Treatment

Working Phase Counseling Tasks

1. Monitor quality of the working alliance. *Diversity considerations:* Adapt and interpret transference within cultural and gender norms, avoiding interpretations or other comments that may be experienced as shameful to client or his family.

   a. *Assessment Intervention:* Monitor and work through transference and countertransference using a safe, non-shaming approach.

2. Monitor progress toward goals. *Diversity considerations:* To avoid attempts to please counselor or otherwise "be successful," counselor will obtain feedback on progress verbally and in writing, emphasizing the importance of honesty over success in this context.

   a. *Assessment Intervention:* Monitor for changes in behavior and relationships in- and outside of session, asking for specific examples of progress outside and directly asking about progress in session. Outcome Questionnaire to measure client progress.

Working Phase Client Goals

1. Decrease use of denial, repression, and suppression of emotions and vulnerable parts of self to reduce depression, substance use, suicidal thinking.

   Interventions:

   a. Interpretation of the role of defense mechanisms in managing emotions and how they developed in early childhood experiences and are being inappropriately used currently; include discussion of cultural and immigration influences.

   b. Analysis of relational matrix in AM's habits of managing emotions including cultural, gender, and professional influences.

2. Increase ego strength and self-coherence to reduce depression and suicidal behavior.

   Interventions:

   a. Mirroring and empathy to strengthen AM's ability to maintain ego strength in the face of strong emotion and stress.

   b. Dream interpretation and free association to bring sources of inner conflict to conscious awareness.

(continued)

3. Increase sense of personal agency informed by emotional intelligence to reduce avoidance of pleasurable social activities.

   Interventions:

   a. Intersubjective responding and analysis of transference/countertransference to increase client's awareness of self in sessions vs. various emotional-relational contexts.

   b. Working through resistance to translating insight into action and fear about taking risks in personal relationships.

Closing Phase of Treatment

Closing Phase Counseling Task

1. Develop aftercare plan and maintain gains. *Diversity considerations:* Consider cultural and gender issues related to endings; consider potential resource in Japanese American community.

   Intervention:

   a. Analyzing transference and abandonment issues as impending termination approaches.

Closing Phase Client Goals

1. Decrease internal conflicts between socially imposed shoulds and personal desire while increasing personality integration to reduce potential for depression and substance use relapse.

   Interventions:

   a. Dream analysis, free association, and analysis of transference to identify internal conflicts generally and to those related to ending treatment.

   b. Enable client to identify, consciously contain, and successfully manage internal conflicts related to success and failure to allow for fuller personality integration.

2. Increase ability to experience mature dependency and intimacy to reduce social isolation.

   Interventions:

   a. Analyze transference and work through resistance to intimacy, in in-session and out-of-session relationships.

   b. Intersubjective responding to critically examine the unconscious organizing principles the client uses to relate to others.

PROGRESS NOTE FOR CLIENT #13009

Date: August 24, 2013 **Time:** 6:00 ❑ am/☒ pm **Session Length:** ☒ 45 min. ❑ 60 min. ❑ Other: _______ minutes

Present: ☒ Adult Male ❑ Adult Female ❑ Child Male ❑ Child Female ❑ Other: ______________

Billing Code: ❑ 90791 (eval) ☒ 90834 (45 min. therapy) ❑ 90837 (60 min. therapy) ❑ 90847 (family)

❑ Other: ______________

Symptom(s)	Duration and Frequency Since Last Visit	Progress
1: Suicidal thinking	Denies for this week	Progressing
2: Depresssed mood	Moderate; Most days	Progressing
3: Percocet	6 of 7 days; reduced dosage	Progressing

Explanatory Notes on Symptoms: AM denies suicidal thinking and reports mood has been slightly better; choosing more proactive activities in the evening; contacted friend to share current struggle. AM reports asking mother to not do laundry and clean this week to "get some space." AM reports using Percocet within prescribed limits, but is trying to reduce use when possible.

In-Session Interventions and Assigned Homework

Continued exploration of repressed emotions and parts of the self and explored the dual nature of helping him to succeed professionally but not in personal life. AM able to verbalize desire for an intimate partner and family; but strong sense of hopelessness and "it's too late for me." Explored culture, gender, and age issues and unconscious organizing principles that have got him this far.

Client Response/Feedback

AM curious and engaged in understanding underlying dynamics, although often feels disheartened with new insight initially.

Plan

☒ Continue with treatment plan: plan for next session: Continue to explore defenses and object-relations patterns.

❑ Modify plan: ______________

Next session: Date: August 31, 2013 Time: 6:00 ❑ am/☒ pm

Crisis Issues: ☒ No indication of crisis/client denies ☒ Crisis assessed/addressed: describe below

Reports adhering to harm reduction plan and medication management plan.

______________, ______________ ______________

Clinician's Signature License/Intern Status Date

Case Consultation/Supervision ❑ Not Applicable

Notes: Supervisor reviewed safety plan and medication misuse plan; recommended coordinating with MD again. Provided insight into object-relations patterns.

(continued)

Collateral Contact ❑ Not Applicable

Name: Dr. Rosetti Date of Contact: August 15, 2013 Time: 9:00 ☒ am/❑pm

☒ Written release on file: ☒ Sent/ ❑ Received ❑ In court docs ❑ Other: ________

Notes: Consulted with MD on medication use and potential misuse; MD wants to continue with reduced Rx for Percocet before changing medications. Will also refer to physical therapist for pain management.

________, ________ ________

Clinician's Signature License/Intern Status Date

________, ________ ________

Supervisor's Signature License Date

CHAPTER

9

Individual Psychology and Adlerian Counseling

Lay of the Land

Arguably one of the least acknowledged founders of the field, Alfred Adler's work laid the foundation for most forms of modern counseling. Even when not directly cited, elements of his ideas are identifiable in object relations, self psychology, humanistic, cognitive, behavioral, family systems, feminist, multicultural, and postmodern approaches. His approach has been characterized as an analytic-behavioral-cognitive approach that also incorporates systemic elements (Mosak & Maniacci, 1999). A contemporary of Freud and Jung who also worked at the University of Vienna, Adler developed a unique approach to counseling that is distinct from the psychoanalysis of Freud. Although modern practitioners have adapted his work for current times (Carlson, Watts, & Maniacci, 2006; Sweeney, 2009), for the most part Adler's Individual Psychology is practiced using the same key principles and practices identified by Adler in the 1910s. Adler's work has also been applied to group counseling and education (Adler, 1978; Carlson et al., 2006; Sweeney, 2009).

In a Nutshell: The Least You Need to Know

Adlerian counselors believe that in striving for *superiority* and betterment of self, each person develops a *style of life* or *lifestyle*, a characteristic set of attitudes and assumptions that help a person make sense of life (Adler, 1978). This style of life clearly emerges in the first six years of life, but later development and events also shape a person's lifestyle. A person's style of life is the template through which all life events are interpreted; faulty interpretations and mistaken notions cause problems and difficulties. The process of counseling aims to help people correct these *basic mistakes* or faulty notions, enabling them to *consciously choose* a new style of life (you can now understand why Adler and Freud had bitter disagreements over espresso and strudel at Cafe Landtmann).

The counseling process itself is brief (generally less than 20 sessions; Bitter & Nicolls, 2000), present- and future-oriented (with some assessment of the past), and directive (Carlson et al., 2006). The counselor's primary role is *educational*—the counselor helping clients to understand the mistaken beliefs that inform their lifestyle and to help them improve their social relatedness, strive for goals that have meaning, and for mastery of the self. Counselors use *encouragement* to help clients move in the direction of their goals. Through a process of understanding *early recollections*, *the family constellation*, *sibling position*, and *style of life*, clients gain insight and self-understanding. Once insight is achieved, counselors help clients develop the courage to take new action and make new decisions in their life and relationships.

The Juice: Significant Contributions to the Field

If there is one thing you remember from this chapter, it should be ...

Social Interest and Community Feeling

Adlerians believe that humans are innately social creatures (modern translation "genetically wired") (Adler, 1924, 1959; Dreikurs, 1950/1989). As a species, humans need each other to survive. *Social interest* or *community feeling* (literal translation of the German *Gemeinschaftsgefühl*) refers to a person subjectively experiencing a sense that he or she has something in common with other people, is a part of a community, and benefits from cooperating with others in the community (Mosak & Maniacci, 1999). Moreover, Dreikurs (1958) emphasized that it is more than just the feeling of belonging: "The ideal expression of social interest is the ability to play the game [of life] with existing demands for cooperation and to help the group to which one belongs in its evolution closer toward a perfect form of social living. This implies progress without creating unnecessary antagonism" (p. 8).

In part, social interest is demonstrated by a willingness to *give more to the community than one receives in return* (i.e., have a generous spirit; Dreikurs, 1950/1989). More important, the draw toward connection is a central organizing value in a well-adjusted person's life. In contrast, those who "measure their happiness and satisfaction only by what they get ... pay [for their error] in unhappiness and suffering" (p. 6). Laying the foundation for social justice and multicultural awareness, Dreikurs (in translating Adler's words) acknowledges that "sometimes the interests of various groups conflict. In such perplexing situations the social interest causes us to see that the interests of the super-ordinate group, which are justified on the ground of objective needs, have the first claim on us. We certainly want to do what we can to help men to found a society embracing the whole human race" (p. 8).

Assessing for Social Interest

When assessing for social interest, Adlerian counselors listen carefully to how clients describe their lives and problems. The three general types of social interest are as follows (Sweeney, 2009):

	Organizing Question	*Content of Conversation*
High Social Interest	*What* am I doing?	Sharing, enjoying, creating
Low Social Interest: "Successful person"	*How* am I doing?	Power, position, possessions
Low Social Interest: "Failure"	*How* am I doing?	Complaining, blaming, fears, excuses

Big Picture: Overview of Counseling Process

Adlerian counseling involves four stages (Sweeney, 2009):

- *Phase 1: Establish an Egalitarian Relationship*
- *Phase 2: Assess Style of Life and Private Logic*
- *Phase 3: Encourage Insight and Self-Understanding*
- *Phase 4: Educate and Reorientate*

Phase 1: Establish an Egalitarian Relationship

The first phase, described in detail in the "Making Connection" section below, involves making a positive, warm connection with clients in which the counselor focuses on strengths and abilities. Adlerian counselors have utmost hope that every person can find better ways of coping, improve their sense of belonging, and become meaningful contributors to the community.

Phase 2: Assess Style of Life and Private Logic

In the second phase, counselors assess clients' style of life and private logic, which is described in detail in "The Viewing: Case Conceptualization" section below. Typically, the assessment period involves reviewing:

- Level of social interest
- Style of life and private logic
- The family constellation and sibling position
- Early recollections
- DSM diagnosis

Phase 3: Encourage Insight and Self-Understanding

In the third phase, counselors help clients gain better self-understanding, promoting *insight*, albeit a different form of insight than is typical in psychoanalytic approaches. In Adlerian work, counselors use insight as an *impetus* and source of positive motivation to take action and make changes, rather than insight being an end in itself. In this phase, the counselor offers possible *interpretations* of behavior by identifying underlying motivations for problems, such as feelings of inferiority motivating a person's avoidance of commitment in a love relationship. Unlike Freudian interpretation, Adlerians *collaboratively* work with clients to find useful, meaningful interpretations of client motivations rather than relying on the counselor's objective perspective to determine the correct interpretation.

Phase 4: Educate and Reorientate

The final phase involves taking action! Counselors challenge clients to develop the *courage* it takes to make life changes based on their insights. These changes in behavior are referred to as a *reorientation*, referring to the fact that a person must "reorient" to life by correcting *basic mistakes* in their *style of life*. This phase involves primarily motivating the client to take action based on education about more accurate and effective approaches to life.

Making Connection: Counseling Relationship

Egalitarian

Taking a radical position during a time when psychoanalysis dominated the field, Adler promoted *egalitarian* relationships with clients that allowed them to maintain a sense of agency and choice (Sweeney, 2009). Counselors should not see themselves as superior even though they are in a helping position. Instead, Adlerian counselors—who do offer interpretations and education—approach clients from a more humble position of having something of potential usefulness for clients, understanding that what is offered may or may not be actually useful in the client's subjective world.

Encouragement

One of its most distinguishing elements, "The Adlerian approach is characterized by its deliberate efforts to encourage the patient" (Dreikurs, 1950/1989, p. 88). However, Adlerian encouragement should not be confused with a Pollyanna, cheerleader-ish, "Just Do It" form of encouragement. Instead, Adlerian encouragement comes from a philosophical presupposition that life problems are not the result of personal failure or innate character flaws—as it may seem to a person experiencing a sense of *personal inferiority*—but rather they are the result of mistaken beliefs about life (a position also adopted in cognitive counseling). Thus, Adlerians are optimistic and hopeful about helping clients resolve their problems, and thus they believe beyond a shadow of a doubt that clients can improve their lives and therefore encourage them to do so.

Described as "a friendly, jovial, concerned person, filled with common sense, an ideal 'uncle'" (Manaster & Corsini, 1982, p. 168), Adler's style of encouraging fuses warmth, honesty, and practicality. To effectively convey encouragement, counselors must do it both verbally and nonverbally, which includes smiling, listening attentively, being patient, and taking action when needed (Sweeney, 2009). In the case study at the end of this chapter, the counselor uses encouragement extensively to help Helga, who was sexually abused as a child and currently experiences panic and agoraphobia, take risks and develop stronger social connections.

Empathy and Social Interest

Counselors should be role models for social interest (see detailed definition below), which Adler defined as inherently requiring empathy. Adler refers to an unidentified "English author" who provides the best definition of social interest and social feeling that he could find at that time: "To see with the eyes of another, to hear with the ears of another, to feel with the heart of another" (Ansbacher & Ansbacher, 1956, p. 135). Carlson et al. (2006) liken this quality of social interest on the part of the counselor to Carl Rogers's empathy (see Chapter 10). Similarly, Carlson et al. (2006) link Adler's concept of encouragement to Rogers's core condition of unconditional positive regard, because both approaches share a fundamental assumption: valuing clients for their humanity.

Directive

The final aspect of the counseling relationship initially seems at odds with the preceding three. Adlerian counselors are directive (Carlson et al., 2006). How can a counselor be egalitarian and at the same time be directive? The catch is that their directiveness comes in the form of *education*: providing practical and helpful information. The key is a teaching style that is "encouraging" and nonhierarchical. The underlying message is: "I am offering you some information I believe to be useful; you can take it or leave it." Thus, they are not pushy salespeople. They educate with enthusiasm and hope, and thus, their clients are generally willing pupils.

The Viewing: Case Conceptualization

Social Interest (also see "The Juice") and Individual Inferiority

Adler explains that a sense of *individual inferiority* impairs a person's social interest. *Individual inferiority* is one of three forms of inferiority posited by Adler (Dreikurs, 1950/1989):

1. *Biological inferiority:* Based on the need to form groups for physical survival; this form of inferiority promotes social interest.
2. *Cosmic inferiority:* Recognizing the inevitable death and the limitations of human existence; this form of inferiority also promotes social interest.
3. *Personal inferiority:* Feeling less powerful, able, or valued than others; this form of inferiority *inhibits* social interest because one does not feel as if he/she belongs to the community.

This sense of personal inferiority is the source of a client's presenting problem: "any person who labors under a sense of inferiority always tries to obtain power of some kind in order to cancel the supposed superiority of other people. His feeling of inferiority impels him to strive for significance" (p. 22); when this becomes a pattern, it is called an *inferiority complex*, a term that has trickled into popular vernacular (Mosak & Maniacci, 1999).

People respond to inferiority in two primary ways: (a) to gain significance by achievement or (b) to avoid obligation, risky decisions, and connection with others. The pursuit of outstanding achievement can contribute to society even if fueled by fear; however, people who are ruthless and unethical in these pursuits waste their lives on what Adler terms "the useless side of life" (p. 24). The counselor's role is to encourage people to transform their sense of inferiority to more effectively promote their social interest and eventually to reduce their overall sense of inferiority.

Lifestyle Assessment

Lifestyle assessment is the heart of Adlerian assessment and case conceptualization. Mosak and Maniacci (1999) define lifestyle as "the individual's characteristic way of thinking, seeing, and feeling toward life and is synonymous with what other theorists call 'personality.'" (p. 31). Adler used style of life liberally and variously to refer to the self, personality, unity of the personality, individuality, method of facing problems, opinion of self, view of life problems, and general attitude toward life (Ansbacher & Ansbacher, 1956). Most commonly, in modern Adlerian counseling, a person's style of living refers to their fundamental beliefs about what is valuable in life, what is ideal, and what is to be avoided. Adler cautions that a person's style of living is not immediately apparent: "As long as a person is in a favorable situation, we cannot see his style of life clearly. In new situations, however, where he is confronted with difficulties, his style of life appears clearly and distinctly" (Ansbacher & Ansbacher, 1956, p. 173). Adler believed that a person's style of life becomes fixed by age five, and general research on personality development supports this claim (Manaster & Corsini, 1982).

Both Sweeney (2009) and Carlson et al. (2006) have developed contemporary approaches to lifestyle assessment. Typically, the following areas are assessed:

- *Parenting Style*
- *Family Constellation and Birth Order*
- *Early Recollections*
- *Basic Mistakes*
- *Organ Inferiority or Physical Weak Points*
- *"The Question": Function of Symptom*
- *Dreams*

Parenting Style

Adler was particularly concerned about two parenting styles: pampering and neglect, with the former having more detrimental effects than the latter (Mosak & Maniacci, 1999). His concern with pampered children was that they are accustomed to "getting," and that they demand whatever they want and thus develop low levels of social interest and do not thrive as adults. In contrast, a neglected child may suffer but is more likely to develop social interest and pursue self-improvement. However, he noted that children were not passive recipients, but rather, children and parents mutually shaped each others' behavior. Adler believed that it was the child's *subjective* perception of the parenting style that ultimately most affected a person's style of life.

Family Constellation and Birth Order

Debated for over 134 years, little consensus has emerged on the effect of birth order on personality (Hartshorne, Salem-Hartshorne, & Hartshorne, 2009). Nearly 200 empirical studies on birth order have yielded significant results; however, it is extremely difficult to control for other variables, such as age, age differences between siblings, the family's social status, ethnic background, and so on (Mills & Mooney, 2013). Issues such as only children, twins, divorce, and blended families have rarely been addressed at all in this literature (Mills & Mooney, 2013).

Adler considered birth order an important—but not determining—variable in understanding human behavior (Sweeney, 2009). However, research over the years has yielded no definitive answer as to whether and how birth order affects development, in part because many past studies did not control for socioeconomic status and ethnicity, both of which are frequently correlated with larger family size (Hartshorne et al., 2009; Sweeney, 2009). However, better-controlled research on birth order continues. For example, a recent study supports the idea that people are more likely to form close friendships and romantic relationships with persons of the same birth order (Hartshorne et al., 2009).

- *Oldest Child:* The oldest child generally begins life as the center of attention and typically learns to take the "newcomers" in stride if the parents provide encouragement for them to recognize their place in the family structure (Sweeney, 2009). Oldest children tend to relate well with adults, assume social responsibility, and develop socially appropriate forms of coping. Their lifestyle often includes striving for superiority, which may be a problem if not moderated over time.
- *Second Child:* The second child will typically pursue an opposite position than the first, because that is the role most readily available to them. On average, they may be less responsible, more independent, or more demanding than their older sibling.

In some cases, the second child strives to be number one, creating *sibling rivalry*, especially if parents do not discourage the competition and comparisons. Some give up in discouragement, while others are socially productive even though they are motivated by the mistaken belief that their value comes from their achievements.

- *Middle Child:* Families of three or more have middle children, who may feel "squeezed" between the others. Being neither the first nor youngest child, many feel like they do not have a clear or unique role to play in the family. Similar to second children, middle children generally tend to define themselves in the opposite direction of their older sibling(s). They may be more independent, sensitive, or even rebellious, and some may directly ask parents for reassurance of their love. A benefit of their position, many learn to be skilled mediators, cope well with social stress, and learn from the mistakes of others (namely their older siblings)—often with minimal gloating or name calling.
- *Youngest Child:* Perhaps the most frequently referred-to family role, the "baby of the family" tends to enjoy being the center of attention and indulgence, given that there are so many people in the family to take care of their needs. Youngest children often grow up to be charming or even manipulative and often avidly seek life's pleasures. If the parents emphasize achievement, they may work hardest of all to prove their place and ultimate worth.
- *Only Child:* Only children are much like older children except that they are never dethroned and generally do not have the pressure of a close competitor. Only children tend to be inducted into the adult world early, becoming responsible, cooperative, and mature for their age. However, many have difficulty relating to their peers, especially in the area of sharing.

Try It Yourself

Find a partner and discuss how you and your siblings fit or do not fit these roles.

Early Recollections

Adler used early childhood recollections as a means for understanding a person's style of life (Ansbacher & Ansbacher, 1956). *Early recollections* refer to a person's earliest clear memories of an event or situation. Often these reveal the source of fundamental beliefs about one's values, others, or life more generally. They tend to be definitive moments that often play a mythic role in a person's life: feeling left out at the playground, picking apples with your mother, or going for a car ride with dad. Generally, a minimum of three memories is required to identify a pattern. However, depending on the complexity of themes, more may be necessary to get to obtain a clearer understanding of how various elements of the lifestyle were developed.

Basic Mistakes

Basic mistakes are faulty assumptions that develop in childhood as children make sense of their experiences, such as loneliness, parental anger, disappointment, traumas, and loss. To some extent, everyone enters adulthood with mistaken notions. However, when basic mistakes lead to a sense of *inferiority* and *low social interest*, a person is more likely to develop symptoms and end up in a counselor's office.

Mosak and Maniacci (1999) elaborate on this by identifying five types of basic mistakes:

1. *Overgeneralizations:* People who overgeneralize tend to exaggerate contextual truths into global all-or-nothing truths (e.g., "my boyfriend cheated on me" gets translated into "men can't be trusted").
2. *False or impossible goals of security:* Some people try to find ways to remove all risk from life, often making unreasonable demands on others (e.g., "If you love me you will never hurt me"—even unintentionally—a great romantic ideal but difficult to achieve if flesh-and-blood humans are involved. Virtual realities may eventually hold different possibilities).

3. *Misperceptions of life and life's demands:* Some basic mistakes boil down to not really understanding the inescapable rules of life: people die, survival takes effort, survival requires cooperation, kindness matters, laws of nature apply evenly, hurting another ultimately hurts you, life doesn't come with guarantees, and so on (e.g., "I want to fall in love with someone who I know won't hurt me": again, a Labrador Retriever may be your best option).
4. *Minimization or denial of one's basic worth:* In other cases, a person has gladly owned their sense of personal inferiority and has come to deny their own intrinsic worth (e.g., "Why would anyone want to love me; I am inherently flawed").
5. *Faulty values:* Alternately, some people cope with life by identifying with faulty values, values that are not in line with social interest but instead with self-promotion (e.g., "If I am successful enough and achieve enough, people will *have to* love me").

Assessing a person's basic mistakes is tricky in that there isn't a simple set of questions to ask. The counselor must tease it out by asking about the family constellation, early recollections, and current problems. However, a careful and thoughtful initial assessment process with an eye toward identifying basic mistakes generally makes this process far easier.

Organ Inferiority or Physical Weak Points

Odd to the modern English ear, *organ inferiority* is the term used by Adler to refer to physically weak points in the body. They are the physical parallel to the basic mistake: "what organ inferiorities are to the body, basic mistakes are to the mind" (Carlson et al., 2006, p. 90). Either actual physical problems or the belief that one is physically inferior can have significant impacts on one's style of life. When Adler used the term he typically referred to children who were blind, had physical deformities, or chronic illnesses that characterized the turn of the 20th century. In modern contexts, these physical issues often include a person's perception of weight, looks, or athletic ability in comparison to peers—or in the case of most young American women, airbrushed supermodels.

Dream Analysis

Like Freud, Adler believed dream analysis provided insight into a client's inner processes; however, unlike Freud, he didn't believe they were related to infantile sexual wishes (Ansbacher & Ansbacher, 1956). Instead, he used the themes of dreams as clues to help analyze a client's style of life and to help identify potential solutions to problems. Furthermore, Adler believed that *the meaning of a dream was specific to the dreamer* and that the counselor was not in the position to have the final determination of their interpretation. For example, people who have dreams with themes of being hampered by obstacles unable to reach destinations or meet up with an important person will likely have similar themes of feeling that the *world* [not their choices or actions] is keeping them from achieving their goals.

"The" Question: Purpose of Symptom

Saving the best for last, *The Question* is used to assess the underlying purpose and need for the symptom (Ansbacher & Ansbacher, 1964; Carlson et al., 2006). The question is as follows:

"The" Question

"What would be different in your life if you didn't have this problem" (Carlson et al., 2006, p. 110).

Try It Yourself

Answer this question as it relates to a current challenge in your life. Do it with a partner verbally or alone in writing.

The client's response often provides clues as to what is being avoided by having the symptoms. For example, one depressed person may say that he would be more successful at work while another may state that she would "be the old self" again who used to spend time with friends. The first response belies insecurities in his ability to succeed at work, and in the second she may fear that enjoying herself apart from her family reflects on her poorly as a mother and wife. More recently, solution-based counselors use the *miracle question*, which is a variation of Adler's original question (see Chapter 13). In the case study at the end of this chapter, the counselor uses "the question" to assess the purpose of Helga's panic and agoraphobia.

Psychodynamic Formulation

When assessing a person's style of life, Adlerians also consider basic psychodynamic formulation in the function of symptom (Carlson et al., 2006). They use three general categories for clients in their psychodynamic formulation: neurotic (emotional disturbance expressed through physical or mental disturbance; behavior is generally within social norms); psychosis (loss of contact with reality); or personality disorder (chronic behavioral pattern that significantly impedes relationships). Adlerians use the basic guidelines for understanding the client's style of life.

Type of Person	Response to Challenge
Encouraged person	"Can-do" attitude. Able to take needed action without worrying about what others think.
Persons with neurotic symptoms	"Yes-but" attitude: "I would take action if I didn't have this problem." They use their symptoms to get away with doing what they want (avoiding social interest) while still receiving social approval ("my symptom is the problem").
Persons with psychotic symptoms	Escapist attitude. They live in fantasy rather than reality to escape life's demands. They say "no" to society's demands.
Persons with personality disorders	"My way or the highway" attitude. They try to convince others that their way is the right way, regardless of what others want or evidence to the contrary: "I'll cooperate if we use my rules."

Life Tasks

Adlerian assessment also involves identifying a person's level of social interest in the six life tasks (Ansbacher & Ansbacher, 1956; Carlson et al., 2006; Dreikurs & Mosak, 1967; Mosak & Dreikurs, 1967; Sweeney, 2009):

- *Work:* Not limited to gainful employment, "work" refers to a person's primary means of being a contributing member of society and can include education, household chores, child care, homemaking, and volunteer activities.
- *Communal life and friendship:* Connecting socially with others and enjoying connections with others is an important life task and measure of a person's social interest.
- *Love relationships:* Perhaps the most challenging of all, love relationships require courage and the greatest level of social interest to sustain.
- *Self-acceptance:* A modern addition that is implied in Adler's original work, developing an accepting relationship of the self, as well as self-awareness, is foundational to successful relating to others.
- *Spirituality:* More recently, Adlerians have added developing a relationship to something greater than the self as a critical life task.

- *Parenting:* Although not applicable to everyone, parenting requires a particular set of social skills and functioning that should be assessed separately from others.

A balanced life involves active and successful involvement in all of these areas of life. Thus, in assessment, counselors should identify the areas in which a person functions best and areas where there are the most problems. In treatment planning, specific goals should be written for each area. Manaster and Corsini (1982) have their clients rate the percentage of happiness in each area before and after counseling to measure progress.

Targeting Change: Goal Setting

Long-Term Goal: The Courage to Develop Social Interest

Adler defined *normal adjustment* as having "enough energy and courage to meet the problems and difficulties of life as they come along" (Ansbacher & Ansbacher, 1956, p. 154). Life difficulties can occur within any of the six life tasks: work, love, friendship, spirituality, self-acceptance, or parenting. Greater levels of social interest improve functioning in each of these areas (Dreikurs, 1950/1989). Thus, Adlerian counseling requires clients to develop the *courage* they need to face their insecurities and go to the places and do the things that they fear most; the counselor's role is to encourage clients to take the risks needed to develop the social interest needed to fulfill their life tasks.

Wellness, Positive Psychology, and Social Interest

Modern Adlerians have explored the links between social interest and positive psychology wellness research (Carlson et al., 2006; Leak & Leak, 2006; Myers, 2009). Both Adlerian theory and positive psychology emphasize building upon and developing strengths (rather than remedying weaknesses) as the preferred approach to addressing strengths. In addition, both approaches set long-term goals of *wellness* as opposed to health—wellness referring to a state of physical, emotional, and social well-being that is achieved through conscious effort, and health referring to a more neutral state in which one is not ill and that does not require effort (Myers, 2009). The Adlerian primary goal of developing social interest correlates with positive psychologists' findings that social connection, altruism, empathy, and social consciousness are highly correlated with happiness (Leak & Leak, 2006). Similarly, Adlerian theory's emphasis on developing social interest within the six life tasks aligns with positive psychology research that emphasizes that meaningful relationships, satisfying work, self-acceptance, and spirituality are all strongly linked to life satisfaction (Myers, 2009). Thus, when setting goals, Adlerian counselors can also draw upon a wellness perspective that emphasizes personal choices and positive actions that lead to a sense of sustainable wellness; simply reducing symptom frequency is only a first step in achieving this long-term goal. Furthermore, like Adlerian counseling, wellness counseling involves psychoeducation in positive psychology and the correlates of happiness.

Developing Adlerian Goal Statements

General Principles Adlerian theory provides clear guidelines for how to develop early, working, and closing phase goals.

- *Early Phase Goals:* Address initial crisis symptoms.
- *Working Phase Goals:* Reduce symptoms related to presenting problem; increase social interest and functioning in life tasks most closely related to the problem.
- *Closing Phase Goals:* Increase social interest and functioning in other key areas of functioning.

Examples of Early and Middle Phase Goals Early and middle phase goals aim to reduce insecurities and basic mistakes that are fueling the presenting problem(s).

- "Reduce insecurities that lead to depressive thinking."
- "Reduce insecurities that fuel jealousy in relationship."
- "Reduce insecurities that lead to underfunctioning at work."
- "Develop more realistic expectations of performance at work."

- "Reduce the tendency to overgeneralize that leads to arguments with spouse."
- "Increase ability to take risks in relationships, to increase sense of intimacy."
- "Reduce tendency to calculate self-worth based on work performance."

Examples of Late Phase Goals Late phase goals aim to take the client beyond basic health (lack of symptoms) and toward developing habits of living that promote wellness and social interest in all six areas of functioning: work, friendship, love, self-acceptance, spirituality, and parenting.

- "Increase intimacy and connection with family of origin."
- "Increase sense of connection with friends and local community."
- "Increase sense of connection to divine by reconnecting with spiritual practice."
- "Increase self-acceptance related to sexual orientation."
- "Increase emotional connection and redefine relationships with adult children."
- "Take steps to pursue line of work (or volunteering) that is personally satisfying."

The Doing: Interventions

Psychoeducation and Task Setting

Perhaps their predominant type of intervention, Adlerians use psychoeducation in all phases of counseling (Carlson et al., 2006). Psychoeducation involves providing clients with psychological information that they can use to change their thoughts, feelings, and/or behaviors. For psychoeducation to be practically useful, counselors need to follow up by setting up specific tasks based on the new information (Sweeney, 2009). In the case study at the end of this chapter, the counselor uses psychoeducation to help Helga understand her diagnosis of Panic with Agoraphobia, to develop a sense of safety that was lost after being sexually abused, and to develop effective social and intimate relationships.

Phase 1 Topics for Psychoeducation: Establish an Egalitarian Relationship

- Describing client's role and rights in the counseling process, including when setting goals and deciding what to discuss.
- Explaining how Adlerian counseling can address the presenting problem and how it works.
- Defining social interest and its role in the client's problem.

Phase 2 Topics for Psychoeducation: Assess Lifestyle and Private Logic

- Providing a rationale for the assessment process.
- Defining lifestyle and describing how private logic develops and how it is related to the presenting problem.

Phase 3 Topics for Psychoeducation: Encourage Insight and Self-Understanding

- Offering information and research results that counter the inaccurate and/or unrealistic private logic that fuels the problem.
- Providing an explanation of the style of life psychological processes based on Adlerian theory.

Phase 4 Topics for Psychoeducation: Education and Reorientation

- Providing convincing research and theoretically based information to motivate clients to take new action related to a specific problem.
- Offering specific instructions on how best to approach changing behaviors or habits of thought.

Interpretation of Symptoms

During the third phase of Adlerian counseling, counselors "interpret" the purpose of symptoms to provide the client's insight into their situation. Distinct from psychoanalytic forms of interpretation, Adlerian interpretation attempts to identify *the purpose of the symptom* and its role in the client's style of life (Ansbacher & Ansbacher, 1956; Sweeney, 2009).

For example, based on the lifestyle assessment, a counselor may interpret a person's procrastination as a way of avoiding taking a risk and possibly failing. General guidelines for offering Adlerian interpretations include:

- *Purpose Focused:* The interpretation should focus on the *goal* or *purpose* of a *behavior* (e.g., procrastination) and avoid globally labeling the person (e.g., lazy, fearful, lacking drive, and such).
- *Tentatively Offered:* Interpretations should be offered *tentatively* rather than as unquestionable truths (e.g., "Could it be that you procrastinate to avoid taking the risk of failing"?).
- *Open to Revision:* Counselors should encourage and allow the client to rephrase or even correct the counselor (e.g., "It's not so much that I am avoiding risk as much as I am simply afraid to fail" or "No, I don't think that is my issue. I think I am saying yes to things I don't want to do").
- *Strengths Emphasis:* The overall tone of the interpretation process should be encouraging, highlighting potential strengths, hope, and resilience (e.g., "So in some ways the procrastination has served to create a sense of safety; but it seems that you may not need that as much as you did in the past.").

Self-Concept Statements

Adlerians listen for *self-concept statements*, which are statements client make that reveal how they see themselves. Carlson et al. (2006) identify three types of self statements that counselors target for intervention:

1. *Inferiority-Based Self Statements:* The client's self-concept falls short of his/her *personal* self-ideal (e.g., "I am stupid, worthless, etc.).
2. *Inadequacy-Based Self Statements:* The client's self-concept falls short of what the client believes is the "worldview" or cultural values (e.g., "I am incompetent, a fool, a loser, etc.").
3. *Guilt-Based Self Statements:* The client's self-concept falls short of ethical or moral beliefs (e.g., I'm bad, evil, unforgivable, etc.).

When counselors hear these types of statements, they help the client explore the comparison process and how to develop more useful, fair, and accurate comparisons. In some cases, clients are making poor decisions about which they feel guilty; the counselor then helps them identify how this happened and how to remedy it. In other cases, clients rigidly try to apply unrealistic standards of superiority; counselors can help these clients explore how they developed these and replace them with more realistic and fair evaluations of themselves. In the case study at the end of this chapter, the counselor uses self statements to help Helga regain her confidence and self-esteem, which diminished greatly after she was sexually abused as a child.

Challenging and Reframing Basic Mistakes and Private Logic

Once clients have achieved sufficient insight, counselors may directly *challenge* the logic or realism of a person's private logic or more gently *reframe* belief so that it is more useful. An example of challenging basic mistakes, counselors may ask clients who believe they must be superior to others "what would happen if everyone had that belief?" (Carlson et al., 2006, p. 140). Counselors can then follow up with questions that highlight the impossibility of a world in which all people are better than everyone else and the ugliness of a world in which everyone lived by this belief. Similarly, in many cases negative situations can be *reframed* in more positive ways. For example, "The upside of worrying is that you tend to be good with details." Counselors can use positive reframing to simultaneously encourage clients and undo basic mistakes.

Natural and Logical Consequences

Introduced by Dreikurs, consequences take two forms in Adlerian counseling—natural and logical—and are primarily used with children (Mosak & Maniacci, 1999; Sweeney, 2009). *Natural consequences* require no conscious human intervention; they occur as part of the physical or social environment. If a child does not do his homework, he loses points, does not learn, and his grades suffer. If you say harsh words to your friend, you weaken or lose the friendship. Whenever possible, Adlerian counselors encourage parents to use natural consequences to help children and others learn from experience. However, if natural consequences are not readily apparent or sufficient, then logical consequences are used instead to *encourage* children to make better decisions (e.g., if you are unable to keep your toys neat and tidy, then you have more toys than you can manage, and some will be taken away until you can manage what you have effectively). Such consequences and encouragement are preferred to behavioral systems of punishment and reward.

Antisuggestion

A classic Adlerian technique, the *antisuggestion* is a type of *paradoxical technique*. The antisuggestion involves the counselor taking the paradoxical position of discouraging change and/or encouraging the symptom, particularly when the client claims that a symptom is "uncontrollable" (e.g., worrying or getting nervous; Ansbacher & Ansbacher, 1956; Carlson et al., 2006; Sweeney, 2009). Antisuggestions can be used in session or out of session. For example, in situations where this is appropriate and safe, the counselor can suggest that the client practice exaggerating a symptom, such as spending extra time worrying every morning:

> "For the next week, I want you to set a timer and worry for ten minutes before you leave the house. If you find you run out of things to worry about after a few minutes, I want you to really try to find more things to worry about. If you want to worry later in the day, that is fine, too. But I want you to schedule ten minutes each morning and do it whether you feel like it or not."

Clients who follow through on this task will quickly gain insight into how they generate worry and anxiety. When asked to worry on cue, it is difficult, even for those with an anxiety disorder. In the process of "forcing" the symptom, the client gains more and more control over it; thus, when it spontaneously occurs, clients are better able to consciously stop worrying.

Spitting in the Soup

An attention-grabbing name for a counseling technique and more hygienic than it sounds, *spitting in the soup* refers to making overt the covert benefits and hidden power of having a symptom. Once the ulterior benefits of the symptoms are revealed, the symptom leaves a "bad taste." Here are some examples:

- "The one benefit of depression is that you have gotten everyone in your family to pay more attention to you."
- "You must have reached near rock-star status to have everyone in the subway looking at you."
- "The nice part about panic is that you get your wife to end the shopping trip early—it even saves you money."
- "It must be very rewarding to know that no other mother at the school worries this much about her children."
- "The great part about temper tantrums is that it fills up your toy chest fast."

Reflecting As If

A contemporary intervention based on Adler's original work, *reflecting as if* is used to help clients deconstruct and shift their mistaken beliefs (Watts, 2013). In the first of three phases, the counselor uses reflective questions to help the client identify how they would be acting differently if they were more the person they hope to be.

Reflecting As If Questions: Phase 1

- If you were behaving more like the person you would like to be, how would you be acting differently? Describe your actions to me as if we were watching it on video.
- What are some indications that you are headed in the right direction?

- If a person met you a few months from now, when you are more like the person you want to be, what would they notice about you?

The counselor writes down the client's response to these questions without critique. In some cases, counselors may need to prompt for more specific answers, such as when a client simply says they will be "happier"; the clinician might then follow up with: "Describe what you will be doing differently when you are happier."

In the second phase, the counselor and client start listing the "as if" behaviors that are associated with moving toward the client's goals. This list is then rank-ordered from easiest to most difficult. Then, in the third phase, the client and counselor begin identifying the easier behaviors to start implementing. Encouragement is prominent in this phase, as clients implement increasingly difficult behaviors associated with their desired goals.

Putting It All Together: Adlerian Case Conceptualization and Treatment Plan Templates

Theory-Specific Case Conceptualization: Adlerian

The prompts below can be used to develop a *theory-specific case conceptualization* using Adlerian theory. The cross-theoretical case conceptualizations at the end of each theory chapter provide examples for writing a conceptualization that includes key elements of this theory-specific conceptualization. Comprehensive examples of theory-specific case conceptualizations are available in *Theory and Treatment Planning in Counseling and Psychotherapy* (Gehart, 2016).

Lifestyle assessment includes the following:

- *Social interest and inferiority*
  - *High social interest:* generally has few symptoms or mild presenting issues
  - *Low social interest, successful person:* power, position, possessions
  - *Low social interest, failure:* complaining, blaming, fears, excuses
- *Parenting style:* Describe:
  - General character of each parent (primary caregivers), including personalities, trauma histories, values, ethnic/religious background, and such.
  - Quality of client's relationship with parents (primary caregivers) and their parenting styles.
  - Whether physical, psychological, and emotional needs were taken care of.
  - How client got what he/she wanted from parents.
- *Family constellation and birth order:* Describe family organization, including:
  - Client's birth order: oldest, second, middle, youngest, or only child.
  - Role of siblings in client's and family's life.
- *Earliest recollections:* Describe two to five of the client's earliest recollections, including:
  - Memory narrative
  - Most vivid moment of the memory
  - Predominant feeling associated with the memory
- *Organ inferiority or physical weak points:* Describe any physical weaknesses or limitations.
- *Role of symptom:* Describe the client's answer to the question: what would be different in your life if you didn't have the problem?
- *Basic mistakes:* Describe the client's basic mistake beliefs, including those related to:
  - Overgeneralization
  - False or impossible goals of security
  - Misperceptions of life and life's demands
  - Minimization or denial of one's basic worth
  - Faulty values

- *Style of life theme:* Describe basic theme of client's style of life:
  - *Control*
  - *Superiority*
  - *Pleasing*
  - *Comfort*
- *Life tasks:* Describe level of social interest and general functioning in each of the life task areas:
  - Work
  - Communal life and friendship
  - Love relationships
  - Self-acceptance
  - Spirituality
  - Parenting

Treatment Plan Template: Adlerian

Use this treatment plan template for developing a plan for clients with depressive, anxious, or compulsive types of presenting problems. Depending on the specific client, presenting problem, and clinical context, the goals and interventions in this template may need to be modified only slightly or significantly; you are encouraged to significantly revise the plan as needed. For the plan to be clinically useful, goals and techniques should be written to target specific beliefs, behaviors, and emotions that the client is experiencing. The more specific the plan, the more helpful it will be to informing the counseling process.

Treatment Plan

Initial Phase of Treatment

Initial Phase Counseling Tasks

1. Develop working counseling relationship. *Diversity considerations:* Describe how you will specifically adjust to respect cultured, gendered, and other styles of relationship building and emotional expression.
   Relationship-building approach/intervention:
   a. Use encouragement, empathy, and education to create an egalitarian relationship in which the client has a sense of free will.
2. Assess individual, systemic, and broader cultural dynamics. *Diversity considerations:* Describe how you will specifically adjust assessment based on cultural, socioeconomic, sexual orientation, gender, and other relevant norms.
   Assessment strategies:
   a. Assess lifestyle, basic mistakes, parenting style, family constellation, early recollections, organ inferiority, and dreams.
   b. Use "the question" to help determine purpose of symptom and goals for treatment.
3. Identify and obtain client agreement on treatment goals. *Diversity considerations:* Describe how you will specifically modify goals to correspond with values from the client's cultural, religious, and other value systems.
   Goal-making intervention:
   a. Identify strategies for how best to enhance social interest and overall well-being, including crisis and symptom reduction and long-term wellness.
4. Identify needed referrals, crisis issues, and other client needs. *Diversity considerations:* Describe diversity issues related to specific crisis issues and referral options.

(continued)

a. *Crisis assessment intervention(s):* Use "the question" to identify crisis issues and psychoeducation to manage crises.
b. *Referral(s):* Refer to psychoeducation and support groups as necessary.

Initial Phase Client Goal

1. Decrease insecurities and basic mistake assumptions that fuel crisis thinking and behaviors to reduce [specific crisis symptoms].
   Interventions:
   a. Psychoeducation on how to manage [crisis behavior]; encouragement to follow through with new response to feelings that signal crisis.
   b. Challenge basic mistake and assumptions related to crisis thoughts and behaviors.

Working Phase of Treatment

Working Phase Counseling Tasks

1. Monitor quality of the working alliance. *Diversity considerations:* Describe how you will specifically adapt expectations for age, gender, cultural, sexual orientation, socioeconomic status, and other norms for relating.
   a. *Assessment Intervention:* Monitor for signs that client has a sense of equality and ownership in relationship.
2. Monitor progress toward goals. *Diversity considerations:* Describe how you will specifically adapt the monitoring of progress for age, ethnicity, educational level, language, etc.
   a. *Assessment Intervention:* Ask client about perceived progress; monitor development of social interest; use Outcome Questionnaire to measure client progress.

Working Phase Client Goals

1. Decrease insecurities that lead to [specific dynamic or problem] to reduce [specific symptoms: depression, anxiety, etc.].
   Interventions:
   a. Psychoeducation to correct basic mistake belief: [specify].
   b. Psychoeducation to correct basic mistake belief: [specify].
2. Decrease tendency to value self based on external achievements and approval from others to reduce [specific symptoms: depression, anxiety, etc.].
   Interventions:
   a. Challenging basic mistake belief that self-worth is based on performance and approval from others.
   b. Alter self-concept statements to reflect a more realistic valuing of self that focuses on "what am I doing?" rather that "how am I doing?".
3. Decrease avoidance of life tasks and/or social connections in [specify: work, relationship, communal, etc.] to reduce [specific symptoms: depression, anxiety, etc.].
   Interventions:
   a. Interpretation of avoidance behaviors in terms of how they enable client to avoid misguided childhood fears, social contact, key life tasks, etc.
   b. Spitting in soup and antisuggestion techniques to unmask how symptoms allow client to avoid feared life tasks.

(*continued*)

Closing Phase of Treatment

Closing Phase Counseling Task

1. Develop aftercare plan and maintain gains. *Diversity considerations:* Describe specific diversity considerations and unique resources for the ending treatment and sustaining gains posttreatment.
   Intervention:
   a. Psychoeducation on wellness and positive psychology to identify key components to maintaining happiness and well-being.

Closing Phase Client Goals

1. Increase self-acceptance and overall sense of wellness to reduce potential for relapse of symptoms.
   Interventions:
   a. Psychoeducation on social interest and positive psychology to develop habits of wellness, such as a strong social network, gratifying activities, and optimistic basic assumptions.
   b. Examine natural consequences of acting from social interest vs. basic mistake assumptions.
2. Increase social connections in intimate relationships and work contexts [and/or parenting, spiritual contexts] to reduce potential for relapse of symptoms.
   Interventions:
   a. Psychoeducation on importance of functioning in all life tasks to achieve balance.
   b. Develop homework and life habits that support social interest in all areas of living.

Digital Download Download from CengageBrain.com

Tapestry Weaving: Working with Diverse Populations

Ethnic and Racial Diversity

Although one of the oldest approaches, Adlerian theory has had from its inception surprisingly modern feminist and multicultural values (Mansager, 2008; Newlon & Arciniega, 1983). Alfred Adler defined mental health as having high levels of social interest, community feeling, and empathy for others, even those others who are quite unlike oneself (Ansbacher & Ansbacher, 1956). He clearly and frequently referred to the subjugation of women and their unfair treatment and considered this in his assessment and diagnosis; although such practices seem commonplace today, it was a radical stand for social justice in the 1910s. More recently, Adlerians have also been advocates for gay, lesbian, bisexual, and transgendered individuals (Mansager, 2008; see Sexual Identity Diversity section below).

Several of the theory's central concepts make Adlerian Individual Psychology particularly well suited for working with diverse clients:

- *Social Interest:* The emphasis on social interest is particularly appropriate for traditional and collectivist cultures that value family and community over individuality and independence. Furthermore, the primary goal of the approach is to help people develop a greater sense of "community feeling" and connection with one's broader community; this is exceptionally important for marginalized populations, whether ostracized due to their sexual orientation, language abilities, physical abilities, or ethnic origin. By definition, the primary means of reducing a sense of marginalization is to create a feeling of belonging. As the default goal of this approach, it is a natural fit for persons who feel marginalized from specific communities or dominant society.

- *Superiority, Racism, and Other -isms:* Adler viewed any attempts to see oneself as superior to another human being as a sign of maladjustment, thus providing a strong antiracist, antisexist, and antiheterosexist foundation to his theory (Mosak & Maniacci, 1999).
- *Spirituality:* Whereas many theories either ignore or are suspicious of religion and spirituality, the Adlerian theory views a person's relationship to something greater as an important relationship to cultivate (Carlson et al., 2006; Sweeney, 2009). This emphasis on spirituality is consistent with values in many traditional cultures and ethnic groups.
- *Social Factors Impacting Mental Health:* Adler carefully assessed and considered the impact of broader social and family factors in the development of problems. Individuals and their symptoms were considered in the context of the *environment*, an important practice when working with persons from minority and marginalized groups.

When working with diverse clients, Adlerian counselors consider some of the following when establishing a counseling relationship, assessing, designing treatment, and intervening; these points can be identified, when appropriate, in the "diversity note" section of the treatment plan.

Developing and Monitoring the Counseling Relationship with Diverse Clients

Expression of Encouragement How a client receives a counselor's expression of "encouragement" very much depends on multiple dynamics in the relationship: the age and gender of each; the ethnicity and social class of each; as well as the perceived disparity in general functioning. For example, men with a more traditionally defined sense of masculinity, those with cultural norms that value saving face, or clients whose counselor is significantly younger may find certain expressions of encouragement (e.g., "I know you can do it") as off-putting or even offensive. Whereas the same words between a different configuration of client-counselor may be very effective. Thus, Adlerian counselors carefully attend to variables such as age difference, cultural norms, and gender dynamics when they express encouragement with their clients, to ensure that their expression of encouragement strengthens rather than jeopardizes the counseling relationship.

Examples of Noting this Diversity Dynamic in Treatment Planning

- Offer expressions of encouragement that allow client to still feel sense of competence/save face.
- Avoid expressions of encouragement that may be experienced as emasculating.
- Ensure that expressions of encouragement show respect for client's achievements and maturity.

"Egalitarian" Relationships with Diverse Clients The Adlerian value of creating an egalitarian relationship with clients quickly becomes complicated when working with diverse clients. For counselors with liberal or modern sensibilities, it may be surprising to learn that not all clients appreciate an egalitarian relationship with their counselor or therapist. Many traditional cultures see "healers" such as doctors and counselors as having a special and higher position in the community, and therefore clients may be more comfortable with the counselor taking an expert position (Qureshi, & Collazos, 2011). Furthermore, even when striving toward equality, it is arguably difficult to declare any relationship as truly "egalitarian" because of the many forms of social power at play; this dynamic is even more pronounced between counselors and clients with diverse backgrounds (Monk, Winslade, & Sinclair, 2008).

Thus, when developing relationships with clients using the Adlerian concept of egalitarianism, counselors consider an appropriate form and expression of this theoretically grounded value. Most critically, when a counselor from a more privileged social position (such as a particular ethnic/racial background, gender, sexual orientation, or social class) works with clients from more marginalized social positions, the counselor must consider the unique client needs and how to best promote the client's sense of agency, which is the underlying purpose of the egalitarian position (Sweeney, 2009). In some cases, promoting agency may involve emphasizing the egalitarian nature of the relationship by frequently inviting client expertise into the conversation to actively undo a perceived status difference, such as social class or age. With other clients, the counselor may best achieve a sense of egalitarianism by honoring a cultural preference for a more formal counselor-client relationship with some elements of hierarchy, while still promoting a sense of client agency through more subtle expressions of encouragement. In sum, the best measure of whether the relationship is appropriately egalitarian is whether the client feels a sense of agency in session and is able to transfer this to his or her everyday life.

Examples of Noting this Diversity Dynamic in Treatment Planning

- Build sense of egalitarianism due to age/gender [or list other differences] differences by frequently asking for client perspectives rather than providing expert answers.
- Use self-deprecating humor to increase sense of egalitarianism in relationship.
- Balance client's desire for "expert" help with reflections that build client sense of agency, by asking for input and preference.

Assessing Individual, Systemic, and Broader Cultural Dynamics with Diverse Clients

Superiority, Racism, and Other –isms Adler viewed any attempts to see oneself as superior to another human being as a sign of maladjustment, thus providing a strong antiracist, antisexist, and antiheterosexist foundation to his theory (Mosak & Maniacci, 1999). These forms of attempted superiority stem from an underlying sense of inferiority, basic mistakes, and low social interest. Thus, when assessing clients, counselors attend to where and how clients may be marginalized in one way or another by such views.

Examples of Noting this Diversity Dynamic in Treatment Planning

- Assess for how client may be experiencing [racism, sexism, heterosexism, ageism, etc.] in their personal, professional, and/or community contexts.
- Assess for contexts in which client may be experiencing harassment and marginalization due to [sexual orientation, race, immigration status, social class, etc.].

Lifestyle Assessment with Diverse Clients The assessment of lifestyle, with its emphasis on childhood experiences and early recollections, may not seem relevant to people who prefer a more pragmatic approach or who do not share the dominant Western assumption that these events shape a person's personality. Therefore, counselors may want to take time to explain the rationale for such assessment and/or limit it when working with clients who may not see its value.

Furthermore, to properly assess a diverse client's style of life, counselors should take time to educate themselves about the culture, including cultural values, immigration patterns, class differences, and acculturation patterns. For example, Reddy and Hanna (1998) describe how Hindu women are shifting from a more traditional pleasing and dependent lifestyle to a more contemporary style of interdependence and assertiveness, especially in upper classes more likely to emigrate. Similarly, Duffey, Carns, Carns, and Garcia (1998) describe how middle-class Mexican American women are combining traditional Mexican cultural values with contemporary values, becoming both collaborative and self-promoting. Finally, Chung and Bernak (1998) provide insight into the lifestyles of immigrant Vietnamese women, who must try to bridge two vastly different cultures, often in the context of significant preemigration trauma.

Examples of Noting this Diversity Dynamic in Treatment Planning

- Focus lifestyle assessment on better understanding client's cultural/ethnic background [and/or immigration or marginalization experience].
- Ensure client is comfortable with and values exploring past as part of lifestyle assessment.
- Provide explanations for purpose of discussing childhood experiences if client uninterested or resistant.

Spirituality Whereas many theories either ignore or are suspicious of religion and spirituality, the Adlerian theory views a person's relationship to "something greater than the self" as an important relationship to cultivate (Carlson et al., 2006; Sweeney, 2009). This emphasis on spirituality is consistent with values in many traditional cultures and ethnic groups, and thus it can be an area of particular focus when working with clients from diverse populations.

Examples of Noting this Diversity Dynamic in Treatment Planning

- Include detailed assessment of potential religious/spiritual resources, including community support and spiritual practices that promote well-being and help cope with stress.
- Include assessment of client's religious community and its role in personal and family life.

Setting Goals and Monitoring Progress with Diverse Clients

Social Interest as a Value The Adlerian goal of developing social interest is particularly salient for cultures and subcultures that value family and community over individuality. In such cases, social interest coincides with many traditional cultural values and thus may be a welcomed and particularly salient long-term goal. Furthermore, the goal of developing a greater sense of "community feeling" and connection with one's broader community is often important for the long-term well-being of marginalized populations, whether due to their sexual orientation, language abilities, physical abilities, or ethnic origin.

Nonetheless, it is important to remember that the particular form of expression of social interest may vary dramatically across cultures, social classes, age groups, genders, religious groups, and even personalities. All clients may not agree to goals that relate to increasing social interest across all areas identified as salient to Adlerians: communal life, work, love relationships, self-acceptance, spirituality, and parenting (Carlson et al., 2006; Sweeney, 2009). Therefore, when setting goals and monitoring progress, counselors may need to adjust these to meet specific client values and beliefs.

Examples of Noting this Diversity Dynamic in Treatment Planning

- Inquire about client views and values related to life tasks and social interest.
- Identify forms of social interest appropriate to cultural/religious background.
- Adjust goals to coincide with cultural/religious values.
- Check to ensure that client progress coincides with client views/goals.

Developing Plans for Aftercare and Maintaining Gains

Building Community and Social Interest The emphasis on social interest in Adlerian counseling provides an excellent foundation for helping clients maintain gains after counseling services end. As repeatedly noted by positive psychologists, people with strong social networks are more likely to report being happy and fulfilled (Leak & Leak, 2006). Thus, by helping clients develop stronger social interest in multiple areas of life, they are more likely to have sufficient social networks to support them going forward without treatment. Of particular importance, many clients who are part of marginalized communities often have access to particularly supportive and readily identifiable support networks, such as support groups, social networks, and formal organizations. Counselors should familiarize themselves with local resources and work with clients to identify suitable connections, to ensure that clients are well connected before ending counseling services.

Examples of Noting this Diversity Dynamic in Treatment Planning

- Help client connect with support network through religious organization.
- Help client connect with support in gay/lesbian community.
- Help client connect with support offered by extended family.

Sexual Identity Diversity

Although ahead of his time in terms of gender and socioeconomic injustices, Adler was not as forward-thinking on the issue of sexual orientation. Similar to psychodynamic theory, theory historically conceptualized same-sex attraction as a form of neurosis (Chernin & Holden, 1995; Mansager, 2008). However, contemporary Individual Psychology practitioners have gone to significant lengths to correct this history. Most notably, contemporary Adlerians have formally (a) admitted that historically this approach has unfairly and inaccurately pathologized same-sex attraction, (b) publically apologized to any LGBT individuals who have been hurt by these erroneous theoretical conceptualizations, (c) amended the work of Individual Psychology to correct and improve the theory, and (d) assured professionals and the public that Individual Psychology affirms and promotes the well-being of LGBT individuals (Mansager, 2008).

As part of the theory's reconceptualization of same-sex attraction, Fisher (1993) identifies three issues that are unique to working with gay and lesbian couples using Alderian theory:

- *Feelings of Inferiority Projected onto Self and Relationship:* Because gay and lesbian individuals experience profound and multiple forms of societal rejection, their style of life is typically dominated by feelings of inferiority both personally and about their relationships; this self-hatred is often referred to as homophobia. These feelings of inferiority are extremely detrimental to relationships, often the source of conflict for the couple.
- *Lack of Positive Role Models:* Gay and lesbian couples often lack positive role models to guide them in forming mutually satisfying relationships. Often they resort to modeling their relationship on their parents' heterosexual relationship, which typically is ineffective and problematic.
- *Lack of Social Interest If "Closeted":* If one or both partners are "closeted," cultivating social interest—which is correlated to well-being—is extremely difficult to cultivate. Because their focus is on protecting the self from society, closeted individuals have greater difficulty attending to the needs of their partner or the community more broadly. Couples who are out of the closet to different degrees are also likely to experience tension and conflict over these differences, too.

When conducting a lifestyle assessment with gay and lesbian clients, Fisher (1993) recommends adding the following questions:

- When did you first remember having same-sex attractions? Can you describe the experience and how you felt about it?
- What were your mother's views about same-sex attraction? Your father's? Siblings?
- How did you first know you were gay/lesbian/bisexual? Did you tell anyone, and, if so, how did they respond? How did you feel about yourself initially?
- How did you feel about gay/lesbian/bisexuals in general at that time? How do you feel now?
- Have you ever known anyone who is LGB that you loved and respected?
- To whom have you "come out" and why? Who have you chosen to not come out to and why?
- What qualities do you seek in a partner? Who do you use as a model for healthy relationships?

Research and the Evidence Base

Adlerian counseling has not been examined carefully in clinical trials due to difficulties in operationalizing terms, such as social interest, and because of a general sense on the part of practitioners that their theory works (Sweeney, 2009). However, *Systematic*

Training for Effective Parenting (STEP) is a notable exception; this Adlerian-based parenting program is listed as "promising" evidence-based treatment for parent training.

Research studies on Adlerian theory have focused on parent-child and teacher-child relations. For example, McVittie and Best (2009) conducted a study on the effectiveness of an Adlerian-based parenting program; their large-scale, self-report study indicated that parents reported setting clearer limits, increasing their sense of positive connection, and decreasing harshness. Similarly, Kelly and Daniels (1997) studied the effect of teachers using praise versus encouragement on children in fourth through tenth grade; they found that teachers who used encouragement were viewed as more potent than those using praise. Pilkington, White, and Matheny (1997) studied the correlation of birth order on coping resources in school-aged children and found some support for differences between the oldest and middle children, with the former having the highest level of coping and the latter the lowest. Despite these initial studies, Adlerian theory and practice would benefit from more detailed research studies on the methods and effectiveness of this approach.

Evidence-Based Treatment: Systematic Training for Effective Parenting (STEP)

Systematic Training for Effective Parenting (STEP) is a promising evidence-based parenting program based on Adlerian principles (Dinkmeyer & McKay, 2007). The STEP program has been researched for almost four decades (Gibson, 1999) and is currently listed as a "promising practice" by state and federal agencies. Using Adlerian principles, the STEP program is an extremely positive parenting approach that uses encouragement, appreciation, and motivation to improve child behaviors and parent-child relations. At its heart, it helps parents develop social interest and cooperative behaviors and directly addresses the classic Adlerian concept of developing the "courage to be imperfect." The programs include a specific program for children under six (Dinkmeyer & McKay, 2008) and one for teens (Dinkmeyer, McKay, & McKay, 2007).

The program includes lessons on:

- Understanding yourself and your child
- Understanding beliefs and feelings
- Encouraging your child and yourself
- Listening and talking to your child
- Helping children learn to cooperate
- Discipline that makes sense
- Choosing your approach

Questions for Personal Reflection and Class Discussion

1. Which ideas from this chapter do you find most personally relevant? Why?
2. Which ideas from this chapter do you think you will be most helpful in working with clients?
3. What are the possibilities and limitations for using this approach with diverse clients? How might you address the limitations?
4. Do you agree with Adler's thoughts on social interest and its importance for emotional well-being? Why or why not?
5. What real-life examples do you have of an inferiority complex? How did it affect the person's life and relationships?
6. What are the key elements of your style of life? How would you characterize your way of viewing and approaching life?
7. Do you believe birth order is useful to consider? Why or why not?
8. For which clients and/or presenting problems do you think this approach would be most appropriate? Least appropriate?

9. Which case conceptualization concept seems most useful for understanding a client's problem?
10. Which intervention do you think would be the most useful?
11. Do you think this approach is a good fit for you as a counselor or therapist? Why or why not?
12. In what ways would you need to grow or what would you need to learn to be able to use this approach well?

Online Resources

Journal

Journal of Individual Psychology
www.utexas.edu/utpress/journals/jip.html

Associations and Societies

International Association of Individual Psychology
www.iaipwebsite.org/

North American Society of Alfred Adler
www.alfredadler.org/

Select Training Institutes

Adler Graduate School (Minnesota)
www.alfredadler.edu/

Adler School of Professional Psychology (Chicago)
www.adler.edu/

Adlerian Training Institute
www.adleriantraining.com

Alfred Adler Institute of New York
www.alfredadler-ny.org/

Alfred Adler Institute of San Francisco and Northwest Washington
http://pws.cablespeed.com/~htstein/

Link to More Resources

Link to Additional Resources from the Adler Graduate School
www.alfredadler.edu/resources/adlerianlinks.htm

References

*Asterisk indicates recommended introductory readings.

Adler, A. (1924). *The practice and theory of individual psychology* (P. Radin, trans.). New York: Harcourt, Brace & Company.

Adler, A. (1959). *Understanding human nature* (C. Brett, trans.). New York: Hazeldon Press.

Adler, A. (1978). *The education of children.* Chicago, IL: Regnery. Original work published 1930.

American Psychiatric Association. (2000). *Diagnostic and statistical manual for mental disorders* (4th ed., Text Revision). Washington, DC: Author.

*Ansbacher, H. L., & Ansbacher, R. R. (Eds.). (1956). *The individual psychology of Alfred Adler* (5th ed.). New York: Basic Books.

*Ansbacher, H. L., & Ansbacher, R. R. (Eds.). (1964). *Superiority and social interest, a collection of later writings.* Evanston, IL: Northwestern University Press.

Bitter, J. R., Christensen, O. C., Hawes, C., & Nicoll, W. G. (1998). Adlerian brief therapy with individual, couples, and families. *Directions in Clinical and Counseling Psychology*, *8*(8), 95–111.

Bitter, J., & Nicolls, W. (2000). Adlerian brief therapy with individuals: Process and practice. *Journal of Individual Psychology*, *56*(1), 31–44.

Carlson, (n.d.) Jon Carlson Homepage. Retrieved May 18, 2010, from http://www.joncarlson.org

Carlson, J., Watts, R., & Maniacci, M. (2006). *Adlerian therapy: Theory and practice.* Washington, DC: American Psychological Association. doi:10.1037/11363-000

Chernin, J., & Holden, J. (1995). Toward an understanding of homosexuality: Origins, status, and relationship to individual psychology. *Individual Psychology: Journal of Adlerian Theory, Research & Practice*, *51*(2), 90–101.

Chung, R., & Bemak, F. (1998). Lifestyle of Vietnamese refugee women. *Journal of Individual Psychology, 54*(3), 373–384.

*Dinkmeyer, D. C., & McKay, G. D. (2007). *The parent's handbook: Systematic training for effective parenting.* Bowling Green, KY: STEP Publishers.

*Dinkmeyer, D. C., & McKay, J. L. (2008). *Parenting young children: Systematic training for effective parenting (STEP) of children under six.* Bowling Green, KY: STEP Publishers.

*Dinkmeyer, D. C., McKay, G. D., & McKay, J. L. (2007). *Parenting teenagers: Systematic training for effective parenting of teens.* Bowling Green, KY: STEP Publishers.

*Dreikurs, R. (1950/1989). *Fundamentals of Adlerian psychology.*Oxford, England: Greenberg. (Original publication in 1933; Translated by Dreikurs from Adler's German.)

Dreikurs, R. (1958). *The challenge of parenthood.* New York: Duell, Sloan and Pierce.

Dreikurs, R. (1968). *Psychology in the classroom.* New York: HarperCollins College.

Dreikurs, R., & Loren, G. (1968). A new approach to discipline: Logical consequences [you will find this very interesting. The 1999 publication changed the two phrases all the way around]. New York: Meredith Press.

Dreikurs, R., & Mosak, H. H. (1967). The tasks of life: II. The fourth task. *The Individual Psychologist, 4*, 51–55.

Duffey, T. H., Carns, M. R., Carns, A. W., & Garcia, J. L. (1998). The lifestyle of the middle-class Mexican American female. *Journal of Individual Psychology, 54*(3), 399–406.

Gehart, D. (2016). *Theory and treatment planning in counseling and psychotherapy* (2nd ed.). Pacific Grove, CA: Brooks Cole.

Gibson, D. G. (1999). *A monograph: Summary of the research related to the use and efficacy of the systematic training for effectiveness program* 1976–1999. Circle Pines, MN: American Guidance Services, Inc.

Fisher, S. (1993). A proposed Adlerian theoretical framework and intervention techniques for gay and lesbian couples. *Individual Psychology: Journal of Adlerian Theory, Research & Practice, 49*(3–4), 438–449.

Hartshorne, J., Salem-Hartshorne, N., & Hartshorne, T. (2009). Birth order effects in the formation of long-term relationships. *Journal of Individual Psychology, 65*(2), 156–176.

Kelly, F., & Daniels, J. (1997). The effects of praise versus encouragement on children's perceptions of teachers. *Individual Psychology: Journal of Adlerian Theory, Research & Practice, 53*(3), 331–341.

Kottman, T., Lingg, M., & Tisdell, T. (1995). Gay and lesbian adolescents: Implications for Adlerian therapists. *Individual Psychology: Journal of Adlerian Theory, Research & Practice, 51*(2), 114–128.

Leak, G. K., & Leak, K. C. (2006). Adlerian social interest and positive psychology: A conceptual and empirical integration. *Journal of Individual Psychology, 62*, 207–233.

*Manaster, G. J., & Corsini, R. J. (1982). *Individual psychology: Theory and practice.* Chicago, IL: Adler School of Professional Psychology.

Maniacci, M. (2002). The DSM and individual psychology: A general comparison. *Journal of Individual Psychology, 58*(4), 356–362.

Mansager, E. (2008). Affirming lesbian, gay, bisexual, and transgender individuals. *Journal of Individual Psychology, 64*(2), 124–136.

McVittie, J., & Best, A. (2009). The impact of Adlerian-based parenting classes on self-reported parental behavior. *Individual Psychology: Journal of Adlerian Theory, Research & Practice, 65*(3), 264–285.

Mills, K. J., & Mooney, G. A. (2013). Methods of ranking birth order: The neglected issue in birth order research. *Journal of Individual Psychology, 69*(4), 357–370.

Monk, G., Winslade, J., & Sinclair, S. (2008). *New horizons in multicultural counseling.* Thousand Oaks, CA: Sage.

Mosak, H. H., & Di Pietro, R. (2006). *Early recollections: Interpretative method and application.* New York: Routledge.

Mosak, H. H., & Dreikurs, R. (1967). The tasks of life: III. The fifth task. *The Individual Psychologist, 5*, 16–22.

*Mosak, H. H., & Maniacci, M. P. (1999). *Primer of Adlerian psychology: The Analytic-Behavioural-Cognitive Psychology of Alfred Adler.* New York: Brunner/Routledge.

Mosak, H. H., & Sculman, B. H. (1988). *Lifestyle inventory.* Muncie, IN: Accelerated Development.

Myers, J. E. (2009). Wellness through social interest. In T. J. Sweeney (Ed.), *Adlerian counseling and psychotherapy: A practitioner's approach* (5th ed., pp. 33–44). New York: Routledge.

Newlon, B. J., & Arciniega, M. (1983). Respecting cultural uniqueness: An Adlerian approach. *Individual Psychology: Journal of Adlerian Theory, Research & Practice, 39*(2), 133–143.

Pilkington, L., White, J., & Matheny, K. (1997). Perceived coping resources and psychological birth order in school-aged children. *Individual Psychology: Journal of Adlerian Theory, Research & Practice, 53*(1), 42–57.

Qureshi, A., & Collazos, F. (2011). The intercultural and interracial therapeutic relationship: Challenges and recommendations. *International Review of Psychiatry, 23*(1), 10–19. doi:10.3109/09540261.2010.544643

Reddy, I., & Hanna, F. J. (1998). The lifestyle of the Hindu woman: Conceptualizing female clients of Indian origin. *Journal of Individual Psychology, 54*(3), 385–398.

*Sweeney, T. J. (2009). *Adlerian counseling and psychotherapy: A practitioner's approach* (5th ed.). New York: Routledge/Taylor & Francis Group.

Watts, R. E. (2013, April). Reflecting as if. *Counseling Today.* Retrieved from http://ct.counseling.org/2013/04/reflecting-as-if/

Adlerian Case Study: Trauma and Immigration

The daughter of German immigrants, Helga, 34, is still struggling with recovery from childhood sexual abuse by her babysitter's husband when she was 7–8 years old. She recently broke up with her boyfriend, which has triggered old childhood fears of being inherently "flawed" and isolated from anyone who really cares. She maintains a good job as a store manager, but has begun avoiding friends and staying at home since the breakup. She reports having a sense of panic when in public places, which she experienced as a teen. She says she has come to the conclusion that it's best and safest for her to be alone.

After an initial consultation, an Adlerian counselor develops the following case conceptualization.

CASE CONCEPTUALIZATION

Date: August 27, 2013 **Clinician:** Charmain **Client/Case #:** **9005**

I. Introduction to Client

Identify primary client and significant others

Client

Adult Female Age: 34 European American Single heterosexual Occupation/Grade: Manager, Children's clothing store Other identifier: Parents immigrated from Germany

Significant Others

Client's Mother Age: 65 European American Married heterosexual Occupation/Grade: Retired grocery clerk

Other identifier: Post-war German immigrant

Client's Father Age: 72 European American Married heterosexual Occupation/Grade: Retired office manager

Other identifier: Post-war German immigrant

Select Person Age: ____________ Select Ethnicity Select Relational Status Occupation/Grade: ____________

Other identifier: ____________

Select Person Age: ____________ Select Ethnicity Select Relational Status Occupation/Grade: ____________

Other identifier: ____________

Others: ____________

II. Presenting Concern(s)

Client Description of Problem(s): After her recent breakup with the man she thought she was going to marry, AF says she has come to the conclusion that she is best off alone and is happiest when alone. AF believes her panic attacks and fear of being in public stem from her childhood experiences of having hardworking parents who did not have much time for her and her childhood sexual abuse from age 7–8.

(continued)

Significant Other/Family Description(s) of Problems: AF has not told her parents much about her personal life, panic, or avoidance of friends. She tells them she is too busy to see them due to work. Her parents see her as too shy for her own good and say she has always worried too much about what other people think about her.

Broader System Problem Descriptions: Description of problem from referring party, teachers, relatives, legal system, etc.:

Ex-boyfriend: Found it hard to feel emotionally connected to AF (as reported by AF).

Name: ______

III. Background Information

Trauma/Abuse History (recent and past): From ages 7–8, AF was sexually molested by her babysitter's husband several times per month. The abuse ended when her parents moved to a different city. She has never told her parents about the abuse.

Substance Use/Abuse (current and past; self, family of origin, significant others): AF denies using alcohol or other substances other than occasional social drinking.

Precipitating Events (recent life changes, first symptoms, stressors, etc.): AF broke up with her boyfriend after two years of dating because he no longer felt a connection to her. AF was surprised by the breakup and has retreated from what was already a limited social network, making excuses to avoid getting together with friends. Shortly after the breakup, she began having panic attacks, which she also had in high school. These have made it increasingly difficult for her to leave the house, which she has to "force" herself to do.

Related Historical Background (family history, related issues, previous counseling, mental health history, etc.): AF worked through her panic episodes with her parents' insistence that she "pull herself together." She was an only child, her parents working long hours to make ends meet. They encouraged her to excel in school, which she did. She rarely made any waves at home, playing for hours by herself. She suffered through her sexual abuse by her babysitter's husband without telling anyone about it for years; she finally told a girlfriend in college.

IV. Client Strengths and Diversity

Client Strengths

Personal: AF is a hard worker, diligent, and can "get herself" to do what needs to be done. She is kind and patient in relationships.

Relational/Social: AF's parents want the best for her and support her in the ways they know how; AF has two girlfriends in whom she can confide.

Spiritual: AF does not have any strong spiritual traditions but does use poetry as an outlet for exploring life and its greater meaning.

(*continued*)

Diversity: Resources and Limitations

Identify potential resources and limitations available to clients based on their age, gender, sexual orientation, cultural background, socioeconomic status, religion, regional community, language, family background, family configuration, abilities, etc.

Unique Resources: AF lives in the same town as her parents and can easily access them as a support system; in many ways embodies German values of strong work ethic, sense of self-discipline, independence, and organization. Family emphasized academic and professional success.

Potential Limitations: AF's family of origin places high value upon marriage and family and puts pressure on her to "find a good man to marry before it is too late." In addition, their immigration experience has created a general sense of fear related to not being able to survive or have enough resources; this fuels their strong work ethic.

Complete One or More of the Following Sections (V–IX) Based on the Theory (IES) You Plan to Use for Your Treatment Plan.

V. Psychodynamic Conceptualization

Psychodynamic Defense Mechanisms

Check 2–4 most commonly used defense mechanisms

❑ Acting Out: *Describe:* __________

❑ Denial: *Describe:* __________

❑ Displacement: *Describe:* __________

❑ Help-Rejecting Complaining: *Describe:* __________

❑ Humor: *Describe:* __________

❑ Passive Aggression: *Describe:* __________

❑ Projection: *Describe:* __________

❑ Projective Identification: *Describe:* __________

☒ Rationalization: *Describe:* AF rationalizes why she does not want future relationships and why it is "normal" to stay at home and avoid social contact.

❑ Reaction Formation: *Describe:* __________

☒ Repression: *Describe:* AF represses most strong, negative feelings, afraid that they will overwhelm her, especially those related to the abuse.

❑ Splitting: *Describe:* __________

❑ Sublimation: *Describe:* __________

❑ Suppression: *Describe:* __________

☒ Other: Self-blame: AF often copes by blaming herself and finding herself at fault for the events in her life.

Object Relational Patterns

Describe relationship with early caregivers in past: AF's parents worked long hours throughout her childhood and she was often placed in the care of babysitters while her parents were at work.

(*continued*)

Was the attachment with the mother (or equivalent) primarily:

❑ Generally Secure ❑ Anxious and Clingy ☒ Avoidant and Emotionally Distant ❑ Other: ________

Was the attachment with the father (or equivalent) primarily:

❑ Generally Secure ❑ Anxious and Clingy ☒ Avoidant and Emotionally Distant ❑ Other: ________

Describe present relationship with these caregivers: AF keeps her parents at a distance and avoids interaction by telling them she is too busy with work. Her parents are supportive in the best way they know how, however, AF feels they put pressure on her to get married and be more social.

Describe relational patterns with partner and other current relationships: AF recently broke up with her boyfriend and states this was because he no longer felt a connection to her.

Erickson's Psychosocial Developmental Stage

Describe development at each stage up to current stage

Trust vs. Mistrust (Infant Stage): AF seems to lack a basic sense of trust in self and other, which may stem from her mother's absence due to working even during her infancy.

Autonomy vs. Shame and Doubt (Toddler Stage): AF remembers being frequently criticized by her parents as a child and still carries a strong sense of shame and doubt.

Initiative vs. Guilt (Preschool Age): AF remembers frequent criticism during the preschool phase, saying her parents parented primarily through guilt.

Industry vs. Inferiority (School Age): AF was rewarded for being industrious; her desire for approval was compounded by sexual abuse during this stage, resulting in a strong need to "achieve" to be worthwhile.

Identity vs. Role Confusion (Adolescence): During teen years, AF continued to excel scholastically to define herself, resulting in the development of panic symptoms.

Intimacy vs. Isolation (Young Adulthood): AF has had difficulty developing intimate relationships, especially with men, resulting in her current resolution that isolation is her best option.

Generativity vs. Stagnation (Adulthood): ________

Ego Integrity vs. Despair (Late Adulthood): ________

Adlerian Style of Life Theme

☒ Control: AF has managed her life by tightly controlling behaviors and avoiding dangerous situations.

❑ Superiority: ________

❑ Pleasing: ________

❑ Comfort: ________

Basic Mistake Misperceptions: AF wants to avoid being hurt, finding life and relationships to be dangerous and unpredictable: "it's better to play it safe."

(continued)

VI. Humanistic-Existential Conceptualization

Expression of Authentic Self

Problems: Are problems perceived as internal or external (caused by others, circumstances, etc.)?

❑ Predominantly internal

☒ Mixed

❑ Predominantly external

Agency and Responsibility: Is self or other discussed as agent of story? Does client take clear responsibility for situation?

❑ Strong sense of agency and responsibility

☒ Agency in some areas

❑ Little agency; frequently blames others/situation

❑ Often feels victimized

Recognition and Expression of Feelings: Are feelings readily recognized, owned, and experienced?

❑ Easily expresses feelings

❑ Identifies feelings with prompting

☒ Difficulty recognizing feelings

Here-and-Now Experiencing: Is the client able to experience full range of feelings as they are happening in the present moment?

❑ Easily experiences emotions in present moment

❑ Experiences some present emotions with assistance

☒ Difficulty with present moment experiencing

Personal Constructs and Facades: Is the client able to recognize and go beyond roles? Is identity rigid or tentatively held?

❑ Tentatively held; able to critique and question

☒ Some awareness of facades and construction of identity

❑ Identity rigidly defined; seems like "fact"

Complexity and Contradictions: Are internal contradictions owned and explored? Is client able to fully engage the complexity of identity and life?

❑ Aware of and resolves contradictions

☒ Some recognition of contradictions

❑ Unaware of internal contradictions

Shoulds: Is client able to question socially imposed shoulds and oughts? Can client balance desire to please others and desire to be authentic?

❑ Able to balance authenticity with social obligation

☒ Identifies tension between social expectations and personal desires

❑ Primarily focuses on external shoulds

List shoulds: ____________________

Acceptance of Others: Is client able to accept others and modify expectations of others to be more realistic?

❑ Readily accepts others as they are

☒ Recognizes expectations of others are unrealistic but still strong emotional reaction to expectations not being met

❑ Difficulty accepting others as is; always wanting others to change to meet expectations

(continued)

Trust of Self: Is client able to trust self as process (rather than a stabile object)?
❑ Able to trust and express authentic self
☒ Trust of self in certain contexts
❑ Difficulty trusting self in most contexts

Existential Analysis
Sources of Life Meaning (as described or demonstrated by client): AF finds meaning in her life at work. She has been employed at the children's clothing store for 8 years and takes pride in her job.

General Themes of Life Meaning:
☒ Personal achievement/work
❑ Significant other
❑ Children
❑ Family of origin
❑ Social cause/contributing to others
❑ Religion/spirituality
❑ Other: __________

Satisfaction with and clarity on life direction:
❑ Clear sense of meaning that creates resilience in difficult times
❑ Current problems require making choices related to life direction
☒ Minimally satisfied with current life direction; wants more from life
❑ Has reflected little on life direction up to this point; living according to life plan defined by someone/something else
❑ Other: __________

Gestalt Contact Boundary Disturbances
❑ *Desensitization:* Failing to notice problems
❑ *Introjection*: Take in others' views whole and unedited
❑ *Projection*: Assign undesired parts of self to others
❑ *Retroflection*: Direct action to self rather than other
☒ *Deflection*: Avoid direct contact with another or self
❑ *Egotism:* Not allowing outside to influence self
❑ *Confluence:* Agree with another to extent that boundary blurred

Describe: AF avoids social interaction to prevent herself from getting hurt by other people.

VII. Cognitive-Behavioral Conceptualization

Baseline of Symptomatic Behavior

Symptom #1 (behavioral description): Panic Attacks

Frequency: 1–2 times per week

Duration: 15 minutes

Context(s): "out of the blue"

Events Before: Difficult to identify; often within 24 hours of hanging out with friends.

Events After: Goes home, reads books or watches television to get mind off things.

(*continued*)

Symptom #2 (behavioral description): Avoids social activities

Frequency: Most days of the week

Duration: Entire weekends

Context(s): NA

Events Before: Receives calls/emails from friends; either does not respond or makes an excuse.

Events After: Stays at home; reads books or watches television.

A-B-C Analysis of Irrational Beliefs

Activating Event ("Problem"): Invited by friends to go to dinner.

Consequence (Mood, behavior, etc.): Feels hopeless; makes excuse to stay home.

Mediating Beliefs (Unhelpful beliefs about event that result in C):

1. Worries she will be embarrassed
2. Worries people will think she is a loser because her boyfriend broke up with her.
3. Worries no one really likes her.

Beck's Schema Analysis

Identify frequently used cognitive schemas:

❑ *Arbitrary inference:*

❑ *Selective abstraction:*

❑ *Overgeneralization:*

☒ *Magnification/Minimization:* Magnifies smallest imperfections in self; believes others will reject her for them.

❑ *Personalization:*

☒ Absolutist/dichotomous thinking: Tends to see self as all worthy or not worthy; life is all good or all bad.

❑ *Mislabeling:*

❑ *Mindreading:*

VIII. Family Systems Conceptualization

Family Life Cycle Stage

☒ Single adult
❑ Marriage
❑ Family with Young Children
❑ Family with Adolescent Children
❑ Launching Children
❑ Later Life

Describe struggles with mastering developmental tasks in one of these stages: AF struggles to maintain intimate relationships which has prevented her from getting married, something that she would like for herself in the near future.

(*continued*)

Boundaries with

Parents ❑ Enmeshed ☒ Clear ❑ Disengaged ❑ NA: *Describe:* Parents care, but maintain a measured distance.

Significant Other ❑ Enmeshed ❑ Clear ☒ Disengaged ❑ NA: *Describe:* AM reported never feeling deeply connected to AF; however, she felt they had a connection.

Children ❑ Enmeshed ❑ Clear ❑ Disengaged ☒ NA: *Describe:* ______

Extended Family ❑ Enmeshed ❑ Clear ❑ Disengaged ☒ NA: *Describe:* ______

Other: Name ❑ Enmeshed ❑ Clear ❑ Disengaged ❑ NA: *Describe:* ______

Typical style for regulating closeness and distance with others: Her family tended to connect by sharing "work" stories; valued each other for work contributions more than personal contributions; avoided direct and expressive sharing of emotions.

Triangles/Coalitions

❑ Coalition in family of origin: *Describe:* ______

❑ Coalitions related to significant other: *Describe:* ______

❑ Other coalitions: ______

Hierarchy between Self and Parent/Child ❑ NA

With own children ❑ Effective ❑ Rigid ❑ Permissive

With parents (for child/young adult) ❑ Effective ☒ Rigid ❑ Permissive

Complementary Patterns with AM:

❑ Pursuer/distancer

❑ Over-/under-functioner

☒ Emotional/logical

❑ Good/bad parent

❑ Other: *Describe*

Example of complementary pattern: AM was emotionally expressive and engaged; AF was the "logical" one in relationship.

Intergenerational Patterns

Substance/Alcohol Abuse: ☒ NA ❑ History: ______

Sexual/Physical/Emotional Abuse: ❑ NA ☒ History: Sexually abused from 7–8 by babysitter's husband.

Parent/Child Relations: ❑ NA ☒ History: Tradition of parenting that focused on prompting child's success in school and work.

Physical/Mental Disorders: ❑ NA ☒ History: History of depression in parents' families.

Family strengths: Describe: Strong work ethic; family members care for each other; want to help each other succeed in all areas of life.

(*continued*)

IX. Solution-Based and Cultural Discourse Conceptualization (Postmodern)

Solutions and Unique Outcomes

Attempted Solutions that DIDN'T or DON'T work:

1. "Forcing" self to see friends and family
2. Watching television drama and police reality shows
3. Ruminating about why AM left her

Exceptions and Unique Outcomes: Times, places, relationships, contexts, etc. when problem is less of a problem; behaviors that seem to make things even slightly better:

1. Feels most connected with talking to two best girlfiends and mother on the phone
2. Writing poetry makes her feel better about life generally
3. Least panicky in familiar public places; is able to go to the grocery store and bank and do "basic" (work-like) errands in public places without a sense of panic

Miracle Question Answer: If the problem were to be resolved overnight, what would client be doing differently the next day? (Describe in terms of doing X rather than not doing Y).

1. She would be spending time out having fun with friends and family
2. She would be more outgoing in social situations
3. She would be in a loving romantic relationship

Dominant Discourses informing definition of problem:

- *Ethnic, Class and Religious Discourses: How do key cultural discourses inform what is perceived as a problem and the possible solutions?* AF comes from an immigrant, working-class, German family with only childhood exposure to the Lutheran church. She continues the work-focused values that her parents taught her, which are compounded by immigration and the need to work harder to survive in a new country. Her family did not value displays of affection or emotions. Her family does place high value upon marriage. AF's family did not have strong social ties outside of work, and AF also continues this approach to organizing her life.
- *Gender and Sexuality Discourses: How do the gender/sexual discourses inform what is perceived as a problem and the possible solutions?* In large part due to her sexual abuse as a child, AF feels very vulnerable as a woman, especially with strangers and in strange places. She almost always worries about her safety, both physically and emotionally. She has adopted the stereotypical female coping strategy of controlling herself internally in order to please others and prevent them from hurting her.
- *Community, School, and Extended Family Discourses: How do other important community discourses inform what is perceived as a problem and the possible solutions?* AF feels confident at work and is well respected at work, which is her safe haven in many ways.

Identity Narratives: How has the problem shaped each client's identity? The breakup and return of panic has led AF to believe that she should just focus on work and give up on intimate relationships and her dream of

(continued)

having a family. She tries to console herself by saying, "being successful at work is more success than many others have." However, the panic is making it harder to do her job, which is why she is seeking help.

Local or Preferred Discourses: What is the client's preferred identity narrative and/or narrative about the problem? Are there local (alternative) discourses about the problem that are preferred? As AF tends to blame herself for her situation and to see it as "inevitable," she has a difficult time generating alternative narratives to the problem-saturated narrative. However, at times, she believes that maybe she could learn to be less shy and that may help her.

CLINICAL ASSESSMENT

Clinician: Charmain	Client ID #: 9005	Primary configuration: ☒ Individual ❑ Couple ❑ Family	Primary Language: ☒ English ❑ Spanish ❑ Other: German

List client and significant others

Adult(s)

Adult Female Age: 34 European American Single heterosexual Occupation: Store manager; children's clothing store

Other identifier: ______

Select Gender Age: _____ Select Ethnicity Select Relational Status Occupation: ______ Other identifier: ______

Child(ren)

Select Gender Age: ______ Select Ethnicity Grade: Select Grade School: ______ Other identifier: ______

Select Gender Age: ______ Select Ethnicity Grade: Select Grade School: ______ Other identifier: ______

Others: ______

Presenting Problems

		Complete for children:
☒ Depression/hopelessness	❑ Couple concerns	❑ School failure/decline performance
☒ Anxiety/worry	❑ Parent/child conflict	❑ Truancy/runaway
❑ Anger issues	❑ Partner violence/abuse	❑ Fighting w/peers
☒ Loss/grief	❑ Divorce adjustment	❑ Hyperactivity
❑ Suicidal thoughts/attempts	❑ Remarriage adjustment	❑ Wetting/soiling clothing
☒ Sexual abuse/rape	❑ Sexuality/intimacy concerns	❑ Child abuse/neglect
❑ Alcohol/drug use	❑ Major life changes	❑ Isolation/withdrawal
❑ Eating problems/disorders	❑ Legal issues/probation	❑ Other: ______
❑ Job problems/unemployed	☒ Other: Panic	

Mental Status Assessment for Identified Patient

Interpersonal	❑ NA	❑ Conflict ❑ Enmeshment ☒ Isolation/avoidance ❑ Harassment ☒ Other: Overly shy
Mood	❑ NA	☒ Depressed/Sad ☒ Anxious ❑ Dysphoric ❑ Angry ❑ Irritable ❑ Manic ❑ Other: ______
Affect	❑ NA	☒ Constricted ❑ Blunt ❑ Flat ❑ Labile ❑ Incongruent ❑ Other: ______
Sleep	❑ NA	❑ Hypersomnia ❑ Insomnia ❑ Disrupted ☒ Nightmares ❑ Other: ______

(continued)

Eating	☒ NA	❑ Increase ❑ Decrease ❑ Anorectic restriction ❑ Binging ❑ Purging ❑ Other: ______
Anxiety	❑ NA	❑ Chronic worry ☒ Panic ❑ Phobias ❑ Obsessions ❑ Compulsions ❑ Other: ______
Trauma Symptoms	❑ NA	❑ Hypervigilance ❑ Flashbacks/Intrusive memories ❑ Dissociation ☒ Numbing ☒ Avoidance efforts ☒ Other: Dreams/nightmares
Psychotic Symptoms	☒ NA	❑ Hallucinations ❑ Delusions ❑ Paranoia ❑ Loose associations ❑ Other: ______
Motor Activity/ Speech	☒ NA	❑ Low energy ❑ Hyperactive ❑ Agitated ❑ Inattentive ❑ Impulsive ❑ Pressured speech ❑ Slow speech ❑ Other: ______
Thought	❑ NA	☒ Poor concentration ❑ Denial ☒ Self-blame ❑ Other-blame ☒ Ruminative ❑ Tangential ❑ Concrete ❑ Poor insight ❑ Impaired decision making ❑ Disoriented ❑ Other: ______
Socio-Legal	☒ NA	❑ Disregards rules ❑ Defiant ❑ Stealing ❑ Lying ❑ Tantrums ❑ Arrest/incarceration ❑ Initiates fights ❑ Other: ______
Other Symptoms	☒ NA	______

Diagnosis for Identified Patient

Contextual Factors considered in making diagnosis: ☒ Age ☒ Gender ☒ Family dynamics ☒ Culture ❑ Language ❑ Religion ❑ Economic ❑ Immigration ❑ Sexual/gender orientation ☒ Trauma ❑ Dual diagnosis/comorbid ❑ Addiction ❑ Cognitive ability ❑ Other: ______

Describe impact of identified factors on diagnosis and assessment process: Considered trauma issues related to abuse and immigration, as well as cultural norms for emotional expession and individual autonomy.

DSM-5 Code	Diagnosis with Specifier *Include V/Z/T-Codes for Psychosocial Stressors/Issues*
1. F43.10	1. Posttraumatic stress disorder with panic attacks
2. F40.00	2. Agoraphobia
3. Z62.810	3. Personal history of sexual abuse in childhood
4. ______	4. ______
5. ______	5. ______

Medical Considerations

Has patient been referred for psychiatric evaluation? ☒ Yes ❑ No

Has patient agreed with referral? ❑ Yes ☒ No ❑ NA

(continued)

Psychometric instruments used for assessment: ❑ None ☒ Cross-cutting symptom inventories

❑ Other: ____

Client response to diagnosis: ☒ Agree ❑ Somewhat agree ❑ Disagree ❑ Not informed for following reason: ____

Current Medications (psychiatric & medical) ❑ NA

1. Xanax; dose 4 mg; start date: August 1, 2013
2. ____; dose ____mg; start date: ____
3. ____; dose ____mg; start date: ____
4. ____; dose ____mg; start date: ____

Medical Necessity: *Check all that apply*

☒ Significant impairment ❑ Probability of significant impairment ❑ Probable developmental arrest

Areas of impairment:

☒ Daily activities ☒ Social relationships ❑ Health ❑ Work/School ❑ Living arrangement

❑ Other: ____

Risk and Safety Assessment for Identified Patient

Suicidality	Homicidality	Alcohol Abuse
☒ No indication/Denies	☒ No indication/Denies	☒ No indication/denies
❑ Active ideation	❑ Active ideation	❑ Past abuse
❑ Passive ideation	❑ Passive ideation	❑ Current; Freq/Amt: ____
❑ Intent without plan	❑ Intent without means	**Drug Use/Abuse**
❑ Intent with means	❑ Intent with means	☒ No indication/denies
❑ Ideation in past year	❑ Ideation in past year	❑ Past use
❑ Attempt in past year	❑ Violence past year	❑ Current drugs: ____
❑ Family or peer history of completed suicide	❑ History of assaulting others	Freq/Amt: ____
	❑ Cruelty to animals	❑ Family/sig.other use

Sexual & Physical Abuse and Other Risk Factors

☒ Childhood abuse history: ☒ Sexual ❑ Physical ❑ Emotional ❑ Neglect

❑ Adult with abuse/assault in adulthood: ❑ Sexual ❑ Physical ❑ Current

❑ History of perpetrating abuse: ❑ Sexual ❑ Physical ❑ Emotional

❑ Elder/dependent adult abuse/neglect

❑ History of or current issues with restrictive eating, binging, and/or purging

❑ Cutting or other self harm: ❑ Current ❑ Past: Method: ____

❑ Criminal/legal history: ____

❑ Other trauma history: ____

❑ None reported

(*continued*)

Indicators of Safety

❑ NA

☒ At least one outside support person

❑ Able to cite specific reasons to live or not harm

❑ Hopeful

☒ Willing to dispose of dangerous items

☒ Has future goals

❑ Willingness to reduce contact with people who make situation worse

☒ Willing to implement safety plan, safety interventions

❑ Developing set of alternatives to self-/other harm

☒ Sustained period of safety: No history of attempts

❑ Other: ______

Elements of Safety Plan

❑ NA

❑ Verbal no harm contract

❑ Written no harm contract

☒ Emergency contact card

☒ Emergency therapist/agency number

☒ Medication management

❑ Plan for contacting friends/support persons during crisis

❑ Specific plan of where to go during crisis

☒ Specific self-calming tasks to reduce risk before reach crisis level (e.g., journaling, exercising, etc.)

❑ Specific daily/weekly activities to reduce stressors

❑ Other: ______

Legal/Ethical Action Taken: ☒ NA ❑ Action: ______

Case Management

Collateral Contacts

- Has contact been made with treating *physicians or other professionals*: ❑ NA ☒ Yes ❑ In process. Name/Notes: Dr. Grossman; psychiatrist. Consultation about medication compliance and progress updates.
- If client is involved in mental health *treatment elsewhere*, has contact been made? ☒ NA ❑ Yes ❑ In process. Name/Notes: ______
- Has contact been made with *social worker*: ☒ NA ❑ Yes ❑ In process. Name/Notes: ______

Referrals

- Has client been referred for *medical assessment*: ☒ Yes ❑ No evidence for need
- Has client been referred for *social services*: ☒ NA ❑ Job/training ❑ Welfare/Food/Housing ❑ Victim services ❑ Legal aid ❑ Medical ❑ Other: ______
- Has client been referred for *group* or other support services: ❑ Yes: ______ ❑ In process ☒ None recommended
- Are there anticipated *forensic/legal processes* related to treatment: ☒ No ❑ Yes; describe: ______

Support Network

- Client social support network includes: ☒ Supportive family ❑ Supportive partner ☒ Friends ❑ Religious/spiritual organization ☒ Supportive work/social group ❑ Other: ______

(*continued*)

- Describe anticipated effects treatment will have on others in support system (Children, partner, etc.): Parents may be surprised if AF starts wanting more direct emotional connection and/or becomes more socially engaged with them or others.
- Is there anything else client will need to be successful? Connection with friends

Expected Outcome and Prognosis

☒ Return to normal functioning ☐ Anticipate less than normal functioning ☐ Prevent deterioration

Client Sense of Hope: 4

Evaluation of Assessment/Client Perspective

How were assessment methods adapted to client needs, including age, culture, and other diversity issues? Family system and cultural issues considered in assessment of affect and relational functioning.

Describe actual or potential areas of client-clinician agreement/disagreement related to the above assessment: Client in agreement; has been diagnosed with panic disorder before.

_______________________, _____________ _________

Clinician Signature | License/Intern Status | Date

_______________________, _____________ _________

Supervisor Signature | License | Date

TREATMENT PLAN

Date: 07/02/13 Case/Client #: 9005

Clinician Name: Charmain Theory: Adlerian

Modalities planned: ☒ Individual Adult ❑ Individual Child ❑ Couple ❑ Family ❑ Group: ________

Recommended session frequency: ☒ Weekly ❑ Every two weeks ❑ Other: ________

Expected length of treatment: 6 months

Initial Phase of Treatment

Initial Phase Counseling Tasks

1. Develop working counseling relationship. *Diversity considerations:* Mindful of abuse background and German immigrant norms that may require extra attention to personal space and privacy.

   Relationship-building approach/intervention:

   a. Used warmth, encouragement, and empathy to create sense of safety and place where AF felt she could speak as an equal in the process.

2. Assess individual, systemic, and broader cultural dynamics. *Diversity considerations:* Assess impact of parents' immigration, including potential associated traumas. Inquire about extended family or "adopted" family here in the states.

   Assessment strategies:

   a. Assess lifestyle, basic mistake, parenting style, family constellation, early recollections, organ inferiority, and dreams, and how abuse, only-child status, and German ethnicity and immigration dynamics shaped lifestyle.

   b. Ask "the question" to help determine role of panic and agoraphobia in maintaining her sense of physical and emotional safety.

3. Identify and obtain client agreement on treatment goals. *Diversity considerations:* Ensure client has sense of personal agency when identifying goals.

   Goal-making intervention:

   a. Work with client using psychoeducation to set goals to not only reduce panic and agoraphobia but also increase social interest and connection.

4. Identify needed referrals, crisis issues, and other client needs. *Diversity considerations:* Consider potential ties to German/Lutheran local community; assess for location of extended family and/or "adopted" family in the states.

   a. *Crisis assessment intervention(s):* Refer and consult with psychiatrist regarding panic and agoraphobia.

   b. *Referral(s):* Provide psychoeducation information for AF; most likely to use Internet or written resources.

(continued)

Initial Phase Client Goal

1. Decrease insecurities that lead to AF feeling fearful of social contact to reduce panic and agoraphobia.

   Interventions:

   a. Psychoeducation on stress response, panic, and agoraphobia, discussing best ways to handle.

   b. Challenge basic mistake beliefs about needing control to be safe and needing approval from others to be okay.

Working Phase of Treatment

Working Phase Counseling Tasks

1. Monitor quality of the working alliance. *Diversity considerations:* Respect need for personal space and privacy.

   a. *Assessment Intervention:* Monitor for AF increasing engagement in process; signs of feeling a sense of equality in process.

2. Monitor progress toward goals. *Diversity considerations:* Adapt social interest goals to account for sexual abuse and family of origin/cultural relational patterns.

   a. *Assessment Intervention:* Ask client about perceived progress and monitor development of social interest; Outcome Questionnaire to measure overall distress pre and post.

Working Phase Client Goals

1. Decrease insecurities about physical and emotional safety in the world to reduce avoidance of social contact.

   Interventions:

   a. Identify and challenge basic beliefs, especially those affected by abuse, to develop a realistic and balanced view of when and how to care for her safety and when it is safe to trust and relax.

   b. Psychoeducation on physical and emotional safety to help AF establish age and gender appropriate expectations for self and other.

2. Decrease avoidance of relational life tasks and overemphasis on work tasks to reduce social isolation.

   Interventions:

   a. Challenge belief that "I am better off alone" and encourage AF to continue pursuing social relationships.

   b. Interpretation of social avoidance behaviors to identify the role they play in creating an illusion of safety.

3. Decrease reliance on work and relational success to define self-worth to reduce social avoidance.

   Interventions:

   a. Identify origin of and challenge belief that value is determined by work contributions while being respectful of family and cultural beliefs.

   b. Alter self statements to increase valuing of self based on "what" rather than "how" she is doing, developing a greater internal locus of evaluation.

(*continued*)

Closing Phase of Treatment

Closing Phase Counseling Task

1. Develop aftercare plan and maintain gains. *Diversity considerations:* Consider potential resources in local German and/or Lutheran communtiy.

   Intervention:

   a. Psychoeducation on social interest and positive psychology to develop habits of wellness, such as a strong social network, gratifying activities, and optimistic basic assumptions while respecting and integrating family and cultural values.

Closing Phase Client Goals

1. Increase self-acceptance and overall sense of wellness to reduce relapse of panic and social avoidance.

   Interventions:

   a. Psychoeducation on the importance of social relationships for well-being, habits of wellness, and activities that support happiness.

   b. Encourage AF to strengthen social network of friends and family and deepen those relationships.

2. Increase AF's ability to emotionally connect with and trust intimate partner to reduce isolation.

   Interventions:

   a. Encourage AF to pursue dating relationships with realistic beliefs and a willingness to connect more deeply once in a safe relationship.

   b. Psychoeducation on how to establish, maintain, and troubleshoot relationships.

PROGRESS NOTE FOR CLIENT #9005

Date: 09/05/13 **Time:** 9:00 ☒ am/❑ pm **Session Length:** ❑ 45 min. ☒ 60 min. ❑ Other: ______ minutes

Present: ❑ Adult Male ☒ Adult Female ❑ Child Male ❑ Child Female ❑ Other: ______________

Billing Code: ❑ 90791 (eval) ❑ 90834 (45 min. therapy) ☒ 90837 (60 min. therapy) ❑ 90847 (family)

❑ Other: ______________________________

Symptom(s)	Duration and Frequency Since Last Visit	Progress
1: Panic	1 mild episode; 5 minutes	Progressing
2: Agoraphobia	2 mild episodes; 4–6 hours	Progressing
3: Social isolation	Moderate, most days	Progressing

Explanatory Notes on Symptoms: AF reports following up on homework to make contact with "safe" friends to go to low-key social activities. Reports she is able to manage panic relatively well with medication and deep breathing. Although she feels like isolating, especially on weekends, pushes self to go out; having "homework" from session helps.

In-Session Interventions and Assigned Homework

Follow-up on prior week's homework; AF reported making calls to friends and accepting invitations to go to low-key events two nights during weekend. In session, continued to challenge basic beliefs about needing to control self at all times, needing to hide feelings from others, and always playing it safe; used recent events with friends to challenge these beliefs. Continued psychoeducation on evaluating safety in relationships and knowing when to take risks. Continue with homework to do something with "safe friends" on Fri and Sat.

Client Response/Feedback

AF finds challenge of homework motivating to make changes. AF responsive to psychoeducation and arguments that draw parallels between work and social life.

Plan

☒ Continue with treatment plan: plan for next session: Follow up on weekly tasks.

❑ Modify plan: ______________________________

Next session: Date: 09/12/13 Time: 9:00 ☒ am/❑ pm

Crisis Issues: ☒ No indication of crisis/client denies ❑ Crisis assessed/addressed: describe below

Reports panic is managable with medication.

______________________, ______________________ ______________________

Clinician's Signature, License/Intern Status Date

Case Consultation/Supervision ❑ Not Applicable

Notes: Supervisor encouraged working toward family session.

(*continued*)

Collateral Contact ❑ Not Applicable

Name: Dr. Grossman Date of Contact: 09/04/2013 Time: 1:15 ❑am/☒pm

☒ Written release on file: ☒ Sent/❑ Received ❑ In court docs ❑ Other: ____________

Notes: Consulted with psychiatrist on medication compliance; update on progress.

______________________, ______________________ ______________________

Clinician's Signature, License/Intern Status Date

______________________, ______________________ ______________________

Supervisor's Signature, License Date

CHAPTER

10

Humanistic-Existential Counseling Approaches

Lay of the Land

Grounded in phenomenological philosophy, humanistic-existential counseling approaches are some of the most widely used and influential counseling approaches. Although humanistic and existential approaches initially developed as distinct counseling therapies, contemporary practitioners typically draw freely from at least three humanistic-existential approaches:

- *Person-Centered Counseling:* Person-centered counseling—also known as client-centered or Rogerian counseling—is a quintessential counseling approach. Developed by Carl Rogers (1942, 1951), this approach is based on the assertion that three core conditions—accurate empathy, counselor genuineness, and unconditional regard—are sufficient to promote client change. The focus is on the emotional and relational processes that promote change rather than the use of specific techniques to achieve desired outcomes. This approach assumes that people tend *naturally* toward positive growth.
- *Gestalt Counseling:* Similar to person-centered, Gestalt counseling is a humanistic approach that focuses on helping people to self-actualize or to become more fully themselves. However, the techniques are more emotionally provocative and confrontational than the person-centered approach.
- *Existential Counseling:* Existential counseling is grounded in existential philosophy, which has more neutral assumptions about the human condition in comparison to the more optimistic humanistic foundations of person-centered counseling. Existential counseling posits that clients experience symptoms and distress because they are avoiding or need to more effectively deal with broader existential issues, such as each human's ultimate separation from others, death, loss, and existential anxiety. This approach emphasizes insight and reflection on existential issues to more effectively resolve the underlying anxiety that fuels a client's presenting concern.

Digital Download Download from CengageBrain.com

This chapter covers person-centered and gestalt counseling; the existential module is available for download from CengageBrain.com.

Person-Centered Counseling

In a Nutshell: The Least You Need to Know

Arguably one of the most influential theories in the field of counseling and psychotherapy (Kirschenbaum & Jourdan, 2005), person-centered counseling is a process-focused approach to helping people become more fully themselves. Developed by Carl Rogers (1942, 1951, 1961, 1981)—thus, it is often referred to as Rogerian counseling or its early term of client-centered counseling—person-centered counseling is based on the radical and startling proposition that the necessary and sufficient elements of therapeutic change are (a) counselor congruence or genuineness, (b) accurate empathic understanding of the client, and (c) unconditional positive regard. Rogers asserted that if these three things were in place, over time the client would become more fully themselves and eventually the problems they came to counseling for would resolve. Person-centered counseling *does not* develop treatment plans to directly address the presenting problems clients report, such as depression, conflict with a spouse, or indecision about career direction. Instead, the counseling focuses on helping clients to experience their in-the-moment internal experiences to expose the facades they live behind and the socially imposed shoulds that may be organizing their lives. As clients are able to more accurately and deeply experience themselves *while in relationship to the counselor*, they become better at making decisions that need to be made, experiencing themselves more fully and accurately, and relating to others, all of which works together to help them resolve the issues that brought them to counseling in the first place. Thus, techniques are avoided in favor of the counselor promoting a basic process of becoming more fully and accurately aware of one's inner world.

The Juice: Significant Contributions to the Field

If you remember one thing from this chapter, it should be ...

Core Conditions

The necessary and sufficient conditions of personality change boldly identified by Carl Rogers (1957/2007) are arguably some of the most influential ideas put forth in the field of counseling and psychotherapy (Kirschenbaum, 2004; Kirschenbaum & Jourdan, 2005). In his 1957/2007 article, Rogers identifies six conditions necessary for constructive personality change over a period of time:

1. Two persons are in psychological contact.
2. The first, whom we shall term the client, is in a state of incongruence, being vulnerable or anxious.
3. The second person, whom we shall term the therapist, is *congruent* or integrated in the relationship.
4. The therapist experiences *unconditional positive regard* for the client.
5. The therapist experiences an *empathic understanding* of the client's internal frame of reference and endeavors to communicate this experience to the client.
6. The communication to the client of the therapist's empathic understanding and unconditional positive regard is—to a minimal degree—achieved. (Rogers, 1957/2007, p. 241; italics added).

In later writings these six conditions are boiled down into three conditions that the therapist must create in the counseling relationship:

1. Congruence or genuineness of the counselor,
2. Unconditional positive regard, and
3. Accurate empathy.

These three conditions are the heart of person-centered counseling. Rogers (1957/2007) believed these to be necessary and sufficient for personality change, regardless of the counselor's theory of choice or the client's presenting problem; he clearly states this is his hypothesis until empirically proven otherwise. Rogers researched the hypothesis put forth in his 1957 article for the subsequent three decades, and many after him have continued to test and refine his hypothesis (Kirschenbaum & Jourdan, 2005). Nonetheless, the debate rages on as to whether his hypothesis is correct (Brown, 2007; Hill, 2007; Kirschenbaum & Jourdan, 2005; Mahrer, 2007; Wachtel, 2007). At present, most would agree that the conditions outlined by Rogers in 1957 are *neither* sufficient *nor* necessary but there is a substantial body of evidence to indicate that they are clearly *facilitative* and "crucial," meaning they are *helpful* to *extremely helpful* in promoting change (Kirschenbaum & Jourdan, 2005). Translated even more simply: although there are some documented exceptions, in most cases the conditions identified by Rogers are highly correlated with positive counseling outcomes; *no research has identified a specific population or problem for which these conditions are counterindicated* (inappropriate). The common factors movement is an outgrowth of the research that indicates the qualities advocated by Rogers are highly correlated with positive therapeutic outcome, more so than the counselor's choice of theory. To boil it down even further, although they may not be necessary and sufficient for all clients in all cases, they are extremely crucial for positive outcomes, regardless of the counseling theory you choose to work from—so read the following sections closely, it's probably the most important part of this book in terms of being a great counselor.

Genuineness or Congruence The first condition is counselor *genuineness* (Rogers, 1957/2007), later referred to as *congruence*, which refers to the counselor's outer expressions being "congruent' with his/her inner experience (Rogers, 1961). In 21st-century vernacular, we call this "being real." However, Rogers is referring to a humanistic, philosophical definition of what it means to be real, whole, and integrated—not what popular culture might define as real. Rogers's definition emphasizes being freely and deeply one's self while able to *accurately* "take in" what is experienced, and simultaneously remaining aware of one's internal processing of that experience. Rogers explained congruence, stating that "by this we mean that the feelings the therapist is experiencing are available to him[/her], available to his[/her] awareness, and he[/she] is able to live these feelings, be them, and able to communicate them if appropriate. No one fully achieves this condition, yet the more the therapist is able to listen acceptingly to what is going on within himself[/herself], and the more he is able to be the complexity of his feelings, without fear, the higher the degree of his congruence" (Rogers, 1961, p. 61). Thus, congruence/genuineness is an idealized goal to which counselors continually aspire to more fully achieve. Far from an all-or-nothing state of affairs, it is a continually evolving and ever-deepening process.

Another way to understand Rogers's definition of genuineness is to approach it from its opposite, which is playing a role or having a facade (Rogers, 1957/2007), including the role of "professional." Being congruent means that one does not try to "act" professional, "be" helpful, or otherwise take on a role or mask. This is a fine distinction, because in some ways there are professional boundaries that need to be maintained: this is not a friendship but a helping relationship that has certain legal and ethical constraints. On the other hand, the typical slightly detached professional role, especially at the time Rogers was developing his ideas, is also not appropriate. Much like Goldilocks, there is a place in the middle that is just right—and the actual contours of this middle ground often vary from client to client.

Finally, I should mention that it is very difficult to be genuine in this way when first starting out, simply because the new counselor has too many other things to think about: getting informed consent, conducting a mental status interview, assessing for danger, making a diagnosis, using new interventions, and so on. The more a counselor's mind is trying to remember these things, the less able the counselor is able to be genuine, because too much focus is elsewhere. With time, these other tasks become second nature, and it becomes easier to be genuine. Perhaps one of the best indicators that a counselor is being genuine is a pervading sense of inner calm and centeredness, no matter what the client says or does.

Unconditional Positive Regard Unconditional positive regard is what it sounds like: valuing your clients no matter what they say or do (Rogers, 1957/2007) and has also been described as warm acceptance, nonpossessive warmth, prizing, affirmation, respect, support, and caring (Hill, 2007). This sounds a bit like Pollyanna, so let's try to analyze what Rogers really meant by this. The underlying attitude here is not a one-dimensional belief that "all people are good" and that good counselors "love everybody." After all, counselors work with some of the most difficult, angry, and mean people in society: child molesters, criminals, divorcing spouses, gang members, negligent parents, substance abusers, and others. If you have developed unconditional positive regard based on the Pollyanna notion that all people are good, it is going to fail you with these clients. Instead, unconditional positive regard needs to be built upon a more subtle and reflected philosophical premise.

Unconditional positive regard is founded upon the idea that we are all human and we all suffer and therefore have the capacity for good and evil (or destructive behavior if you prefer). If you see yourself as far superior to the pedophile, vengeful divorcee, or gang-banger, you are probably unaware of the darker potentials that lie within each of us. Thus, unconditional positive regard is best motivated by a deep sense of compassion for how hard it is to be human—and for how easy it is to get off track and make bad decisions. When you view clients from this perspective, you can still hold them accountable for their past and current decisions and yet have compassion and hope for their current situation and future.

Accurate Empathy Rogers defines *empathy* as being able "to sense the client's private world as if it were your own, but without ever losing the "as if" quality" (Rogers, 1957/2007, p. 243). In the practice of counseling, empathy involves not only the ability to accurately perceive the internal world of the client but also the ability to meaningfully share this understanding with the client. Rogers explains, "To sense the client's anger, fear, or confusion as if it were your own, yet without your own anger, fear, or confusion getting bound up in it, is the condition we are endeavoring to describe. When the client's world is this clear to the therapist, and he moves about in it freely, then he can both communicate his understanding of what is clearly known to the client and can also voice meanings in the client's experience of which the client is scarcely aware" (Rogers, 1957/2007, p. 243). Doing this requires the counselor being keenly in tune with his or her internal world while having clear enough boundaries to perceive how another person's internal world hangs together.

Once the counselor has a sense of what the client *might* be feeling, the counselor then *reflects* (see below) this back to the client to (a) indicate that the counselor has understood, (b) check to make sure the counselor has understood correctly, and (c) provide the client with an opportunity to reflect on his/her internal experience in a slightly different context—namely, in external dialogue in the words of another person. Having one's intimate, private world described by someone else is often a profoundly moving experience that often transforms one's experience, perception, and/or understanding of one's own experience. *That* is where the counseling comes in. For this reason, the question "how does that make you feel?" is generally not as helpful as being able to convey accurate empathy.

Empathy should be conveyed tentatively, and the counselor should create space in the relationship for the client to say, "No, that is not how I feel" and not get into a tug-of-war over who's right about how the client feels. To be sure, there will be times when the counselor's reflection is accurate and yet the client denies it. If this is the case, the counselor may want to rephrase it in a less dramatic version (e.g., rather than "you are angry at your mother" to say "you didn't like what your mother said yesterday") and then allow the client to further explore this *at her or his own pace*. The good news about empathy is that you don't have to get it right every time. If you have established a strong relationship and frequently seem to understand, then the times when you don't the client feels safe enough to correct you. In fact, when working with clients who tend toward people pleasing, I do not believe a rapport has been established until a client feels safe enough to tell me that I got it wrong. Only then do I know that they have dropped the people pleasing facade and feel safe enough to be real with me. All that said, indeed, there are times, once you have a strong rapport, when it is effective to ask that oft-mocked question, "How does that make you feel?"

Cultural and Gender Considerations Although in theory it is simple enough, demonstrating appropriate empathy is far more difficult than it initially sounds, because culture and gender greatly affect how one expresses empathy and what a person experiences as empathic. For example, some people expect heartfelt, warm expressions of empathy: "You feel deeply betrayed by your daughter's choice," while others find such empathic statements shameful and insensitive because they lose face or think you are putting words into their mouth. Such persons may experience a subtle or even nonverbal expression of empathy as more sincere and meaningful: a silent nod with a look of understanding. Thus, counselors need to become skilled in different ways of conveying empathy. In the case study at the end of this chapter, the counselor adapts the core conditions to work with Shandra, an African American woman who is struggling with anxiety and perfectionism, by using culturally sensitive expressions of warmth and reflecting her experiences of marginalization as a professional African American woman in the business world.

Big Picture: Overview of Counseling Process

Person-centered counseling is a *process*-oriented approach, meaning that the counselor's attention is on the *how* things happen (process) rather than *what* happens (content). As the name implies, the focus is on *persons*—most notably their inner processes—rather than on their problems (Rogers, 1961). As a humanistic approach, counselors' primary aim is to help the client become more fully themselves, more authentic, and less attached to social roles and expectations. The person-centered counselor has a strong belief that symptoms will resolve themselves as clients become more self-actualized, because they will view problems differently and take more responsibility for their emotions and life situations.

The process of self-actualization is not as easy or smooth as it initially sounds. In session, the counselor pays less attention to the content of the client's life—which is almost always less anxiety-provoking to discuss—and instead focuses on *how* the client interacts with self, others, and life challenges: Does the client tend to blame others or does the client take responsibility for his/her life? Does the client focus on details of external events or is the client able to identify what is going on within him/herself? Does the client have realistic expectations of self and others? The process is not always easy, as the counselor will gently "confront" attitudes, beliefs, and inconsistencies that keep the client from becoming more self-actualized. Throughout this process, the counselor gently and consistently redirects the client to more clearly articulate thoughts, feelings, and longings, especially those that may be difficult to admit to self or others, such as embarrassment, anger, shame, resentment, and such. Through this process, the client begins to integrate contradictory and less-than-perfect parts of the self, reducing defensiveness and increasing their openness to experience. The counselor's primary role is to help the client remove the barriers—most of which the client has erected—to their own self-actualization.

Rogers (1961) describes seven stages of the change process a person typically experiences, from the time of entering counseling to achieving—at least to some degree—self-actualization.

Seven Stages of the Change Process

1. **First Stage:** In this stage, a person's personality seems fixed, personal problems are not acknowledged, there is a remoteness of experiencing, and there is little desire to change; the person is not likely to voluntarily enter counseling.
2. **Second Stage:** If a person in the first stage is able to feel "received" by the counselor, they begin to loosen up and are more open to seeing problems, which are viewed as external to the self ("bad things happen to me"), with little sense of personal responsibility.
3. **Third Stage:** If clients continue to feel accepted and understood by the counselor, they become more able to express past feelings and personal meanings.
4. **Fourth Stage:** If clients continue to feel safe with the counselor, they begin to become more open to reconsidering their constructs about self and others and are increasingly able to verbalize deep emotions.
5. **Fifth Stage:** As clients continue to explore themselves in the safety of the counseling relationship, they are increasingly able to verbalize in-the-moment emotions and experiences and an increasing desire to be the "real me."
6. **Sixth Stage:** Rogers describes a distinct shift in the sixth stage, where the person is now able to experience difficult emotions as they arise in the present moment with

acceptance rather than fear, denial, or struggle.[1] Once this change happens, it tends to be irreversible, meaning that the client will continue to accept even the most difficult emotions rather than deny them.

7. **Seventh Stage:** In this stage it is no longer necessary for the client to be received by the counselor in order to self-actualize, although it is still helpful, because the client has learned how to sustain the process of self-actualization without outside help. This stage generally occurs outside the counseling relationship.

Making Connection: Therapeutic Relationship

Relationship as Change Agent

Unlike most psychotherapies, person-centered counselors view the counseling relationship as the primary vehicle for change—*not* the counselor's interventions. They believe that it is through the authentic, human relationship between the counselor and client that the client is able to progress through the seven stages described above and become more authentically themselves (Rogers, 1961). This is different from psychodynamic approaches in which the client is "working through" their issues in the therapeutic relationship and the counselor is interacting from a therapeutic role to "repair" and "correct." Instead, the person-centered counselor views the relationship as two authentic humans in relationship; when the client experiences being allowed to be fully themselves in relationship, their inherent tendency to strive for positive growth is activated.

Therapeutic Presence and the Core Conditions

As discussed above—and as we will continue to repeat throughout this section—Carl Rogers (1961, 1981) based his person-centered approach on three counselor qualities used to promote change in clients, the core conditions: (a) congruence or genuineness of the counselor, (b) accurate empathy, and (c) unconditional positive regard. These are the heart of the counseling relationship, but they are not an end in themselves. They are best thought of as the key ingredients in a chemical reaction that, when mixed together, create something far greater and more powerful than the inert ingredients alone. The result of this chemical experiment in this case is called *therapeutic presence* (Gehart & McCollum, 2008; Geller & Greenberg, 2002; McDonough-Means, Kreitzer, & Bell, 2004). Therapeutic presence is a quality of being, having intrapersonal, interpersonal, and transpersonal elements, including empathy, compassion, charisma, spirituality, transpersonal communication, client responsiveness, optimism, and expectancy, making it an elusive and difficult-to-operationalize concept. That said, research indicates that clients know it when they feel it.

Clients tend to accurately sense how much and what type of information to share with counselors based on their quality of presence (Geller & Greenberg, 2002; McDonough-Means et al., 2004). If a counselor exudes even the slightest bit of anxiety while a person retells a tale of sexual abuse or trauma or judgment while sharing about a relationship or drinking episode, the client is likely to edit, recast, or simply cut short their relaying of experience. If the counselor is uncomfortable with sharing their emotions about what is going on in the present moment (i.e., immediacy, see below), the client will be, too. As counselors become more experienced in session while also practicing personal reflection and self-care, the quality of their therapeutic presence is likely to become more noticeable and facilitative.

The Viewing: Case Conceptualization

When Carl Rogers talked with people, he didn't just experience unconditional positive regard and empathy. He also carefully observed what they spoke about and how they spoke, in order to assess to what extent they were in touch with their authentic selves.

---

[1]This acceptance of immediate experience is the goal of mindfulness meditation, which has been most fully developed in cognitive, behaviorally oriented therapies discussed in Chapter 11; humanistic counselors also integrate mindfulness to cultivate the type of lived experience described by Rogers in this stage.

He developed a seven-stage model (Rogers, 1961) that described how he saw people moving along a continuum from a rigid definition of self to a more flowing and ever-changing experience of self. Rather than simply change the definition of self—from one static identity to another—Rogers (1961) came to believe that self-actualization involves a process of letting go of static definitions of self and increasingly embracing a fluid experience of self in lieu of a singular identity.

In the early stages, people are unaware of their feelings, speak more about others than themselves, and often feel more like the victim than the protagonist in their life stories. As people experience the effect of the core conditions in the counseling, these things change. People begin to experience their emotions as they are happening in the moment; they are able to readily identify what they are feeling; they take greater responsibility for what happens in their life and how they respond emotionally. These stages are used to conceptualize where the client is along the continuum of self-actualization. Rogers maintained that people generally hovered around a single stage in all areas of functioning, although minor exceptions may be noted at a particular time or in a specific context. Table 10.1 illustrates the changes as people move through the stages.

TABLE **10.1**
Seven Stages of Rogers's Change Process

	Stage 1	Stage 2	Stage 3	Stage 4	Stage 5	Stage 6	Stage 7
Experience and Communication of Self	Communication about externals.	Able to discuss non-self topics.	Expression of self as object; self-experiences as objects.	Increased awareness of self.	Desire to be "real me."	Self as object tends to disappear.	Self as process.
Recognition of Feeling	Unrecognized or not owned.	Described as unwanted or past objects.	Little acceptance of feelings.	Feelings described as objects in present.	Begin owning feelings.	Feelings readily accepted.	Feelings accepted and owned.
Expression of Feelings	Little to none.	May be exhibited but not owned.	Description of feelings.	More intense description of past feeling.	Expressed freely in present.	Full; physical loosening.	Full and flowing.
Present Moment Experiencing	Little to none.	Bound by structure of the past.	Bound by past primarily.	Less bound by past, less remote.	More immediate, but still somewhat surprising.	Immediate and rich. Process quality. Physiological loosening.	Immediate and rich in and out of session.
Personal Constructs	Extremely rigid. Black/white.	Considered "facts."	Rigid but recognized as constructs.	Discovery of constructs.	Critical examination of constructs.	Dissolve in experiencing moments.	Tentatively held.
Complexity and Contradiction	Unrecognized.	Expressed but unrecognized.	Recognition of contradictions.	Concern about incongruence.	Surprise and fright as feelings bubble through; more acceptance.	Vividly experienced, and dissolve in congruence.	Acceptance and ownership of changing feelings.
Perception of Problems; Responsibility for Situation	Unrecognized.	External to self. No sense of personal responsibility.	Personal choices seen as ineffective.	Some self-responsibility in relation to problems.	Increased responsibility.	No longer external or internal. Problem not perceived as object.	Full responsibility for self and emotions; confident about self as process.

Experience and Communication of Self

As people become more self-actualized, *how* they experience themselves changes. The sense of self evolves from a static entity to one where the self is more of a process that is constantly unfolding and changing. Paradoxically, rather than "discovering" a constant self, a person discovers that the self is constantly in flux and unfolding.

Recognition of Feelings

Rogers theorized that the more self-actualized a person is, the better that person can identify and own emotion. In assessing clients, counselors look for whether clients can identify a range of emotions when they discuss the concerns they bring to counseling. Can they identify feelings of anger, hurt, joy, fear? In most cases that warrant seeking counseling, a wide range of emotions is present to some degree or another. In some cases, a client has great difficulty identifying any emotion; in others, there is a particular favorite, such as anger or hurt, that is primarily felt. The more self-actualized a person is, the greater the range of emotion and the greater their ability to "own" that emotion as one that they feel without shame, fear, or embarrassment.

Expression of Emotion

In the process of self-actualization, people become better able to, and more comfortable with, expressing their full range of emotions. Early in the process, people may not express any emotion: they appear almost emotionless, and therefore at times they appear to themselves and others as having "everything under control." However, that sense of control is extremely fragile. Through the counseling process, people become more aware of their feelings, initially describing them as if they were happening to someone else. As they continue, they become able to describe both past and present emotions fully and in a way that is flowing and natural.

Gender and ethnic background often significantly impact which emotions are expressed and how they are expressed. For example, in most cultures, women are allowed to more freely express emotion than men. All cultures have values related to emotional expression that define where, how, and with whom emotion is best expressed and also which emotions are socially acceptable in which situation. For example, Japanese culture values emotional restraint in most public settings whereas Mediterranean cultures, such as the Greeks and Italians, value relatively bold expression of emotion in the same situations. Thus, counselors need to carefully consider gender and culture, as well as age and socioeconomic status, to fairly interpret a person's emotional expression.

Present Moment Experiencing

Present moment experiencing refers to the ability to mindfully experience emotions in the present moment. When experiencing emotions in the here-and-now, a person is able to (a) actually feel the emotion and (b) reflectively articulate the emotion (e.g., "I am feeling angry" rather than launch into an angry tirade that blames others). The more a person can experience intense, difficult emotions in the present while still being able to productively talk about them, the greater their level of self-actualization. Initially, most clients have little present moment experiencing; most of their experience is related to thoughts and worries about the past or future. Through the counseling process, clients become increasingly able to feel their feelings in the present moment *and be aware of this experience*, experiencing and witnessing their experience at the same time.

Personal Constructs and Facades

Rogers (1961) often described inauthentic living as living behind a "mask" or facade. These facades are the *personal constructs* we use to tell us who we are, how we should behave, and what we are worth. In contrast, authentic living refers to living in the process of being human, accepting the varied flow of experience that cannot be captured by a single construct or definition of who we are. For example, if a person maintains the construct that she is a "nice" person, she will have to suppress, ignore, or otherwise disregard the very real and normal human reactions, such as anger, disappointment, boredom, and dislike; she will have to disregard parts of herself, some vital, in order to maintain the facade. Initially, a person's personal constructs are rigid and black-and-white: *I am X, not Y.* As people become more self-actualized and begin to experience themselves more as an unfolding process than a static entity, these constructs become less and less important and instead people simply experience themselves as complex beings having a series of unfolding life experiences, a process that involves a fluid and adapting sense of self. In the case study at the end of this chapter, the counselor helps Shandra become less identified with her professional facade, allowing herself to increasingly experience herself as a constantly evolving process.

Complexity and Contradictions

Humanistic counselors also assess for a person's ability to engage the complexities and contradictions that characterize one's internal lives and life more generally. We often believe that humans are "logical" creatures that make sense, have singular opinions, and emotions that are rational. This is one myth that is quickly busted if you ever decide to practice mindfulness meditation for even 60 seconds. The Buddhists liken the mind to a monkey that jumps from tree to tree, up and down, here and there in an erratic, unpredictable pattern. The mind similarly jumps from topic to topic, past to future, thought to feeling, without necessarily being consistent or coherent. In fact, the more complex the topic, the more likely a person has contradictory thoughts and emotions: both loving and resenting a significant other; both liking and hating one's career, for example.

Early in the counseling process, most people are totally unaware of their own contradictory thoughts and feelings. As they become more aware, they become increasingly concerned about the lack of congruence. Rather than "pick a side" and end contradiction, the process of self-actualization moves toward greater acceptance of these contradictions as part of the complexity and "messiness" of being human. The greater a person's ability to accept these inherent contradictions in oneself, others, and life, the more resourceful one will be in managing life stressors.

Perception of Problems and Responsibility

In the early stages, problems are perceived as primarily caused by the outside world: others, circumstances, and so on. As people progress through the stages, there is an increasing awareness of one's responsibility and agency in every situation, and therefore problems are increasingly described with an emphasis on how one is contributing and/or perpetuating the situation. For example, rather than complain, "my wife is always nagging me," or "my husband never helps out around the house," clients increasingly say the problem is "I have a hard time motivating myself to get things done" or "my expectations are too high for myself and others."

Often in life, it feels like life happens "to us": people do things to make us angry, hurt us, or prevent us from getting what we want. It may be a lover who says something thoughtless, a boss who passes us up for a promotion, or a parent who doesn't have time for us. The more self-actualized a person becomes, the greater the awareness that life is a two-way street. In most cases, how we interact with another contributes to how they respond to us. In all cases, we have control of how we decide to respond, in terms of actions, words, and even emotions. When clients describe the problems in terms of being agents of their own lives, they take responsibility for their part in creating the problem situation and are quick to assume full responsibility for resolving the problem, no matter the source. In contrast, clients with lower levels of agency tend to feel victimized and often are mystified about how to go about solving problems.

Peak Experience and Flow

Rogers describes the self-actualized self as "fluid" and "flowing." Recent positive psychology researchers also describe peak experience as a "*flow*" state, a unique quality of experience in which a person feels fully present, in sync, and immersed in a challenging activity for which one has sufficient skill. Typically, during flow experiences, time seems to be moving more slowly and activity seems to happen without effort or thought. A classic example is the football quarterback making a seemingly impossible pass to another player; often, when interviewed afterward, the athlete will describe the event as though he, the ball, and the receiver were one. Other common flow experiences involve playing music, cooking, writing, running, dancing, and similar activities. Flow experiences typically are associated with activities that require effort and practice. After a certain level of mastery, the activity takes on an effortless, automatic, and fully alive quality for distinct periods of time. These are a type of peak experience that is associated with the humanistic view of being self-actualized. Counselors can ask about the frequency and quality of these flow experiences in assessing a client's level of functioning. For example, depression is typically an experience in which there are few if any experiences of flow; as people begin to recover, they often find that flow experiences return.

Targeting Change: Goal Setting

Self-Actualization: "Becoming That Self Which One Truly Is"

It's easy to write the final goal on a person-centered treatment plan because the overarching goal in person-centered counseling is consistent with most other humanistic approaches: to promote *self-actualization*. Self-actualization refers to fulfilling one's potential and living an authentic, meaningful life, or, as Rogers explains: "To be that self which one truly is" (1961, p. 163). Self-actualization is correlated with Rogers's (1961) Stage 7 level of development. Unlike existentialists, Rogers firmly believed that humans *naturally* tend toward positive, prosocial growth; the counselor's primary job is to provide the correct environment that fosters this growth (i.e., the core conditions). Maslow (1954) also identified self-actualization as the highest order in his hierarchy of human needs, coming only after more basic physiological, safety, social, and self-esteem needs are met.

Self-actualization (Rogers, 1961) is characterized by:

- Openness to present moment experiencing of emotions
- Trust in self
- Internal locus of evaluation and control
- Living without roles, facades, shoulds, or social expectation
- Being a complex, dynamic, and unfolding process (rather than a static entity)
- Openness to experience
- Acceptance of others

Self-actualization is always a long-term, late phase goal: the broad, overarching direction for counseling. Unfortunately, it is a vague goal unless smaller goals that address impediments are used in the middle phase.

Process Goals

It's well established that self-actualization is a BIG goal. However, most of the work in counseling occurs in smaller goals along the way that address *process* issues: a person's internal process. Here is where your case conceptualization comes into play. You can identify areas of growth and turn these into middle phase goals. For example, if a woman describes her life as unfairly limited by all the things she *should do* to be a "good wife," counselors write a goal to "increase living by conscious choice rather than a list of shoulds." Similarly, if a man reports wanting to constantly please others, to his own detriment, a process goal would be to "reduce attempts to please others in ways that are detrimental to personal needs."

Example of goals related to specific areas of functioning

Emotional Expression and Here-and-Now Experiencing

- "Increase ability to identify emotions in present moment."

Victimization and Experience of Problems

- "Increase sense of responsibility for own problems and their resolution."

Agency

- "Increase sense of agency and proactive behavior in work life."

(continued)

Facades and Masks

- "Reduce use of facades in personal relationships to increase experience of intimacy."

Peak Experience and Flow

- "Increase frequency of peak experience and flow in work life."

Perfectionism and Unrealistic Expectations

- "Increase ability to set realistic expectations for self and other to increase acceptance."

Trust Self

- "Increase ability to trust the evolving and changing nature of the self."

The Doing: Interventions

Self of the Counselor and the Core Conditions

The fundamental "instrument" of intervention in person-centered counseling is the "self" of the counselor: the counselor's way of being in the world. It's hard to get more nebulous than that, so you will find a list of other "techniques" in the rest of this section that are all trying to cultivate this one essential instrument of change: the counselor. As a highly relational form of counseling, person-centered counseling relies on the personhood of the counselor to bring a quality of presence that helps clients to transform and become more comfortable with experiencing their authentic selves. In a smaller nutshell, the self of the counselor is the vehicle through which the core conditions are established. Thus, in many ways the crux of change in person-centered counseling is the quality of the relationship between the counselor and counselee.

In practical terms, using the self of the counselor/counselor could involve a wide range of activities, including expressing empathy, using humor, and self-disclosure. What is demanded of the counselor changes based on the client, the problem, the topic of conversation, and the goals for counseling. Ultimately, it is the clearly communicated authenticity of the counselor that sets the stage for clients to identify, explore, and freely express their authentic selves. Knowing how to use one's personhood to facilitate authenticity in others requires significant maturity, self-awareness, and reflection on the part of the counselor: you can't learn it from a book or by practicing deeper levels of empathy. It's a way of being that take time—and an excellent supervisor—to cultivate.

Focused Listening or Attending

"*Very early in my work as a therapist, I discovered that simply listening to my client, very attentively, was an important way of being helpful. So when I was in doubt as to what I should do in some active way, I listened*" (Rogers, 1981, p. 137). This is an excellent piece of advice that is useful not just in counseling contexts but most every sphere of life: *when in doubt, listen.* Still not sure? Listen some more.

One of the first skills new counselors learn is listening. Listening in person-centered counseling has a very specific form based on its philosophical foundation in phenomenology. As you might remember from the beginning of the chapter, phenomenology encompasses the study of the internal, subjective world. Thus, when a person-centered counselor listens to clients share their stories, they are listening for and attending to descriptions of the persons *internal world*, most notably their emotions and logic that connects this affective inner world. For example, if a woman begins to describe how she no longer feels loved by her husband, the counselor does not focus on what the husband is doing, what she can behaviorally do differently, or how she could reframe what is going on. Instead, the counselor is curious about the contours of her internal life. Does she feel betrayed, hopeless, rejected, ugly, angry, or sad? The counselor listens for a rich and nuanced description of her internal emotional experience and selects these descriptions to comment on or ask about.

Summarizing

For those of us who expect life to be hard and difficult and assume that effective counseling must be hard, summarizing as a counseling intervention can be difficult to understand. How can simply restating what a person has just said be helpful and worth paying for? Basically, most of us aren't listening carefully when we speak; even if we are, it sounds very different when someone else says it, especially if it is about a difficult topic. For example, many people frequently make fun of themselves or put themselves down. But when someone else says the same thing—or simply agrees with what was just said, they feel offended, hurt, or angry. That is the same principle at work when summarizing. When counselors paraphrase back the essence of what a client just said, it helps clients to hear what they said in a different way. In most cases, it hits home harder than when they said it themselves. When another person skillfully summarizes emotionally difficult material, clients often hear and feel things in a new way: the reality of a situation often comes into bold relief.

For summarizations to be effective, they need to be (a) well timed, (b) about emerging insights (not just anything the client says), (c) in the client's language, and (d) not biased by the counselor's values, assumptions, or desires. For example, if a woman is going on about all the ways she is not happy with her boyfriend that she was planning to marry and states that she knows the relationship is doomed, she is likely to find a summarization from a counselor helpful in crystallizing her insight: "Even though you initially thought he was the one you would marry, you have begun to realize during the events of the past few months that this relationship will not work for you long-term." If the client is struggling against this reality, it can help to recast the summary in the form of a question: "It sounds like you are beginning to question whether this relationship will work for you based on the events of the past few months?"

Try It Yourself

Find a partner, share a recent event, and practice summarizing. Notice how you respond to having your experience summarized in someone else's words.

Clarifying

Similar to summarizing, clarifying statements and questions are not glamorous. They seem so simple-minded, you sometimes wonder if it is worth asking. Nonetheless, clarifying questions are some of the most important because often what seems simple and obvious is not. Just as the name implies, clarifying questions involve querying clients to provide more detail or explanation about what they are talking about. Clarifying questions can be categorized into two types, with each playing an important role. The first type of clarifying questions addresses factual issues: who, what, where, and how. These clarifying questions are not considered therapeutic in and of themselves in person-centered counseling, and if overused they actually distract from the counseling process. However, these can be important questions, especially when working with persons from diverse backgrounds. Counselors use fact-focused clarifying questions to ensure that they understand the basic information that comprises the client's experience. These questions help counselors avoid bias by ensuring that they don't project their assumptions onto clients. These questions help clients share their story: Who else was there? When did this happen? What happened next?

The other type of clarifying questions focus on the client's emotional process. These questions help the client more clearly articulate and conceptualize their internal process and are essential in promoting self-actualization. These clarifying questions are used to help the client more deeply probe and explore their internal emotional life. For example, "you say you are 'upset.' Can you say more about what you mean by this?" Or "There is a lot to be sad about in this situation, can you share what saddens you the most?"

These questions help clients sharpen their ability to identify, name, and share their emotions and thereby better understand and accept their inner life.

Reflecting Feelings

One of the most readily identifiable things that a person-centered counselor does, *reflecting feelings* refers to identifying feelings that the client just described or that seem to underlie what the client just said. For example, if a client complains about an incident at work, rather than focusing on who did what to whom, the counselor listens for the client's emotional experience, which may be one of being betrayed, taken advantage of, or loss—or even all three. This technique highlights and amplifies clients' awareness of their emotions, reactions, and feelings so that they can more consciously experience them. This technique is especially useful in the earlier stages of actualization when emotions are more difficult to identify, access, and experience. Even with clients who are skilled at identifying their emotions, having another person describe your emotional state can be a powerful experience that provides new experiencing and insight into one's subjective experience.

Process Questions

Process questions refer to questions or comments that direct clients' focus toward their inner process rather than on content. In everyday conversation, people tend to ask follow-up questions about the content of what happened: who said what to whom when. The conversation stays at a more factual-level description of what happened. Speculation as to why things happen distracts from a client's inner process. In contrast, counselors use process questions to help clients focus on the inner experience, emotions, and subjective reality—broadly speaking, to get them out of their heads and into their heart and bodies. Thus, the focus is on inner *emotional process* rather than factual description or rational analysis of what happened. Process questions can include the following:

- Can you describe what was going on inside of you when you heard the news?
- When you heard the door shut, what was going on inside for you?
- As you are telling me the story now, what types of feelings are coming up? Are these the same or different from what you experienced when things were happening?

Carkhuff's Core Conditions

Robert Carkhuff (1969, 2000; Truax & Carkhuff, 1976) extended Rogers's research by studying the observable and measurable behaviors that facilitated change in counseling. Researching a variety of facilitative conditions, Carkhuff identified several core conditions that are often used to help new counselors develop basic counseling skills. They include:

- Empathy (similar to Rogers's accurate empathy)
- Authenticity and Genuineness (similar to Rogers's authenticity)
- Respect (similar to Rogers's unconditional positive regard)
- Concreteness and Specificity
- Self-Disclosure
- Confrontation
- Immediacy

As the first three have been discussed at length above, we will just focus on the last four here.

Concreteness and Specificity

Carkhuff identified concreteness and specificity as counselor behaviors that facilitate the counseling process. Counselors demonstrate concreteness and specificity with questions and statements that help clients to clarify what is vaguely expressed. For example, to describe oneself as "upset" is really not saying much. For some this means to feel angry, others sad, and yet others anxious. Similarly, to say, "My mother's death made me sad" is also quite vague if it isn't followed up with more; such a major loss can be sad in many different ways. Counselors can help clients increase their inner awareness by asking questions that help them to be more concrete and specific about their subjective experiences.

Self-Disclosure

Self-disclosure is a bit like saffron. One of the most valued spices, in large quantities or in the wrong dish saffron is a culinary disaster that cannot be fixed. So, too is self-disclosure in counseling. It is so difficult to get right I often caution new counselors to not use it until after their first year of training. This is not always possible, and in some senses is impossible if you take into account that wearing a wedding band, your style of clothes, and your choice of mobile phone are all forms of disclosure at some level. However, what person-centered counselors more generally refer to as self-disclosure involves sharing *relevant* personal experience—generally personal struggles that are similar to what the client is dealing with—with the client *for the sole purpose of helping the client achieve their goals.* Self-disclosures may serve several clinical purposes: providing a role model, offering hope, or normalizing the client's experience. All of these are valid uses of self-disclosure and are highly effective when used with the right person at the right time. *However*—and this is a big however—when used at the wrong time with the wrong client, the damage done to the therapeutic relationship is often irreparable because once you reveal personal information, it cannot be taken back or undone. If there is a miscommunication, that can be cleared up. But if your client begins to doubt your credibility, was offended in some way, or has any of an infinite number of interpretations, it may be difficult or impossible to repair the counseling relationship, greatly reducing the chance of a positive outcome. Thus, self-disclosure requires excellent judgment in determining what will be most helpful to clients.

Confrontation

One of the more often misunderstood techniques, affective confrontation—especially when done in person-centered counseling—is not a harsh, critical confrontation but rather the counselor's effort to address discrepancies in verbalizations, perception, and/or body language. In the first case, the counselor points out that what the client just said does not jive with what was said earlier, either in this or another conversation: "you are saying now that you don't care, but earlier you said you were angry." The counselor may also point out discrepancies in terms of how another person is "all to blame" and the client an innocent victim in a situation where each played a part: "you say you don't like how your husband spoke to you; can you also describe how you spoke to him?" Alternatively, the counselor can comment on how the client's body language (e.g., on the edge of tears) is not congruent with what the client is saying (e.g. "I'm fine"). The spirit of these confrontations, unlike Gestalt, is generally one of curiosity and support rather than challenge.

Immediacy

Immediacy refers to when the counselor and client are able to discuss the client's immediate emotional state, which can be related to (a) an outside topic, (b) in-session behaviors, or (c) the counselor-client relationship. The ability to feel and immediately reflect upon and discuss the emotion of the moment is considered a higher-ordered level of emotional expression and a sign of increasing levels of self-actualization, the ultimate goal of counseling. Counselors can facilitate immediacy in several ways. One is to comment on an emotion that the counselor can clearly observe: "It seems as though you were offended by the comment I just made." Alternatively, counselors can prompt clients to try to identify what they are feeling in the moment: "What emotions are you feeling as you tell me about the car accident you saw on the way to the appointment *or* as we discuss your thoughts about ending the marriage?" Immediacy is intense and intimate, and thus must be used with caution. The client can feel put on the spot, attacked, or belittled if the counseling alliance isn't strong enough. It is not a technique to use frequently in most cases—even once a session can be too much for some clients. Additionally, it must be well timed, in a moment where the client is open to feeling vulnerable and exposed.

Try It Yourself

Find a partner and use immediacy to share your present emotional state; if possible, share your experience about your present-moment experiencing of your partner.

Gestalt Counseling

In a Nutshell: The Least You Need to Know

Pioneered by Fritz Perls—a dynamic counselor who is known for his often flamboyant and controversial style—and further developed by numerous others (Woldt & Toman, 2005; Yontef, 1993), Gestalt counseling is a phenomenological approach that emphasizes that people must be understood holistically and contextually—or in Perls's native German, as a *Gestalt*. Similar to person-centered counselors, Gestalt counselors help people become more of who they really are by helping them to stop trying to be what they are not. Gestalt counselors achieve this end by enabling clients to develop present moment awareness of and direct contact with their internal world (including parts of the self that have been cut off) and the environment (significant others, society, etc.). Gestalt counselors believe neuroses and other problems develop when a person avoids direct contact with the environment or parts of the self. The in-session, present moment experiences facilitated by counselors enable people to reintegrate these cutoff parts of the self to create an increasingly greater sense of *wholeness*.

Gestalt counseling methods are active, provocative, and experiential. Counselors in this approach interact as a whole person, using their emotional responses to clients as part of the process. Some Gestalt counselors use a more theatrical, cathartic style, while others use a more person-to-person approach (Yontef, 1993). Through the Gestalt process of reintegrating cutoff parts of the self and increasingly making authentic contact with the environment, a person becomes a more vibrant and self-actualized person who is fully aware of and responsive to what is going on in their emotions, body, and relationships, resulting in a *natural flow of being*. Gestalt practitioners went through a more extreme "anything goes," antitheoretical phase in the 1960s but "sobered up" in the 1970s with a greater focus on a more supportive dialogical engagement with clients (Yontef, 1993).

The Juice: Significant Contributions to the Field

If you remember one thing from this chapter, it should be ...

Body Awareness

Gestalt counselors believe that every emotion has a physiological component (Perls, 1973; Polster & Polster, 1973). When a person is cut off from the awareness of an emotion or part of the self, this becomes expressed in the body, usually as a tightening or dysfunction somewhere. Gestalt counselors are masters at picking up information from a person's body posture, fidgeting, tone of voice, and movements: "how a person sits ... tells so much about the contact he is willing to make" (Polster & Polster, 1973, p. 161). For example, a tight jaw may indicate holding back something a person wants to say and wringing of hands the suppression of what a person might want to do. Similarly, covering the abdomen may signal a sense of vulnerability, while stiff movements may be part of an attempt to hold oneself together. The Gestalt view that the repressed and suppressed emotions become expressed in the body is similar to Freud's; however, Perls believed that awareness of the *process of repression* was the key to integration, whereas psychoanalysts believed interpretation of the *content of repression* was the primary goal.

Gestalt counselors help clients increase their awareness of their bodies and the emotions expressed through the body. Bringing a person's attention to body movements that are expressing repressed emotion is risky business: the mind has put a lot of energy into remaining unaware of the emotions, so you should proceed with caution and gentleness—or you may encounter quite a bit of resistance. Typically, Gestalt counselors approach bodily awareness by creating a *safe emergency*, which involves increasing the client's affective intensity while still supporting the client with affirmation (Yontef & Jacobs, 2000). In the case study at the end of this chapter, the counselor uses body awareness to help Shandra more effectively manage the anxiety and perfectionism she is experiencing in relation to her new job.

Specific techniques for this include:

- *Where do you feel X in your body?* When a person is talking about a difficult emotion or situation, the counselor can ask: Where do you feel the sadness [anger, hurt, disappointment, etc.] in your body?
- *What would [body part/movement] say if it had a voice?* If the counselor has noticed a particular movement or body part that seems to be holding repressed emotion, the counselor could ask: If that clenched fist could speak, what would it say?
- *Exaggerate a movement:* If clients are having a difficult time understanding a particular body movement or expression, the counselor may direct them to exaggerate the movement to increase awareness: Can you try to make yourself as stiff as you can? Exaggerate the stiffness. Feel and notice what emotions, memories, or thoughts emerge as you do this.

Big Picture: Overview of Counseling Process

Layers of Neurosis

The Gestalt counseling process aims to help people achieve a greater sense of wholeness, awareness, and aliveness. Perls (1973) describes the process of becoming more authentic as a five-part process that he likens to the peeling of an onion:

1. **Phony Layer:** At this point, a person lives according to shoulds and habit, living an inauthentic life (e.g., an engaged woman who becomes fixated on having the perfect wedding, perfect dress, and perfect partner).
2. **Phobic Layer:** In the phobic layer or stage, a person begins to become worried and fearful that something is amiss; they may feel helpless but work hard to keep their feelings hidden (e.g., the soon-to-be bride starts having second thoughts and doubts).
3. **Impasse Layer:** At the point of impasse, a person begins to feel stuck, not knowing which way to go, and thus becomes more open to seeking help, preferably from someone who will tell them the "right" answer (e.g., the bride-to-be begins asking for advice from family, friends, religious support persons, and/or a counselor).
4. **Implosive Layer:** In this next phase, the phony layer begins to collapse and the person feels empty inside and lost, which makes them more open to present moment awareness and experiences (e.g., the soon-to-be bride loses touch with why she wanted to get married and have a wedding in the first place and begins to ask herself and her fiancé some difficult and discerning questions).
5. **Explosive Layer:** In this final period, the person lets go of old pretenses, releasing a burst of new energy for authentic action (e.g., the young woman decides with a new sense of clarity that she wants to be married and designs a wedding that uniquely expresses who she and her partner are, without relying on empty traditions or the latest fads).

Integration Sequence

The Polsters describe a similar change process, which they call the *integration sequence* (Roberts, 1999).

1. *Discovery:* In the discovery phase, the client comes to new realizations about the self in which new "figures" emerge from the ground. Often the counselor is instrumental in helping the client make discoveries through interventions and experiments.
2. *Accommodation:* In the next phase, the client begins to accommodate this new perception and to behave in the world based on the discovery; the client may feel awkward and clumsy in their interactions.

3. *Assimilation:* In this third phase, the novel self becomes more representative of who the client is: "feels like me."
4. *Integration:* In the final phase, the new behavior fits seamlessly with the person's sense of self and seems effortless.

Making Connection: Therapeutic Relationship

Person of Counselor: Being Fully Human

The person of the counselor is the primary vehicle for change in Gestalt counseling (Perls, Hefferline, & Goodman, 1951; Yontef, 1993). The counselor uses his or her whole personhood to make a real and authentic contact with the client. More so than in most of the forms of counseling, the Gestalt counselor engages the client without professional pretense or role. Thus, counselors freely share their thoughts, perceptions, and feelings as they occur in session, in order to rattle and awaken the client's authentic self. In short, the counselor is fully human, expressing a full range of emotion and openly admitting to mistakes and failings.

Here-and-Now, Presence, and Spontaneity

One of the primary experiences Gestalt counselors offer clients is their *presence* in *here-and-now* experiences (Polster & Polster, 1973). The counselor is fully in the present moment with the client, living in the *now*, where past and future fade away: "Since neurotic living is basically anachronistic living, any return to present experience is in itself a part of the antidote to neurosis" (p. 11). Polster and Polster further define the counseling process as "an exercise in unhampered living *now*," and therefore the counselor's primary role is to help clients more fully experience themselves—all aspects of themselves—as they arise moment-to-moment in session. Thus, counselors encourage clients to explore the tightness in their breathing, the spontaneous feelings that arise as they share what is on their mind, and whatever seems to bubble up during the counseling hour. The counselor does not try to "make sense of it all" or even connect early comments in session with contradictory later ones; instead, the focus is on becoming aware and fully experiencing and expressing the client's flow of consciousness.

Imperfect Role Model

Many people (including counselors) expect counselors to be nearly perfect, rarely getting angry, having happily-ever-after relationships, and everlasting good hair days. Many of us enter the field with the secret hope that maybe, just maybe, by reading enough books and learning how to help others through their problems, we won't have any of our own. It's tempting to hope for such bliss. Arguably, through popular books and media, the field frequently implies that such happiness and bliss are possible if you do enough positive self-talk, creative visualization, and feeling of emotion. But Gestalt counselors would argue that such problem-free living is a dangerous myth—so dangerous, in fact, that they are willing to be a role model for imperfection and thus a role model for the processes of integrating polarities. Consequently, they do not hide behind a professional veneer; instead, they boldly go where many counselors will not go. For example, they will freely comment on how a person's weight or grooming may be part of the reason getting a date is difficult, or confront a person who was victimized as a child and who copes by feeling victimized by everyone and everything. Similarly, they may share their own frustrations, struggles, or failures to provide clients with more realistic expectations.

Dialogic Engagement

Drawing on the work of Buber (1958), more recent Gestalt applications include *dialogic engagement*: "the dialogic view of reality is that all reality is relating" (Yontef, 1993, p. 33). Thus, growth happens "between" people and is best promoted in relationship rather through than individual's awareness. The counselor's role is to engage the client fully, genuinely, and openly, willingly exploring despair, love, anger, joy, humor, and sensuality. This dialogic openness requires discrimination on the part of the counselor to share personal feelings and information appropriately.

In dialogic approaches, the counselor uses the relationship as the primary context for making contact (Hycner, 1995). In the encounters between counselor and client, clients are able to develop awareness and differentiate self from nonself. Counselors use their authentic selves to help clients more clearly and safely experience what is self and nonself so that they can more freely experience here-and-now experiences.

Confirmation and Inclusion

Gestalt counselors believe "people become unique selves by the confirmation of other people" (Yontef, 1993, p. 36). *Inclusion* is considered the highest form of confirmation, when a person "feels into" the other's worldview while still maintaining a clear sense of self. The counselor practicing inclusion sees the world, life, and the client's situation through the eyes of the client as much as possible (Hycner, 1995). Since I know you'd ask, Yontef (1993) distinguishes inclusion from empathy by emphasizing that inclusion moves farther on the pole of really "feeling" another's world, while simultaneously demanding greater awareness of self, than empathy typically does. Generally, Gestalt counselors criticize empathy because it often leads to a confluence or blurring between self and other.

The Viewing: Case Conceptualization

Assessing the Field

Contemporary Gestalt counselors used Kurt Lewin's *field theory* as a primary tool for viewing clients and their lives (Parlett & Lee, 2005; Yontef, 1993). Similar to Gestalt psychology, field theory shares the view that a figure is intimately connected with its background. Field theory further posits greater and more dynamic interrelationships between figure and background than traditional Gestalt psychology does. In field theory, the figure/background are viewed as a systematic web of relationships that forms a unitary whole: "everything affects everything else in the field" (Yontef, 1993, p. 297). Field theory can be applied to a variety of counseling phenomena: the client as a whole, the counseling relationship, and how clients perceive their situations. In every case, the counselor is part of the field, affecting what is being observed; simply asking clients about their situations affects their situations (Parlett & Lee, 2005). Thus, counselors remain cognizant of how their questions and presence shape and affect clients' lived experience.

Assessing the field requires investigation of the ever-fluctuating dynamics of the field and invites nondichotomous thinking, examining how each part affects the others (Lobb & Lichtenberg, 2005). For example, if a client complains that her partner has hurt her, the counselor explores not only how the client feels hurt, but also how she may have contributed to her partner hurting her and how the client may have contributed to hurting her partner.

Questions to Consider When Assessing the Field

- What was your experience?
- How did you contribute to creating your experience?
- What were the experiences of others? How did you contribute to their experience?
- What other factors may have contributed to your experience? How might have you affected these factors?
- How is the sharing of this situation in the counseling encounter affecting your experience of this situation?

Try It Yourself

Find a partner and discuss a recent life experience using these questions to assess the field.

Contact Boundaries and Encounters

Gestalt counselors view each moment of lived experience primarily in terms of a form of *contact* between the self (organism) and outside world (others and environment) (Perls et al., 1951; Yontef, 1993). If a person is able to make direct contact and authentically *encounter* the outside world, the person is living a fully and authentic life. However, for a variety of reasons—early life lessons, fears, social dictates—people avoid genuine contact to protect themselves. These *contact boundary disturbances* refer to distortions in perceptions of self or others.

An encounter involves a continuum of seven phases, beginning with initial perception, moving toward direct encounter, and ending in withdrawal. The human experience involves an endless ebb and flow of making contact with one person/object/idea and then withdrawing; then making contact and withdrawing from another; in an endless series of connections and disconnections. A person can avoid contact at any of the seven phases using specific resistance processes at each stage (Woldt & Toman, 2005):

Continuum Phase	Resistance Process	Example of Resistance
1. *Sensation/Perception:* Organism perceives input from environment.	*Desensitization:* Failing to notice problems.	Ignoring increasing violence by partner in fights.
2. *Awareness:* One's lived experience becomes focused on the environmental sensation.	*Introjection*: Take in others' views whole and unedited.	Becoming what your parents wanted you to be.
3. *Excitement/Mobilization:* The organism mobilizes to prepare for contact.	*Projection*: Assign undesired parts of self to others.	Rejecting sexual aspects of self and then perceiving others as "oversexed."
4. *Encounter/Action:* The organism takes action to engage the other.	*Retroflection*: Direct action to self rather than others.	Rather than creating conflict with others, focus criticism on self.
5. *Interaction/Full Contact:* A back and forth exchange happens; the self becomes part of "we."	*Deflection*: Avoid direct contact with another or self.	Working long hours to avoid spouse or avoiding own emotions.
6. *Assimilation/Integration:* The organism takes in and integrates new information, behavior, etc.	*Egotism:* Not allowing outside to influence self.	Claiming to be "in love," but not being open to changing self to meet needs of relationship.
7. *Differentiation/Withdrawal:* The organism withdraws from contact and returns to its individual state.	*Confluence*: Agree with another to the extent that boundary blurred.	Agreeing with spouse to the extent that one no longer allows self to have a divergent opinion.

When assessing clients, Gestalt counselors look for where their clients are "stuck" in the cycle of making contact, and they direct their interventions to encourage clients to make contact and complete the encounter cycle.

Polarities and Disowned Parts

Gestalt counselors view people as a never-ending sequence of *polarities* or complementary parts, as Adult versus Child, Strong versus weak, Loving versus Hateful, and so on (Polster & Polster, 1973). When a person is rigidly polarized—always acts like an adult; always strong; always loving, and such—they typically have disowned the opposite quality, for example, childishness, weakness, or hatefulness. On the surface, this may not seem like much of a problem. The problem is that we are talking about members of the human species, who are human after all. Being human, each person experiences, at some level, the full range of human emotion. Thus, although a person may be very responsible in their day job, the ability to be playful like a child is an important counterbalance.

People may accomplish extensive personal growth to feel emotionally strong, but will still encounter difficult moments, loss, tragedy, and trauma, and during these times they will need to allow themselves to feel their weakness. Similarly, a person may engage in religious and spiritual practices to become more loving, but may also experience loss, victimization, or trauma that elicits feelings of animosity and hate; that is part of the human experience. The person doesn't need to *act* on this hate, but it is important to be accepting of having such feelings. When such feelings are *disowned*, the person must develop elaborate avoidance strategies, which impede a person's ability to be fully who he or she is. Thus, the Gestalt counselors try to identify the polarities within a person that may be contributing to the presenting problem. Common problematic polarities include:

- Social self versus natural self
- Adult versus child
- Perfect versus failure
- Emotional versus logical
- Shallow versus deep
- Responsible versus carefree

In the case study at the end of this chapter, the counselor helps Shandra, a high achiever who helped raise her four younger siblings, integrate disowned polarities, including the parts related to being a child and carefree.

"Shoulds"

Gestalt counselors listen carefully for clients using "shoulds" to justify and explain their behavior and choices (Yontef, 1993). They believe that people who routinely organize their lives by doing what they "should" do rather than what they want to do, what they value, and so on, are not living authentically and are in fact *avoiding* taking existential responsibility for their lives (for example, "I am doing what others have told me to do rather than decide for myself what I want to be doing, believe in, etc.). Counselors view "shoulds" as a form of *neurotic self-regulation*, meaning that a person is regulating emotions in unhealthy ways. Gestalt counselors confront persons living by "shoulds" and encourage them to make more authentic choices that are not fear-based or based on social pressure.

Unfinished Business

Like it sounds, *unfinished business* refers to any incompletely expressed feeling, which most often takes the form of resentment (Yontef, 1993). Gestalt counselors help clients identify unfinished business by playing the following game:

Unfinished Business Assessment Game

"For the next two (choose a time) minutes, I want you to list out as many things that you are feeling resentful about as you can. You can do this by starting your statements with: "I resent...." Just keep going and try to identify as many as you can, no matter how silly they may seem. Have fun with it, and we will talk about it when you are done. Any questions? Ready? Go."

Try It Yourself

Whether at home or as part of a class activity, pull out a timer and see what forms of unfinished business turn up for you.

Targeting Change: Goal Setting

Awareness

"In Gestalt, the only *goal* is *awareness*" (Yontef, 1993, p. 150). The counselor's primary goal is to help clients increase their awareness of their experiences so that they can make direct contact with the environment without resistance. The ability to be aware and in contact requires (a) organismic self-regulation, (b) acceptance of what is, and (c) the integration of polarities.

Organismic Self-Regulation

Perls (1973) described the long-term goal of counseling as helping clients to become *organismically self regulating* rather than "*shouldistic*," meaning ruled by cognition and lists of "shoulds." Yontef (1993) defines organismic self-regulation (and, yes, it is hard not to slip up and say orgasmic) as "choosing and learning happen holistically, with a natural integration of mind and body, thought and feeling, spontaneity and deliberateness" (p. 143). Vibrant and alive, such a person lives in a dynamic, responsive relationship with the environment, embracing the ebb and flow of life, including the more difficult moments, while responding authentically. An organismically self-regulated person has the courage to make "contact" with people and situations without having to rely on resistance processes to protect the self, thus trusting the self and life itself. This type of person takes responsibility for their relationships with others and the world and is able to *creatively adapt* to situations (Yontef, 1993). Furthermore, an organismically self-regulated person is *self-supporting*, meaning that this person can provide basic support for the self and does not need to manipulate others to meet personal needs.

Accepting "What is": Paradoxical Theory of Change

Beisser (1970) posited a paradoxical theory of change that has been adopted by contemporary Gestalt counselors: the more one tries to change (and be who one is not), the more one stays the same. Thus, paradoxically, the long-term goals in Gestalt are less about correcting personal defects and more about removing barriers to experiencing who one already is. Alternatively stated, the goal is to accept that what is "*is*," and to make peace with who and what one is. When a person is able to make contact with "what is," change spontaneously happens (Yontef, 1993). For example, many clients refuse to "make contact" with the "what is" of their body: they may believe they are not pretty or thin enough, be afraid of their sexuality or impulses, or be frustrated by pain or a debilitating condition. If the counselor can help clients make direct contact with "what is" by removing resistance barriers, clients' relationships with their bodies automatically transform to be more accepting, less fearful, and less judgmental. This paradoxical theory has been compared with Taoist and Buddhist "non-doing" and mindfulness practices (Smith, 1976).

Integration of Polarities

Another long-term goal in Gestalt counseling is *integrating polarities*, which involves accepting differences within the self and between self and the environment. In practice, integration takes the form of becoming less dogmatic, less rigid, and, quite simply, more complex as a human being, because the person has accepted and integrated more aspects of the self. For example, if a man enters counseling defining his value in terms of his career achievements, the process of integration will involve accepting the "relaxed," "less than ideal," and less dominant parts of himself. Through this process, he may continue to excel at work but now also create time for a romantic relationship, hobbies, and "wasting time" with chit-chat.

Early and Middle Phase Goals

Early and middle phase goals in Gestalt counseling address the blockages to experiencing this integrated sense of self and generally address the presenting symptoms more directly.

Examples

- Increase awareness of suppressed anger that fuels depression.
- Decrease avoidance of difficult interpersonal exchanges and increase expression of feelings in situations where client fears negative rejection from others (or increase assertiveness with others).

- Decrease angry outbursts and hurtful comments with wife and children and increase ability to express more vulnerable emotions.
- Increase ability to identify and separate own feelings from those of others and ability to act on these feelings.

Closing Phase Goals

The closing phase goals address the longer-term issues of (a) organismic self-regulation, (b) making contact with what is, and (c) integrating polarities.

Examples

- Increase organismic self-regulation in marriage to increase emotional intimacy.
- Increase acceptance of "driven" versus "relaxed" polarities to create better work-home balance.
- Increase capacity to make direct contact with family of origin.
- Increase ability to accept "what is" related to loss of mother.

The Doing: Interventions

Body Awareness (see "The Juice" above)

Gestalt Experiment and Empty Chair

A Hollywood favorite for mocking counselors, the Gestalt empty chair involves having clients pour out their hearts to an empty chair and then turn around and respond from the empty chair, having a conversation with themselves. Although this technique looks strange and even silly from the outside, when you are the one speaking, it is rarely a joke—it is challenging and powerful. This technique enables clients to have conversations with people and parts of themselves that they would otherwise never be able to have.

Gestalt counselors use the empty chair and similar Gestalt experiments because they prefer action over talk. Thus, their characteristic technique is the *Gestalt experiment*, which involves inviting the client to take action in the room by creating a "safe emergency" (Polster & Polster, 1973). An experiment may involve having an "empty chair" conversation by speaking aloud to an imagined person in an empty chair, sharing things the person is too afraid to say to the person directly. For example, if a person is angry with his boss but afraid to speak to her, the counselor may ask him to speak aloud what he has been too afraid to say to this person. The purpose of this empty chair encounter is *not* to rehearse for an actual confrontation or to "vent" feelings, but rather "to relate to reality out there by expressing his needs at that moment in time" and experience "in the present what it is like for him to flow from awareness to experimental action" (p. 235). This safe opportunity to experience acting and speaking from one's immediate lived experience makes it easier and more likely that the client will do so outside of the session. In most cases, the person's actions outside the session will not be a replica of what occurred in counseling (most of us tone it down in the real world). The Gestalt experiment is *not* an "acting out" of emotion, but rather a safe context for experimenting with authentic expression.

Gestalt experiments can take many forms (Polster & Polster, 1973):

- Enactment of an unfinished business situation from the distant past
- Enactment of a contemporary unfinished business situation
- Enactment of a characteristic (desired or undesired)
- Enactment of a polarity (both sides)

Yontef (1993) lists the purposes of experiments, including:

- To expand a person's repertoire of behaviors outside the session and stimulate experiential learning.
- To create conditions in which the client can see life as his/her own creation and also take ownership of the counseling process.
- To complete unfinished business, overcome blockages in awareness, and integrate polarities.
- To stimulate a sense of strength, competencies, self-support, and responsibility.

Successfully staging an experiment involves several steps:

1. Through dialogue, the counselor and client identify areas of unfinished business, polarities, resistance, etc. (e.g., unexpressed anger at mother).
2. The counselor then invites the client into the experiment by specifically *directing* the client to experiment by speaking to an empty chair, saying something aloud, or taking physical action of some form (e.g. "I want you to pretend for a moment that your mother is in the chair next to you. Go ahead and speak to her, saying those things you wish you would have said the last time you saw her").
3. During the experiment, the counselor may encourage the client to address specific areas or take certain actions (e.g., "Why don't you address what happened during the divorce, too?").
4. After the experiment, the counselor focuses on helping the client identify the here-and-now experiencing of the experiment (e.g., "What were you feeling inside when you were talking to your mother? Did any particular part of your body react? What are you feeling like now that you said that aloud?").

Try It Yourself

Find a partner and try the empty chair technique for a polarity related to your experience of becoming a professional counselor and psychotherapist, such as perfection/failure, parent/child, social/natural self, or such.

Semantics and Language Modification

Gestalt counselors direct clients to modify their language to highlight their autonomy, choice, and responsibility. Common examples include:

- *"Questions to Statements":* Gestalt counselors ask clients to change questions to statements, because questions are often disguised statements or demands for support from others (Yontef, 1993).
- *"I versus You or It statements":* Rather than describing someone else as the agent in a situation ("*you* made me do X") or in a passive voice ("*it* just makes me feel X"), Gestalt counselors have clients rephrase a statement beginning with "I": "*I* decided to do X" or "I chose to feel X."
- *"Choose versus Can't":* When a client says I "can't" but there is an element of choice, the counselor has the client restate their position acknowledging their choice: "I choose to spend time at work to make a deadline rather than come home on time."
- *"Want versus Have to":* Similarly, Gestalt counselors have clients clearly distinguish between "having to do something" (which is ultimately extremely rare) and wanting to do something: "I want to pay taxes to avoid being pursued by the IRS" rather than "I have to pay taxes." By constantly highlighting that we all have free choice in most all life circumstances, *choose* increases a person's sense of freedom, will, and responsibility, even if the life choices remain the same ("I am going to choose to keep paying taxes").
- *"But":* Another word Gestalt counselors watch for is "but," which is typically followed by excuses, polarity, or a double message. Instead, clients are encourage to develop integration by replacing "but" with "and."

Staying with Feelings

To increase awareness, Gestalt counselors often encourage clients to "stay with" difficult feelings, coaching them through the continuum of contact: sensation, awareness, excitement, encounter, integration, assimilation, and withdrawal (see Contact Boundaries and Encounters above). The counselor encourages the client in each phase to move through resistances to have direct experiences. Much like the experiment, encouraging clients to stay with feelings helps them develop the skills and courage to do this outside of session.

Dream Work

Gestalt counselors use a unique approach to dreams. They see them as attempts to integrate parts of the self and/or as an existential message, and the counselor is not assumed to know the true interpretation better than the client (Yontef, 1993). Gestalt counselors view each character in the dream as a part of the self. For example, if a person is being chased in the dream, both the pursuer and the one fleeing are viewed as different aspects of the self. The counselor and client can explore how these parts interact, what each might represent, and how they have been neglected or emphasized in the person's life.

Putting It All Together: Humanistic Case Conceptualization and Treatment Plan Templates

Theory-Specific Case Conceptualization: Humanistic

The prompts below can be used to develop a *theory-specific case conceptualization* using humanistic theory. The cross-theoretical case conceptualizations at the end of each theory chapter provide examples for writing a conceptualization that includes key elements of this theory-specific conceptualization. Comprehensive examples of theory-specific case conceptualizations are available in *Theory and Treatment Planning in Counseling and Psychotherapy* (Gehart, 2015).

- *Describe client's areas of functioning based on Rogers's stages of change process:*
  - *Stage of Change Process:* Describe client's approximate stage in the change process (Stages 1–7).
  - *Experience of Problems:* Are problems perceived as internal or external (caused by others, circumstance, etc.)?
  - *Agency and Responsibility:* Is self or other discussed as agent of story? Does client take clear responsibility for situation? Does client frequently describe self as victim of others or life?
  - *Recognition and Expression of Feelings:* Are feelings readily recognized, owned, and experienced?
  - *Here-and-now Experiencing:* Is the client able to experience full range of feelings as they are happening in the present moment?
  - *Personal Constructs and Facades:* Is the client able to recognize and go beyond roles? Is identity rigid or tentatively held?
  - *Complexity and Contradictions:* Are internal contradictions owned and explored? Is client able to fully engage the complexity of identity and life?
  - *"Shoulds":* Is client able to question socially imposed "shoulds" and "oughts"? Can client balance desire to please others and desire to be authentic?
  - *Acceptance of Others:* Is client able to accept others and modify expectations of others to be more realistic?
  - *Trust of Self:* Is client able to trust self as process (rather than a stabile object)?
- *Meaning, Meaningless, and Life Purpose:* Describe sources of meaning for client; may involve the following themes:
  - Personal achievement and work
  - Significant other
  - Children
  - Family of origin
  - Social cause/contributing to others
  - Religion/spirituality
- *Contact Boundaries and Encounters:* Describe typical contact boundary pattern:
  - *Desensitization:* Failing to notice problems
  - *Introjection:* Taking in others' views whole and unedited
  - *Projection:* Assigning undesired parts of self to others

- *Retroflection:* Directing action to self rather than other
- *Deflection:* Avoiding direct contact with another or self
- *Egotism:* Not allowing outside to influence self
- *Confluence:* Agreeing with another to the extent that boundary blurred

- *Polarities and Disowned Parts:* Describe polarities and disowned parts, which may include:
  - Social self versus natural self
  - Adult versus child
  - Perfect versus failure
  - Emotional versus logical
  - Shallow versus deep
  - Responsible versus carefree
- *Shoulds:* Describe problematic shoulds that relate specifically to the problem and those that more generally organize the client's life.
- *Unfinished Business:* Identify any unfinished business, such as resentments and guilt, that client has yet to deal with.

Theory-Specific Treatment Plan: Humanistic

Use this treatment plan template for developing a plan for clients with depressive, anxious, or compulsive types of presenting problems. Depending on the specific client, presenting problem, and clinical context, the goals and interventions in this template may need to be modified only slightly or significantly; you are encouraged to significantly revise the plan as needed. For the plan to be useful, goals and techniques should be written to target specific beliefs, behaviors, and emotions that the client is experiencing. The more specific, the more useful it will be to you.

Treatment Plan

Initial Phase of Treatment

Initial Phase Counseling Tasks

1. Develop working counseling relationship. *Diversity considerations:* Describe how you will specifically adjust to respect cultured, gendered, and other styles of relationship building and emotional expression.
   Relationship-building approach/intervention:
   a. Confirmation of client's **unique self** while counselor is also expressing authentic self.
2. Assess individual, systemic, and broader cultural dynamics. *Diversity considerations:* Describe how you will specifically adjust assessment based on cultural, socioeconomic status, sexual orientation, gender, and other relevant norms.
   Assessment strategies:
   a. Assess client's ability to make **authentic contact** with others and environment.
   b. Identify **polarities, disowned parts, shoulds, and unfinished business**.
3. Identify and obtain client agreement on treatment goals. *Diversity considerations:* Adapt goals to be culturally and gender-appropriate, relative to expectations for **independence** and **emotional expression**.
   Goal-making intervention:
   a. Involve client in identifying goals for greater **self-regulation** and **wholeness**.

(continued)

4. Identify needed referrals, crisis issues, and other client needs. *Diversity considerations: Describe diversity issues related to specific crisis issues and referral options.*
   a. *Crisis assessment intervention(s):* **Body awareness** to help client identify emotions that fuel crisis.
   b. *Referral(s):* To process groups as needed, to increase capacity for authentic relating.

Initial Phase Client Goal

1. Increase tolerance of difficult emotions and **unwanted parts of self** that fuel crisis to reduce [specific crisis symptoms].
   Interventions:
   a. **Body awareness** exercises to help client identify and more effectively manage crisis emotions.
   b. Encourage client to **"stay with" difficult feelings** that fuel crisis and coach client through experiencing these emotions to defuse crisis.

Working Phase of Treatment

Working Phase Counseling Tasks

1. Monitor quality of the working alliance. *Diversity considerations:* Adapt relationship to be responsive to gender and cultural forms of **emotional expression** and **contact norms.**
   a. *Assessment Intervention:* Monitor frequency of **here-and-now experiencing**, willingness to tolerate differences between self and other, and **authentic expression of self**; use Session Rating Scale.
2. Monitor progress toward goals. *Diversity considerations: Describe how you will specifically adapt the monitoring of progress for age, ethnicity, educational level, language, etc.*
   a. *Assessment Intervention:* Monitor ability to increasingly experience and express all aspects of self; use Outcome Questionnaire to measure client progress.

Working Phase Client Goals

1. Increase **integration of polarities** between [X] and [Y] to reduce [specific symptom: depression, anxiety, etc].
   Interventions:
   a. **Gestalt experiments** and **empty chair** exercises to facilitate awareness and integration of polarities
   b. **Modify language** to allow for both/and acceptance of polarities.
2. Increase ability to **self-regulate** in [X: specific context, relationship, problem, etc.] to reduce [specific symptom: depression, anxiety, etc].
   Interventions:
   a. Coach client on **staying with difficult feelings** to increase ability to self-regulate.
   b. **Gestalt experiments** with alternative behaviors to increase self-regulation skills.
3. Increase ability to **accept "what is"** in relation to [unchangeable situation] to reduce [specific symptom: depression, anxiety, etc].
   Interventions:
   a. **Dream analysis** to better understand resistance to and rejection of what is.
   b. **Language modification** to reduce "shoulds" in relation to "what is."

(continued)

Closing Phase of Treatment

Closing Phase Counseling Task

1. Develop aftercare plan and maintain gains. *Diversity considerations: Describe specific diversity considerations and unique resources for the ending treatment and sustaining gains posttreatment.*
   Intervention:
   a. Increase capacity for **organismic self-regulation** in relation to potential future stressors.

Closing Phase Client Goals

1. Increase capacity to **self-regulate** and expand **here-and-now experiencing** to be primary mode for daily living in all contexts to reduce potential for relapse in [specific symptom: depression, anxiety, etc].
   Interventions:
   a. Increasingly challenging **Gestalt experiments** to integrate spontaneity into all aspects of daily living.
   b. **Dream work** to identify more subtle resistance and **polarities** that impeded full authenticity in daily living.
2. Increase **self-regulation** and **authentic expression of self** in intimate relationships while simultaneously allow for another's authenticity to reduce potential for relapse in [specific symptom: depression, anxiety, etc].
   Interventions:
   a. **Empty chair** experiments to develop awareness and skills for authentic relating.
   b. **Gestalt experiments** in significant relationships that help to build capacity for authentic intimacy.

Digital Download Download from CengageBrain.com

Tapestry Weaving: Working with Diverse Populations

Cultural, Ethnic, and Gender Diversity

Used with a wide range of clients, experiential approaches value clear, congruent emotional expression and the willingness to be vulnerable. Therefore, when working with populations that have different attitudes toward emotional expression and/or are in a treatment context where such vulnerability feels unsafe, counselors need to proceed thoughtfully. For example, the emotional expression often promoted in the experiential approaches may not be comfortable for some men or East Asian Americans (Wang, 1994), populations that generally value less dramatic and more indirect emotional expression; thus, they should be used with caution. That said, one recent study found that expressive writing was found to be beneficial for most people but especially those of Asian origin (Lu & Stanton, 2010). Similarly, in another study both Asian and female college students rated experiential therapy approaches more positively than cognitive-behavioral or psychodynamic (Yu, 1998).

Culturally Competent Person-Centered Counseling

Based on his careful review of literature on person-centered therapy with diverse clients, Quinn (2013) hypothesizes that two specific adaptations are necessary to provide culturally competent person-centered therapy:

- Counselor congruence with the client's illness myth (i.e., belief or theory about the problem)
- Counselor empathic understanding of the client's perception of and attitude toward the counselor

The first, understanding the client's illness myth—which is a mental health disorder in dominant Western discourses—involves both (a) having an awareness of and familiarity with the common cultural beliefs from the client's background (not client-specific), and (b) listening carefully for the client's personal interpretations of the problem situation (client-specific). This occurs through a recursive process of frequently checking the accuracy of the counselor's understanding with the client. When the counselor maintains a nonjudgmental stance and unconditional positive regard for the client, this exploration allows for counselor congruence with the client's illness myth.

The second adaption is more challenging. Multicultural clients, especially those with less acculturation, may be slower to trust expressions of "genuine caring" from a counselor. The task of the person-centered counselor is to tolerate the ambiguity of allowing trust to build cross-culturally rather than switch to a more directive style, which would be less anxiety-provoking for both parties. Thus, when the counselor perceives reticence or other hesitation on the part of the client, the counselor empathically and nonjudgmentally responds:

> "I would like to hear about you, but I suspect that it may be hard to trust me with certain things. You may not think I will be able to understand; that is a fair and reasonable concern to have. In fact, I might not. But I can assure you that I want to not only understand you but be helpful to you. I am willing to take this at a pace that feels comfortable to you."

By using the facilitative conditions, the person-centered counselor allows for trust to build across cultural differences, to safely emerge for clients in a form and pace that is right for them.

Asian Americans and Gestalt Empty Chair

Cheung and Nguyen (2012) have explored the possibility of using the Gestalt empty chair technique with Asian Americans. In adapting this intervention for working with Asians, they identified four characteristics of the population observed in research that they used to frame their approach:

1. Connecting the meaning of shame in therapeutic interventions
2. Avoiding the loss of "face" in confronting relatives and friends
3. Using alternative and complementary means to replace traditional therapy and direct confrontation
4. Using inner control and spirituality in resolving interpersonal guilt and conflict (Cheung & Nguyen, 2012, p. 54)

The empty chair technique allows some Asian clients to more easily express their emotions because they do not need to make direct eye contact (with counselor or family member) and they need not fear losing face or being disrespectful.

Cheung and Ngyuen (2012) describe three steps to using the Gestalt chair with Asian Americans:

Step 1: Introduce the function of the empty chair: Introduce the chair as an "exercise" with a concrete function or goal, such as helping to address a conflict with a specific person. Clients should never be forced to use the chair, but instead encouraged to explore any concerns or resistance if they are voiced. Often, if the conflict is with an authority figure, Asian clients will mention that it feels disrespectful; in such cases, the counselor can describe how the chair exercise will allow them to safely explore the conflict without being disrespectful or with anyone losing face.

Step 2: Engage the client in the therapeutic process: Once the client has agreed, the counselor's job is to facilitate the change process in a form that is comfortable to the client. In addition to more traditional empty chair techniques, adaptations that may work for Asian American clients include:

1. Imagining the chair: Starting without an empty chair; simply imagining the person is in the room.
2. Using imagery: Having the client imagine a specific time in the past when there was conflict.

3. Using direct dialogue: Once the client begins to talk to the person, direct the client to talk to the chair.
4. Role-playing: If the client does not want to look at the chair, the client can speak to the counselor instead.
5. Swapping chairs: The counselor can pretend to be the client in the dialogue, and the client can sit in what would otherwise be the empty chair; then the counselor and client can swap chairs again, allowing the client to speak from his/her own position in the next round.
6. Telling one thing: Have the client identify one thing that the other person might say (that the client wishes the other would say, something that might be helpful, for example) and then also invite the client to respond to this "one thing."
7. Telling a story: Have the client and the imagined other (role-played by counselor) tell a story together.
8. Native language: If the client has a native language, speak for the imagined other in that native language and respond in that language.

Step 3: Debriefing: After finishing one or more of the above exercises, the counselor should take time to reflect on what happened using a transition statement, such as, "Now, let's come back to this room with just you and me. What was that experience like for you?" (Cheung & Nguyen, 2012, p. 58). With Asian American clients, it may be helpful to also include concrete follow-up questions, such as: What did you learn from this exercise? Can you see a way to apply this knowledge to future situations?

Gender

In addition to cross-cultural differences, emotional expression is also a concern related to the client's and therapist's genders. In particular, counselors need to critically examine their expectations for the client's emotional expression based on the client's gender. In one study, nontraditional female clients who had experience with both male and female counselors reported that they believed female counselors expected them to express their emotions in a particular gendered way. These clients felt judged and misunderstood by female counselors because they did not subscribe to stereotyped modes of gendered emotional expression (Gehart & Lyle, 2001). Male clients in the same study reported feeling safer sharing more vulnerable emotions with female counselors. Both male and female clients reported feeling that male counselors were more interested in solutions and practical matters than in emotions. Thus, with same-gendered and opposite-gendered clients, counselors need to be aware of how cultural norms for emotional expression potentially shape or impede the humanistic-experiential counseling process. Thus, as part of working sensitively with gender, counselors should be careful to (a) avoid inaccurate assessment due to different cultural and gender norms and values concerning emotional expression, (b) adjust the level of intimacy in the therapeutic alliance to fit with the client's level of comfort, and (c) choose interventions that actively engage clients at their comfortable level.

Sexual Identity Diversity

Grounded in their values of authentic self-expression, humanistic-existential counselors avoid conceptualizations of sexuality that are based on norms and performance (Kleinplatz, 1996). Thus, humanistic-existential approaches have been widely used with lesbian, gay, bisexual, transgendered, and questioning (LGBTQ) clients (Davies, 2000). The phenomenological emphasis on describing subjective lived experience and avoiding pathologizing make humanistic-existential counseling approaches a viable option for LGBTQ clients (Milton, 2000). More specifically, the coming out process can be viewed as a critical part of the self-actualizing process and desire for congruence described by Rogers and other humanists (Bean, 1981; Davies, 2000).

Within the humanistic counseling community, there has been debate about what it means to be a "gay affirmative therapy" (Langdridge, 2007; Milton, 2000). Ethically affirmative, the "weaker" form of gay affirmative therapy, honors the lived realities of LGBTQ clients using fundamental phenomenological and humanistic approach (Milton, 2000). In contrast, the stronger form, simply referred to as gay affirmative, involves certain prescribed views and practices on the part of the counselor, including advocacy and positive affirmation to directly ameliorate the effect of society's heterosexism. Although this advocate stance is well intended, it is ultimately an expert position, one that does not privilege the client's lived subjective experience but rather foregrounds political and societal realities. Thus, gay affirmative humanistic counselors must strive to carefully balance working within the client's subjective worldview (a more "pure" humanistic approach) with addressing and potentially countering strong internalized messages of heterosexism while working within the assumptions of the model (a more political activist position).

When considering the experience of LGBTQ clients, humanistic counselors can choose to focus on the burden of societal rejection of the client's authentic self, and help clients move toward finding safe ways and contexts to express their true selves (Pachankis & Bernstein, 2012). Humanistic counselors should also consider how clients' social contexts may seriously constrain their communication styles, both in their intimate relationships, with supportive versus nonsupportive family members, as well as with colleagues and strangers. Experiential practices, such as Satir's Parts Party and family reconstruction, have been used in gay and lesbian group programs to allow them to reexperience support and their family-of-origin relationships in new and more empowering ways (Picucci, 1992).

Research and the Evidence Base

Carl Rogers (1961, 1981) was initially a leader in psychotherapy and counseling research. He developed person-centered counseling based on extensive and ongoing research. However, by the mid-1970s, research on person-centered counseling essentially ended after the deaths of Rogers and Truax (Quinn, 2013). Gestalt and existential approaches have had even less systematic research than person-centered approach (McLeod, 2002). With the notable exception of emotionally focused couples therapy (Johnson, 2004), an empirically supported treatment for distressed couples (see Chapter 12), contemporary humanistic approaches have not been on the forefront of the evidence-based therapy movement. However, one of the most significant and robust findings in the field of counseling and psychotherapy research is the importance of the counseling relationship: the evidence provides strong and consistent support for many of Rogers's ideas about what is helpful in the counseling relationship.

In his 1957 article "The necessary and sufficient conditions of therapeutic change," Carl Rogers set forth a research hypothesis that would define his career and redefine the landscape of psychotherapy for generations to come. In the decades that followed that publication, he pursued a meticulous research agenda that attempted to determine whether his core conditions were (a) necessary and/or (b) sufficient. In his search for answers, Carl Rogers was the first researcher to record counseling sessions (Brazier, 1996), providing the technological and ethical foundation for *process research*, the study of in-session counseling processes that promote or hinder change. Consistently, the vast majority of studies over the past four decades have found that the *client's* perception of the core conditions—more so than the counselor's or neutral third party's—is correlated with positive outcome (Kirschenbaum & Jourdan, 2005). However, although there is strong support for the importance of empathy, positive regard, and congruence, most concede that the core conditions may be neither necessary nor sufficient (Kirschenbaum & Jourdan, 2005). Nonetheless, they are considered "extremely helpful" with virtually all clients.

Common factors research has reintroduced and recontexualized the importance of Rogers's core conditions (Miller, Duncan, & Hubble, 1997). Rather than particular models accounting for change, the common factors movement posits that similarities rather than differences across models are more closely correlated with successful counseling outcomes, with the counseling relationship accounting for 30% of outcome variance (Miller et al., 1997). These findings continue to be replicated in large-scale studies that compare person-centered with cognitive-behavioral and psychodynamic counseling (Stiles, Barkham, Mellor-Clark, & Connell, 2008). Thus, although there has been a revival of Rogers's work, it is likely that the person-centered model will be practiced in combination with other humanistic, experiential, and/or existential approaches (Kirschenbaum & Jourdan, 2005).

Furthermore, there is a significant stream of research that supports experiential counselors' claims that emotional expression promotes well-being (Stanton & Low, 2012). In particular, writing to express emotions has been found to transform meaning and increase positive emotion related to an event (Langens, & Schüler, 2007). Of particular interest, constructive expression of emotion characterizes more satisfying intimate relationships (Yoshida, 2011). Additionally, young families with a positive attitude toward emotional expression also reported a greater sense of social support, suggesting that such an attitude may strengthen relationships on multiple levels (Castle, Slade, Barranco-Wadlow, & Rogers, 2008). In sum, although the specific interventions and overall outcome have not received significant research support, the principles and practices behind the humanistic approach to counseling relationships and to facilitating emotional expression have strong, consistent support.

Questions for Personal Reflection and Class Discussion

1. Which ideas from this chapter do you find most personally relevant? Why?
2. Which ideas from this chapter do you think will be most helpful in working with clients?
3. Do you agree with humanists who believe that all people naturally tend toward positive growth? Why or why not?
4. What are your thoughts about being an "imperfect role model" for clients? In what ways might this be useful or potentially harmful?
5. What are the possibilities and limitations for using this approach with diverse clients? How might you address the limitations?
6. What specific problems do you see arising when working with clients of different genders and ethnicity around issues of emotional expression? How might you address these concerns?
7. Describe a situation in which you were able to be "immediate" with someone. How did it feel to discuss emotions in the present moment? What helped you to do this?
8. For which clients and/or presenting problems do you think this approach would be most appropriate? Least appropriate?
9. Which case conceptualization concept seems most useful for understanding a client's problem?
10. Which intervention do you think would be the most useful?
11. Do you think this approach is a good fit for you as a counselor or therapist? Why or why not?
12. In what ways would you need to grow, or what would you need to learn, to be able to use this approach well?

Online Resources

Associations and Training Institutes

Association for the Development of the Person-Centered Approach
www.adpca.org

Association for Humanistic Psychology
www.ahpweb.org/

American Psychological Association, Division 32: Humanistic Psychology
www.apa.org/divisions/div32/

Carl Rogers Website
www.carlrogers.info

Erickson Institute: Resources on Erick Erickson's Work
www.erikson.edu

Esalen Institute, Big Sur California
www.esalen.org

Natalie Rogers: Expressive Arts Therapy
www.nrogers.com

New York Institute for Gestalt Therapy
www.newyorkgestalt.org/

Gestalt Institute of Cleveland
www.gestaltcleveland.org/

Gestalt Institute of San Francisco
http://gestaltinstitute.com/enter/

Gestalt Institute of the Rockies
www.gestaltoftherockies.com/

Gestalt Therapy Institute of Philadelphia
www.gestaltphila.org/

International Society for Existential Psychotherapy and Counseling
www.existentialpsychotherapy.net

Pacific Gestalt Institute
www.gestalttherapy.org/

World Association for Person Centered & Experiential Psychotherapy & Counseling
www.pce-world.org/

Journals

British Gestalt Journal
www.britishgestaltjournal.com

Gestalt Review
www.gestaltreview.com

International Gestalt Journal
www.gestalt.org/igipromo

International Journal of Existential Psychology and Psychotherapy
www.meaning.ca/ijepp.htm

Journal of Humanistic Psychology
www.ahpweb.org/pub/journal/menu.html

Journal of the World Association for Person-Centered and Experiential Psychotherapy and Counseling
www.pce-world.org/pcep-journal.html

Person-Centered Journal
www.adpca.org/Journal/journalindex.htm

References

*Asterisk indicates recommended introductory readings.

Beane, J. (1981). "I'd rather be dead than gay": Counseling gay men who are coming out. *Personnel & Guidance Journal, 60*(4), 222–226. doi:10.1002/j.2164-4918.1981.tb00286.x.

Beisser, A. (1970). The paradoxical theory of change. In J. Fagan & I. Shepherd (Eds.), *Gestalt therapy now* (pp. 77–80). New York: Harper.

Brazier, D. D. (1996). The post-Rogerian therapy of Robert Carkhuff. *Amida Trust*. Retrieved from http://www.amidatrust.com/article_carkhuff.html

Brown, L. S. (2007). Empathy, genuineness—and the dynamics of power: A feminist responds to Rogers. *Psychotherapy: Theory, Research, Practice, Training, 44*(3), 257–259. doi: 10.1037/0033-3204.44.3.257.

Buber, M. (1958). *I and Thou* (R. G. Smith, Trans.). New York: Collier Books. (Original work published in 1923).

Carkhuff, R. (1969). *Helping and human relations: A primer for lay and professional helpers*. New York: Holt, Rinehart and Winston.

Carkhuff, R. (2000). *The art of helping* (8th ed.). Amherst, MA: Human Resource Development Press.

Castle, H., Slade, P., Barranco-Wadlow, M., & Rogers, M. (2008). Attitudes to emotional expression, social support and postnatal adjustment in new parents. *Journal of Reproductive and Infant Psychology*, *26*(3), 180–194. doi:10.1080/02646830701691319.

Cheung, M., & Nguyen, P. V. (2012). Connecting the strengths of Gestalt chairs to Asian clients. *Smith College Studies in Social Work*, *82*(1), 51–62. doi:10.1080/00377317.2012.638895.

Davies D. (2009). Person-centered therapy. Therapeutic perspectives on working with lesbian, gay and bisexual clients [e-book]. Maidenhead, BRK, England: Open University Press; pp. 91–105. Available from: PsycINFO, Ipswich, MA. Accessed January 12, 2015.

Gehart, D. (2015). *Theory and treatment planning in counseling and psychotherapy* (2nd ed.). Pacific Grove, CA: Brooks Cole.

Gehart, D. R., & Lyle, R. R. (2001). Client experience of gender in therapeutic relationships: An interpretive ethnography. *Family Process*, *40*, 443–458.

Gehart, D., & McCollum, E. (2008). Teaching therapeutic presence: A mindfulness-based approach. In S. Hick & T. Bien (Eds.), *Mindfulness and the therapeutic relationship* (pp. 176–194). New York: Guilford.

Geller, S. M., & Greenberg, L. S. (2002). Therapeutic presence: Therapists' experience of presence in the psychotherapy encounter. *Person-Centered and Experiential Psychotherapies*, *1*, 71–86.

Hill, C. (2007). My personal reactions to Rogers (1957): The facilitative but neither necessary nor sufficient conditions of therapeutic personality change. *Psychotherapy: Theory, Research, Practice, Training*, *44*, 260–264. doi: 10.1037/0033-3204.44.3.260.

Hycner, R. (1995). The dialogic ground. In R. Hycner & L. Jacobs (Eds.), *The healing relationship in Gestalt therapy* (pp. 3–30). Highland, NY: Gestalt Journal Press.

Johnson, S. M. (2004). *The practice of emotionally focused marital therapy: Creating connection* (2nd ed.). New York: Brunner/Routledge.

Kirschenbaum, H. (2004). Carl Rogers's life and work: An assessment on the 100th anniversary of his birth. *Journal of Counseling and Development*, *82*, 116–124.

Kirschenbaum, H., & Jourdan, A. (2005). The current status of Carl Rogers and the Person-Centered Approach. *Psychotherapy: Theory, Research, Practice, Training*, *42*, 37–51.

Kleinplatz, P. J. (1996). Transforming sex therapy: Integrating erotic potential. *The Humanistic Psychologist*, *24*(2), 190–202. doi:10.1080/08873267.1996.9986850.

Langdridge, D. (2007). Gay affirmative therapy: A theoretical framework and defence. *Journal of Gay & Lesbian Psychotherapy*, *11*(1–2), 27–43. doi:10.1300/J236v11n01_03.

Langens, T. A., & Schüler, J. (2007). Effects of written emotional expression: The role of positive expectancies. *Health Psychology*, *26*(2), 174–182. doi:10.1037/0278-6133.26.2.174.

Lobb, M. S., & Lichtenberg, P. (2005). Classic Gestalt therapy theory: Field theory. In A. L. Woldt & S. M. Toman (Eds.), *Gestalt therapy: History, theory, and practice* (pp. 21–39). Thousand Oaks, CA: Sage.

Lu, Q., & Stanton, A. L. (2010). How benefits of expressive writing vary as a function of writing instructions, ethnicity and ambivalence over emotional expression. *Psychology & Health*, *25*(6), 669–684.

Mahrer, A. (2007). To a large extent, the field got it wrong: New learnings from a new look at an old classic. *Psychotherapy: Theory, Research, Practice, Training*, *44*, 274–278. doi: 0.1037/0033-3204.44.3.274.

Maslow, A. (1954). *Motivation and personality*. New York: Harper.

McDonough-Means, S. I., Kreitzer, M. J., & Bell, I. R. (2004). Fostering a healing presence and investigating its mediators. *Journal of Alternative and Complementary Medicine*, *10*, S25–S41.

McLeod, J. (2002). Research policy and practice in person-centered and experiential therapy: Restoring coherence. *Person-Centered and Experiential Psychotherapies*, *1*(1–2), 87–101.

Miller, S. D., Duncan, B. L., & Hubble, M. (1997). *Escape from Babel: Toward a unifying language for psychotherapy practice*. New York: Norton.

Milton, M. (2000). Existential-phenomenological therapy. In D. Davies & C. Neal (Eds.), *Therapeutic perspectives on working with lesbian, gay and bisexual clients* (pp. 39–53). Maidenhead, BRK, England: Open University Press.

Pachankis, J. E., & Bernstein, L. B. (2012). An etiological model of anxiety in young gay men: From early stress to public self-consciousness. *Psychology of Men & Masculinity*, *13*(2), 107–122. doi:10.1037/a0024594.

Parlett, M., & Lee, R. G. (2005). Contemporary Gestalt therapy: Field theory. In A. L. Woldt & S. M. Toman (Eds.), *Gestalt therapy: History, theory, and practice* (pp. 41–63). Thousand Oaks, CA: Sage.

Perls, F. (1973). *The Gestalt approach and eyewitness to therapy*. Palo Alto, CA: Science and Behavior Books.

Perls, F., Hefferline, R. F., & Goodman, P. (1951). *Gestalt therapy: Excitement and growth in the human personality*. New York: Julian Press.

Picucci, M. (1992). Planning an experiential weekend workshop for lesbians and gay males in recovery. *Journal of Chemical Dependency Treatment*, *5*(1), 119–139. doi:10.1300/J034v05n01_10.

Polster, E., & Polster, M. (1973). *Gestalt therapy integrated*. New York: Brunner/Mazel.

Quinn, A. (2013). A person-centered approach to multicultural counseling competence. *Journal of Humanistic Psychology*, *53*(2), 202–251. doi:10.1177/0022167812458452.

Roberts, A. (1999). *From the radical center: The heart of Gestalt therapy: Selected writings of Erving and Miriam Polster*. Cleveland, OH: Gestalt Institute of Cleveland Press.

Rogers, C. (1942). *Counseling and psychotherapy: Newer concepts in practice*. New York: Houghton Mifflin.

Rogers, C. (1951). *Client-centered counseling*. Cambridge, MA: Riverside Press.

*Rogers, C. (1957/2007). The necessary and sufficient conditions of personality change. *Psychotherapy: Theory, Research, Practice, Training*, *44*, 240–248. doi: 10.1037/

0033-3204.44.3.240. (Originally published in 1957 in the *Journal of Consulting Psychology*, 21(2), 95–103).

*Rogers, C. (1961). *On becoming a person: A counselor's view of psychocounseling*. London: Constable.

Rogers, C. (1981). *Way of Being*. Boston, MA: Houghton Mifflin.

Smith, E. W. L. (1976). The roots of Gestalt therapy. In E. W. L. Smith (Ed.), *The growing edge of Gestalt therapy* (pp. 3–36). Highland, NY: Gestalt Journal Press.

Stanton, A. L., & Low, C. A. (2012). Expressing emotions in stressful contexts: Benefits, moderators, and mechanisms. *Current Directions in Psychological Science, 21*(2), 124–128. doi:10.1177/0963721411434978.

Stiles, W., Barkham, M., Mellor-Clark, J., & Connell, J. (2008). Effectiveness of cognitive-behavioural, person-centred, and psychodynamic therapies in UK primary-care routine practice: Replication in a larger sample. *Psychological Medicine: A Journal of Research in Psychiatry and the Allied Sciences, 38*(5), 677–688. doi:10.1017/S0033291707001511.

Truax, C. B., & Carkhuff, R. R. (1976). *Towards effective counseling and psychotherapy*. Chicago, IL: Aldine.

Wachtel, P. L. (2007). Carl Rogers and the larger context of therapeutic thought. *Theory, Research, Practice, Training, 44*(3), 279–284. doi: 10.1037/0033-3204.44.3.279.

Wang, L. (1994). Marriage and family therapy with people from China. *Contemporary Family Therapy: An International Journal, 16*(1), 25–37. doi:10.1007/BF02197600.

Woldt, A. L., & Toman, S. M. (Eds.) (2005). *Gestalt therapy: History, theory, and practice*. Thousand Oaks, CA: Sage.

Yontef, G. (1993). *Awareness dialogue and process: Essays on Gestalt therapy*. Highland, NY: Gestalt Journal Press.

Yontef, G., & Jacobs, L. (2000). Gestalt therapy. In R. J. Corsini & D. Wedding (Eds.), *Current psychotherapies* (6th ed., pp. 303–339). Itasca, IL: Peacock Publishers.

Yoshida, T. (2011). Effects of attitudes toward emotional expression on anger regulation tactics and intimacy in close and equal relationships. *The Japanese Journal of Social Psychology, 26*(3), 211–218.

Yu, J. (1998, November). Asian students' preferences for psychotherapeutic approaches: Cognitive-behavioral, process-experiential and short-term dynamic therapies. *Dissertation Abstracts International*, 59, 2444.

Humanistic Case Study: Perfectionism and Anxiety

Shandra, a 30-year-old, single, African American woman, has been experiencing severe anxiety since starting her new marketing job. She has always been successful at work, but this latest position has her highly anxious about failure. She works long hours at night to stay ahead, constantly reviews her schedule to avoid missing appointments, and never turns off her smartphone. She recently stopped going to church on Sundays, telling her family and friends she was too tired and busy, which is when they told her she really needed to get help. Shandra is the eldest of five children, spending most of her childhood helping to raise her younger brothers and sisters so her parents could work. She excelled in school and stayed out of trouble and tried to keep the peace at home when her parents would argue and sometimes physically fight. She has always been prone to perfectionism and worry, but it has gotten out of hand in the past couple of months.

After an initial consultation, a humanistic counselor develops the case conceptualization shown on the next page.

CASE CONCEPTUALIZATION

Date: October 23, 2013 **Clinician:** Shizue **Client/Case #:** 10008

I. Introduction to Client

Identify primary client and significant others

Client

Adult Female Age: 30 African American Single heterosexual Occupation/Grade: Marketing; pharmaceutical sales

Other: Lives near parents and siblings

Significant Others

Client's Mother Age: 48 African American Married heterosexual Occupation/Grade: Waitress

Other: ______

Client's Father Age: 52 African American Married heterosexual Occupation/Grade: Construction

Other: ______

Select Person Age: ____ Select Ethnicity Select Relational Status Occupation/Grade: ______ Other: ______

Select Person Age: ____ Select Ethnicity Select Relational Status Occupation/Grade: ______ Other: ______

Others: ______

II. Presenting Concern(s)

Client Description of Problem(s): AF says that she probably does worry too much and works too hard. But she wants to be a success and says she can't count on Prince Charming to show up.

Significant Other/Family Description(s) of Problems: AF's parents are increasingly worried about AF's overemphasis on work and failing to put much energy into her personal life. She has only had two boyfriends, with the longest relationship lasting only a year. They sometimes feel guilty that maybe they put too much adult pressure on her as she was growing up and she never learned to live and have fun. Nonetheless, they are very proud of her for being a successful college graduate and role model for her siblings.

Broader System Problem Descriptions: Description of problem from referring party, teachers, relatives, legal system, etc.:

Friends: AF's friends reportedly tell her that she works too much and doesn't know how to have fun. They think she needs to learn to make her social life and finding a boyfriend a priority.

______: ______

III. Background Information

Trauma/Abuse History (recent and past): AF witnessed her parents fight verbally when she was growing up; at times they threw things at each other and slapped each other. During these times, AF would focus

(continued)

on shielding the other children from their fights by taking them to the park or up into their rooms. AF denies any direct abuse to herself. AF reports mild experiences of racism, mostly from her school years.

Substance Use/Abuse (current and past; self, family of origin, significant others): AF reports only periodic social drinking, never trying any illegal substance, and no notable substance abuse issue in her family of origin.

Precipitating Events (recent life changes, first symptoms, stressors, etc.): A marketing major in college, AF recently got a high-pressure position in pharmaceutical sales. She has been working increasingly long hours to ensure her success, including reviewing materials, double-checking appointments, and staying connected 24/7 with her smartphone. She has spent less and less time with family, friends, and her church community. Although most of the worrying is currently about her job, she admits that she has always made "mountains out of mole hills" and been a perfectionist.

Related Historical Background (family history, related issues, previous counseling, etc.): When AF was a child, her parents worked long hours to support their five children. As long as she can remember, she was helping her parents take care of her siblings. She was reliably the "responsible one," never in trouble in school, and always had "worries beyond her years."

IV. Client Strengths and Diversity

Client Strengths

Personal: AF is intelligent, hard-working, and loyal to family and friends.

Relational/Social: AF comes from a family with strong bonds and an extended family/friend support network.

Spiritual: AF has always been active in her church, where she finds great comfort and shelter from her worries.

Diversity: Resources and Limitations

Identify potential resources and limitations available to clients based on their age, gender, sexual orientation, cultural background, socioeconomic status, religion, regional community, language, family background, family configuration, abilities, etc.

Unique Resources: AF has a large support system through her family, friends, and church. Her religious beliefs provide her with a sense of peace and purpose in her life.

Potential Limitations: As an African American female, AF states that at times she feels she has to work harder than others, in particular the Caucasian males who dominate the pharmaceutical company she works for. AF feels she needs to prove herself as a successful African American businesswoman.

Complete All of the Following Sections for a Complete Case Conceptualization or Specific Sections for Theory-Specific Conceptualization.

(continued)

V. Psychodynamic Conceptualization

Psychodynamic Defense Mechanisms

Check 2-4 most commonly used defense mechanisms

❑ Acting Out: *Describe:* ______

❑ Denial: *Describe:* ______

❑ Displacement: *Describe:* ______

❑ Help-Rejecting Complaining: *Describe:* ______

❑ Humor: *Describe:* ______

❑ Passive Aggression: *Describe:* ______

❑ Projection: *Describe:* ______

❑ Projective Identification: *Describe:* ______

❑ Rationalization: *Describe:* ______

❑ Reaction Formation: *Describe:* ______

☒ Repression: *Describe:* AF often represses her more vulnerable feeling and needs.

❑ Splitting: *Describe:* ______

☒ Sublimation: *Describe:* AF redirects her frustrations and lack of fulfillment in her personal life into her work.

☒ Suppression: *Describe:* AF tries to push out of her mind "selfish" and "unrealistic" desires, such as longing for a husband, vacations, and the "good life."

❑ Other: ______

Object Relational Patterns

Describe relationship with early caregivers in past: AF's parents worked long hours to support her and her siblings. She spent little time interacting with her mother and father as a child. From a very young age AF was parentified and expected to help raise her younger siblings.

Was the attachment with the mother (or equivalent) primarily:

❑ Generally Secure ❑ Anxious and Clingy ☒ Avoidant and Emotionally Distant ❑ Other: ______

Was the attachment with the father (or equivalent) primarily:

❑ Generally Secure ❑ Anxious and Clingy ☒ Avoidant and Emotionally Distant ❑ Other: ______

Describe present relationship with these caregivers: AF is close with her parents and states that her current relationship with both her mother and father is supportive and positive.

Describe relational patterns with partner and other current relationships: N/A

Erickson's Psychosocial Developmental Stage

Describe development at each stage up to current stage

Trust vs. Mistrust (Infant Stage): AF's grandmother took care of her in her first two years of life; they were very close until her death when AF was 22.

(*continued*)

Autonomy vs. Shame and Doubt (Toddler Stage): AF began helping out with her siblings when she was only 3; she developed a sense of responsibility and duty at this age that seems to be fueled by doubt and fear.

Initiative vs. Guilt (Preschool Age): AF was forced to take initiative and responsibility before she was developmentally ready and seems to be plagued by guilt and fear of doing things wrong.

Industry vs. Inferiority (School Age): During school years, AF was highly industrious both at home and at school but did not learn to counterbalance this with a healthy sense of fun and play.

Identity vs. Role Confusion (Adolescence): AF's identity has always been closely tied to taking care of her siblings, never defining herself in terms of her interests, dreams, desires, etc.

Intimacy vs. Isolation (Young Adulthood): AF is struggling with developing intimate relationships as an adult outside of her childhood friends and family.

Generativity vs. Stagnation (Adulthood): ____________

Ego Integrity vs. Despair (Late Adulthood): ____________

Adlerian Style of Life Theme

☒ Control: AF's life has been organized around having to control and deny herself so that she could care for others.

❑ Superiority: ____________

❑ Pleasing: ____________

❑ Comfort: ____________

Basic Mistake Misperceptions: Early in life, AF learned that she had to sacrifice herself to make life better for others; she also learned that her value was in what she did, not in who she was.

VI. Humanistic-Existential Conceptualization

Expression of Authentic Self

Problems: Are problems perceived as internal or external (caused by others, circumstance, etc.)?

❑ Predominantly internal
☒ Mixed
❑ Predominantly external

Agency and Responsibility: Is self or other discussed as agent of story? Does client take clear responsibility for situation?

☒ Strong sense of agency and responsibility
❑ Agency in some areas
❑ Little agency; frequently blames others/situation
❑ Often feels victimized

Recognition and Expression of Feelings: Are feelings readily recognized, owned, and experienced?

❑ Easily expresses feelings
❑ Identifies feelings with prompting
☒ Difficulty recognizing feelings

(*continued*)

Here-and-Now Experiencing: Is the client able to experience full range of feelings as they are happening in the present moment?

❑ Easily experiences emotions in present moment

☒ Experiences some present emotions with assistance

❑ Difficulty with present moment experiencing

Personal Constructs and Facades: Is the client able to recognize and go beyond roles? Is identity rigid or tentatively held?

❑ Tentatively held; able to critique and question

☒ Some awareness of facades and construction of identity

❑ Identity rigidly defined; seems like "fact"

Complexity and Contradictions: Are internal contradictions owned and explored? Is client able to fully engage the complexity of identity and life?

❑ Aware of and resolves contradictions

☒ Some recognition of contradictions

❑ Unaware of internal contradictions

Shoulds: Is client able to question socially imposed shoulds and oughts? Can client balance desire to please others and desire to be authentic?

❑ Able to balance authenticity with social obligation

❑ Identifies tension between social expectations and personal desires

☒ Primarily focuses on external shoulds

*List shoulds:*____________________________

Acceptance of Others: Is client able to accept others and modify expectations of others to be more realistic?

❑ Readily accepts others as they are

☒ Recognizes expectations of others are unrealistic but still strong emotional reaction to expectations not being met

❑ Difficulty accepting others as is; always wanting others to change to meet expectations

Trust of Self: Is client able to trust self as process (rather than a stabile object)?

❑ Able to trust and express authentic self

☒ Trust of self in certain contexts

❑ Difficulty trusting self in most contexts

Existential Analysis

Sources of Life Meaning (as described or demonstrated by client): AF's religious beliefs give her a sense of purpose and represent a significant piece of her identity. She also places a great deal of value in work and believes that one's work and personal acheivements are indicative of success or failure of a person.

General Themes of Life Meaning:

☒ Personal achievement/work

❑ Significant other

❑ Children

❑ Family of origin

❑ Social cause/contributing to others

☒ Religion/spirituality

❑ Other:____________________________

(continued)

Satisfaction with and clarity on life direction:

❑ Clear sense of meaning that creates resilience in difficult times

❑ Current problems require making choices related to life direction

☒ Minimally satisfied with current life direction; wants more from life

❑ Has reflected little on life direction up to this point; living according to life plan defined by someone/something else

❑ Other: ______

Gestalt Contact Boundary Disturbances

❑ *Desensitization:* Failing to notice problems

❑ *Introjection*: Take in others' views whole and unedited

❑ *Projection*: Assign undesired parts of self to others

❑ *Retroflection*: Direct action to self rather than other

❑ *Deflection*: Avoid direct contact with another or self

❑ *Egotism:* Not allowing outside to influence self

❑ *Confluence*: Agree with another to extent that boundary blurred

Describe: AF uses work to avoid relationships and the part of herself that longs for a family of her own.

VII. Cognitive-Behavioral Conceptualization

Baseline of Symptomatic Behavior

Symptom #1 (behavioral description): Worrying about multiple details of life

Frequency: Daily

Duration: Several hours each day

Context(s): Worse when home at night; better at work

Events Before: Driving home with extra time to think

Events After: Checking email; making lists; studying documents; generally performs well at work

Symptom #2 (behavioral description): Avoiding social relationships

Frequency: More often than not over course of month; approx 6 out of 8 social invitations

Duration: 1-2 weeks at a time

Context(s): Family, extended family, friends, church

Events Before: Busy with work; tired; overwhelmed; worrying at its worst

Events After: Spends time catching up and/or getting ahead with work

A-B-C Analysis of Irrational Beliefs

Activating Event ("Problem"): Compares her sales records to those of established persons in her region

Consequence (Mood, behavior, etc.): Feels embarrassed; works harder

Mediating Beliefs (Unhelpful beliefs about event that result in C):

1. I must be the best to be good enough.
2. I cannot fail at anything.
3. ______

(continued)

Beck's Schema Analysis

Identify frequently used cognitive schemas:

❑ *Arbitrary inference:* ______

☒ *Selective abstraction:* Compares self with well-established sales persons, filtering out the need for her to learn the position and get up to speed.

❑ *Overgeneralization:* ______

☒ *Magnification/Minimization:* Magnifies importance of small tasks that do not contribute substantially to life goals.

☒ *Personalization:* Personalizes what others say, her work performance as measuring value of self

☒ *Absolutist/dichotomous thinking:* Either success or failure; does not see anything in between

❑ *Mislabeling:* ______

❑ *Mindreading:* ______

VIII. Family Systems Conceptualization

Family Life Cycle Stage

☒ Single adult
❑ Marriage
❑ Family with Young Children
❑ Family with Adolescent Children
❑ Launching Children
❑ Later Life

Describe struggles with mastering developmental tasks in one of these stages: AF struggles to find a balance between work and making time to start a family of her own. She would like to get married and start a family; however, views work and independent success as being more important and practical.

Boundaries with

Parents ☒ Enmeshed ❑ Clear ❑ Disengaged ❑ NA: *Describe:* AF was parentified to the point of not experiencing age-appropriate social relationships and activities.

Significant Other ❑ Enmeshed ❑ Clear ❑ Disengaged ❑ NA: *Describe:* ______

Children ❑ Enmeshed ❑ Clear ❑ Disengaged ❑ NA: *Describe:* ______

Extended Family ☒ Enmeshed ❑ Clear ❑ Disengaged ❑ NA: *Describe:* More like a mother than sister to siblings

Other: Name ❑ Enmeshed ❑ Clear ❑ Disengaged ❑ NA: *Describe:* ______

Typical style for regulating closeness and distance with others: ______

Triangles/Coalitions

☒ Coalition in family of origin: *Describe:* AF triangulated into parents' marriage to stabilize their conflict, esp. when younger.

❑ Coalitions related to significant other: *Describe:* ______

❑ Other coalitions: ______

(*continued*)

Hierarchy between Self and Parent/Child ❑ NA

With own children ❑ Effective ❑ Rigid ❑ Permissive

With parents (for child/young adult) ☒ Effective ❑ Rigid ❑ Permissive

Complementary Patterns with Siblings:

❑ Pursuer/distancer

☒ Over-/underfunctioner

❑ Emotional/logical

❑ Good/bad parent

❑ Other: *Describe*

Example of complementary pattern: AF takes responsibility for her siblings and enables them to overly rely on her.

Intergenerational Patterns

Substance/Alcohol Abuse: ☒ NA ❑ History: ______

Sexual/Physical/Emotional Abuse: ❑ NA ☒ History: Witnessed parents' emotional and physical abuse with one another.

Parent/Child Relations: ❑ NA ☒ History: Parentified child; mother also parentified as a child.

Physical/Mental Disorders: ☒ NA ❑ History: ______

Family strengths: Describe: Strong extended family ties; parents have stayed together and get along better now; family very involved in church.

IX. Solution-Based and Cultural Discourse Conceptualization (Postmodern)

Solutions and Unique Outcomes

Attempted Solutions that DIDN'T or DON'T work:

1. Working harder to alleviate fears has only perpetuated the problem.
2. Avoiding church has not reduced stress.
3. ______

Exceptions and Unique Outcomes: Times, places, relationships, contexts, etc. when problem is less of a problem; behaviors that seem to make things even slightly better:

1. AF does make it to church at least once a month and generally feels better afterwards.
2. AF makes it to birthdays and major holiday events.
3. AF is able to relax when she goes to yoga, works out, or hangs out with high school friends.

Miracle Question Answer: If the problem were to be resolved overnight, what would client be doing differently the next day? (Describe in terms of doing X rather than not doing Y).

1. She would be spending more time interacting with family and friends.
2. She would start dating and begin to think more seriously about finding a boyfriend/husband.
3. She would feel "successful" at work and work for reasonable periods of time.

(continued)

Dominant Discourses informing definition of problem:

- *Ethnic, Class and Religious Discourses: How do key cultural discourses inform what is perceived as a problem and the possible solutions?* AF feels connected to and is proud of her African American community, especially her church. She feels the pressure of being marginalized and responds by working harder than others to ensure her success. As the eldest daughter, she has sacrificed her personal happiness to take care of her siblings and support her working-class parents in providing for the family. She carries with her a sense of burden of struggling to survive in a hostile environment.
- *Gender and Sexuality Discourses: How do the gender/sexual discourses inform what is perceived as a problem and the possible solutions?* AF has taken on a motherly caretaking role in her family to the extent that she has failed to allow herself to enjoy life herself. Like many modern African American women, she has led her life assuming she must be self-sufficient and not rely on a man or anyone else to take care of her.
- *Community, School, and Extended Family Discourses: How do other important community discourses inform what is perceived as a problem and the possible solutions?* AF is in a sales job where her "value" and worth is measured by her productivity; she has bought into this to the extent that it creates extreme anxiety and hardship for her.

Identity Narratives: How has the problem shaped each client's identity? Worry and perfectionism has been so central to AF's identity and survival, she does not see her current situation as problematically as her family and friends do. Although a part of her is disappointed, most of her believes that she does not have time for a personal life because work is too important.

Local or Preferred Discourses: What is the client's preferred identity narrative and/or narrative about the problem? Are there local (alternative) discourses about the problem that are preferred? AF admits to longing for a husband, a family of her own, and a home where she can really relax. She just feels hopeless about finding such things any time soon.

CLINICAL ASSESSMENT

Clinician: Shizue	Client ID #: 10008	Primary configuration: ☒ Individual ❑ Couple ❑ Family	Primary Language: ☒ English ❑ Spanish ❑ Other: ______

List client and significant others

Adult(s)

Adult Female Age: ____ African American Single heterosexual Occupation: Marketing; pharmaceutical sales

Other identifier: ______

Select Gender Age: ____ Select Ethnicity Select Relational Status Occupation: ____ Other identifier: ____

Child(ren)

Select Gender Age: ____ Select Ethnicity Grade: Select Grade School: ____ Other identifier: ____

Select Gender Age: ____ Select Ethnicity Grade: Select Grade School: ____ Other identifier: ____

Others: ______

Presenting Problems

		Complete for children:
☒ Depression/hopelessness	❑ Couple concerns	❑ School failure/decline performance
☒ Anxiety/worry	❑ Parent/child conflict	❑ Truancy/runaway
❑ Anger issues	❑ Partner violence/abuse	❑ Fighting w/peers
❑ Loss/grief	❑ Divorce adjustment	❑ Hyperactivity
❑ Suicidal thoughts/attempts	❑ Remarriage adjustment	❑ Wetting/soiling clothing
❑ Sexual abuse/rape	❑ Sexuality/intimacy concerns	❑ Child abuse/neglect
❑ Alcohol/drug use	☒ Major life changes	❑ Isolation/withdrawal
❑ Eating problems/disorders	❑ Legal issues/probation	❑ Other: ______
☒ Job problems/unemployed	❑ Other: ______	

Mental Status Assessment for Identified Patient

Interpersonal	❑ NA	❑ Conflict ❑ Enmeshment ☒ Isolation/avoidance ❑ Harassment ❑ Other: ______
Mood	❑ NA	❑ Depressed/Sad ☒ Anxious ❑ Dysphoric ❑ Angry ❑ Irritable ❑ Manic ❑ Other: ______
Affect	❑ NA	☒ Constricted ❑ Blunt ❑ Flat ❑ Labile ❑ Incongruent ❑ Other: ______
Sleep	❑ NA	❑ Hypersomnia ☒ Insomnia ❑ Disrupted ❑ Nightmares ❑ Other: ______

(*continued*)

Eating	☒ NA	❑ Increase ❑ Decrease ❑ Anorectic restriction ❑ Binging ❑ Purging ❑ Other: ______
Anxiety	❑ NA	☒ Chronic worry ❑ Panic ❑ Phobias ❑ Obsessions ❑ Compulsions ❑ Other: ______
Trauma Symptoms	☒ NA	❑ Hypervigilance ❑ Flashbacks/Intrusive memories ❑ Dissociation ❑ Numbing ❑ Avoidance efforts ❑ Other: ______
Psychotic Symptoms	☒ NA	❑ Hallucinations ❑ Delusions ❑ Paranoia ❑ Loose associations ❑ Other: ______
Motor Activity/ Speech	❑ NA	❑ Low energy ☒ Hyperactive ❑ Agitated ❑ Inattentive ❑ Impulsive ❑ Pressured speech ❑ Slow speech ❑ Other: ______
Thought	❑ NA	❑ Poor concentration ❑ Denial ❑ Self-blame ❑ Other-blame ☒ Ruminative ❑ Tangential ❑ Concrete ❑ Poor insight ❑ Impaired decision making ❑ Disoriented ❑ Other: ______
Socio-Legal	☒ NA	❑ Disregards rules ❑ Defiant ❑ Stealing ❑ Lying ❑ Tantrums ❑ Arrest/ incarceration ❑ Initiates fights ❑ Other: ______
Other Symptoms	☒ NA	______

Diagnosis for Identified Patient

Contextual Factors considered in making diagnosis: ❑ Age ☒ Gender ❑ Family dynamics ☒ Culture ❑ Language ☒ Religion ☒ Economic ❑ Immigration ❑ Sexual/gender orientation ☒ Trauma ❑ Dual diagnosis/comorbid ❑ Addiction ❑ Cognitive ability ❑ Other: ______

Describe impact of identified factors on diagnosis and assessment process: Considered environmental and social stressors that are typical for African Americans in region, including marginalization experiences

DSM-5 Code	Diagnosis with Specifier *Include V/Z/T-Codes for Psychosocial Stressors/Issues*
1. F41.1	1. Generalized Anxiety Disorder
2. ______	2. ______
3. ______	3. ______
4. ______	4. ______
5. ______	5. ______

Medical Considerations

Has patient been referred for psychiatric evaluation? ☒ Yes ❑ No

Has patient agreed with referral? ❑ Yes ☒ No ❑ NA

(continued)

Psychometric instruments used for assessment: ☒ None ❑ Cross-cutting symptom inventories ❑ Other: AF wants to try counseling before medications.

Client response to diagnosis: ☒ Agree ❑ Somewhat agree ❑ Disagree ❑ Not informed for following reason: ________

Current Medications (psychiatric & medical) ☒ NA

1. ________; dose ________ mg; start date: ________
2. ________; dose ________ mg; start date: ________
3. ________; dose ________ mg; start date: ________
4. ________; dose ________ mg; start date: ________

Medical Necessity: *Check all that apply*

☒ Significant impairment ❑ Probability of significant impairment ❑ Probable developmental arrest

Areas of impairment:

☒ Daily activities ☒ Social relationships ☒ Health ☒ Work/School ❑ Living arrangement ❑ Other: ____________

Risk and Safety Assessment for Identified Patient

Suicidality	Homicidality	Alcohol Abuse
☒ No indication/Denies	☒ No indication/Denies	☒ No indication/denies
❑ Active ideation	❑ Active ideation	❑ Past abuse
❑ Passive ideation	❑ Passive ideation	❑ Current; Freq/Amt:
❑ Intent without plan	❑ Intent without means	**Drug Use/Abuse** ____________
❑ Intent with means	❑ Intent with means	☒ No indication/denies
❑ Ideation in past year	❑ Ideation in past year	❑ Past use
❑ Attempt in past year	❑ Violence past year	❑ Current drugs: ____________
❑ Family or peer history of completed suicide	❑ History of assaulting others	Freq/Amt: ____________
	❑ Cruelty to animals	❑ Family/sig. other use

Sexual & Physical Abuse and Other Risk Factors

☒ Childhood abuse history: ❑ Sexual ❑ Physical ❑ Emotional ❑ Neglect

❑ Adult with abuse/assault in adulthood: ❑ Sexual ❑ Physical ❑ Current

❑ History of perpetrating abuse: ❑ Sexual ❑ Physical ❑ Emotional

❑ Elder/dependent adult abuse/neglect

❑ History of or current issues with restrictive eating, binging, and/or purging

❑ Cutting or other self harm: ❑ Current ❑ Past: Method: ____________

❑ Criminal/legal history: ____________

❑ Other trauma history: ____________

❑ None reported

(*continued*)

Indicators of Safety

❑ NA

☒ At least one outside support person

☒ Able to cite specific reasons to live or not harm

❑ Hopeful

❑ Willing to dispose of dangerous items

☒ Has future goals

❑ Willingness to reduce contact with people who make situation worse

❑ Willing to implement safety plan, safety interventions

❑ Developing set of alternatives to self/other harm

☒ Sustained period of safety: No Hx of self-harm

❑ Other: ______

Elements of Safety Plan

❑ NA

❑ Verbal no harm contract

❑ Written no harm contract

☒ Emergency contact card

☒ Emergency therapist/agency number

❑ Medication management

❑ Plan for contacting friends/support persons during crisis

❑ Specific plan of where to go during crisis

☒ Specific self-calming tasks to reduce risk before reach crisis level (e.g., journaling, exercising, etc.)

☒ Specific daily/weekly activities to reduce stressors

❑ Other: ______

Legal/Ethical Action Taken: ☒ NA ❑ Action: ______

Case Management

Collateral Contacts

- Has contact been made with treating *physicians or other professionals*: ☒ NA ❑ Yes ❑ In process.
  Name/Notes: ______
- If client is involved in mental health *treatment elsewhere*, has contact been made? ☒ NA ❑ Yes ❑ In process.
  Name/Notes: ______
- Has contact been made with *social worker*: ☒ NA ❑ Yes ❑ In process. Name/Notes: ______

Referrals

- Has client been referred for *medical assessment*: ❑ Yes ☒ No evidence for need
- Has client been referred for *social services*: ☒ NA ❑ Job/training ❑ Welfare/Food/Housing ❑ Victim services ❑ Legal aid ❑ Medical ❑ Other: ______
- Has client been referred for *group* or other support services: ☒ Yes:______ ❑ In process ❑ None recommended
- Are there anticipated *forensic/legal processes* related to treatment: ☒ No ❑ Yes; describe: ______

Support Network

- Client social support network includes: ☒ Supportive family ❑ Supportive partner ☒ Friends ☒ Religious/ spiritual organization ❑ Supportive work/social group ❑ Other: ______
- Describe anticipated effects treatment will have on others in support system (Children, partner, etc.): AF may be seen as abandoning family if focuses more on personal needs.
- Is there anything else client will need to be successful? NA

(continued)

Expected Outcome and Prognosis

☒ Return to normal functioning ☐ Anticipate less than normal functioning ☐ Prevent deterioration

Client Sense of Hope: 6

Evaluation of Assessment/Client Perspective

How were assessment methods adapted to client needs, including age, culture, and other diversity issues? Considered cultural norms of emotional expression, effects of oppression, experience of marginalization, typical family roles, female roles in African American families, ratio of available AA men to women when identifying "normal" worry and stress from clinical levels.

Describe actual or potential areas of client-clinician agreement/disagreement related to the above assessment: AF wants to try counseling before using medication to manage worry.

____________________, __________ ________

Clinician Signature License/Intern Status Date

____________________, __________ ________

Supervisor Signature License Date

TREATMENT PLAN

Date: 11/04/13 Case/Client #: 10008

Clinician Name: Shizue Theory: Humanistic (integration of person-centered, existential, and Gestalt)

Modalities planned: ☒ Individual Adult ❑ Individual Child ❑ Couple ❑ Family ❑ Group: ________

Recommended session frequency: ☒ Weekly ❑ Every two weeks ❑ Other: ________

Expected length of treatment: 12 months

Initial Phase of Treatment

Initial Phase Counseling Tasks

1. Develop working counseling relationship. *Diversity considerations:* Ensure counselor's expression of emotion and empathy are received as supportive and culturally relevant.

   Relationship-building approach/intervention:

   a. Use warmth, unconditional positive regard, authenticity, and culturally sensitive empathy; attend to cross-cultural communication issues.

2. Assess individual, systemic, and broader cultural dynamics. *Diversity considerations:* Adapt norms to address culture, social class, and gender.

   Assessment strategies:

   a. Assess for ability to identify, express, and experience emotions in present moment.

   b. Identify polarities, disowned parts, shoulds, life purpose and meaning.

3. Identify and obtain client agreement on treatment goals. *Diversity note:* Consider cultural and community resources and values; ensure goals related to self-actualization match client's value system.

   Goal-making intervention:

   a. Collaboratively with client identify areas of life in which she can be more of her authentic self.

4. Identify needed referrals, crisis issues, and other client needs. *Diversity note:* Identify community resources such as church resources to support client.

   a. *Crisis assessment intervention(s):* Summarize, clarify, and reflect feelings to help client identify source of emotions that create sense of worry and overwhelm.

   b. *Referral(s):* Encourage client to access support groups in her church community and/or process groups.

Initial Phase Client Goal

1. Decrease overidentification with and defining self by work performance to reduce chronic worry.

   Interventions:

   a. Identify, accept and own feelings of inadequancy and fear that fuel worry.

   b. Body awareness exercises to help AF manage worry in everyday situations.

(continued)

Working Phase of Treatment

Working Phase Counseling Tasks

1. Monitor quality of the working alliance. *Diversity considerations:* Directly address and discuss cultural and class differences between counselor and client as they arise.
   a. *Assessment Intervention:* Directly ask about satisfaction with sessions and watch for nonverbal communication to monitor quality of relationship and I-Thou encounters.

2. Monitor progress toward goals. *Diversity considerations:* Invite client to evaluate progress using her values while also addressing tendency for perfection.
   a. *Assessment Intervention:* Include perspectives of friends and family members in measuring progress; invite client to periodically evaluate her own progress.

Working Phase Client Goals

1. Increase ability to identify significant sources of purpose and life meaning, especially those related to personal life to reduce social withdrawal.

   Interventions:
   a. Help client identify and express hopes and dreams for personal life and encourage client to take responsibility to achieving these goals.
   b. Help client explore how childhood role as caretaker for siblings has contributed to overemphasis on responsibility and an underemphasis on taking care of personal needs and dreams.

2. Increase ability to recognize authentic self without facade of "professional" and "provider" to reduce worry.

   Interventions:
   a. Process questions to enable client to clarify inner experience of self, including the pressures of being the eldest child and being a professional African American woman.
   b. Immediacy to help client experience self in relationship to counselor.

3. Increase ability to experience and express emotions as they arise in the present moment to reduce insecurity-based worry.

   Interventions:
   a. Gestalt experiments to identify the needs of each part of self and begin to see how each is an important part of her life experience.
   b. Modify language to allow AF to accept both the capable and needy parts of self.

Closing Phase of Treatment

Closing Phase Counseling Task

1. Develop aftercare plan and maintain gains. *Diversity considerations:* Strengthen connection with existing support system, including church, community, and family.

(continued)

Intervention:

a. Process questions to help client identify how best to manage potential future challenges; terminate only after client has developed ability to reflect on self without assistance.

Closing Phase Client Goals

1. Increase experience and acceptance of self as an unfolding, evolving process to reduce potential for relapse of worry and anxiety.

   Interventions:

   a. Unconditional positive regard to enable client to also accept all elements of self.

   b. Gestalt experiments to experience authentic self in various contexts and relationships.

2. Increase self-regulation and authentic expression of self in intimate relationships while simultaneously allowing for another's authenticity to reduce social withdrawal.

   Interventions:

   a. Relate to client using genuineness and authenticity to create context in which it is safe for her to do the same; encourage AF to translate these skills to outside relationships.

   b. Encourage AF to pursue goal of having a husband and family, creating space to share fears of not finding a man given the sociopolitical realities.

PROGRESS NOTE FOR CLIENT #13099

Date: 11/04/2013 **Time:** 3:30 ❑ am/☒ pm **Session Length:** ☒ 45 min. ❑ 60 min. ❑ Other: ______ minutes

Present: ❑ Adult Male ☒ Adult Female ❑ Child Male ❑ Child Female ❑ Other: ______________

Billing Code: ❑ 90791 (eval) ☒ 90834 (45 min. therapy) ❑ 90837 (60 min. therapy) ❑ 90847 (family)

❑ Other: ______________________________

Symptom(s)	Duration and Frequency Since Last Visit	Progress
1: Anxiety/worry	4 days; 1-2 hours; milder	**Maintained**
2: Social withdrawal	Mild; attended church; no other activities	**Maintained**
3: Overfunctioning	Limited self to 1 hour of work after hours; 4 days	**Progressing**

Explanatory Notes on Symptoms: ______________________________

In-Session Interventions and Assigned Homework

Continued exploring fears and pressure that fuel AF's drive for work success as well as the parts of herself that she hides from others; continued connecting childhood responsibilities and experience of marginalization to current fanatical and fear-based approach to work. Used body awareness exercises to have AF experience fears and anxiety in present moment and learning to tolerate and accept them.

Client Response/Feedback

AF began session somewhat resistant to exploring sources of anxiety but quickly relaxes into process and expresses relief at simply putting fears into words.

Plan

☒ Continue with treatment plan: plan for next session: Continue to increase ability to experience emotions in present moment; connect with disowned parts of self.

❑ Modify plan: ______________________________

Next session: Date: 11/11/2013 Time: 3:30 ❑ am/☒ pm

Crisis Issues: ☒ No indication of crisis/client denies ❑ Crisis assessed/addressed: describe below

______________________, ______________________ ______________________

Clinician's Signature License/Intern Status Date

Case Consultation/Supervision ❑ Not Applicable

Notes: Supervisor encouraged use of in-session exercises to experience anxiety and disowned parts of self.

Collateral Contact ❑ Not Applicable

Name: Johanna White Date of Contact: 11/04/2013 Time: 1:30 ❑ am/☒pm

☒ Written release on file: ☒ Sent/❑ Received ❑ In court docs ❑ Other: ______________

(*continued*)

Notes: Contact Ms. White who is leading women's group at church to review goals of tx and coordinate with group process.

_______________, _______________ _______________
Clinician's Signature License/Intern Status Date

_______________, _______________ _______________
Supervisor's Signature License Date

CHAPTER

11

Cognitive-Behavioral Approaches

Lay of the Land

Behavioral, cognitive, and cognitive-behavioral approaches are a group of related counseling methods that emphasize using active techniques and psychoeducation to achieve changes in behaviors, cognition, and affect. Third-party payers, such as insurance companies, often favor them because they are brief, they target medical symptoms rather than broader personality issues, and they are based in a strong research tradition. These approaches can be divided into three streams of practice:

- *Behavioral Approaches:* Using classical conditioning, operant conditioning, and social learning theory, behavioral approaches focus on analyzing and intervening upon observable measurable behaviors; in this approach, thought is conceptualized as a covert behavior that operates according to standard behavioral principles (Skinner, 1974). The evolution of behavioral approaches occurred in three waves (Hayes, 2004):
    1. *The First Wave of Behaviorism:* The original "pure" behavioral approaches, based on classical conditioning, operant conditioning, and social learning theory (see Case Conceptualization below).
    2. *The Second Wave of Behaviorism:* Integration of cognitive approaches with behavioral, which, before the 1980s was generally considered a separate stream of research and practice.
    3. *The Third Wave of Behaviorism:* In the 21st century, mindfulness approaches are transforming behavioral practices to use compassionate acceptance of thoughts and feelings to paradoxically promote change.
- *Cognitive Approaches:* Developed independently from behavioral approaches by Aaron Beck, cognitive approaches are based on the premise that (a) psychological disorders are characterized by dysfunctional thinking based on dysfunctional beliefs, and (b) improvement results from modifying dysfunctional thinking and beliefs (Beck, 1991, 1997). Cognitive theory can be used (a) separately from behaviorism, (b) as part of an integrated cognitive-behavioral practice, or (c) as *metatheory* for a general integrative approach (Alford & Beck, 1997)
- *Cognitive-Behavioral Approaches:* The mainstay of many contemporary practitioners, cognitive-behavioral approaches integrate both behavioral and cognitive techniques for changing problem thoughts, behaviors, and feelings. This chapter will focus on this commonly practiced combined approach.

Numerous distinct forms of cognitive-behavioral approaches have been developed over the years, with some of the more prominent being:

- *Rational Emotive Behavior Therapy:* Developed by Albert Ellis, REBT counselors use "A-B-C" analysis to help clients identify the *"B"elief* that results in symptomatic *"C"onsequences* in response to an *"A"ctivating event.* This approach uses a confrontational style to dispute irrational beliefs.
- *Multimodal Therapy:* An approach that uses an eclectic set of interventions, Arnold Lazarus's multimodal therapy is based on assessment of the BASIC-ID: behavior, affect, sensation, imagery, cognition, interpersonal relationships, and drug treatment.
- *Reality Therapy:* More philosophical than other cognitive-behavioral approaches (and not always considered a CBT approach), William Glasser's (1975, 1997) reality theory is based on the premise that people are driven by five basic needs—survival, love, power, freedom, and fun—and emphasizes how people *choose everything* they do, including feeling miserable.
- *Mindfulness-Based Therapies:* Employing mindfulness meditation practices, mindfulness-based therapies are group educational approaches based on Kabt-Zinn's (1990) mindfulness-based stress reduction curriculum. Specific programs have been developed for physical health, anxiety, depression, addictive behaviors, eating disorders, parents, and nondistressed couples.
- *Mindfulness-Informed Therapies (DBT & ACT):* The most recently developed, mindfulness-informed approaches, most notably *Dialectical Behavior Therapy (DBT)* and *Acceptance and Commitment Therapy (ACT)*, use principles from mindfulness practice—most significantly, accepting and observing problematic thoughts and feelings—to reduce their intensity.

Cognitive-Behavioral Approaches

In a Nutshell: The Least You Need to Know

Cognitive-behavioral counselors have a no-nonsense, matter-of-fact approach to helping clients that is based on logic and education. Judith Beck (2005) wraps up cognitive approaches thusly, "In a nutshell, the *cognitive model* proposes that distorted or dysfunctional thinking (which influences the patient's mood and behavior) is common to all psychological disturbances. Realistic evaluation and modification of thinking procedures produces an improvement in mood and behavior" (p. 1; italics in original). More simply stated, cognitive counselors believe unhelpful thoughts are the source of emotional and behavioral problems. Behaviorists add that maladaptive behavioral reinforcement also results in problem symptoms.

Cognitive-behavioral counselors use behavioral and cognitive techniques to directly treat symptoms, either by creating new behavioral associations or by helping clients think and feel differently. More so than any other approach, they rely heavily on psychoeducation to help clients change their thinking and behavioral habits. The role of counselors is educational, using their expertise to help clients learn how to manage their thoughts, feelings, and emotions more effectively. Clients are actively engaged by performing homework tasks out of session. Unlike psychodynamic and humanistic approaches, the overarching goal is not personality change; instead, cognitive-behavioral counselors have the more modest goal of helping clients learn how to better manage troubling symptoms. Developed using the scientific method, cognitive-behavioralists have a strong research tradition, generating a solid evidence base for its effectiveness with a wide range of clinical concerns.

The Juice: Significant Contributions to the Field

If you remember one thing from this chapter, it should be ...

A-B-C Theory

Originally developed by Albert Ellis (1962, 1996) using Beck's (cognitive theory, 1976), the A-B-C theory is the centerpiece of rational emotive behavioral therapy. This model highlights the essence of all cognitive approaches: our *thoughts about a situation*—not the situation itself—are the source of emotional and behavioral problems. When you truly and deeply understand the wisdom in this statement, your life will never be the same—and you will be in a much better position to help others. So, to help lock this into your mind, I am going to put it in another one of those grey boxes:

> Our *thoughts about a situation*—not the situation itself—are the source of emotional and behavioral problems.

If you still need convincing, ponder how certain prisoners of war respond to torture. They experience forms of suffering far greater than most counselors and their clients face in the 21st century, making common presenting problems, such as having a critical parent or breaking up with a boyfriend, hard to label as a problem. For example, there are numerous Tibetan monks and nuns who were brutally tortured by the Chinese in the 1960s and 1970s and, when eventually released, did not report symptoms of trauma (Hayward & Varela, 1992). In fact, some described having compassion for those who tortured them *while being tortured*. Such responses defy Western psychological theories about trauma, until the mediating beliefs are considered: these Buddhist practitioners have a different set of beliefs about "human rights" and maintain religious beliefs that emphasize compassion for one's enemies and acceptance of difficulty. Their beliefs shaped their response. Similarly, Viktor Frankl, whom we learned about in Chapter 10, also noted that the attitude of prisoners in Nazi concentration camps dramatically affected their mental and physical survival, with those able to make meaning better able to survive the most horrifying of circumstances. These are extreme examples of how a person's thoughts shape emotional and behavioral responses to an event. The event itself is not the cause.

However, for most of us mere mortals, when we experience an adverse event *it seems as though* it is clearly the cause of negative thoughts and feelings, because the beliefs silently mediate the response in the background. Ultimately, cognitive-behavioralists argue, it is the individual who is responsible for choosing thoughts and beliefs that result in healthy behaviors and positive emotions. Let's not kid ourselves: that is quite a challenge.

So, let's explore the other end of the spectrum and consider a mundane, nonclinical illustration. I feel hurt when you insult me, saying, "Your last example about the Tibetans and Nazis is moronic." Common sense (in Western cultures, after all, common sense is always culturally defined) would hold that feeling hurt after being insulted is "normal." However, that is not the cognitive-behavioral approach. Instead, the question would be: What belief do I hold that results in my feeling hurt? In this case, I would have to answer that based on my culture, class, age, and education, I believe that a person should not harshly criticize another even if there is disagreement; the person should find a more polite way to say it (i.e., "your example did not convince me"), not say anything at all, or find an academic source to refute my claim. However, a cognitive-behavioralist would be quick to point out that my feeling hurt is the result of *my beliefs*, not your comment. To further complicate matters, another person with slightly different but similar beliefs may feel angry, ashamed, or embarrassed. How one feels is a result of their belief, not the comment. The comment is only the trigger.

Cultural Considerations At this point you may be wondering when is a comment fairly labeled "an insult," "rude," or "appropriate." The general answer is that it depends on a complex matrix of age, social class, gender, education, ethnicity, ability, and sexual orientation, as well as the level of intimacy of the persons involved. The cognitive-behavioralist would add that a person should opt to not blindly follow a belief that doesn't work for them (Ellis, 1994). Thus, even if a person comes from a cultural context in which insults are considered rude and a reason to be hurt or angry, that person should consider adopting new beliefs that do not result in negative emotions. From this perspective, although culture influences our every thought, action, and feeling, each person still has choice in terms of *how*. It should be noted that this highly individualistic belief is not shared in all cultures, and counselors must consider this when working with diverse clients (see Tapestry Weaving: Working with Diverse Populations below). Perhaps now, you have a better sense why cross-cultural communication becomes tricky quickly.

Clinical Applications Finally, let's also consider the type of beliefs you are likely to work with in session, beliefs that fuel depression, anxiety, substance abuse, eating disorders, and so forth. The basic rule still applies: beliefs are the missing link between a situation and the resulting feelings and behaviors. For example, many people experience the feelings and behaviors that characterize depression, such as feeling sad, avoiding once pleasurable activities, and difficulty getting out of bed in the morning. Many beliefs can fuel these feelings, such as "I am worthless," "No one cares about me," or "I will never achieve my dreams" (note: you will read about Beck's and Ellis's specific cognitive theories on depression in "Case Conceptualization" below). The counselor's job is to help clients realize that it was not the specific event, such as losing a job or girlfriend, that caused these feelings; instead, it is the belief that they have about these events that are causing the symptoms (e.g., "without that job or girlfriend, I am worthless").

Ellis developed the A-B-C model to illustrate how humans create their difficulties by the beliefs they hold. In this model, A is the "activating event" (the problem person, situation, etc.), B is the "belief" about the meaning of that event (that one is generally not aware of until a counselor points it out), and C is the emotional or behavioral "consequence" based on the belief (the symptoms).

A-B-C Model

A = Activating event → B = Belief about A → C = Emotional & Behavioral Consequences

(Trigger event or person) (Symptoms)

Most clients come in able to see only the connection between A and C, and thus report A *causes* C: "I am depressed *because* my boyfriend broke up with me" or "I am angry *because* my boss favors my coworker." The counselor's job is to help the client identify the "B" belief that the client does not put into the equation, such as "I am worthless if a man decides not to be with me" or "I need to be the best in the office." These *irrational beliefs* are identified in assessment and targeted for change in the intervention phase by disputing these beliefs and adopting more realistic ones. If you are wondering, identifying the dysfunctional beliefs is far easier than changing them, but it is the requisite first step.

Try It Yourself

Identify a recent stressful situation. Identify the activating events, consequences, and mediating belief(s). If you are struggling with the belief(s), ask a friend or partner for input.

Big Picture: Overview of Counseling Process

The cognitive-behavioral approach involves four basic phases or steps:

- *Step 1: Assessment:* Counseling begins by obtaining a detailed behavioral and/or cognitive assessment of *baseline functioning*, including frequency, duration, and context of problem behaviors and thoughts.
- *Step 2: Target Behaviors/Thoughts for Change:* Cognitive-behavioral counselors identify specific behaviors and thoughts for intervention (e.g., rather than the general goal of "improve mood," the counselor would target "increasing engagement in pleasurable activities," "initiating social contact," and so on).
- *Step 3: Educate:* Counselors educate clients about their irrational thoughts and dysfunctional patterns, helping to motivate them to make changes.

- *Step 4: Replace and Retrain:* Finally, specific interventions are designed to replace dysfunctional behaviors and thoughts with more productive ones. Once the presenting symptoms have dissipated, treatment is ended.

Making Connection: Counseling Relationship

Educator and Expert

"REBT has always been very forceful, confrontative, and opposed to namby-pamby methods of therapy. It has particularly encouraged therapists to take the risks of quickly showing clients how they defeat themselves, rather than taking a long time to get to this point and rather than allowing clients to be evasive and defensive." (Ellis, 2003, p. 232).

Although the affective quality of connection exhibited by cognitive-behavioral counselors varies greatly—from cool and detached to warm and friendly to forceful and confrontative (but never namby-pamby)—the primary role of the counselor is the same: to serve as an expert who *directs* and *educates* the client and family on how to better manage their problems (Ellis, 2003). Especially in the working phase of counseling, the counselor's primary role is to educate clients on better ways to think and behave. Some cognitive-behavioral counselors, such as Ellis and Glasser, conceive of their role primarily as educators and adopt a highly directive approach. Others, such as Aaron Beck (1976), Judith Beck (2005), and Arnold Lazarus (1981), advocate a much warmer approach that "educates" using questions in Socratic style that require clients to critically and logically analyze their situation, offering a gentler means of guidance.

Empathy in Cognitive-Behavioral Counseling

True to their research foundations, cognitive-behavioral counselors increasingly use empathy, warmth, and a nonjudgmental stance to build a counseling alliance based on research results that indicate these counselor qualities predict positive outcomes (Meichenbaum, 1997). However, *the reason a cognitive-behavioral counselor uses empathy is quite different from the reason a humanistic counselor uses empathy*. This is frequently misunderstood, so I am going to say it again in case your mind was wandering: *cognitive-behavioral counselors use empathy for entirely different reasons than humanistic counselors.* Cognitive-behavioral counselors use empathy to create *rapport*, which then allows them to get to the "real" interventions that will change clients' behaviors, thoughts, and emotions. In dramatic contrast, for an experiential counselor, empathy *is* the intervention: they maintain that empathy is a curative process in and of itself (Rogers, 1961). The cognitive-behavioral counselor who uses empathy should not be seen as "manipulative" because in most cases the idea is to make the client feel more comfortable with the process, not to trick them. They should also not be seen as "integrating" experiential concepts, because they are not using an experiential concept in the way an experiential counselor would use it. Instead, they are *adapting* it to work within their philosophical assumptions about counseling and the change process.

Contemporary Cognitive-Behavioral Alliance

Judith Beck (2005) describes five practices for fostering the counseling alliance that reflect more contemporary sensibilities:

1. *Actively collaborate with the patient:* Decisions about counseling should be jointly made with the client.
2. *Demonstrate empathy, caring, and understanding:* Expressing empathy helps clients trust the counselor.
3. *Adapt one's counseling style:* Interventions, self-disclosure, and directiveness should be adjusted for each client based on personality, presenting problem, and so such.
4. *Alleviate distress:* Demonstrating clinical effectiveness by helping clients solve problems and improving their moods enhances the counseling relationship.
5. *Elicit feedback at the end of the session:* By asking clients "how did it go?" at the end of each session, counselors can intervene early in cases of alliance rupture.

By building a collaborative and engaged alliance, counselors are more likely to be effective and work through possible dysfunctional beliefs the client may have about counseling or the counselor that interfere with the process, such as "My counselor doesn't understand me" or "This will never work."

Written Contracts

Cognitive-behavioral counselors are perhaps the most businesslike when it comes to a counseling relationship (Holtzworth-Munroe & Jacobson, 1991), at least in terms of how they write about it on paper. And, they are actually the most likely to write about it on paper. They frequently use *written contracts* spelling out the goals and expectations to help structure the relationship and to increase motivation and dedication with clients. By putting the goals and agreement in writing and having clients sign that they agree can be a very motivating experience for clients, creating a sense of commitment to the process.

The Viewing: Case Conceptualization

Baseline Functioning

At the beginning of treatment, sometimes even before the first session, cognitive-behavioral counselors conduct a baseline assessment of functioning, which provides a starting point for measuring change. They ask clients to log the (a) frequency, (b) duration, and (c) severity of specific behavioral symptoms, such as depression, anxiety, panic, anger, social withdrawal, or conflict. Counselors may also include in the log identifying *antecedent* events that may have triggered the symptoms. Although it may seem that relying on clients' verbal recall of their symptoms is sufficient, most always a baseline assessment provides more detailed and accurate information than recall alone. In the case study at the end of this chapter, an assessment of baseline functioning is used to assess Roberta's bipolar episodes.

A baseline log may look like this:

Problem Behavior	When?	How Long?	How Severe?	Events Before?	Events After?
Binging and purging	Monday evening, 7 pm; after a stressful day	1 hour	7 (on scale 1–10)	No breakfast; did not sleep well night before; tension with boss.	Surfed Internet to distract self.
Binging and purging	Friday night, 1 am; after date	2 hours	9+	Fight with boyfriend during date; felt fat when saw other girls at club.	Slept in next day; called boyfriend to make up.

Cognitive-Behavioral Functional Analysis

Originally a purely behavioral assessment technique that was also later adopted for cognitions, *functional analysis* involves careful analysis of the antecedents and consequences of problem thoughts and behaviors in order to identify naturally occurring triggers, rewards, and punishments, in order to clearly identify cause-and-effect patterns (Meichenbaum, 1977). Counselors use functional analysis to examine what a person was doing and thinking as well as what was going on in the environment *before*, *during*, and *after* an episode of the symptom. For example, if a person reports cutting to manage stress, the counselor would ask about what she was thinking and doing before the episode as well as ask about what was happening in her life at the time: the who, what, where, when of her life. Similar questions are used to assess what she was feeling and thinking during and after cutting and what was going on in her life. The counselor does this with several episodes early in treatment to identify patterns of what triggers and what reinforces the cutting. Functional analysis makes it easy to design successful interventions that are likely to quickly modify the problem behavior and thoughts.

Questions for Cognitive-Behavioral Functional Analysis

- What were you doing before (during and after) the episode? Where were you? Who was around? What time of day?
- What were you thinking before (during and after) the episode? Describe your inner conversation—thought by thought.
- What was going on in your life at the time (during and after)? What were the normal activities? What were atypical stressors?
- Repeat the above sequence of questions for "during" and "after" the episode.

Try It Yourself

Identify a recent stressful situation and use functional analysis to examine it.

Schemas and Core Beliefs

The cognitive approach of Aaron Beck (1976, 1997) focused on identifying and changing *schemas* and *core beliefs* that fuel problems in clients' lives, such as the belief that one must be perfect or that life should be fair. As the foundation for *dysfunctional thinking*, dysfunctional schemas are the root source of psychopathology; for the gains in counseling to be long-term, the counseling process must modify core schemas, not just specific thoughts about a particular issue (Beck, 1997).

Schemas are the deepest of four levels in Beck's conceptualization of cognitions:

1. *Automatic Thoughts:* These thoughts are "knee-jerk" reactions to distressing situations that run through a person's mind and that the person can generally identify, for example, "If my friend does not return my call in 24 hours, she does not really like me."
2. *Intermediate Beliefs:* Extreme or absolute rules that are more general and shape automatic thoughts, i.e., "Good friends always return calls quickly."
3. *Core Beliefs:* Also global and absolute, core beliefs are about *ourselves*, such as "I am worthless." Beck identifies two general unifying principles or themes that underlie most core beliefs: (a) autonomy (beliefs about being effective and productive versus helpless) and (b) sociotropic (beliefs about being lovable or unlovable).
4. *Schemas:* The deepest level of the cognitive structure, schemas are cognitive frameworks in the mind, organizing and shaping thoughts, feelings, and behaviors. Developed in childhood and informed by numerous other factors, including family, culture, gender, religion, and occupation, schemas may lie dormant until triggered by a specific event, such as "I am utterly worthless if even my best friend won't take the time to call me; no one really cares about me at all; what is the point of even trying to have friends if they only call when it's convenient for *them*." Once triggered, information tends to be filtered to support the premise of the schema and valid evidence to the contrary is ignored; that is, even when the friend calls apologizing that she didn't call back sooner because she felt ill, this is only seen as an excuse and further confirmation of being unlovable.

Assessing and correctly identifying schemas take more time than assessing automatic thoughts and intermediate beliefs and add greater depth to the counseling process. In the case study at the end of this chapter, the counselor identifies the core beliefs and schemas that fuel Roberta's bipolar episodes and those that developed in response to her childhood sexual abuse.

Distorted Cognitions

Changing schemas is the ultimate goal in Beck's (1997) cognitive approach. To achieve this end, counselors often begin by identifying common *distortions* in automatic thoughts and intermediate beliefs, which can then be changed using thought records (see The Doing below). These include:

1. *Arbitrary Inference:* A belief based on little evidence (e.g., assuming your partner is cheating on you because she does not answer the phone immediately).
2. *Selective Abstraction:* Focusing on one detail while ignoring the context and other obvious details (e.g., believing your boss/supervisor/instructor thinks you are incompetent because they identified areas for improvement in addition to strengths).
3. *Overgeneralization:* Just like it sounds, generalizing one or two incidents to make a broad sweeping judgment (e.g., believing that because your son listens to acid rock he not going to college and will end up on drugs).
4. *Magnification and Minimization:* Going to either extreme of overemphasizing or underemphasizing based on the facts (e.g., ignoring two semesters of your child's poor grades is minimizing; hiring a tutor for one low test score is magnification).
5. *Personalization:* A particular form of arbitrary influence that is especially common in intimate relationships where external events are attributed to oneself (e.g., my spouse has lost interest in me because she did not want to have sex tonight).
6. *Dichotomous thinking:* All-or-nothing thinking: always/never, success/failure, or good/bad. (e.g., if my husband isn't "madly in love" with me, then he really doesn't love me at all).
7. *Mislabeling:* Assigning a personality trait to someone based on a handful of incidents, often ignoring exceptions (e.g., saying one's husband is lazy because he does not help immediately upon being asked).
8. *Mindreading:* A favorite in families and couple relationships, mindreading is believing you know what the other is thinking or will do without any supporting evidence, and it becomes a significant barrier to communication, especially when related to disagreements and hot topics such as sex, religion, money, and housework, among others (e.g., before your spouse says a word, you are defending yourself).

In addition, Beck (1997) has identified dysfunctional schemas that are commonly associated with specific personality disorders:

- *Dependent:* "I am helpless."
- *Avoidant:* "I might get hurt."
- *Passive-aggressive:* "I might get stepped on."
- *Paranoid:* "People are out to get me."
- *Narcissistic:* "I am special."
- *Histrionic:* "I need to impress others."
- *Compulsive:* "Errors are bad."
- *Antisocial:* "People are there to be taken."
- *Schizoid:* "I need plenty of space."

Irrational Beliefs: The Three Basic Musts

Similar to assessing schemas in Beck's cognitive approach, Ellis (1994, 2003) assesses for *irrational beliefs*, which are typically flagged by words such as "should," "ought," and "must." These are preferences that get exaggerated into absolutist, extreme thinking and unrealistic beliefs that lead to depression, anxiety, and a host of other unpleasant experiences. Over the years, Ellis (2003) has collapsed what were originally eleven categories into three basic categories of irrational beliefs:

1. **Perfection-Based Worth:** "'I must be thoroughly competent, adequate, achieving, and lovable at all times, or else I am an incompetent worthless person.' This belief usually leads to feelings of anxiety, panic, depression, despair, and worthlessness" (p. 236).

2. **Justice for Me:** "'Other significant people in my life, must treat me kindly and fairly at all times, or else I can't stand it, and they are bad, rotten, and evil persons who should be severely blamed, damned, and vindictively punished for their horrible treatment of me.' This leads to feelings of anger, rage, fury, and vindictiveness and to actions like feuds, wars, fights, genocide, and ultimately, an atomic holocaust" (pp. 236–237).
3. **Effortless Perfection:** "'Things and conditions absolutely must be the way I want them to be and must never be too difficult or frustrating. Otherwise, life is awful, terrible, horrible, catastrophic and unbearable.' This leads to low-frustration tolerance, self-pity, anger, depression, and to behaviors such as procrastination, avoidance, and inaction" (p. 237).

Negative Cognitive Triad

Beck's (1972, 1976) theory of depression describes a *negative cognitive triad* that characterizes depressed thinking. This triad consists of three sets of negative thoughts that characterize the thinking of the person who is depressed:

1. Negative thoughts about the self (e.g., "I am worthless").
2. Negative thoughts about the world/environment (e.g., "life is unfair"), and
3. Negative thoughts about the future (e.g., "things will never get better").

Typically, people who are clinically depressed report having negative thoughts in all three areas rather than just one or two. For example, pessimism is defined by negative thoughts about the future, but does not automatically lead to depression unless the personal also has negative thoughts about self and the world.

BASIC-ID

Designed to be a brief, solution-oriented, yet comprehensive approach, Lazarus's (1981) *multimodal therapy* is "best described as *systematic eclecticism*" (p. 4) and is organized around the seven-pronged assessment of the BASIC-ID: behavior, affect, sensation, imagery, cognition, interpersonal relationships, and drugs/biology. The BASIC-ID questions can be used for a general global assessment or around a specific problem or symptom (p. 17).

BASIC-ID Assessment for General Mental Health

- *Behavior:* What behaviors are getting in the way of your happiness? What behaviors do you want to stop or start doing and/or do more of?
- *Affect:* What makes you laugh? Cry? What makes you mad, sad, glad, scared? Are you troubled by any particular emotions?
- *Sensation:* What do you especially like/dislike to see, hear, taste, touch, and smell? Do you experience frequent unpleasant sensations (such as pain, dizziness, tremors, etc.)? What are some sensual and sexual turn-ons and turn-offs for you?
- *Imagery:* What do you picture yourself doing in the immediate future? How would you describe your self-image? Body image? What do you like/dislike about these images? How do they influence your life?
- *Cognition:* What are some of your most cherished beliefs and values? What are your main shoulds, oughts, and musts? What are your intellectual interests and pursuits? How do your thoughts affect your emotions?
- *Interpersonal relationships:* Who are the most important people in your life? What do they expect from you and you of them? How do they affect you and you affect them?
- *Drugs and Biology:* Do you have any medical concerns? What are your diet and exercise habits? What type of medications do you use? Do you drink, smoke, or use recreational drugs? How much, how often?

BASIC-ID can also be used to assess a specific area or problem:

- *Behavior:* What are you doing in relation to the problems? (e.g., frequent crying, insomnia, bathing less often)
- *Affect:* What are your problematic emotional states? (e.g., depressed mood; no enthusiasm for or interest in favorite activities, worry).
- *Sensation:* What physiological sensations are you experiencing in relation to the problem? (tight back and jaw, abdominal discomforts, exhaustion, tightness in chest).
- *Imagery:* What images or metaphors do you associate with the problem? (e.g., nightmares of being chased, daydreams of quitting job).
- *Cognition:* What thoughts and beliefs are associated with the problem? (e.g., catastrophic thinking, self-blame, perfectionistic thinking).
- *Interpersonal relationships:* Which of your relationships impact and are affected by the problem? (e.g., shutting out boyfriend, drifting away from friends, avoiding family).
- *Drugs and Biology:* What medications and physical conditions impact and are affected by the problem? (e.g., gaining weight, on antidepressants for two months, minimal progress).

A client-focused approach, multimodal assessment is used to fit the treatment to the client rather than requiring the client adapt to the treatment (Lazarus, 1981). Lazarus tailors treatment by *tracking* the clients' modality *firing order* or preferences and then sequences techniques accordingly. For example, if a client primarily describes the problem in behavioral terms, behavioral interventions will be the first line of intervention; then, if imagery were the second-most salient, it would be targeted next, and so forth. To keep treatment brief, Lazarus (1997) recommends using one of six modalities (B, S, I, C, I, D; basically, any modality *except* Affect) to treat an issue "because affect cannot be directly modified but has to be accessed through one or more of the other six modalities" (p. 88). Lazarus contends that any shift in one area affects shifts in all the areas, because they are interrelated.

Choice Theory

Developed from his early *control theory* that conceptualized people as driven by inner control systems, Glasser's (1975, 1998, 2000) *choice theory* posits that the choices people make determine the quality of their lives. Glasser believed that five basic needs motivate the choices people make: (a) belonging/relationships, (b) power/achievement, (c) fun, (d) freedom/independence, and (e) survival. The choices people make inform behaviors, which Glasser conceptualized as *total behavior* that incorporates acting, thinking, feeling, and physiology. Using the metaphor of four car wheels, any one behavior is inherently connected to all other elements. For example, a person cannot decide to get drunk (or stay sober) without the choice impacting thoughts, feelings, and physiology. Similar to behavioralists and solution-focused counselors (see Chapter 13), Glasser believed that when a person wants to change, *action* is generally the easiest and most effective place to start. Thus, when assessing clients, counselors use choice theory to identify the actions clients choose that drive the negative thoughts, feelings, and physical symptoms (e.g., nagging a partner or not giving one's best at the office) and then target these for later intervention. In the case study at the end of this chapter, the counselor uses choice theory to help Roberta make better choices about money, which she has a history of recklessly spending during manic phases.

DSM Diagnosis

Of all the mental health treatment approaches, cognitive-behavioral counseling is most closely aligned with the medical model, and thus counselors organize treatment using

DSM-5 diagnosis (see Chapter 3). Beck (1997) developed specific cognitive approaches for working with different diagnoses, such as depression, anxiety, eating disorders, substance abuse, and so on, having identified common dysfunctional cognitive patterns associated with each. Similarly, specific behavioral approaches have been developed for phobias, panic, depression, and various anxiety issues. Glasser (2003) is a notable exception, arguing that mental health symptoms are not "diseases" per se and that they can be changed when clients are supported in making new choices.

Targeting Change: Goal Setting

"When people accept the fact that they largely control their own emotional and behavioral destiny, and that they can make themselves undisturbed or less disturbed mainly by acquiring realistic and sensible attitudes about the undesirable things that occur or that they make occur in their lives, they then usually have the ability and power of changing their belief system, making it more functional, and helping themselves to feel and to behave in a significantly less disturbed fashion" (Ellis, 2003, p. 220).

Symptom and Problem Resolution

Unlike depth psychology and humanistic approaches, cognitive-behavioral counselors' primary goal is to reduce presenting symptoms and problems. Symptom resolution is considered a sufficient goal in and of itself, and broader, growth-oriented goals are not considered necessary. Furthermore, cognitive-behavioral counselors do not have a laundry list of "normal" thoughts and behaviors that all clients should exhibit to be considered healthy; instead, they work with clients to identify which beliefs and actions are resulting in problems and change *those and only those*, not adding other long-term goals based on a theory of personality or health.

Independent Problem Solvers

The long-term vision in cognitive-behavioral approaches is to enable clients to independently solve their own problems by recognizing dysfunctional thoughts and behaviors early enough to keep them from creating unnecessary emotional distress (Beck, 1997; Ellis, 2003). This goal is conceptually quite different from psychodynamic and humanistic goals that target personality change. Aspiring to be realistic, cognitive-behavioral counselors do not promise dramatic changes in the structure of the psyche, but rather they measure success by a client's ability to handle life stressors better, not perfectly. They also do not expect that life will be without future challenges, and instead see the goal as preparing clients to better manage these on their own.

Behavioral and Measurable Goals

Specific treatment goals are identified through the above assessment procedures. Goals are stated in *behavioral* and *measurable* terms, such as "reduce arguments to no more than one per month." Once clear goals are agreed upon, counselors also obtain a commitment from the client to follow instructions and complete out-of-session assignments in order to achieve the agreed-upon goals. This agreement is often written down in the form of a written counseling contract. Getting client "buy-in" to complete assignments immediately upon setting goals greatly increases the likelihood of client follow-through.

Examples of middle phase cognitive-behavioral goals:

- Reduce episodes of cutting and self-harm.
- Replace perfectionist beliefs about work performance.
- Reduce generalizations and mindreading with partner.

Examples of late phase cognitive-behavioral goals:

- Increase engagement in enjoyable activities, hobbies, and relationships.
- End use of substances to manage difficult moods; manage moods using healthy coping skills.
- Redefine "I must be perfect to be loved" schema to increase capacity for intimacy.

The Doing: Interventions

Psychoeducation

A hallmark of cognitive-behavioral counseling, psychoeducation involves teaching clients psychological principles and using them to handle problems (Ellis & Dryden, 1997; Lazarus, 1981). Psychoeducation can be done in individual or group sessions. The content typically falls into four categories:

- *Problem-Oriented:* Information about the patient's diagnosis and/or situation, such as ADHD, schizophrenia, alcohol dependence, depression, and others. Counselors use this type of education to motivate clients toward taking new action.
- *Change-Oriented:* Information about how to reduce problem symptoms, such as improve communication, reduce anger, decrease depression, and so forth. Counselors use this type of education to help clients actively solve their problems. For such education to be successful, clients must be highly motivated, and counselors need to introduce the new behavior in small, practical steps using everyday language.
- *Bibliotherapy:* Bibliotherapy is a fancy term for assigning clients readings that will be (a) motivating and/or (b) instructional for dealing with their presenting problem. Typically, counselors assign cognitive-behavioral self-help books, such as *Feeling Good* (Burns, 1988) or *The Worry Cure* (Leahy, 2005) to reinforce what is learned in session, but fiction or professional literature may also be assigned.
- *Cinema Therapy:* Similar to bibliotherapy, cinema therapy involves assigning clients to watch a movie that will speak to the problem issues (Berg-Cross, Jennings, & Baruch, 1990).

Tips for Effectively Providing Psychoeducation and Task Setting *(Yes, these are similar to those used by Adlerians in Chapter 9)*

- *Practice!* Yes, I'm serious. There aren't too many counseling skills I recommend new counselors "practice" on family and friends, but psychoeducation is the major exception. Try explaining concepts and research outcomes to people who haven't read books like this one. Notice the types of questions they ask after you explain a concept. That will help you learn what you might be leaving out, what type of jargon needs defining, and what people actually find useful.
- *Ask first.* Perhaps the single-greatest secret to making psychoeducation work is *timing:* providing information when the client is in a receptive state. How do you know when they are ready? Ask them. "Would you be open to learning more about X?" If you fail to ask, you may not find a receptive audience. Alternatively, master the REBT style of confrontation and forget about timing.
- *Keep it very, very brief.* During a 50-minute session, I recommend keeping total psychoeducation time to one to two minutes—that's the max—and I am not exaggerating. Any other brilliant information you have to share should be saved for the following week, because most clients cannot meaningfully integrate and act upon more than a single principle at once.
- *Make one point—and one point only.* Only try to teach one concept, point, or skill in a session. Anything else is too much to be *practically* useful. (See Judith Beck's recommendations for Thought Records below.)
- *Ensure understanding and acceptance:* After briefly providing information, *directly ask* if clients understand and if they believe it is useful and realistic for their life.
- *Apply it immediately.* After you provide information, immediately identify how it can be practically applied in the clients' life to address a problem that occurred in the past week or upcoming week.
- *Step-by-step tasks:* After offering two minutes of psychoeducation, the following 48 minutes involve step-by-step instructions on how to apply the information to solve

(*continued*)

a current problem. Get specific: who does what, when, where, and how often, and any resistance or potential roadblocks.

- *Follow up on tasks:* The next time you meet, ask the client if they used the information to any extent. If not, why not? If so, what happened?

Socratic Method and Guided Discovery

Using the *Socratic method,* sometimes referred to as *guided discovery* or *inductive reasoning*, to gently encourage clients to question their own beliefs, cognitive counselors use open-ended questions that help clients "discover" for themselves that their beliefs are either illogical (i.e., contrary to obvious evidence) or dysfunctional (i.e., not working for them; Beck, 2005). A less confrontational approach than other techniques, when questioning the validity of belief, counselors generally take a relatively neutral stance, allowing the client's own logic, evidence, and reason to do the majority of convincing. Although the term "change" is used to describe what happens, in actuality tightly held beliefs are slowly eroded over time by the client questioning and requestioning their validity in different situations.

Questions for Evaluating the Validity of Beliefs

- What evidence do you have to support your belief? What evidence is there to the contrary? So, what might be a realistic middle ground?
- What does respected person X (Y, and Z) say about your situation? How could they all be wrong?
- If your child [or another significant person] were to say the same thing, how would you respond?
- What is the realistic likelihood that things will really go *that* badly? What is a more realistic outcome?
- You bring up one possible reason for X. Have you considered another explanation? Perhaps ... ?
- How likely is it that Person X's behavior was 100% directed at you? What else might have played a role in his/her behavior?

Try It Yourself

Using a problematic belief from an earlier exercise in this chapter (or any other), use these questions to evaluate the validity of the belief.

Thought Records

Cognitive counselors use thought records (Beck, 1995) to help clients learn how to better respond to automatic thoughts (the most readily accessible dysfunctional thoughts); see Schemas and Core Beliefs above. By completing thought records, clients can use Socratic questions to help them counter their own negative thinking and develop more adaptive responses. Thought records involve identifying:

- *The triggering situation:* Event that triggered negative emotions and physical reactions
- *The automatic thought and strength of belief in terms of a percentage*
- *The resulting negative emotions and percentage of severity*
- *An alternative adaptive response:* Alternative interpretation of the event
- *The alternative outcome:* How much does the client believe the alternative interpretation and how does it change things in terms of percentage of belief, intensity of emotion, and new action?

To generate an alternative adaptive response, Beck (1995) recommends having clients ask themselves all of the following questions:

- What is the evidence that the automatic thought is true? Not true?
- Is there an alternative explanation for the situation?
- What's the worst that could happen? Could I live through it? What's the best that could happen? What's the most realistic outcome?
- What's the effect of my believing the automatic thought? What could be the effect of my changing my thinking?
- What should I do about it?
- If _____were in the situation and had this thought, what would I tell him/her? (or what would he/she do?; p. 126)

One of the keys to the technique is to use *percentage* to measure *how much a person believes* an automatic thought and *how strong the emotions are.* By using percentage of emotion and belief, clients can begin to see how dysfunctional beliefs wax and wane and that not all negative emotions are as devastating as others. Simply noting the variability in symptom severity generates hope, a greater sense of control, and motivation to change; "third wave" behaviorists using mindfulness and solution-focused counselors also focus on using these small indicators of control, change, and improvement to effect change.

Sample Thought Record

Trigger Situation: In department meeting, boss praised Greg endlessly.
Automatic Thought with Strength of Thought in Percentage

- Thought 1: My boss likes Greg better than me: 90%
- Thought 2: I will never get anywhere in this company: 80%
- Thought 3: I am a loser: 70%.

Emotions with Strength of Emotion in Percentage

- Angry (at boss): 75%
- Helpless: 100%
- Hopeless: 80%

Adaptive Response

- Greg works harder and builds relationships better; I could do the same; I am a loser only if I don't give my personal best: 80%

Outcome

- Changes to belief in thoughts 1, 2, and 3: 20%; 30%; 20%
- Changes to emotions:
  - Angry (at self) 50%
  - Helpless 20%
  - Hopeless 10%
  - Motivated 50%
- Changes in behavior: Get to work earlier; goof off less; talk with boss

The most important role is for counselors to *motivate* clients to use these outside of session instead of falling back into old patterns. Judith Beck (1995, p. 127) recommends the following to ensure success with this relatively involved homework task:

- Counselors need to develop competence using thought records *personally* before asking clients to do so.
- Before introducing the thought record, the counselors should determine if the client understands and responds well to the basic principles of the cognitive model.
- Before introducing the thought record, clients should (a) demonstrate an ability to readily identify automatic thoughts and (b) have had a positive experience with *successfully reducing negative emotions* using a *verbal* variation of this intervention or Socratic questioning.

- The counselor should introduce thought records in two stages: describing how to identify the automatic thought in the first session, and then, in the second session, how to generate adaptive responses.
- Clients should successfully identify automatic thoughts in several situations before moving on to identifying adaptive responses.
- If the client fails to complete thought records once properly introduced, the counselor should explore automatic thoughts related to doing the homework, such as believing "these will not make a difference" or "I don't have time in my busy schedule."

Disputing Beliefs and the REBT Self-Help Form

Ellis's A-B-C Theory has a part two: you guessed it, D-E-F, which describes the interventions for "D"isputing irrational beliefs and the new "E"ffects and "F"eelings (see The Juice above for A-B-C; Ellis, 1994, 2004). The D-E-F intervention is used both in and out of session to help clients dispute troubling beliefs and replace them with new ones. Not attacking any or all beliefs, cognitive-behavioral counselors specifically target "hot" beliefs, the ones that are the most emotionally charged, rather than "warm" or "cool" beliefs that tend to cause fewer problems (Ellis, 2003).

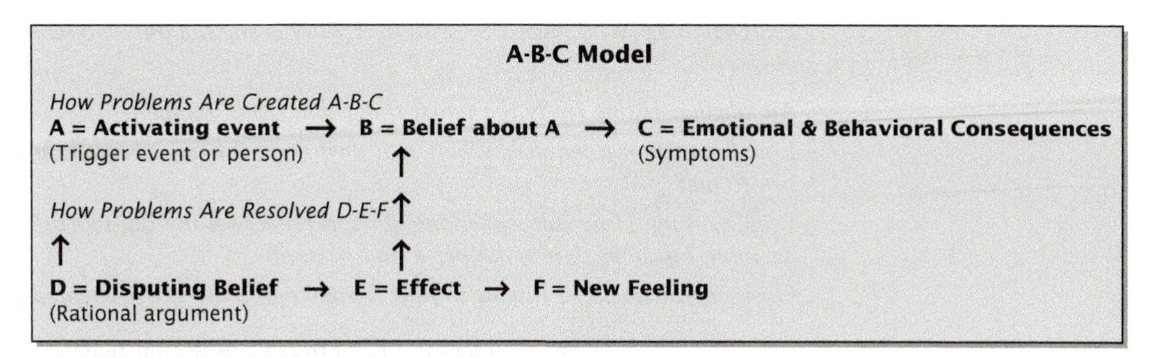

A-B-C Model
How Problems Are Created A-B-C
A = Activating event → B = Belief about A → C = Emotional & Behavioral Consequences
(Trigger event or person)
(Symptoms)
How Problems Are Resolved D-E-F
D = Disputing Belief → E = Effect → F = New Feeling
(Rational argument)

Counselors use the ABCDEF model to provide clients a means to analyze their own cognitions and behaviors and develop more adaptive responses. Before assigning this as homework, counselors usually practice in session on a whiteboard to demonstrate the process. Clients are then asked to do the exercises on their own over the week as distressing events arise. Over the years, several REBT Self-Help Forms have been available (Ellis & Dryden, 1997), the most recent of which is an interactive online version available from the Rational Emotive Therapy Network website (Ross, 2006). The REBT Self-Help Form walks clients through the A–E process. In the case study at the end of this chapter, the counselor uses the REBT self-help form to help Roberta dispute irrational beliefs that she learned from being sexually abused and from her experiences of bipolar disorder.

Step1: Identify "A," the Activating or Trigger Event

What situation are you upset about?

Ex. My girlfriend cheated on me.

Step 2: Identify "C," Unhealthy Negative Emotional and Behaviors and Consequences

What negative feelings and behaviors you are experiencing in response to this event?

Unhealthy Emotions	*Unhealthy Behaviors*
Ex: I feel hurt, angry, vengeful, depressed, jealous, and plain sad.	*Ex:* I yelled at her; broke up with her; can't sleep or eat; don't want to see anyone.

(*continued*)

Step 3: Identify "B," Irrational Beliefs

What beliefs do you have that led you to interpret the event so that you feel and behave the way you do? Include unrealistic demands, awfulizing, low frustration tolerance, people rating, and overgeneralizing (one or more) beliefs as well as demanding to (a) be approved of to feel self-worth, (b) be treated fairly, and (c) for life to be effortless.

Ex. Demands: I must be with Yvonne; she should not have done this; I can't live without her.

Awfulizing: This is the worst thing in the world that has ever happened to me; my life is over.

Low frustration tolerance: I can't stand being treated like this.

People rating: Her actions prove I am worthless. She is a terrible person.

Overgeneralizing: I will never find anyone like her again.

Step 4: Dispute, "D," Irrational Beliefs Using Disputing Questions

Ex. Demands: Why must I be with her? Why is she the only woman on the planet for me?

Awfulizing: Is this really the worst thing that could happen?

Low frustration tolerance: Where is it written that being cheated on should not happen to me?

People rating: How can something she did reflect on my self-worth? She made a bad decision, but does that make her a bad person?

Overgeneralizing: Do I want to find someone like her if she cheated on me?

Step 5: Identify "E," Effective, Rational Beliefs

Ex. Demands: I want to be with her—or at least I did want to be with her. I would have preferred having her in my life if she could have been faithful.

Awfulizing: Although this hurts, there are many things far worse that could happen to me. This only feels like the worst thing in the world. This type of thing has happened to millions of others for centuries; they survived and I shall too.

Low frustration tolerance: I don't want to handle this, but I know that I can.

People rating: Her actions do not reflect on my self worth; only my actions do that. I admire many of her qualities, but obviously she has flaws when it comes to faithfulness.

Overgeneralizing: When I am ready, I will look for someone who I love as much and can be faithful to me.

Step 6: Identify New "F," Feelings and Behaviors, such as "Healthy Negative Emotions" and Self-Helping Behaviors

Healthy Negative Emotions	*Healthy Self-Helping Behaviors*
Ex: I am very disappointed and hurt, but I will be okay. *It may take awhile, but I will find someone else.*	*Ex: I will start hanging out with my best friend to cheer me up; I will talk with people I trust about this; I am will get myself to eat.*

Labeling Cognitions

In addition to Socratic questioning and direct confrontation, some clients find it helpful to identify and label distorted thinking in order to reduce its sway on them. Counselors can help them practice labeling distorted thinking in session so that clients can transfer this skill to their everyday lives. Most frequently, counselors use Beck's (1976) categories of distorted thinking described above in "Case Conceptualization":

- *Arbitrary Inference:* "jumping to conclusions"
- *Selective Abstraction:* "filtering out the positive"
- *Overgeneralization:* "making sweeping conclusions without evidence"
- *Magnification and Minimization:* "emphasizing the negative and ignoring the positive"
- *Personalization:* "exaggerating one's responsibility" and/or "misinterpreting neutral comments"
- *Dichotomous Thinking:* "black-and-white thinking"
- *Mislabeling:* "attaching an extreme or overgeneralized label to a person or situation"
- *Mindreading:* "assuming negative thoughts and intentions on the part of other"
- *Catastrophizing:* "assuming the worst will happen"

Problem Solving and Coping Skills Training

Meichenbaum (1977) noticed that while dysfunctional beliefs were sometimes the problem, at other times clients simply lacked problem solving and coping skills. Thus, in addition to listening for the presence of erroneous beliefs, he listened for the "*absence* of specific, adaptive cognitive skills and responses" (p. 194). In the case of problem solving, the counselor engages in directly teaching clients how to (a) identify problems, (b) identify potential solutions, (c) select and act on a solution, and (d) evaluate the effectiveness of the solution. Similarly, with situations that are not easily solved, such as loss of a loved one or a chronic condition, the counselor helps clients learn coping skills using a similar format: (a) identifying the specific elements where the client could cope better, (b) identifying potential coping strategies, (c) choosing and applying these strategies, and (d) evaluating their effectiveness.

Changing Self-Talk: Stress Inoculation Training

As an alternative to and/or in addition to confronting irrational beliefs, clients can use *stress inoculation training* to help them change their negative *self-talk* and unhelpful inner dialogues and to increase coping skills (Meichenbaum, 1977, 1985). Stress inoculation involves three phases:

1. *Education:* Providing information on negative self-talk and how it creates stress
2. *Training:* Rehearsing and practicing skills that apply to the client's situation
3. *Practice:* Applying skills in real-world situations

The process of stress inoculation training helps clients change their self-talk in all phases of experiencing stress: (a) preparing for a stressor, (b) confronting and handling the stressor, (c) coping with the feeling of being overwhelmed, and (d) reinforcing self statements after stress. In the case study at the end of this chapter, the counselor uses stress inoculation training to help Roberta prevent depressive and manic episodes and recover from the negative self-talk that developed in response to her childhood sexual abuse.

Positive Self-Talk in Stress Inoculation Training (Adapted from Meichenbaum, 1977, p. 155)

Things clients can tell themselves in each phase of coping with a stressor:

Preparing for a stressor

"I can develop a plan to deal with the stress."
"Just think about what I need to do rather than get anxious."
"Don't worry; worry won't help anything."

(*continued*)

Confronting and handling the stressor

"One step at a time; I can handle this."
"Don't think about the fear: just think about what I have to do. Stay relevant. Just do it."
"This anxiety is what the counselor said I would feel; it's a reminder to use my coping skills."

Coping with the feeling of being overwhelmed

"Stay focused in the present. What is it that I have to do?"
"Don't try to eliminate the anxiety; just keep it manageable."
"When fear comes, just breathe."

Reinforcing self statements

"You did it!"
"That wasn't as bad as I thought it would be."
"I am making good progress."

Cost/Benefit Analysis

Another common cognitive-behavioral technique, *cost-benefit analysis* helps confront dysfunctional thinking and create motivation by having clients identify the "costs" of a problematic behavior and the "benefit" (Ellis, 1991, 1994). Many problem behaviors develop by trying to avoid another problem, such as drinking to avoid feeling lonely. The counselor typically works with the client to make a written list of the costs/benefits or the pros/cons. The counselor has the client begin the list and prompts the client to rationally think through the list from both perspectives.

Choice and Responsibility

In reality therapy, counselors analyze behavior to help motivate clients to take responsibility for the quality of their lives and make choices to improve their situations using the WDEP (Wants-Doing-Evaluation-Planning) system (Glasser, 2000; Wubbolding, 2008).

W = Exploring Wants, Needs, and Motivations

Counselors explore clients' wants using a series of questions to assess what clients really want and need in all areas of their lives: family, friends, job, self, health, and so on (Wubbolding, 2008, p. 379):

- What do you want that you *are* getting? What do you want that you *are not* getting? What are you getting that you don't want?
- What are you willing to settle for?
- How much effort are you willing to exert to get what you want? How committed are you?
- What do you have to give up to get what you want? Are you willing to do this?

Doing = Discussing What Clients Are Doing and the Resulting Direction

Compared to thoughts, feelings, and physiology, Glasser believed that behaviors were the easiest things for people to control. Thus, he asked clients to examine their actions and whether or not those were helping them move toward their wants and needs.

- What actions are you taking right now that are helping you fulfill your wants?
- What actions are taking *away from* your wants?
- When you are feeling bad [name the symptom], what actions do you take? What thoughts inform your choice to take this action?

E = Evaluating the Effectiveness of Actions and Choices

Next, counselors encourage clients to *self-evaluate* the effectiveness of their actions and choices. Some ways counselors encourage this is to ask evaluative questions:

- Are these actions helpful or hurtful to you in the short run? Long run?
- Are these actions improving your relationships or destroying them?
- Are these actions your best effort or least effort?

P = Planning a Course of Action

Based on clients' evaluations of their actions, counselors help them develop a doable, realistic plan for getting more of what they want. They strive to keep plans simple and attainable, with measurable goals that are within the clients' control.

Classical Conditioning: Pavlov's Dogs and Relaxation

Frequently used to treat anxiety disorders, classical conditioning was developed by Ivan Pavlov (1932a, 1932b) in his famous experiments with salivating dogs. In these experiments, he was able to train dogs to salivate at the sound of a bell by *pairing* the dog's natural response to salivate at the *sight* of food with the *sound* of the bell. When the bell was rung each time food was presented, the dog learned that the bell signaled that food was coming and began salivating. After enough repetition, the dog began to salivate with just the sound of the bell. This procedure is technically described in terms of *conditioned/unconditioned stimuli and responses.*

Initially, these responses were believed to be purely behavioral and almost involuntary, but later behavioralists found that thought and conscious learning were required even in this most basic form of conditions: "Contrary to popular belief, the fabled reflexive conditioning in humans is largely a myth. *Conditioning* is simply a descriptive term for learning through paired experiences, not an explanation of how the changes come about. Originally, conditioning was assumed to occur automatically. On closer examination it turned out to be cognitively mediated" (Bandura, 1974, p. 859); or, more to the point, "Humans do not simply respond to stimuli: they interpret them" (Bandura, 1977, p. 59). Classical conditioning is used in clinical settings to address phobias, child behaviors, and anxieties.

How Classical Conditioning Works

1. The Natural State of Affairs
Unconditioned Stimulus (UCS) → Unconditioned Response (UCR)

- Pavlov's original research: Dog food → Salivation
- Treating arachnophobia: Deep breathing → Relaxation response (slowed heart rate, decreased arousal)

2. Process of Pairing Conditional Stimulus with Response
UCS + Conditioned Stimulus (CS) → Conditioned Response (CR)

- Dog Food + Bell → Salivation
- Deep Breathing + Spider → Relaxation

3. Resulting Pairing
Conditioned Stimulus (CS) → Conditioned Response (CR)

- Bell → Salivation
- Spider → Relaxation

Operant Conditioning and Reinforcement Techniques: Skinner's Cats

Operant conditioning-based interventions use the principles identified by B. F. Skinner (1953, 1971) to modify human behavior, whether one's own or another's. The essential principle is to reward behavior *in the direction of* the desired behavior using small, incremental steps, a process called *shaping behavior*: "When a bit of behavior is followed by a certain kind of consequence, it is more likely to occur again, and a consequence having this effect is called a reinforcer" (Skinner, 1971, p. 27). Once a certain set of skills has been mastered, the "bar is raised" for which behavior will be reinforced, with ever-closer approximations to the desired behavior. Thus, if parents are trying to teach a child how to complete homework independently, they may begin by overseeing when, where, and how the child completes homework, and reinforcing success and failure under these conditions. Once the child regularly succeeds with full oversight, the child is given an area of responsibility to master—perhaps when the homework is done—and reinforced for success in this area. Next, the child may be rewarded for managing the list of homework assignments without oversight. This process continues until the child completes homework independently, much to the parents' delight. Individual clients can apply operant conditioning to themselves to change habits, such as developing a new exercise regimen, lose weight, reduce anxiety, increase social activity, or any number of behavioral changes.

Forms of Reinforcement and Punishment In operant conditioning, desired behaviors can be positively or negatively reinforced or punished, depending on the desired behavior. The four options below are used alone or in combination to *shape* desired behavior.

Types of Reinforcement and Punishment

- *Positive Reinforcement or Reward:* Rewards desired behaviors by *giving* something desirable (e.g., a treat).
- *Negative Reinforcement:* Rewards desired behaviors by *removing* something undesirable (e.g., relaxing curfew; take a day off from a routine task).
- *Positive Punishment:* Reduces undesirable behavior by *adding* something undesirable (e.g., assigning extra chores; getting yourself to do a disliked task).
- *Negative Punishment:* Reduces undesirable behavior by *removing* something desirable (e.g., grounding; denying self something enjoyable).

To boil it down even more:

	Increase Desired Behavior	Decrease Undesirable Behavior
Add Something	Positive reinforcement; reward	Positive punishment
Remove Something	Negative reinforcement	Negative punishment

Frequency of Reinforcement and Punishment The frequency of reinforcement and punishment is key to increasing or decreasing behavior.

- *Immediacy:* The more immediate the reinforcement/punishment, the quicker the learning, especially with young children.
- *Consistency:* The more consistent the reinforcement/punishment, the quicker the learning. Consistency involves rewarding or punishing a behavior *every time* it occurs or on a consistent schedule (e.g., every other time), creating predictability.
- *Intermittent Reinforcement:* Random and unpredictable reinforcement *increases* the likelihood of a behavior, for better or worse. Thus, if a parent inconsistently reinforces curfew (sometimes enforces it and other times not), the child is *more likely* to break it. Based on the same principle, random positive reinforcement of

well-established desired behaviors helps sustains them (e.g., randomly reinforcing positive grades with an extra privilege or treat).

Point Charts and Token Economies Generally used with younger children but adaptable for adults, point charts (Patterson & Forgatch, 1995) or token economies (Falloon, 1991) are used to shape and reward positive behaviors by building up "points" that can be applied to privileges, treats, or purchases. The rewards must be motivating for the particular person involved; thus, what may work for one person may not work for another (Bandura, 1974, 1986). In addition, the rewards should follow the desired behavior closely in time and should be frequent enough for a person to feel motivated to do more. These principles can be used on children or adults to achieve behavioral change. For example, if parents want to increase a child's independence with homework, they can reward the children with a sticker that is placed on a chart; when the child accrues the target amount (perhaps 5), the parents offer a motivating reward of some kind (e.g., a new book in a favorite series). Similarly, a typically shy adult wanting to increase his social connections could reward himself each time he contacts three friends in a week by buying a favorite CD or book.

Systematic Desensitization

A classic behavioral technique, *systematic desensitization* is a technique frequently used with anxieties and phobias in which a client begins with a low intensity image and increasingly works toward direct contact with the stressful stimulus (Wolpe, 1997). Using classical conditioning, "desensitization" is achieved by pairing relaxation with the stressful stimulus, first in small amounts and then slowly increasing exposure, a process called *reciprocal inhibition*. The underlying assumption is that a person cannot be both anxious and stressed at the same time.

The process involves (a) teaching relaxation techniques, (b) creating a hierarchy of anxiety triggers, and (c) working up the hierarchy until the client no longer experiences anxiety related to the trigger. For practical reasons (such as having to bring spiders and snakes to the office), imagery is used for most of the desensitization process. Adding a cognitive component to this classic behavioral technique, Meichenbaum (1997) found that adding a *coping image*—imagining oneself coping rather than mastering the anxiety-provoking situation—resulted in better and more sustainable outcomes. For example, if a man fears public speaking, a counselor would first teach him how to get into a relaxed state using breathing and visualization techniques. He would also work with the client to create a hierarchy of anxiety-provoking speaking events. Next the counselor would have him get into the relaxed state and then *imagine* himself coping well with making a point during a business meeting; the client would practice doing this until he could imagine it without feeling anxious. The next step would be to have him identify a slightly more anxious situation—such as making a presentation at a meeting—and repeat the procedure. As the client gains confidence, this learning is transferred to real-world situations until the client is able to cope well with speaking in public.

In Vivo Exposure and Flooding

A variation on systematic desensitization, *in vivo exposure* and *flooding* are used to treat anxiety and phobias. In vivo exposure refers to putting the client in real-life (in vivo), anxiety-provoking situations while supporting clients as they face their fears (Spiegler & Guevremont, 2003). Often a hierarchy similar to that used in systematic desensitization is used to expose the client in small doses to the feared situation or object, such as spiders or public speaking. In contrast, flooding refers to intense and prolonged exposure to the anxiety-provoking stimulus, either imagined or in vivo. In flooding, the client is not allowed to engage in the anxiety-reducing behaviors, and the fear generally resolves itself rapidly. Obviously, exposure treatments are appropriate for limited problems and are not appropriate for all clients, but when they are a good fit, they can be very effective in reducing phobias and anxiety.

Eye Movement Desensitization and Reprocessing (EMDR)

A highly specialized technique that requires additional training, EMDR is a form of exposure therapy used with trauma and stress. The procedure involves having clients imagine the traumatic or anxiety-provoking event while using rapid eye movements to create bilateral stimulation of the brain (Shapiro, 2001). During the process, the counselor asks questions about the associated memories that surface. The eye movements are used to help reconnect memory networks with more adaptive semantic memory networks. The EMDR specialist identifies negative and positive cognitions to structure the treatment, using the eye movements to defuse the negative cognition and associated bodily sensations. As this wanes, the client is then asked to "install" new positive cognitions, again using eye movements to affect memory networks. Although its effectiveness is still questioned by some, EMDR is generally recognized as an evidence-based treatment for trauma (Nowill, 2010).

Putting It All Together: Cognitive-Behavioral Case Conceptualization and Treatment Plan Templates

Theory-Specific Case Conceptualization: Cognitive-Behavioral

The prompts below can be used to develop a *theory-specific case conceptualization* using Adlerian theory. The cross-theoretical case conceptualizations at the end of each theory chapter provide examples for writing a conceptualization that includes key elements of this theory-specific conceptualization. Comprehensive examples of theory-specific case conceptualizations are available in *Theory and Treatment Planning in Counseling and Psychotherapy* (Gehart, 2015).

Baseline Assessment of Symptomatic Behavior: Provide a baseline assessment of the symptomatic behavior:

- *Symptom:* Define behaviorally; also include the following:
    - Frequency
    - Duration
    - Context(s)
    - Events before
    - Events after

A-B-C Analysis of Irrational Beliefs: Describe the activating events, consequences, and mediating beliefs related to the problem (or particular incident):

- Activating event ("problem"): ___
- Consequence (mood, behavior, etc.): ___
- Mediating beliefs (unhelpful beliefs about event that result in C):

Schema and Core Beliefs: Describe three to five problematic schemas and core beliefs that relate to the presenting problem(s), which may include:

- Arbitrary inference
- Selective abstraction
- Overgeneralization
- Magnification/minimization
- Personalization
- Absolutist/dichotomous thinking
- Mislabeling
- Mindreading

BASIC-ID: Assess the client in all areas:

- Behavior
- Affect
- Sensation

- Imagery
- Cognition
- Interpersonal relationships
- Drugs and biology

Treatment Plan Template: CBT

Use this Treatment Plan template for developing a plan for clients with depressive, anxious, or compulsive types of presenting problems. Depending on the specific client, presenting problem, and clinical context, the goals and interventions in this template may need to be modified only slightly or significantly; you are encouraged to significantly revise the plan as needed. For the plan to be useful, goals and techniques should be written to target specific beliefs, behaviors, and emotions that the client is experiencing. The more specific, the more useful it will be to you.

Cognitive-Behavioral Treatment Plan

Initial Phase of Treatment

Initial Phase Counseling Tasks

1. Develop working counseling relationship. *Diversity considerations:* Adapt use of warmth, "expertise," and emotional versus rational focus based on ethnicity, gender, age, etc.
   Relationship-building approach/intervention:
   a. Use warmth and **empathy** to build rapport; establish **credibility**.
2. Assess individual, systemic, and broader cultural dynamics. *Diversity considerations:* Determine whether traditional **individualistic goals** are appropriate for client's personal and cultural background.
   Assessment strategies:
   a. Obtain **baseline** of problem behavior; **functional analysis** of problem behaviors and thoughts; DSM-IV diagnosis.
   b. Identify specific **schemas** and **irrational beliefs** related to presenting problem.
3. Identify and obtain client agreement on treatment goals. *Diversity considerations:*
   Goal-making intervention:
   a. Develop **written contract** with specific goals and interventions.
4. Identify needed referrals, crisis issues, and other client needs. *Diversity considerations:*
   a. *Crisis assessment intervention(s):* Use **functional analysis** to assess dangerous behaviors and substance abuse disorders.
   b. *Referral(s):* To **cognitive-behavioral groups** related to presenting problem.

Initial Phase Client Goal

1. Decrease [name specific crisis-related behavior] to reduce [crisis] symptoms.

   Interventions:
   a. Use **functional analysis** to identify one behavior the client is willing to do to reduce severity of symptoms.
   b. Use **control theory** to motivate client to *choose* functional behaviors that move toward desired life goals.

(continued)

Working Phase of Treatment

Working Phase Counseling Tasks

1. Monitor quality of the working alliance. *Diversity considerations:* Ensure goals and premises are a good fit for diverse clients.
   a. *Assessment Intervention:* Use Session Rating Scale; verbally ask clients if sessions are beneficial and if they feel understood by counselor.
2. Monitor progress toward goals. *Diversity considerations:* Use **choice theory** and **cognitive restructuring** to motivate clients toward change.
   a. *Assessment Intervention:* Use Outcome Rating Scale to measure client progress.

Closing Phase of Treatment

Closing Phase Counseling Task

1. Develop aftercare plan and maintain gains. *Diversity considerations:* Include individual, family, and community resources as supports.
   Intervention:
   a. Use **thought records** and **REBT Self-Help Form** for potential future problems.

Closing Phase Client Goals

1. Increase **positive self-talk** about self-worth and expectations from life to reduce feelings of hopelessness, anxiety, fear, etc.
   Interventions:
   a. **Socratic dialogue** to help client develop positive views of self and life.
   b. Use **thought record** to develop realistic self-talk about self and worth.
2. Decrease **dysfunctional schemas** and **core beliefs** about self, others, and life to reduce depressive, anxious, and compulsive symptoms.
   Interventions:
   a. **Dispute three basic musts, negative cognitive triad**, and related core schemas.
   b. **Thought records** to develop alternative, realistic schema and core belief about worth as person and relationships.

Digital Download Download from CengageBrain.com

Mindfulness-Based Approaches

In a Nutshell: The Least You Need to Know

Described as the third wave of behavioral therapy (with "pure" behavioral therapy as the first wave and cognitive-behavioral therapy as the second), mindfulness-based approaches add a paradoxical twist to cognitive-behavioral approaches: *accepting* difficult thoughts and emotions in order to transform them (Hayes, 2004). Counselors using mindfulness-based approaches encourage clients to curiously and compassionately observe difficult thoughts and feelings *without the intention to change them.* By changing *how* clients relate to their problems—with curiosity and acceptance rather than avoidance—they experience new thoughts, emotions, and behaviors in relation to the problem, and thus have many new options for coping and resolving issues. These practices require counselors to have their own mindfulness practice and training before trying to teach clients to do the same.

A Brief History of Mindfulness in Mental Health

Mindfulness has an unusual history as a cognitive-behavioral technique: it was not developed in a researcher's lab or from a Western philosophical tradition. Instead, mindfulness comes from religious and spiritual traditions, making it a surprising favorite for cognitive-behavioral counselors, who traditionally ground themselves almost exclusively in Western scientific traditions. Most commonly associated with Buddhist forms of meditation, mindfulness is found in virtually all cultures and religious traditions, including Christian contemplative prayer (Keating, 2006), Jewish mysticism, and the Islamic-based Sufi tradition. Although it has religious roots, mindfulness entered mental health as a nonreligious "stress reduction" technique and was intentionally separated from religion and spiritual elements and adapted for use in behavioral health settings (Kabat-Zinn, 1990).

Over 30 years ago, Jon Kabat-Zinn (1990) began researching the *Mindfulness-Based Stress Reduction* (MBSR) program at the University of Massachusetts, which has been highly influential in making mindfulness a mainstream practice in behavioral medicine. The MBSR program is an eight-week group curriculum that teaches participants how to practice mindful breathing, mindful yoga postures, and mindful daily activities. Participants are encouraged to practice daily at home for 20–45 minutes per day. MBSR shows great promise as an effective treatment for a wide range of physical and mental health disorders, including chronic pain, fibromyalgia, psoriasis, depression, anxiety, ADHD, eating disorders, substance abuse, compulsive behaviors, and personality disorders (Baer, 2003). Closely related to this treatment, Teasdale, Segal, and Williams (1995) have adapted the MBSR curriculum for depression relapse in their program, *Mindfulness-Based Cognitive Therapy*. With 50% of "successfully" treated cases of depression ending in relapse within a year, MBCT counselors are using mindfulness to reduce the high relapse rate, with promising findings.

In addition to including *Mindfulness-Based Stress Reduction* (Kabat-Zinn, 1990) and *Mindfulness-Based Cognitive Therapy* (Teasdale et al., 1995), mindfulness has been integrated into two counseling approaches—*Dialectic Behavioral Therapy* (Linehan, 1993) and *Acceptance and Commitment Therapy* (Hayes, Strosahl, & Wilson, 1999)—that have also shown great promise in treating a wide range of clinical conditions.

Mindfulness Basics

The most common form of mindfulness involves observing the breath (or focusing on a repeated word, a *mantra*) while quieting the mind of inner chatter and thoughts (Kabat-Zinn, 1990; Stahl & Goldstein, 2010). Focus is maintained on the breath, grounding the practitioner in the present moment *without judging* the experience as good or bad, preferred or not preferred. Usually within seconds, the mind loses focus and wanders off—thinking about the exercise, a fight that morning, to-do lists, past memories, future plans; feeling an emotion or itch; or hearing a noise in the room. At some point, the practitioner realizes that the mind has wandered off and then returns to the object of focus without berating the self for "failing" to focus but rather with compassionate understanding that the loss of focus is part of the process—refraining from beating oneself up is usually the most difficult part. This process of focusing—losing focus—regaining focus—losing focus—regaining focus continues for an established period of time, usually 10–20 minutes.

Specific Mindfulness Approaches

Mindfulness-Based Stress Reduction and Mindfulness-Based Cognitive Therapy

Not primarily about becoming a good meditation practitioner, these mindfulness-based group treatments are designed to help clients change *how they relate to their thoughts and internal dialogue*. Using a highly structured group process, clients are introduced to mindfulness breathing (similar to the instructions above), as well as mindful yoga (stretching) positions, and mindful daily activities (e.g., washing dishes mindfully, walking, and such; Kabat-Zinn, 1990). Depending on the group's focus, clients may be taught to apply mindfulness to physical conditions, difficult emotions, depressive thinking, and so on. The group format is ideal for motivating clients to practice regularly at home and report back to the group on progress.

The eight groups in MBSR cover the following:

Session 1: Introduction to mindfulness: Foundations of mindfulness and body scan meditation

Session 2: Patience: Working with perceptions and dealing with the "wandering mind"

Session 3: Nonstriving: Introduction to breathing meditation; mindful lying yoga; qualities of attention

Session 4: Nonjudging: Responding versus reacting; awareness in breath meditation; standing yoga; research on stress

Session 5: Acknowledgment: Group check-in on progress; sitting meditation

Session 6: Let It Be: Skillful communication; loving kindness meditation; walking meditation; day-long retreat

Session 7: Everyday mindfulness: Mindful movement and everyday applications; practicing on one's own life

Session 8: Practice never ends: Integrating with everyday life

The eight groups of MBCT cover the following (Segal, William, & Teasdale, 2002):

Session 1: Automatic pilot: Introduce mindfulness; eating mindfulness exercise; mindfulness body scan

Session 2: Dealing with barriers: Explore mental chatter using the body scan exercise

Session 3: Mindfulness of the breath: Introduce mindfulness breath focus and 3-Minute Breathing Space exercise

Session 4: Staying present: Link mindfulness to automatic thoughts and depression

Session 5: Allowing and letting be: Introduce acceptance and "allowing" things to just be

Session 6: Thoughts are not Facts: Reframe thoughts as "just thoughts" and not facts

Session 7: How can I best take care of myself? Introduce specific techniques for depressive thoughts

Session 8: Using what has been learned to deal with future moods: Motivate to continue practice.

Through these mindfulness exercises, clients learn to:

- Deliberately direct their attention and thereby better control their thoughts.
- Become curious, open, and accepting of their thoughts and feelings, even those that are unpleasant.
- Develop greater acceptance of self, other, and things as they are.
- Live in and experience themselves in the present moment.

Dialectical Behavior Therapy DBT is a well-regarded, widely used evidence-based treatment for borderline personality disorder (Linehan, 1993). Its primary evidence base has been with borderline personality, but over the years it has been increasingly used with other difficult-to-treatment populations, such as eating disorders, depressive disorders, bipolar disorders, substance use disorders, self-harming adolescents, anger/aggressive behavior, and other personality disorders (Chesin, & Stanley, 2013; Dimeff & Koerner, 2007; Frazier & Vela, 2014; Miller, Rathus, & Linehan, 2007; Safer, Telch, & Chen, 2009; Van Dijk, Jeffrey, & Katz, 2013). Taking a compassionate stance with clients, the overarching goal of DBT is to increase dialectical behavior patterns in order to increase emotional and behavioral regulation.

DBT is delivered through a comprehensive program of individual and group treatment modalities, which includes phone support between sessions and case consultation for practitioners. In most applications, clients are required to attend weekly individual sessions and weekly group sessions (Linehan, 1993). In the individual sessions, the counselor establishes a relationship that constantly balances validating and nurturing clients while also maintaining clear limits and demanding behavioral change. In their group sessions, clients are taught a standard curriculum of psychosocial skills. Mindfulness core skills are foundational to the three sets of skills for specific situations: (a) interpersonal effectiveness, (b) emotion regulation, and (c) distress tolerance. These skills are practiced at home with worksheets and reinforced in individual meeting with counselors. The model is specifically designed to target suicidal behaviors, self-harm, and trauma, which are common in persons diagnosed with borderline personality disorder.

DBT counselors help clients "be with" difficult emotions by encouraging clients to manage dialectic tension, the tension between two polar opposites, such as both loving and hating someone. Rather than retreating to either pole, the counselor encourages clients to experience how they can both simultaneously feel love and dislike by acknowledging the multiple levels of truth and reality in a given situation. These contradictory feelings and thoughts are first tolerated, then explored, and eventually synthesized, so that the reality of both extremes can be recognized. For example, an adult might come to acknowledge both ultimately loving a critical parent but at the same time hating how that parent speaks to her. As the client becomes able to accept having both loving and hateful feelings toward the parent, she will find herself less reactive and emotional about the situation. The process of DBT involves helping clients learn to increase balance in their lives by better managing the inherent dialectic tensions in life:

- Being able to both seek to improve oneself as well as accept oneself.
- Being able to accept life as it is and also seek to solve problems.
- Taking care of one's own needs as well as those of others.
- Balancing independence and interdependence.

Acceptance and Commitment Therapy A behavioral approach that shares philosophical assumptions with postmodern, narrative, and feminist approaches (see Chapter 14), acceptance and commitment therapy (ACT, pronounced "act" not A-C-T) is based on the postmodern premise that we construct our realities through language, which shapes our thoughts, feelings, and behaviors (Hayes et al., 1999; Hayes & Smith, 2005). ACT practitioners believe that human suffering is in large measure created and sustained through language: "It is not that people are thinking the wrong thing—the problem is thought itself and how the verbal community (contemporary culture) supports its excessive use as a mode of behavioral regulation" (Hayes et al., 1999, p. 49). Unlike traditional cognitive-behavioralists, ACT practitioners assert that attempts to control thoughts and feelings and avoid direct experience are the *problem*, not the solution. Instead, they advocate mindfulness-based *experiencing* to promote acceptance of the full range of human emotions: "In the ACT approach, a goal of healthy living is not so much to feel *good*, but rather to *feel* good. It is psychologically healthy to feel bad feelings as well as good feelings" (p. 77).

The same acronym, ACT, is used to outline the process of counseling:

A = Accept and embrace difficult thoughts and feelings

C = Choose and commit to a life direction that reflects who the client truly is

T = Take action steps toward this life direction.

The first phase in ACT is to accept and embrace the very thoughts and feelings clients have been trying to avoid via their symptoms: accepting loss, feeling fear, and acknowledging anger. Counselors caution clients to not "buy into" their thoughts, and challenge them to see the flimsy link between reasons (a.k.a., excuses) and causes of their behavior. At the same time, they help them develop a *willingness* to experience difficult thoughts and feelings with their *observing self*. Through this process of observation, clients are better able to identify their true values and selves, which helps them not only readily identify a life direction but commit to pursuing it. As you might imagine, this is not as simple as it sounds. In the action phase, most clients reexperience the resistance to experience and negative thoughts that brought them to counseling in the first place. However, with increased ability to accept these thoughts, and a renewed commitment to pursue a meaningful life direction, the counselor can work with the client when obstacles arise in pursuing new action.

Tapestry Weaving: Working with Diverse Populations

Ethnic, Racial, and Cultural Diversity

Because CBT defines behavioral norms (e.g., each culture defines "rational" differently), therapists must carefully apply this approach with diverse populations to avoid conflicts in values and relational styles. CBT's emphasis on the expert stance in relation to clients has strengths and weaknesses when working with diverse populations. Men, and certain culture groups such as Latinos, Asians, and Native Americans, often prefer active, directive therapy (Gehart & Lyle, 2001; Pedersen, Draguns, Lonner, & Trimble, 2002). However, hierarchical difference may cause a rebellious reaction in some clients (e.g., highly educated adults or teens) or an overly compliant and withholding response in others (e.g., women who have a habit of people pleasing; Gehart & Lyle, 2001).

Because cognitive-behavioral approaches involve identifying "irrational beliefs" and "problematic behaviors," both of which are culturally and contextually determined, counselors must be particularly alert to unintentionally perpetuating dominant cultural norms with diverse clients. Counselors must carefully evaluate treatment goals prior to intervention to ensure that they do not clash with religious, cultural, racial, socioeconomic, or other values and realities, and they must consider how the various cultures of which a client is a part may have conflicting values. To ensure cultural appropriateness of their methods, researchers have explored the specific effects of ethnicity in CBT practice, identifying in which contexts ethnicity plays the greatest role. For example, initial studies have found no significant difference when using CBT for depression with European Americans, Latinos, and Asian Americans (Marchand, Ng, Rohde, & Stice, 2010), yet another study found that ethnicity played a significant role in the strength of the therapeutic relationship over the course of therapy with perpetrators of domestic violence (Walling, Suvak, Howard, Taft, & Murphy, 2012); thus, ongoing research will further refine our understanding of how best to use CBT with diverse populations. Based on this emerging research and clinical expertise, CBT therapists have begun developing recommendations for specific ethnic groups.

Hispanic and Latinos CBT is generally considered to be culturally consistent and appropriate for working with Hispanic and Latino clients (Organista & Muñoz, 1996). Therapists have developed several suggestions for successfully working with Hispanic and Latino clients using CBT.

- *Addressing language needs:* Language issues are central when working with many immigrant Latino families, who often prefer to discuss private and emotional issues in their native language (most people prefer to discuss emotional issues in their native language, and Spanish speakers are particularly passionate about this). In addition, Spanish-speaking therapists need to consider how to translate not just words but concepts across cultures; for example, in one CBT program for Latinos, the A-B-C method for disputing irrational beliefs was streamlined and translated as the *Si, Pero* (Yes, but ...) technique (Piedra & Byoun, 2012).
- *Increasing experiential components:* When modifying standard CBT curricula, therapists often increase the applied and experiential components: rather than talk about it, do it (Piedra & Byoun, 2012).
- *Respecting cultural value of* familismo: Family is highly valued, with individual interests often placed second to family needs; thus, CBT therapists need to be careful

to avoid labeling a Latino/a's choice to put family above personal needs as "irrational" (Duarté-Vélez et al., 2010; González-Prendes, Hindo, & Pardo, 2011).

- *Respecting cultural value of* personalismo*:* Latino culture values warm and trusting personal relationships, which therapists need to integrate into the therapeutic relationship (González-Prendes et al., 2011). To create a context of *personalismo*, therapists can begin their initial session in "small talk" to share their own background and also learn about the client's (Organista & Muñoz, 1996).
- *Respecting the cultural value of* respecto: Latino families are typically hierarchical, with formal expectations of respect to parents and elders; in addition, clients may prefer to be addressed with formal titles, Señor or Señora (González-Prendes et al., 2011; Organista & Muñoz, 1996).
- *Respecting the cultural value of* machismo*:* Often misunderstood in its negative extreme, *machismo* within its native culture refers to a man's sense of leadership, loyalty, and responsibility to provide and care for the family (Duarté-Vélez et al., 2010; González-Prendes et al., 2011).
- *Working with spirituality:* Many Hispanic/Latino clients have a strong sense of spirituality, most often Roman Catholic (Duarté-Vélez et al., 2010). Prayer, church, and the church community are resources that therapists can tap into; but therapists should also discuss the use of prayer to ensure that it facilitates active problem solving rather than reducing clients' sense of efficacy or responsibility (Organista & Muñoz, 1996).
- *Attitude to gay/lesbian relationships:* Often due to their strong religious beliefs, Hispanic families may have a highly negative response to a child's coming out, often viewing same-sex attraction as a "sin," creating significant cultural dissonance and rejection for gay Latino youth (Duarté-Vélez et al., 2010).
- *Addressing immigration, migration, and acculturation:* Many Hispanic clients have complex immigration and migration patterns, often moving back and forth between cultures multiple times and with family members living in different countries at the same time. In addition, there are often acculturation issues between parents and children that CBT therapists need to help them address (Piedra & Byoun, 2012).

African Americans Many counselors also consider CBT an appropriate choice for working with African Americans because the therapy helps them to directly dispute problematic social beliefs and because it focuses on present behaviors (Kelly, 2006; McNair, 1996). Recommendations for adaptation include:

- *Forming a collaborative relationship:* Clients should be invited to work with the therapist in setting goals, agreeing on time frames; this relationship should be used to foster a greater sense of self-efficacy in the client (Kelly, 2006; McNair, 1996).
- *Focusing on behaviors and skills:* Rather than analyzing the past, therapists should focus on problems that are experienced in the present and are of immediate importance and relevance to the client (McNair, 1996).
- *Empowerment:* CBT therapists can help empower clients by helping them to develop coping and communication skills and to expand the support networks (Kelly, 2006). Furthermore, clients can be taught how to use thought records and other strategies to solve their own problems without the therapist.
- *Disputing stereotypes and expectations:* CBT therapists can use the techniques of the approach to help African Americans identify and logically dispute many of the stereotypes and expectations they have internalized from the broader culture—such as having to be twice as good to be good enough—and to increase their personal sense of purpose and opportunities (McNair, 1996).
- *Addressing discrimination:* Therapists can help African Americans mitigate the effects of discrimination by specifically identifying how they cope with discrimination and how it relates to how they perceive and relate to the world (McNair, 1996).

- *Functional analysis:* Functional analysis that examines the symptom in behavioral terms can help circumvent potential therapist bias and prejudice and can help clients do the same (Kelly, 2006).

Chinese Americans Therapists have also considered how best to use cognitive-behavioral approaches with Chinese Americans (Hwang, Wood, Lin, & Cheung, 2006). Hwang and colleagues (2006) recommend the following:

1. Explicitly educating clients about the process and goals of therapy to increase their understanding and acceptance.
2. Therapist learning more about the client's cultural background and its significance to the client.
3. Clearly establishing goals and measures of improvement early in treatment to reduce confusion about the process.
4. Focusing on psychoeducational aspects and reinforcing efforts to learn to reduce stigma and empower clients.
5. Using *cultural bridging* to link Western psychological concepts to client's cultural beliefs and practices (e.g., discussing Qi (life energy) when discussing depression.
6. Presenting therapist as an expert often is helpful to Chinese American clients.
7. Explicitly discussing therapist-client relationship to clarify roles and set realistic expectations.
8. Attending to cultural differences in communication and deference to authority.
9. Spending extra time joining with client and learning about immigration history and family background.
10. Respecting family orientation of Chinese culture and involving family whenever possible.
11. Being sensitive to social stigma associated with mental illness in Chinese community and the desire to keep diagnosis private.
12. Being patient because Chinese may not be as comfortable discussing emotions.
13. Being aware of the push-pull between client's culture of origin and the culture of therapy.
14. Integrating Chinese cultural healing traditions, such as QiGong or acupuncture, into treatment plan.
15. Being aware of the ethnic differences in expressing distress, with Chinese notion of self involving a closer relationship between mind and body than in Western culture.

Sexual Identity Diversity

Several authors have considered how to adapt CBT for working with lesbian, gay, bisexual, transgendered, and questioning (LGBTQ) clients (Safren & Rogers, 2001). Safren and Rogers (2001) note that it is common that therapists either over- or underestimate the impact that sexual orientation and difference has on a client's presenting problems, and therefore they recommend that therapists begin by examining their own beliefs and schemas related to sexual orientation and identity. Furthermore, Safren and Rogers (2001) encourage CBT therapists to examine the role that societal norms and stigma play in the development of a client's beliefs and schemas.

When working with LGBTQ youth and adults, therapists need to assess additional areas of stress and functioning:

- Overt acts of harassment, abuse, and violence (Safren, Hollander, Hart, & Heimberg, 2001)
- Internalized homophobia (Safren et al., 2001)
- Existence of social support networks (Safren & Rogers, 2001)
- Development of identity as a sexual minority (Safren et al., 2001)
- Disclosure of sexual orientation to family, friends, and others (Safren et al., 2001)
- Development of platonic and romantic relationships with other gay, lesbian, bisexual, or transgendered persons (Safren et al., 2001)
- Stress due to social stigma (Glassgold, 2009)
- Stress due to concealing stigma and distress (Glassgold, 2009)

Mylott (1994) has identified common irrational beliefs with which gay, lesbian, and bisexual adults frequently struggle; these beliefs are largely informed by societal norms and include:

- I need to be loved.
- I can't stand rejection.
- Because people will often accept or reject me on the basis of my physical attractiveness, age, socioeconomic status, masculinity, or femininity, I have to use these same criteria and accept or reject myself.
- It will be awful if I grow old without a lover.
- I can't stand being alone, and since I can't stand being alone, it is better to be in an emotionally and even physically damaging relationship than to be alone.
- When gay people are the victims of homophobia, I have to get very angry and upset about it; I also have to become enraged at homophobic individuals, groups and institutions.
- I can only accept my homosexuality if I know for certain that it is genetically determined, or that "God made me gay." Otherwise, I cannot accept myself.
- It's awful if people (family, friends, the church, etc.) don't accept my homosexuality.

CBT therapists help clients learn how to adapt more realistic beliefs about their life, sexuality, and others by using techniques such as thought records or Socratic dialogue.

Research and the Evidence Base

Due to their conceptual home in experimental psychology, research is part of the culture of cognitive-behavioral counseling (Beck, 1976) and, therefore, they are some of the best-researched approaches in the field. More so than any other approach, cognitive-behavioral counselors integrate research into their conceptualization of theory development and intervention, carefully researching specific interventions for specific populations (Beck, 1997).

With an impressive range of applications, cognitive-behavioral therapies dominate the National Institute for Mental Health's list of evidence-based treatments (empirically supported treatments; Chambless et al., 1996). The list includes but is not limited to:

- Cognitive behavioral therapy for panic disorder
- Cognitive behavioral therapy for generalized anxiety disorder
- Exposure treatment for agoraphobia
- Exposure/guided imagery for specific phobias
- Exposure and response prevention for obsessive compulsive disorder
- Stress inoculation for coping with stressors
- Behavior therapy for depression
- Cognitive therapy for depression
- Cognitive-behavior therapy for bulimia
- Behavior modification for enuresis
- Applied relaxation for panic disorder and generalized anxiety disorder
- Cognitive behavioral therapy for social phobia
- Cognitive therapy for obsessive compulsive disorder
- Exposure treatment for posttraumatic stress disorder
- Stress inoculation training for posttraumatic stress disorder
- Relapse prevention program for obsessive-compulsive disorder
- Behavior therapy for cocaine dependence
- Cognitive therapy for opiate dependence
- Cognitive-behavior therapy for benzodiazepine withdrawal in panic disorder patients
- Trauma-focused cognitive-behavioral therapy

(Detailed descriptions of these and other evidence-based programs can be found on the National Registry of Evidence-Based Practices and Programs website: http://nrepp.samhsa.gov)

Over the years, CBT theorists have modified their approaches based on research outcomes—sometimes dramatically—to incorporate more affective and relational components. Behavioral couples therapy is the premier example of this trend. Because of good short-term but poor long-term outcomes, Neil Jacobson reformulated his couples therapy to include more affective aspects; his new approach is called *integrative behavioral couples therapy* (Jacobson & Christensen, 1996). Similarly, because research indicates that a nonjudgmental therapeutic alliance is crucial, CBT therapists have become increasingly attentive to this aspect of therapy (Beck, 2005).

The meticulous and extensive research efforts of cognitive-behavioralists enable counselors to better know when and how their methods work. In a recent meta-analysis (analysis of the findings from several studies) of well-controlled studies on cognitive-behavioral approaches, Lynch, Laws, and McKenna (2010) found that cognitive-behavioral treatment was not effective in treating or preventing relapse with schizophrenia; it was effective in treating and reducing relapse in depression, although the effect size was small; and it was not effective in preventing relapse in bipolar disorder. To the untrained eye, these may seem like less than flattering findings, but the specificity is unparalleled, with no other approach able to provide similar information or superior findings.

Although CBT has an extensive research history and has the most robust evidence base of any approach, therapists should not assume that it is therefore superior to other approaches in every case or in general. For example, common factors advocates point out that when confounding factors such as researcher allegiance are controlled for, no therapy is consistently found to be superior to any other (Sprenkle & Blow, 2004). Furthermore, for certain concerns such as adolescent conduct issues, systemic approaches have been found to be superior to individual forms of CBT (see Chapter 11). Finally, many therapists have criticized CBT on the basis that its claims to superiority have more to do with the volume of research by CBT proponents than with any substantive advantage (Loewenthal & House, 2010).

Along those lines, Miller (2012) reports that a massive effort to transform all mental health in Sweden to CBT resulted in no effect on overall outcome of those diagnosed with depression and anxiety, with over 25% dropping out of treatment. In addition, a significant number of these clients who were not considered disabled prior to treatment *became* disabled, costing the government more money. The Swedish government soon ended its attempt to systematically institute CBT, encouraging new approaches. Thus, although CBT does have the most extensive evidence base in the field, it is by no means a panacea and has by no means provided a simple answer to the question of what works best in therapy.

Questions for Personal Reflection and Class Discussion

1. Which ideas from this chapter do you find most personally relevant? Why?
2. Which ideas from this chapter do you think will be most helpful in working with clients?
3. What are the possibilities and limitations for using this approach with diverse clients? How might you address the limitations?
4. How do you view thoughts, feelings, and behaviors relating and influencing each other?
5. Describe a time you were able to change a behavior. How did you do it? Describe how feelings and thoughts related to this process.
6. What are your thoughts about assigning clients written homework? Would you be good at completing such assignments if you were a client? For which clients might this be a good option? For which might it be more of a challenge?
7. What are your thoughts about creating a written contract with clients for counseling?

8. For which clients and/or presenting problems do you think this approach would be most appropriate? Least appropriate?
9. Which case conceptualization concept seems most useful for understanding a client's problem?
10. Which intervention do you think would be the most useful?
11. Do you think this approach is a good fit for you as a counselor or therapist? Why or why not?
12. In what ways would you need to grow, or what would you need to learn to be able to use this approach well?

Online Resources

Associations and Training Institutes

Academy of Cognitive Therapy
www.academyofct.org

American Institute for Cognitive Therapy
www.cognitivetherapynyc.com

Association for the Behavioral and Cognitive Therapies
www.abct.org

Beck Institute
www.beckinstitute.org

Mindfulness Awareness Research Center: UCLA
http://marc.ucla.edu

Mindfulness-Based Stress Reduction Clinic: Jon Kabit-Zinn
www.umassmed.edu/cfm/mbsr/

National Association of Cognitive-Behavioral Therapists
www.nacbt.org

Rational Emotive Behavioral Therapy Network
www.rebtnetwork.org

REBT Self-Help Form (Thought record exercise)
www.rebtnetwork.org/library/shf.html

William Glasser Institute
www.wglasser.com

Journals

Behavior Therapy
www.elsevier.com/wps/find/journaldescription.cws_home/707105/description#description

Cognitive Therapy and Research
www.springer.com/medicine/journal/10608

International Journal of Cognitive Therapy
www.guilford.com

International Journal of Reality Therapy
www.journalofrealitytherapy.com

Journal of Behavior Therapy and Experimental Psychiatry
www.sciencedirect.com/science/journal/00057916

Journal of Cognitive Psychotherapy
www.springerpub.com/product/08898391

Journal of Rational Emotive Behavioral Therapy
www.springerlink.com/content/104937/

References

*Asterisk indicates recommended introductory readings.

Alford, B. A., & Beck, A. T. (1997). *The integrative power of cognitive therapy*. New York: Guilford.

*Baer, R. A. (2003). Mindfulness training as a clinical intervention: A conceptual and empirical review. *Clinical Psychology: Science and Practice, 10*(2), 125–143. doi: 10.1093/clipsy.bpg015

Bandura, A. (1974). Behavior theories and the models of man. *American Psychologist, 29*, 859–869. doi 10.1037/h0037514

*Bandura, A. (1977). *Social learning theory*. Englewood Cliffs, NJ: Prentice-Hall.

Bandura, A. (1986). *Social foundations of thought and action: A social cognitive theory*. Englewood Cliffs, NJ: Prentice-Hall.

Beck, A. T. (1972). *Depression: Causes and treatment*. Philadelphia: University of Pennsylvania Press.

*Beck, A. T. (1976). *Cognitive therapy and the emotional disorders*. New York: International Universities Press.

Beck, A. T. (1991). Cognitive therapy: Reflections. In J. K. Zeig (Ed.), *The evolution of psychotherapy: Third conference* (pp. 55–64). New York: Brunner/Mazel.

Beck, A. T. (1997). The past and future of cognitive therapy. *Journal of Psychotherapy Practice and Research, 6*(4), 276–284.

*Beck, J. (1995). *Cognitive therapy: Basics and beyond*. New York: Guilford.

*Beck, J. (2005). *Cognitive therapy for challenging problems: What to do when the basics don't work*. New York: Guilford.

Berg-Cross L., Jennings, P., & Baruch, R. (1990). Cinematherapy: Theory and application. *Psychotherapy in Private Practice, 8*, 135–157.

Burns, D. (1988). *Feeling good: The new mood therapy*. New York: Signet.

Chambless, D. L., Sanderson, W. C., Shoham, V., Johnson, S. B., Pope, K. S., Crits-Christoph, P., Baker, M., Johnson, B., Woody, S. R., Sue, S., Beutler, L., Williams, D. A., & McCurry, S. (1996). An update on empirically validated treatments. *The Clinical Psychologist, 49*(2), 5–18. Available www.apa.org/divisions/div12/journals.html

Chesin, M. S., & Stanley, B. H. (2013). Dialectical behavior therapy for mood disorders. In J. Mann, P. J. McGrath, & S. P. Roose (Eds.), *Clinical handbook for the management of mood disorders* (pp. 280–288). New York: Cambridge University Press. doi:10.1017/CBO9781139175869.021

Dimeff, L. A., & Koerner, K. (2007). *Dialectical behavior therapy in clinical practice: Applications across disorders and settings*. New York: Guilford.

Duarté-Vélez, Y., Bernal, G., & Bonilla, K. (2010). Culturally adapted cognitive-behavioral therapy: Integrating sexual, spiritual, and family identities in an evidence-based treatment of a depressed Latino adolescent. *Journal of Clinical Psychology, 66*(8), 895–906. doi:10.1002/jclp.20710

Ellis, A. (1962). *Reason and emotion in psychotherapy*. New York: Lyle Stuart.

Ellis, A. (1991). Using RET effectively: Reflections and interview. In M. E. Bernard (Ed.), *Using rational emotive therapy effectively* (pp. 1–33). New York: Plenum.

Ellis, A. (1994). *Reason and emotion in psychotherapy* (rev. 2nd ed.). New York: Kensington.

*Ellis, A. (1996). *Better, deeper, and more enduring brief therapy: The rational emotive behavior therapy approach*. New York: Brunner/Mazel.

Ellis, A. (2003). Early theories and practices of rational emotive behavior therapy and how they have been augmented and revised during the last three decades. *Journal of Rational-Emotive & Cognitive Behavior Therapy, 21*(3–4), 219–243. doi:10.1023/A:1025890112319

Ellis, A. (2004). *The road to tolerance: The philosophy of rational emotive behavior therapy*. Amherst, NY: Prometheus Books.

Ellis, A., & Dryden, W. (1997). *The practice of rational emotive behavior therapy* (2nd ed.). New York: Springer.

Frazier, S. N., & Vela, J. (2014). Dialectical behavior therapy for the treatment of anger and aggressive behavior: A review. *Aggression and Violent Behavior, 19*(2), 156–163. doi:10.1016/j.avb.2014.02.001

Gehart, D. (2015). *Theory and treatment planning in counseling and psychotherapy* (2nd ed.). Pacific Grove, CA: Brooks Cole.

Gehart, D. R., & Lyle, R. R. (2001). Client experience of gender in therapeutic relationships: An interpretive ethnography. *Family Process, 40*, 443–458. doi:10.1111/j.1545-5300.2001.4040100443.x

Glasser, W. (1975). *Reality therapy*. New York: Harper & Row.

Glasser, W. (1997). Teaching and learning reality therapy. In J. K. Zeig (Ed.), *The evolution of psychotherapy: Third conference* (pp. 123–130). New York: Brunner/Mazel.

Glasser, W. (1998). *Choice theory: A new psychology of personal freedom*. New York: HarperColins.

Glasser, W. (2000). *Counseling with choice theory: The new reality therapy*. New York: HarperCollins.

Glasser, W. (2003). *Warning: Psychiatry can be hazardous to your mental health*. New York: HarperCollins.

Glassgold, J. M. (2009). The case of Felix: An example of gay-affirmative, cognitive-behavioral therapy. *Pragmatic Case Studies in Psychotherapy, 5*(4), 1–21.

González-Prendes, A., Hindo, C., & Pardo, Y. (2011). Cultural values integration in cognitive-behavioral therapy for a Latino with depression. *Clinical Case Studies, 10*(5), 376–394. doi:10.1177/1534650111427075

Hayes, S. C. (2004). Acceptance and commitment therapy, relational frame theory, and the third wave of behavior therapy.*Behavior Therapeutic, 35*, 639–666.

*Hayes, S. C., & Smith, S. (2005). *Get out of your mind and into your life*. Oakland, CA: New Harbinger.

*Hayes, S. C., Strosahl, K. D., & Wilson, K. G. (1999). *Acceptance and commitment therapy: An experiential approach to behavior change*. New York: Guilford.

Hayward, J. W., & Varela, F. J. (1992). *Gentle bridges: Conversations with the Dali Lama on the Sciences of the mind*. Boston, MA: Shambhala.

Holtzworth-Munroe, A., & Jacobson, N. S. (1991). Behavioral marital therapy. In A. S. Gunman & D. P Kniskern (Eds.), *Handbook of family therapy* (Vol. II, pp. 96–132). New York: Brunner/Mazel.

Hwang, W., Wood, J. J., Lin, K., & Cheung, F. (2006). Cognitive-behavioral therapy with Chinese Americans:

Research, theory, and clinical practice. *Cognitive and Behavioral Practice*, *13*, 293–303.

*Jacobson, N. S., & Christensen, A. (1996). *Integrative couple therapy*. New York: Norton.

Kabat-Zinn, J. (1990). *Full catastrophe living: Using the wisdom of your body and mind to face stress, pain, and illness*. New York: Delta.

Keating, T. (2006). *Open mind, open heart: The contemplative dimension of the gospel*. New York: Continuum International.

Kelly, S. (2006). Cognitive-behavioral therapy with African Americans. In P. A. Hays & G. Y. Iwamasa (Eds.), *Culturally responsive cognitive-behavioral therapy: Assessment, practice, and supervision* (pp. 97–116). Washington, DC: American Psychological Association. doi:10.1037/11433-004

Lazarus, A. A. (1981). *The practice of multimodal therapy: systematic, comprehensive and effective psychotherapy*. New York: McGraw-Hill.

Lazarus, A. A. (1997). Can psychotherapy be brief, focused, solution-oriented, and yet comprehensive? A personal evolutionary perspective. In J. K. Zeig (Ed.), *The evolution of psychotherapy: Third conference* (pp. 83–89). New York: Brunner/Mazel.

Leahy, R. L. (2005). *The worry cure: Seven steps to stop worry from stopping you*. New York: Marmony Books.

*Linehan, M. M. (1993). *Cognitive-behavioral treatment of borderline personality disorder*. New York: Guilford.

Loewenthal, D., & House, R. (2010). *Critically engaging CBT*. Berkshire, UK: Open University Press.

Lynch, D., Laws, K., & McKenna, P. (2010). Cognitive behavioural therapy for major psychiatric disorder: Does it really work? A meta-analytical review of well-controlled trials. *Psychological Medicine: A Journal of Research in Psychiatry and the Allied Sciences*, *40*(1), 9–24. doi: 10.1017/S003329170900590X

Marchand, E., Ng, J., Rohde, P., & Stice, E. (2010). Effects of an indicated cognitive-behavioral depression prevention program are similar for Asian American, Latino, and European American adolescents. *Behaviour Research and Therapy*, *48*(8), 821–825. doi:10.1016/j.brat.2010.05.005

McNair, L. D. (1996). African American women and behavior therapy: Integrating theory, culture, and clinical practice. *Cognitive and Behavioral Practice*, *3*(2), 337–349. doi:10.1016/S1077-7229(96)80022-8

Meichenbaum, D. (1977). *Cognitive behavioral modification: An integrative approach*. New York: Plenum.

Meichenbaum, D. (1985). *Stress inoculation training*. New York: Pergamon Press.

Meichenbaum, D. (1997). The evolution of a cognitive-behavior therapist. In J. K. Zeig (Ed.), *The evolution of psychotherapy: Third conference* (pp. 95–106). New York: Brunner/Mazel.

Miller, A. L., Rathus, J. H., & Linehan, M. M. (2007). *Dialectical behavior therapy with suicidal adolescents*. New York: Guilford.

Miller, S. (2012). *Revolution in Swedish mental health practice: The cognitive behavioral therapy monopoly gives way*. Retrieved from www.scottmiller.com/?q=node%F160.

Mylott, K. (1994). Twelve irrational ideas that drive gay men and women crazy. *Journal of Rational-Emotive & Cognitive Behavior Therapy*, *12*(1), 61–71. doi:10.1007/BF02354490

Nowill, J. (2010). A critical review of the controversy surrounding eye movement desensitisation and reprocessing. *Counselling Psychology Review*, *25*(1), 63–70.

Organista, K. C., & Muñoz, R. F. (1996). Cognitive behavioral therapy with Latinos. *Cognitive and Behavioral Practice*, *3*(2), 255–270. doi:10.1016/S1077-7229(96)80017-4

Patterson, G. R., & Forgatch, M. S. (1995). Predicting future clinical adjustment from treatment outcome and process variables. *Psychological Assessment*, *7*(3), 275–285.

Pavlov, I. P. (1932a). Neuroses in man and animals. *Journal of the American Medical Association*, *99*, 1012–1013.

Pavlov, I. P. (1932b). The reply of a psychologist to psychologists. *Psychological Review*, *39*, 91–127.

Pedersen, P. B., Draguns, J. G., Lonner, W. J., & Trimble, J. E. (Eds.). (2002). *Counseling across cultures* (5th ed.). Thousand Oaks, CA: Sage.

Piedra, L. M., & Byoun, S. (2012). Vida Alegre: Preliminary findings of a depression intervention for immigrant Latino mothers. *Research on Social Work Practice*, *22*(2), 138–150. doi:10.1177/1049731511424168

Rogers, C. (1961). *On becoming a person: A therapist's view of psychotherapy*. Boston, MA: Houghton Mifflin.

Ross, W. (2006). REBT self-help form. http://www.rebtnetwork.org/library/shf.html

Safer, D. L., Telch, C. F., & Chen, E. Y. (2009). *Dialectical behavior therapy for binge eating and bulimia*. New York: Guilford.

Safren, S. A., Hollander, G., Hart, T. A., & Heimberg, R. G. (2001). Cognitive-behavioral therapy with lesbian, gay, and bisexual youth. *Cognitive and Behavioral Practice*, *8*(3), 215–223. doi:10.1016/S1077-7229(01)80056-0

Safren, S. A., & Rogers, T. (2001). Cognitive-behavioral therapy with gay, lesbian, and bisexual clients. *Journal of Clinical Psychology*, *57*(5), 629–643. doi:10.1002/jclp.1033

Segal, Z. V., William, J. M. G., & Teasdale, J. D. (2002). *Mindfulness-based cognitive therapy for depression: A new approach to preventing relapse*. New York: Guilford.

Shapiro, F. (2001). *EMDR as an integrative psychotherapy approach: Experts of diverse orientations explore the paradigm prism*. Washington, DC: American Psychological Association.

Skinner, B. F. (1953). *Science and human behavior*. New York: Macmillan.

Skinner, B. F. (1971). *Beyond freedom and dignity*. New York: Knopf.

Skinner, B. F. (1974). *About behaviorism*. New York: Alfred Knopf.

Spiegler, M. D., & Guevremont, D. C. (2003). *Contemporary behavior therapy* (4th ed.). Pacific Grove, CA: Wadsworth.

Sprenkle, D. H., & Blow, A. J. (2004). Common factors and our sacred models. *Journal of Marital and Family Therapy*, *30*, 113–129.

Stahl, B., & Goldstein, E. (2010). *The mindfulness-based stress reduction workbook*. Oakland, CA: New Harbinger.

Teasdale, J. D., Segal, Z. V., & Williams, J. M. C. (1995). How does cognitive therapy prevent depressive relapse and why should attentional control (mindfulness) help? *Behaviour Research and Therapy*, *33*, 25–39.

Van Dijk, S., Jeffrey, J., & Katz, M. R. (2013). A randomized, controlled, pilot study of dialectical behavior therapy skills in a psychoeducational group for individuals with bipolar disorder. *Journal of Affective Disorders*, *145*(3), 386–393. doi:10.1016/j.jad.2012.05.054

Walling, S., Suvak, M. K., Howard, J. M., Taft, C. T., & Murphy, C. M. (2012). Race/ethnicity as a predictor of change in working alliance during cognitive behavioral therapy for intimate partner violence perpetrators. *Psychotherapy*, *49*(2), 180–189. doi:10.1037/a0025751

Wolpe, J. W. (1997). From psychoanalytic to behavioral methods in anxiety disorders: A continuing evolution. In J. K. Zeig (Ed.), *The evolution of psychotherapy: Third conference* (pp. 107–119). New York: Brunner/Mazel.

Wubbolding, R. (2008). *Reality therapy theory*. Reality therapy. In J. Frew & M. D. Spiegler (Eds.), *Contemporary psychotherapies for a diverse world* (pp. 360–396). Boston, MA: Lakhasa.

Cognitive-Behavioral Case Study: Child Abuse History and Bipolar Disorder

Roberta, a 34-year-old artist, begins session by telling the counselor that her partner says that if she does not change soon, she will leave her. Her partner's demands followed a weekend during which Roberta charged over $20,000 shopping, which led to several weeks of arguing and fighting afterwards. She says prior to her "good week," she had been depressed, not enjoying anything or wanting to get out of bed. She says that as a young adult she was diagnosed with bipolar disorder but stopped taking medication after a couple of months because it took away her creativity. She also mentions that she was molested by her brother as a child but her parents did not do much to protect her and now are apologetic for not doing more. She has a close relationship now with her mother but less so with her father and brother.

CASE CONCEPTUALIZATION

Date: March 11, 2013 **Clinician:** Mary Ellen **Client/Case #:** 10482

I. Introduction to Client

Identify primary client and significant others

Client

Adult Female Age: 34 Caucasian Partnered Gay/Lesbian/Bisexual Occupation/Grade: Self-employed artist (paint, various media) Other: Lives near parents and siblings

Significant Others

Client's Female Partner Age: 36 Caucasian Partnered Gay/Lesbian/Bisexual Occupation/Grade: Immigration attorney Other: ______

Select Person Age: ____ Select Ethnicity Select Relational Status Occupation/Grade: ____ Other: ____

Select Person Age: ____ Select Ethnicity Select Relational Status Occupation/Grade: ____ Other: ____

Select Person Age: ____ Select Ethnicity Select Relational Status Occupation/Grade: ____ Other: ____

Others: ______

II. Presenting Concern(s)

Client Description of Problem(s): States that she is coming to counseling because her girlfriend is tired of the "merry-go-round." She reports that she was diagnosed with bipolar as a young adult and stopped taking mood stabilizers a couple of months after they were prescribed because they dulled her creativity. She admits that she does get depressed, but she uses these times to inspire her art. Although she reports enjoying the "high" times, she is frustrated with some of the consequences, the most recent being a $20,000 credit card bill shopping in one week.

Significant Other/Family Description(s) of Problems: AF34's partner believes that AF34 should be on mood-stabilizing medications, because her life is a series of dramatic ups and downs. She is sympathetic to AF34's fears of losing her creativity, but thinks things have gotten so out of hand that something needs to be done. AF36 believes that if AF34 could learn to love herself better that she won't need all the drama.

Broader System Problem Descriptions: Description of problem from referring party, teachers, relatives, legal system, etc.:

Friends: AF34's friends agree with AF36 that things need to stabilize. They also believe that AF36, who is a highly organized business attorney, overfunctions for AF34, enabling her to be irresponsible.

____:____

III. Background Information

Trauma/Abuse History (recent and past): AF34 reports being sexually molested from age 8-11 by her older brother when her parents would leave for extended periods (3-4 times per year). When she first told her

(*continued*)

parents, they didn't fully believe or support her, saying it was just normal exploratory play, but they did take action to not leave the two alone. Several years later, after some large media cases, her mother finally came around to apologize for not taking her more seriously. Her brother has also apologized as a young adult. Her father now believes this is the reason for her sexual orientation.

Substance Use/Abuse (current and past; self, family of origin, significant others): AF34 describes herself as a social drinker who periodically goes out "partying" with her friends, usually during a manic episode. She reports experimenting with marajuana in her teens but rarely smoking as an adult. She does not report drinking problems in her family of origin or by her partner.

Precipitating Events (recent life changes, first symptoms, stressors, etc.): After her last art show 3 months ago, AF34 started slipping into a depression, not wanting to paint or do anything artistic. During this period, she stayed home, slept in, and managed the laundry and basic household tasks while her partner worked long hours at her law firm. Two weeks ago, an old friend visited and they went on a shopping spree, during which AF34 charged over $20,000 on her credit cards. After this, she and her partner had a series of arguments, which ended in AF36 saying that she would break up with her if AF34 didn't go to counseling and get her act together.

Related Historical Background (family history, related issues, previous counseling, etc.): AF34 was first diagnosed with bipolar disorder in college at age 22. Her psychiatrist prescribed a mood stabilizer, but AF34 refused to take it after a couple of months because "I lost my creativity." Since then, she has had 1–2 cycles per year, with several stabile months in between. She has seen counselors on and off, but reports none have really helped her. She reports that her mother believes her grandmother had similar issues.

IV. Client Strengths and Diversity

Client Strengths

Personal: AF34 is a creative artist who has recently begun showing her work; has a good sense of humor and strong independent streak.

Relational/Social: AF34 has a committed and capable partner; a large network of friends; supportive mother.

Spiritual: AF describes her art as her spiritual practice, which makes her feel alive and connected to something greater than herself.

Diversity: Resources and Limitations

Identify potential resources and limitations available to clients based on their age, gender, sexual orientation, cultural background, socioeconomic status, religion, regional community, language, family background, family configuration, abilities, etc.

Unique Resources: Strong support system within LGBT community as well as art community/culture. Multiple avenues for a sense of connection and acceptance.

(*continued*)

Potential Limitations: Father and brother have been withdrawn since she came out.

Complete All of the Following Sections for a Complete Case Conceptualization or Specific Sections for Theory-Specific Conceptualization.

V. Psychodynamic Conceptualization

Psychodynamic Defense Mechanisms

Check 2-4 most commonly used defense mechanisms

❑ Acting Out: *Describe:* ______

☒ Denial: *Describe:* AF denies the severity of her problems and does not recognize their effects on others.

❑ Displacement: *Describe:* ______

☒ Help-rejecting complaining: *Describe:* When depressed, AF frequently complains about how bad her life is but refuses to accept help or do anything to change the situation.

☒ Humor: *Describe:* AF uses humor to deflect criticism about her manic behaviors.

❑ Passive Aggression: *Describe:* ______

❑ Projection: *Describe:* ______

☒ Projective Identification: *Describe:* After an episode, AF sees others as irresponsible and the reason for her problems.

❑ Rationalization: *Describe:* ______

❑ Reaction Formation: *Describe:* ______

❑ Repression: *Describe:* ______

☒ Splitting: *Describe:* AF often justifies her behavior by villainizing her partner; at other times describes her as a savior.

☒ Sublimation: *Describe:* AF uses her art to channel and process various emotions.

❑ Suppression: *Describe:* ______

❑ Other: ______

Object Relational Patterns

Describe relationship with early caregivers in past: AF's parents were loving and attentive when they were at home. However, her father traveled often for work and her mother began to travel with him as well when the kids got a little older. They left the children in the care of relatives when they were away for extended periods of time. Growing up, AF felt as though her brother was the favorite, especially in the eyes of her father. This feeling intensified after her parents were unsupportive of the reported abuse by her brother.

Was the attachment with the mother (or equivalent) primarily:

☒ Generally Secure ❑ Anxious and Clingy ❑ Avoidant and Emotionally Distant ❑ Other: ______

Was the attachment with the father (or equivalent) primarily: ______

❑ Generally Secure ❑ Anxious and Clingy ☒ Avoidant and Emotionally Distant ❑ Other: ______

(*continued*)

Describe present relationship with these caregivers: AF's relationship with her parents improved after her mother apologized for not being more supportive when the abuse was initially disclosed. Her relationship with her father is still strained since he is very close with her brother and does not completely approve of her sexual orientation.

Describe relational patterns with partner and other current relationships: AF depends on her girlfriend for emotional support; however is quick to distance herself from her if she feels she is not being supportive of her creativity or more relaxed approach to life.

Erickson's Psychosocial Developmental Stage

Describe development at each stage up to current stage

Trust vs. Mistrust (Infant Stage): AF reports "normal" infancy.

Autonomy vs. Shame and Doubt (Toddler Stage): AF reports mother took care of her and brother; father worked and was distant.

Initiative vs. Guilt (Preschool Age): Although shy, AF generally did well socially and in early academic work.

Industry vs. Inferiority (School Age): AF sexually abused by brother during this time, which resulted in her overinvesting in being perfect at school.

Identity vs. Role Confusion (Adolescence): Reports painful adolescence, when she struggled with sexual identity.

Intimacy vs. Isolation (Young Adulthood): During this period "came out" and began having first intimate relationships in college.

Generativity vs. Stagnation (Adulthood): AF currently has periods of great generativity alternated with stagnation.

Ego Integrity vs. Despair (Late Adulthood): ______

Adlerian Style of Life Theme

❑ Control: ______

❑ Superiority: ______

❑ Pleasing: ______

☒ Comfort: AF seeks comfort, fun, and excitement, often at the expense of stability, relationships, and security.

Basic Mistake Misperceptions: AF believes life should take less effort than is realistic; she also minimizes her basic worth.

VI. Humanistic-Existential Conceptualization

Expression of Authentic Self

Problems: Are problems perceived as internal or external (caused by others, circumstance, etc.)?

❑ Predominantly internal

❑ Mixed

☒ Predominantly external

(continued)

Agency and Responsibility: Is self or other discussed as agent of story? Does client take clear responsibility for situation?

❑ Strong sense of agency and responsibility

❑ Agency in some areas

☒ Little agency; frequently blames others/situation

☒ Often feels victimized

Recognition and Expression of Feelings: Are feelings readily recognized, owned, and experienced?

☒ Easily expresses feelings

❑ Identifies feelings with prompting

❑ Difficulty recognizing feelings

Here-and-Now Experiencing: Is the client able to experience full range of feelings as they are happening in the present moment?

❑ Easily experiences emotions in present moment

☒ Experiences some present emotions with assistance

❑ Difficulty with present moment experiencing

Personal Constructs and Facades: Is the client able to recognize and go beyond roles? Is identity rigid or tentatively held?

❑ Tentatively held; able to critique and question

❑ Some awareness of facades and construction of identity

☒ Identity rigidly defined; seems like "fact"

Complexity and Contradictions: Are internal contradictions owned and explored? Is client able to fully engage the complexity of identity and life?

❑ Aware of and resolves contradictions

☒ Some recognition of contradictions

❑ Unaware of internal contradictions

Shoulds: Is client able to question socially imposed shoulds and oughts? Can client balance desire to please others and desire to be authentic?

❑ Able to balance authenticity with social obligation

☒ Identifies tension between social expectations and personal desires

❑ Primarily focuses on external shoulds

List shoulds: ______________________________

Acceptance of Others: Is client able to accept others and modify expectations of others to be more realistic?

❑ Readily accepts others as they are

☒ Recognizes expectations of others are unrealistic but still strong emotional reaction to expectations not being met

❑ Difficulty accepting others as is; always wanting others to change to meet expectations

Trust of Self: Is client able to trust self as process (rather than a stabile object)?

❑ Able to trust and express authentic self

❑ Trust of self in certain contexts

☒ Difficulty trusting self in most contexts

Existential Analysis

Sources of Life Meaning (as described or demonstrated by client): ______________________________

General Themes of Life Meaning:

☒ Personal achievement/work

☒ Significant other

(continued)

❑ Children
❑ Family of origin
☒ Social cause/contributing to others
❑ Religion/spirituality
❑ Other: ______

Satisfaction with and clarity on life direction:
❑ Clear sense of meaning that creates resilience in difficult times
☒ Current problems require making choices related to life direction
❑ Minimally satisfied with current life direction; wants more from life
❑ Has reflected little on life direction up to this point; living according to life plan defined by someone/something else
❑ Other: ______

Gestalt Contact Boundary Disturbances
❑ *Desensitization:* Failing to notice problems
☒ *Introjection*: Take in others' views whole and unedited
❑ *Projection*: Assign undesired parts of self to others
❑ *Retroflection*: Direct action to self rather than other
❑ *Deflection*: Avoid direct contact with another or self
❑ *Egotism:* Not allowing outside to influence self
❑ *Confluence*: Agree with another to extent that boundary blurred

Describe: AF34 is extremely sensitive to criticism, especially from her significant other.

VII. Cognitive-Behavioral Conceptualization

Baseline of Symptomatic Behavior

Symptom #1 (behavioral description): Depressive episodes that involve sleeping 10+ hours per day; increased eating; loss of interest in normal activities; partial withdrawal from friendships; loss of creativity; feeling as though life is pointless.

Frequency: 2-3 times per year

Duration: 1-3 months each

Context(s): Most noticable in work context (lack of productivity).

Events Before: Often after achieving major life goal.

Events After: May have a manic episode afterwards.

Symptom #2 (behavioral description): Manic episodes that involve irresponsible shopping sprees, unusually excessive social activity, excessive talking, requiring less sleep (5 hours or less), more argumentative with partner; more creative and productive with art.

Frequency: 1-2 times per year.

Duration: 3-4 days

Context(s): Affects all areas of functioning: relationship, work, friends, etc.

Events Before: Often preceded by period of depression or feeling "blah"

Events After: Fights with partner; productive period of artistic creativity (working with ideas generated during episode).

(continued)

A-B-C Analysis of Irrational Beliefs

Activating Event ("Problem"): Argument with partner over erratic behavior

Consequence (Mood, behavior, etc.): Angry, defensive, distance in relationship

Mediating Beliefs (Unhelpful beliefs about event that result in C):

1. Anyone who criticizes me does not understand or appreciate what is unique and special about me.
2. Life isn't fun unless I can "let go" and enjoy myself.
3. Everyone is always judging me.

Beck's Schema Analysis

Identify frequently used cognitive schemas:

❑ *Arbitrary inference:* ______

☒ *Selective abstraction:* Finds negative elements in neutral comments

❑ *Overgeneralization:* ______

☒ *Magnification/Minimization:* Overreacts to criticism; minimizes severity of her problems.

❑ *Personalization:* ______

☒ *Absolutist/dichotomous thinking:* Sees situations in black-and-white (e.g., art is great or horrible)

❑ *Mislabeling:* ______

❑ *Mindreading:* ______

VIII. Family Systems Conceptualization

Family Life Cycle Stage

☒ Single adult
❑ Marriage
❑ Family with Young Children
❑ Family with Adolescent Children
❑ Launching Children
❑ Later Life

Describe struggles with mastering developmental tasks in one of these stages: AF34's bipolar disorder at times interferes with her success in her work as an artist as well as her relationship with her partner.

Boundaries with

Parents	☒ Enmeshed	❑ Clear	❑ Disengaged	❑ NA: *Describe:* Generally close but can still be very reactive when father or mother make a critical comment.
Significant Other	☒ Enmeshed	❑ Clear	❑ Disengaged	❑ NA: *Describe:* AF is highly enmeshed with AF36, closely identifying herself with the relationship and very reactive to AF36's opinion of her.
Children	❑ Enmeshed	❑ Clear	❑ Disengaged	❑ NA: *Describe:* ______
Extended Family	❑ Enmeshed	❑ Clear	☒ Disengaged	❑ NA: *Describe:* After abuse with her brother, AF has typically avoided him; they see each other during holidays with minimal exchanges otherwise.
Other: Name ______	❑ Enmeshed	❑ Clear	❑ Disengaged	❑ NA: *Describe:* ______

(*continued*)

Typical style for regulating closeness and distance with others: Makes friends quickly and easily, but when they do not behave as she thinks they should, she "cools" the friendship. This pattern stems from family of origin in which members would act very close and simply avoid each other when there was conflict.

Triangles/Coalitions

☒ Coalition in family of origin: *Describe:* During childhood, AF felt that parents took brother's side; now she believes they are closer to her, especially her mother.

❑ Coalitions related to significant other: *Describe:* ______

❑ Other coalitions: ______

Hierarchy between Self and Parent/Child ☒ NA

With own children ❑ Effective ❑ Rigid ❑ Permissive

With parents (for child/young adult) ☒ Effective ❑ Rigid ❑ Permissive

Complementary Patterns with AF36:

❑ Pursuer/distancer

☒ Over-/underfunctioner

❑ Emotional/logical

❑ Good/bad parent

❑ Other: *Describe*

Example of complementary pattern: AF36 and AF34 have exaggerated over-/underfunctioner patterns with AF36 paying for most expenses and being the responsible one in the relationship. AF36 is also labeled as the logical one, and AF34 the artistic and emotional one.

Intergenerational Patterns

Substance/Alcohol Abuse: ☒ NA ❑ History: ______

Sexual/Physical/Emotional Abuse: ❑ NA ☒ History: AF34 sexually abused by brother from 8–11 years old.

Parent/Child Relations: ❑ NA ☒ History: AF felt estranged from parents from 11–18 when they thought the abuse was more "sexual exploration."

Physical/Mental Disorders: ❑ NA ☒ History: AF's grandmother possibly had bipolar, too.

Family strengths: Describe: AF's family supported her education and artistic talents; they are generally accepting of her sexual orientation; have apologized for abuse issues.

IX. Solution-Based and Cultural Discourse Conceptualization (Postmodern)

Solutions and Unique Outcomes

Attempted Solutions that DIDN'T or DON'T work:

1. Arguing with AF36.
2. AF36 threatening to stop supporting her or breaking up.
3. Avoiding AF36 by hanging out with party friends.

(continued)

Exceptions and Unique Outcomes: Times, places, relationships, contexts, etc. when problem is less of a problem; behaviors that seem to make things even slightly better:

1. AF's mood is always better when her art career is going well.
2. She can "pull herself together" and be responsible for work or when her partner needs her emotional support.
3. Getting regular sleep and exercise seems to reduce mood symptoms.

Miracle Question Answer: If the problem were to be resolved overnight, what would client be doing differently the next day? (Describe in terms of doing X rather than not doing Y).

1. She and her partner would get along more often than not.
2. She would feel more inspired to create art.
3. She would feel more in control over her moods and behaviors.

Dominant Discourses informing definition of problem:

- *Ethnic, Class and Religious Discourses: How do key cultural discourses inform what is perceived as a problem and the possible solutions?* AF's middle-class, Irish-American family did not value talking about emotions, problems, and she has continued this tradition in trying to avoid some of her current issues; her family generally avoids discussing or acknowledging her sexual orientation or bipolar tendencies.
- *Gender and Sexuality Discourses: How do the gender/sexual discourses inform what is perceived as a problem and the possible solutions?* AF spent her teen years struggling with her sexual orientation and came out in her early twenties; she is connected to a strong support group of professional lesbian women, who tend to see her issues as "just being emotional" and part of the stress of being marginalized.
- *Community, School, and Extended Family Discourses: How do other important community discourses inform what is perceived as a problem and the possible solutions?* AF is an aspiring artist and is heavily influenced by the trends, politics, and drama in the local art scene; she tries to impress the critics and key players, often hiding parts of herself to do so.

Identity Narratives: *How has the problem shaped each client's identity?* AF feels increasingly like a child and incompetent because she tends to make bad choices during her episodes. Comparing herself to her partner just makes her feel worse about herself. However, the ups and downs are also closely linked to her sense of being a vibrant and alive artist who feels life deeply and fully.

Local or Preferred Discourses: What is the client's preferred identity narrative and/or narrative about the problem? Are there local (alternative) discourses about the problem that are preferred? AF has mixed emotions about the roller coaster that is her life. At present, she wants to work on making more responsible decisions to feel less like a child in relation to her partner. She also wants to find a way to feel like an inspired artist with less drama in her personal life. She is strongly against using medications.

CLINICAL ASSESSMENT

Clinician: Mary Ellen	Client ID #: 10482	Primary configuration: ☒ Individual ❑ Couple ❑ Family	Primary Language: ☒ English ❑ Spanish ❑ Other: ______

List client and significant others

Adult(s)

Identified Patient: Adult Female Age: 34 Caucasian Partnered Gay/Lesbian/Bisexual Occupation: self-employed; artist Other identifier: ______

Adult Female Age: 36 Caucasian Partnered Gay/Lesbian/Bisexual Occupation: immigration attorney

Other identifier: ______

Child(ren)

Select Gender Age: ______ Select Ethnicity Grade: Select Grade School: ______ Other identifier: ______

Select Gender Age: ______ Select Ethnicity Grade: Select Grade School: ______ Other identifier: ______

Others: ______

Presenting Problems

		Complete for children:
☒ Depression/hopelessness	☒ Couple concerns	❑ School failure/decline performance
❑ Anxiety/worry	❑ Parent/child conflict	❑ Truancy/runaway
❑ Anger issues	❑ Partner violence/abuse	❑ Fighting w/peers
❑ Loss/grief	❑ Divorce adjustment	❑ Hyperactivity
❑ Suicidal thoughts/attempts	❑ Remarriage adjustment	❑ Wetting/soiling clothing
☒ Sexual abuse/rape	❑ Sexuality/intimacy concerns	❑ Isolation/withdrawal
❑ Alcohol/drug use	❑ Major life changes	❑ Other: ______
❑ Eating problems/disorders	❑ Legal issues/probation	
☒ Job problems/unemployed	❑ Other: ______	

Mental Status Assessment for Identified Patient

Interpersonal	❑ NA	☒ Conflict ☒ Enmeshment ❑ Isolation/avoidance ❑ Harassment ❑ Other: ______
Mood	❑ NA	☒ Depressed/Sad ❑ Anxious ❑ Dysphoric ❑ Angry ❑ Irritable ☒ Manic ❑ Other: ______
Affect	❑ NA	❑ Constricted ❑ Blunt ❑ Flat ☒ Labile ❑ Incongruent ☒ Other: **Dramatic**
Sleep	❑ NA	☒ Hypersomnia ❑ Insomnia ❑ Disrupted ❑ Nightmares ❑ Other: ______

(continued)

Eating	❑ NA	☒ Increase ❑ Decrease ❑ Anorectic restriction ❑ Binging ❑ Purging ❑ Other: ______
Anxiety	☒ NA	❑ Chronic worry ❑ Panic ❑ Phobias ❑ Obsessions ❑ Compulsions ❑ Other: ______
Trauma Symptoms	❑ NA	❑ Hypervigilance ❑ Flashbacks/Intrusive memories ❑ Dissociation ❑ Numbing ❑ Avoidance efforts ☒ Other: Dreams; emotional numbness
Psychotic Symptoms	☒ NA	❑ Hallucinations ❑ Delusions ❑ Paranoia ❑ Loose associations ❑ Other: ______
Motor Activity/ Speech	❑ NA	❑ Low energy ☒ Hyperactive ❑ Agitated ❑ Inattentive ❑ Impulsive ❑ Pressured speech ❑ Slow speech ❑ Other: ______
Thought	❑ NA	❑ Poor concentration ☒ Denial ❑ Self-blame ☒ Other-blame ❑ Ruminative ☒ Tangential ❑ Concrete ❑ Poor insight ☒ Impaired decision making ❑ Disoriented ❑ Other: ______
Socio-Legal	☒ NA	❑ Disregards rules ❑ Defiant ❑ Stealing ❑ Lying ❑ Tantrums ❑ Arrest/incarceration ❑ Initiates fights ❑ Other: ______
Other Symptoms	☒ NA	______

Diagnosis for Identified Patient

Contextual Factors considered in making diagnosis: ☒ Age ☒ Gender ☒ Family dynamics ❑ Culture ❑ Language ❑ Religion ❑ Economic ❑ Immigration ☒ Sexual/gender orientation ❑ Trauma ❑ Dual diagnosis/comorbid ❑ Addiction ❑ Cognitive ability ☒ Other: Artists community/culture

Describe impact of identified factors on diagnosis and assessment process: Considered Irish American family dynamics and emotional patterns as well as stereotypical gender/lesbian/artist patterns re: emotional expression; used "clinical impairment" as reported by client and partner as key criteria for determining diagnosis.

DSM-5 Code	Diagnosis with Specifier *Include V/Z/T-Codes for Psychosocial Stressors/Issues*
1. F31.81	1. Bipolar II Disorder
2. Z62.810	2. Personal history (past history) of sexual abuse in childhood
3. ______	3. ______
4. ______	4. ______
5. ______	5. ______

(*continued*)

Medical Considerations

Has patient been referred for psychiatric evaluation? ☒ Yes ❑ No

Has patient agreed with referral? ❑ Yes ☒ No ❑ NA

Psychometric instruments used for assessment: ☒ None ☒ Cross-cutting symptom inventories ❑ Other: ________

Client response to diagnosis: ☒ Agree ❑ Somewhat agree ❑ Disagree ❑ Not informed for following reason: ______

Current Medications (psychiatric & medical) ☒ NA

1. ______; dose ______ mg; start date: ______
2. ______; dose ______ mg; start date: ______
3. ______; dose ______ mg; start date: ______
4. ______; dose ______ mg; start date: ______

Medical Necessity: *Check all that apply*

☒ Significant impairment ❑ Probability of significant impairment ❑ Probable developmental arrest

Areas of impairment: ☒ Daily activities ☒ Social relationships ❑ Health ☒ Work/School ❑ Living arrangement

❑ Other: ____________________

Risk and Safety Assessment for Identified Patient

Suicidality	**Homicidality**	**Alcohol Abuse**
❑ No indication/Denies	☒ No indication/Denies	❑ No indication/denies
❑ Active ideation	❑ Active ideation	❑ Past abuse
☒ Passive ideation	❑ Passive ideation	☒ Current; Freq/Amt: 4-5 drinks when out with friends; 2-3 times per year.
❑ Intent without plan	❑ Intent without means	**Drug Use/Abuse**
❑ Intent with means	❑ Intent with means	❑ No indication/denies
☒ Ideation in past year	❑ Ideation in past year	☒ Past use
❑ Attempt in past year	❑ Violence past year	☒ Current drugs: Marijuana
❑ Family or peer history of completed suicide	❑ History of assaulting others	Freq/Amt: 2-3 times per year
	❑ Cruelty to animals	❑ Family/sig.other use

Sexual & Physical Abuse and Other Risk Factors

☒ Childhood abuse history: ☒ Sexual ❑ Physical ❑ Emotional ❑ Neglect

❑ Adult with abuse/assault in adulthood: ❑ Sexual ❑ Physical ❑ Current

❑ History of perpetrating abuse: ❑ Sexual ❑ Physical ❑ Emotional

❑ Elder/dependent adult abuse/neglect

❑ History of or current issues with restrictive eating, binging, and/or purging

❑ Cutting or other self harm: ❑ Current ❑ Past: Method: ____________

❑ Criminal/legal history: ____________________

❑ Other trauma history: ____________________

❑ None reported

(continued)

Indicators of Safety

❑ NA

☒ At least one outside support person

☒ Able to cite specific reasons to live or not harm

❑ Hopeful

☒ Willing to dispose of dangerous items

☒ Has future goals

❑ Willingness to reduce contact with people who make situation worse

❑ Willing to implement safety plan, safety interventions

☒ Developing set of alternatives to self/other harm

☒ Sustained period of safety: 2 months

❑ Other: ____________

Elements of Safety Plan

❑ NA

☒ Verbal no harm contract

❑ Written no harm contract

☒ Emergency contact card

☒ Emergency therapist/agency number

❑ Medication management

❑ Plan for contacting friends/support persons during crisis

❑ Specific plan of where to go during crisis

☒ Specific self-calming tasks to reduce risk before reach crisis level (e.g., journaling, exercising, etc.)

❑ Specific daily/weekly activities to reduce stressors

❑ Other: ____________

Legal/Ethical Action Taken: ☒ NA ❑ Action: ____________

Case Management

Collateral Contacts

- Has contact been made with treating *physicians or other professionals*: ☒ NA ❑ Yes ❑ In process. Name/Notes: ____________
- If client is involved in mental health *treatment elsewhere*, has contact been made? ☒ NA ❑ Yes ❑ In process. Name/Notes: ____________
- Has contact been made with *social worker*: ☒ NA ❑ Yes ❑ In process. Name/Notes: ____________

Referrals

- Has client been referred for *medical assessment*: ☒ Yes ❑ No evidence for need
- Has client been referred for *social services*: ☒ NA ❑ Job/training ❑ Welfare/Food/Housing ❑ Victim services ❑ Legal aid ❑ Medical ❑ Other: ____________
- Has client been referred for *group* or other support services: ☒ Yes:_______ ❑ In process ❑ None recommended
- Are there anticipated *forensic/legal processes* related to treatment: ☒ No ❑ Yes; describe: ____________

Support Network

- Client social support network includes: ☒ Supportive family ☒ Supportive partner ☒ Friends ❑ Religious/spiritual organization ☒ Supportive work/social group ❑ Other: ____________

(*continued*)

- Describe anticipated effects treatment will have on others in support system (Children, partner, etc.): As AF becomes more functional, this will change the over-/underfunctioning pattern for couple and will shift the balance of power.
- Is there anything else client will need to be successful? May want to try alternative health options since refusing to use medications.

Expected Outcome and Prognosis

☒ Return to normal functioning ❑ Anticipate less than normal functioning ❑ Prevent deterioration

Client Sense of Hope: 5 Moderate hope

Evaluation of Assessment/Client Perspective

How were assessment methods adapted to client needs, including age, culture, and other diversity issues? Included Z62.810 to address any lingering abuse issues that may be affecting client; deferred until bipolar issues are stabilized; carefully considered diversity issues—especially emotional expression biases—before making diagnosis.

Describe actual or potential areas of client-clinician agreement/disagreement related to the above assessment: AF would agree; strong emphasis on not taking medications.

______________________, ______________ ______________

Clinician Signature License/Intern Status Date

______________________, ______________ ______________

Supervisor Signature License Date

TREATMENT PLAN

Date: October 3, 2013 — Case/Client #: 10482

Clinician Name: Mary Ellen — Theory: Cognitive-Behavioral

Modalities planned: ☒ Individual Adult ❑ Individual Child ☒ Couple ❑ Family ❑ Group: ______

Recommended session frequency: ☒ Weekly ❑ Every two weeks ❑ Other: ______

Expected length of treatment: 12 months

Initial Phase of Treatment

Initial Phase Counseling Tasks

1. Develop working counseling relationship. *Diversity considerations:* Ensure client and couple feels understood and accepted as individuals and as couple.

   Relationship building approach/intervention:

   a. Use warmth and empathy to build relationship; establish credibility.

2. Assess individual, systemic, and broader cultural dynamics. *Diversity considerations:* Include assessment of dynamics within network of lesbian friends and art/legal community.

   Assessment strategies:

   a. Obtain baseline of depressive-manic cycle; functional analysis of problem behaviors and thoughts; DSM diagnosis; consult with former psychiatrist and counselors on diagnosis.

   b. Identify schemas and core beliefs related to self-worth and "excitement" in life, noting effects of childhood abuse, sexual marginalization, and Irish American preference to avoid discussing problems.

3. Identify and obtain client agreement on treatment goals. *Diversity note:* ethical issues related to client wish to not be on medication.

   Goal-making intervention:

   a. Develop written contract with goals and investment required to meet goals without using medication to assist.

4. Identify needed referrals, crisis issues, and other client needs. *Note:* Ethical and safety issues related to desire to not use medications.

   a. *Crisis assessment intervention(s):* Discuss safety issues and plan related to history of self-harm and periodic partying. Discuss ethical and medical implications of not taking medications and identify potential alternatives and/or timeline for revisiting topic.

   b. *Referral(s):* Refer to DBT group to develop greater tolerance of contradictory emotions.

(continued)

Initial Phase Client Goal

1. Decrease impulsive decisions regarding money to reduce irresponsible behaviors and manic behaviors.

   Interventions:

   a. Develop contract and plan for how to manage future impulses.

   b. Choice theory to motivate client to make responsible financial decisions.

Working Phase of Treatment

Working Phase Counseling Tasks

1. Monitor quality of the working alliance. *Diversity considerations:* Monitor AF in-session responses to ensure she feels understood; use sensitive and appropriate language.

   a. *Assessment Intervention:* Session Rating Scale; verbally ask about alliance and address any signs of resistance.

2. Monitor progress toward goals. *Diversity considerations:* Consider stressors related to marginalization when assessing progress.

   a. *Assessment Intervention:* Outcome rating scale; symptom checklist.

Working Phase Client Goals

1. Increase ability to question "shoulds" and "oughts" about what others should do to reduce depressive and manic symptoms.

   Interventions:

   a. Dispute irrational beliefs about always being liked by others using REBT Self-Help Form and Thought records; address negative beliefs from abuse.

   b. Alter beliefs about need life to be "exciting" and "dramatic" in order to be a good artist.

2. Increase responsibility and functioning in partnership to reduce reliance on partner to maintain stable life and household (symptom).

   Interventions:

   a. Examine cognitive schemas about self and abilities, including those related to childhood abuse.

   b. Cost/benefit analysis to develop motivation and improve decision making skills.

3. Increase realistic beliefs related to needing drama for life to be exciting and having inspiration for art to reduce depressive episodes.

   Interventions:

   a. Socratic dialogue around core beliefs and schemas related to needing drama to feel valuable and alive.

   b. Thought records to reinforce alternative beliefs about drama.

(continued)

Closing Phase of Treatment

Closing Phase Counseling Task

1. Develop aftercare plan and maintain gains. *Diversity considerations:* Assess progress without medication and revisit the possibility.

   Intervention:

   a. Develop system for identfying warning signs of depression or hypomanic-type behaviors and develop healthy behaviors and thoughts.

Closing Phase Client Goals

1. Increase positive self-talk about worth that is less dependent on artistic creations or relationship status to reduce depressive moods.

   Interventions:

   a. Stress innoculation training to increase positive self-talk related to art critiques and comparison to partner.

   b. Thought records to reinforce positive thoughts about self regardless of performance and feedback from others; address negative thoughts that remain from abuse and/or marginalization related to sexual orientation.

2. Increase ability to recognize slight variations in mood and actions to mitigate to reduce mood cycling.

   Interventions:

   a. Develop active aftercare/maintenance plan that includes quick responses to early depressive and/or hypomanic symptoms; develop motivation related to staying off medication.

   b. Develop mindfulness practice (MBCT class) to better monitor thoughts and emotions to reduce chances of depression relapse.

PROGRESS NOTE FOR CLIENT #10482

Date: March 30, 2013 **Time:** 4:00 ❑ am/☒ pm **Session Length:** ☒ 45 min. ❑ 60 min. ❑ Other: _______ minutes

Present: ❑ Adult Male ☒ Adult Female ❑ Child Male ❑ Child Female ❑ Other: ______________________

Billing Code: ❑ 90791 (eval) ☒ 90834 (45 min. therapy) ❑ 90837 (60 min. therapy) ❑ 90847 (family)

❑ Other: ______________________

Symptom(s)	Duration and Frequency Since Last Visit	Progress
1: Loss of interest/low energy	2 days; mild episodes; managed with self-talk	**Progressing**
2: Magnification	Most days of week; mild epsodes; able to use self-talk to reduce intensity	**Progressing**
3: Irresponsible choices	No significant episodes this week	**Progressing**

Explanatory Notes on Symptoms: AF highly motivated to use skills learned in session to manage mood and behavioral symptoms by monitoring thoughts with self-talk and thought records.

In-Session Interventions and Assigned Homework

Followed up on thought records from last week and added second element of "adaptive response"; AF able to generate alternative perspectives relatively easily; linked to artistic skills of seeing life from other perspectives. Reviewed plan for managing moods and AF's success and struggles with plan; problem solving for managing mood when in large social group. Assigned full thought record this week with adaptive response sections.

Client Response/Feedback

Client is highly motivated to try to manage moods with cognitive strategies; particularly enthusiastic about viewing "adaptive response" as an artisitc rendition of the mundane world.

Plan

☒ Continue with treatment plan: plan for next session: Follow up on thought record

❑ Modify plan: ______________________

Next session: Date: April 7, 2013 Time: 4:00 ❑ am/☒ pm

Crisis Issues: ☒ No indication of crisis/client denies ❑ Crisis assessed/addressed: describe below

______________________, ______________________ ______________________

Clinician's Signature, License/Intern Status Date

Case Consultation/Supervision ❑ Not Applicable

Notes: Supervisor satisfied with progress; recommends preparing client for potential setbacks with self-talk messages to handle setbacks.

(*continued*)

Collateral Contact ❑ Not Applicable

Name: Dr. Dana Rodriguez Date of Contact: March 30, 2012 Time: 2:00 ❑ am/☒ pm

☒ Written release on file: ☒ Sent/❑ Received ❑ In court docs ❑ Other: ______________________

Notes: Spoke briefly with MD to review treatment plan; discuss AF decision to not use medications; discussed safety measures; informed MD no signs of danger presently but has had suicidal thoughts and self-harm in past year. Will call MD if client experiences setbacks.

______________________,	______________________	______________________
Clinician's Signature,	License/Intern Status	Date
______________________,	______________________	______________________
Supervisor's Signature,	License	Date

CHAPTER

12

Systemic Family Counseling and Therapy

Lay of the Land

Systemic counseling approaches were originally developed for work with couples and families. They represent a unique set of theories that conceptualize an individual's symptoms as arising within family and relational dynamics and serving to balance the family dynamics in some way. For this reason, even when a person is presenting with an "individual problem," such as depression or anxiety, systemic counselors often work with significant others in the person's life, such as a partner or family. Developed in the 1960s, systemic approaches represented such a radically new way of working that they inspired a separate discipline and license to support this distinctive approach. In fact, the field of family therapy, which is the focus of those who study to become marriage and family therapists (MFT or LMFT), has enough theories to fill its own textbook; and, as you may already know, there are several on the topic (Gehart, 2014; Goldenberg & Goldenberg, 2012; Nichols, 2012).

Thus, I will not endeavor in this text to scantily cover the same material that fills several others books—that would guarantee my failure *and* a funky treatment plan and would most likely leave even the brightest readers more confused than when they began (I have had several students report hurling confusing texts across the room, so my most modest goal here is to not go splat!). Instead, this chapter will present a *general, integrated systemic counseling approach* that counselors, psychologists, social workers, and family counselors can use as their primary theoretical approach for working with individuals, couples, and families. At the very least, systemic ideas are useful to counselors of any theoretical stripe during the initial case conceptualization process to identify systemic dynamics that may be affecting an individual (see Chapter 2) or when working with couples or families. In short, I hope to provide a meaningful, coherent, integrated systemic counseling approach rather than briefly review each of the 15-plus family therapy approaches that rightly deserve their own book.

In this chapter I distinguish *systemic family counseling* from generic "family counseling," which can refer to a wide range of counseling models, including, Adlerian, solution-focused, or psychodynamic family counseling. I use the term *systemic* as it is generally used in counseling, psychology, and social work, which is quite different from the use of the term systemic within the field of family therapy, where virtually all of the theories are systemic and thus they must make finer distinctions. Translated into the more delicately delineated language in the field of family therapy, this chapter will specifically cover a structural-strategic family therapy approach, which is the most commonly used, especially in newer evidence-based approaches. The other major family therapy schools, Bowen's intergenerational and Satir's human growth model, will be briefly described in clearly marked, special sections, and they are described in greater detail with model-specific treatment plans elsewhere for curious readers (Gehart, 2014).

In a Nutshell: The Least You Need to Know

Systemic counselors always view a person as inherently part of larger *relational systems*, which include the *family of origin* (mother, father, siblings, extended family), *family of procreation* (spouse, partner, children, stepchildren, and so on), social communities (e.g., church, neighborhoods, and even online communities), and broader societal groups (such as gay/lesbian communities, ethnic communities, region, state, nation, and so forth). Systemic counselors radically propose that a person's problems or symptoms are inherently related to the dynamics of these systems; thus, an individual's depression (or fill in the blank with any other symptom) plays a role in maintaining a sense of "normalcy" in the system. *Simultaneously* (and this is critical to the approach's success), systemic counselors maintain a *nonpathologizing* position, not blaming persons within the system or the system itself for the symptoms (Jackson, 1967). Instead, symptoms are viewed more *neutrally* and with curious enthusiasm—much like an anthropologist trying to understand a long-lost culture—as a set of behaviors, feelings, and beliefs that help the system maintain a sense of balance or *homeostasis*. In the tiniest of nutshells, systemic counselors see their jobs as helping individuals and families find new relational patterns that do not require the symptom for the system or its members to feel balanced and connected.

Systemic counselors are the Zen masters of the counseling world: their interventions are rarely logical on the surface, and they get people thinking by using surprising Zen-like koans. Much like a martial artist, they work *with* the symptoms, taking their energy and redirecting them in more productive ways rather than trying to forcefully stop a problem behavior, thought, or feeling. Thus, they *do not* reeducate individuals and families on how to better relate, as do Adlerians and cognitive counselors. Instead, system counselors use a wide variety of techniques to interrupt and redirect problem behavior sequences, often allowing the family to develop its own new ways of responding. They conceptualize families using two basic paradigms: (a) family structure: boundaries, hierarchy, and subsystems, and (b) systemic interaction patterns: repetitive interaction cycles related to the problem. Systemic counselors are *strength-focused*, never seeing individuals or families as dysfunctional, but rather seeing people who need assistance in expanding their repertoire of interaction patterns to adjust to the ever-changing developmental and contextual demands.

The Juice: Significant Contributions to the Field

If there is one thing you remember from this chapter, it should be ...

Enactments

Perhaps the most practical and researched systemic intervention, counselors use *enactments* to redirect symptom-laden interactions toward interaction patterns that are more effective and satisfying (Colapinto, 1991; Minuchin, 1974; Minuchin & Fishman, 1981). Regardless of whichever counseling model you choose to use in the end, you will need to master enactments. Why? Because most couples and families are going to start arguing in your office whether you ask them or not, and even individual clients may need to be coached in how to appropriately communicate. So you'd better be prepared! Enactments are one of the best ways to handle dicey, difficult moments in session (or in the waiting room).

Systemic counselors prefer enactments to talking about interactions because often people describe themselves as one way but behave quite differently (clearly this does not apply to you or me; we are speaking hypothetically, of course). This incongruity is not because people are malicious or hypocritical but because it often is difficult to clearly see how our behavior looks from the outside (Minuchin & Fishman, 1981). Enactments are used to both assess and alter the problematic interactional sequences, allowing the counselor to *map*, *track*, and *modify* the family structure or an individual's interaction patterns.

As a counselor becomes more experienced, it requires only a couple of minutes of listening to an individual recount a problem situation or watching a family interact to quickly know where and how to *restructure* boundaries and other relational structures. Restructuring may take the form of creating a clearer boundary in enmeshed relationships (e.g., stopping people from interrupting and speaking for one another), increasing engagement by encouraging the expression of empathy or direct eye contact, or improving parental effectiveness by helping the parent successfully manage a child's in-session behavior.

An enactment occurs in three phases (Minuchin & Fishman, 1981):

Phase 1: Tracking and Mapping: Observation of Spontaneous Interactions: When talking with an individual or family, the counselor closely follows both content and metacommunication, listening for the assumptions that coordinate the interactions, such as demands for intense intimacy, independence, or control, as well as strengths and abilities (Watzlawick, Bavelas, & Jackson, 1967). When talking with clients, the counselor *tracks actual transactions* (what is done in session) more closely than verbal accounts (Colapinto, 1991). Gathering information for what is observed, the content of what is said, and the metacommunication, the counselor develops a working hypothesis that *maps* the family's boundaries and hierarchy (Minuchin & Fishman, 1981). Once counselors identify an area for change, they are ready to invite the individual or family into the active phase of enactment.

Phase 2: Eliciting Interaction: The Invitation: Counselors issue an "invitation" for an enactment in one of two ways: either by the counselor directly requesting the individual or family to enact a real-world interaction, or by the clients spontaneously engaging in the problematic behavior, usually in the form of an argument or stone-cold silence (Colapinto, 1991). Obviously, the counselor does not need to do much when the client spontaneously begins; otherwise, the counselor must issue an explicit invitation for the client to "show" the problem:

Eliciting Interaction

- "Can you reenact what happened last night?" or
- "Please show me what happens at home when he is 'defiant'; can you act out an incident of defiance that happened last week so I have a good idea of what the problem really is?"

Enactments can also be used with individuals by having them enact their half of the encounter and summarizing—or even using a puppet to say—what the other person said. Using enactments is important when working with individuals because it is easy to collude with them in blaming others. Although it solves nothing and typically makes the situation far worse (see triangulation below), blaming others without being held responsible for one's own half of the dynamic is a favorite recreational sport for many. Counselors can avoid this common helper's pitfall when working with individual clients by using enactments to keep both counselor and client focused on the only element in the system that they can affect: the client.

Phase 3: Redirecting Alternative Transactions: Up to this point, the enactment process has just been the more-of-the-same problem pattern and does not count as an intervention (and actually isn't helpful) until counselors actually help clients *do something different.* Thus, in this phase, the counselor redirects interaction patterns to clarify boundaries, hierarchy, subsystems, and other structural issues. How exactly counselors redirect the interaction depends on the particular dynamics assessed in Phase 1. Some of the more common ways systemic counselors redirect interactions includes:

- *Increase Parental Hierarchy*: Directing a parent to set limits for a child in session (rather than the counselor doing it).
- *Reduce Enmeshment:* Allowing each person to finish speaking and stopping interruptions.
- *Reduce Disengagement:* Encouraging a couple to share thoughts and feelings on difficult topics.
- *Reduce Triangulation:* Asking two people to talk directly to each other while asking a third (typically intrusive person) to remain quiet.
- *Clarify Boundaries:* Rearranging chairs physically to increase or decrease emotional closeness.
- *Alter Pattern with Individual:* Directing them to rephrase or "redeliver" a request or response as if the other person were present.

Minuchin and Fishman (1981) identify several benefits of enactments, including providing real-life practice in new behaviors, shattering the illusion that the problem belongs to "the other" person, and increasing a person's sense of competence and confidence in handling the problem situation better.

Big Picture: Overview of Treatment

Systemic counseling focuses on resolving the presenting problem with the counselor while imposing no other goals or agendas based on theories of normalcy. Systemic counselors view the presenting problem not as an individual problem but as a relational one, specifically an *interactional* one, even if the counselor is working with an individual (Cecchin, 1987; Haley, 1963, 1973, 1987). Systemic counselors conceptualize interaction using two lenses: (a) identifying problematic interaction sequences, and (b) mapping family structure, including boundaries, hierarchy, and coalitions. In this approach, neither an individual nor a relationship is considered "dysfunctional"; instead, the problem is viewed as part of the interactional sequence of behaviors that have emerged through repeated exchanges, with no one person to blame (the sure sign that a counselor does not understand systems theory is when they use the word "dysfunctional" or imply that if only person X changed, everyone else in the system would be fine).

In the early phase, the counselor observes and maps the problem behavior by obtaining a detailed description of the behavioral sequence surrounding the problem and by observing how clients interact. Often counselors achieve this by having them *enact* the problem situation (see The Juice above). Once the counselor has identified the interactional behavioral patterns and meanings associated with the problem, the counselor uses one of many potential interventions to *interrupt* and *alter* this sequence—not necessarily correct it. By simply interrupting highly repetitive and rigid interaction patterns that constitute a problem (a problem wouldn't be a problem if it weren't highly repetitive and resistant to change), the system—which is inherently self-correcting and seeking balance—will effortless reconfigure itself around the new information that has been introduced. For example, if a man complains of frequent arguments with his partner, the counselor does not try to educate him in better communication skills. Instead, the counselor strives to simply *interrupt* the sequence by having him do *one thing different*, often a small, personally symbolic, easily achieved behavioral change—such as scheduling arguments at random times during the week or passing a symbolic object during the argument. Alternatively, the counselor may offer a reframe to give new meaning to the arguments that radically alter how they are viewed, for example, as a way to build connection and in some special way show love. Another option would be an enactment to help the client find new ways to interact more effectively. Any of these tactics of change will interrupt the problem sequence and allow for self-correction, resulting in new actions, thoughts, and behaviors.

Counselors frequently give clients some form of homework, sometimes a specific behavioral task or a cognitive reframing that highlights the systemic nature of the problem. Each week, the counselor follows up on the prior week's homework and then designs another task or reframe based on clients' responses. This continues just as long as is necessary to resolve the presenting problem, and then counseling is terminated. To recap, the general flow of systemic or strategic therapies is as follows:

The Process of Systemic Counseling

Step 1: Assess the Interactional Sequence, Family Structure, and Associated Meanings: Identify interactional behavior sequences that constitute the problem, including the actions and reactions of everyone in the system and the associated meanings; assess boundaries, hierarchy, subsystems, and coalitions (see Case Conceptualization below).

Step 2: Intervene by Interrupting and Redirecting the Interactional Sequence: Using a reframing technique or a task, the counselor interrupts the sequence, allowing the family to reorganize itself in response to the intervention. *The differences between the specific schools of MRI, Strategic, Milan, and Structural are primarily seen in the preferred method of interrupting the interactional sequence.* Contemporary practitioners generally borrow freely from all of these systemic approaches (hence, they are presented together in this chapter).

Step 3: Evaluate Outcome and Client Response: After the intervention, the counselor assesses the client's response and uses this information to design the next intervention.

Step 4: Interrupt the New Pattern: Then, the counselor interrupts the new pattern with another intervention. This continues—interrupting behavioral sequence, allowing family to reorganize and respond, and intervening again—until the problem is resolved.

Who's Involved

When possible, systemic counselors prefer to begin counseling with the persons most significant to the identified client in attendance, often the family or partner, to assess the relational system (Colapinto, 1991). Once the relational system has been assessed, the counselor may meet with specific subsystems and individuals to achieve particular goals. For example, often, sessions with the couple alone are necessary to strengthen the boundaries between the couple and parental subsystems and to sever cross-generational coalitions with children or in-laws. If seeing only an individual, the counselor still assesses the *entire relational system* as much as possible, often using *circular questions* (see interventions below) that trace how each person in the system responds to the other in situations involving the problem.

Making Connection: Counseling Relationship

Joining

Rather than conceptualize the counseling relationship in terms of empathy, transference, or rapport, systemic counselors build relationships with clients by recognizing that they are *joining* with the system that has its own distinct set of rules for communicating, showing respect, and making meaning (Minuchin, 1974; Minuchin & Fishman, 1981; Minuchin & Nichols, 1993). Rather than demonstrate understanding by verbally expressing empathy, systemic counselors "join" a system by accommodating to its style: how people talk, forms of emotional expression, pacing, and so forth. In the historical context of mental health, this is a radical concept in that the counseling relationship accommodates to the client rather than the inverse, making it more adaptable to various cultural groups.

Much like an anthropologist observing and studying a new culture, systemic counselors approach clients with abundant curiosity about how they make meaning, organize their relationships, handle power, solve problems, express love, hang tough, entertain themselves, and otherwise move through life (Minuchin, 1974). The process of joining can also be likened to learning a new dance. Do they talk fast or slow? Do they talk over one another or do they wait for clear pauses to speak? Do they use teasing and humor or are their words gentle and soft? A successful systemic counselor needs to have a wide repertoire of social skills to successfully join with families, especially when working with diverse populations. In the case study at the end of this chapter, the counselor joins with Billy, a young adult whose mother is Sioux, by respecting his preference for not having direct eye contact and by incorporating his religious beliefs and practices into the treatment plan.

Respecting and Trusting the System

Systemic counselors respect the *system* of which the client is a part and view it as an entity that has its unique *epistemology* or way of knowing and understanding the world. Fully and humbly aware that they do not have direct control over a system, systemic counselors have an abiding trust that the system will reorganize itself in new and better ways without the counselor forcing the change. Instead, the counselor provides opportunities—sometimes many opportunities—for the system to reorganize itself, using various interventions that are not designed to be the "solution" for the client but rather are designed to shake the system up and allow it to naturally resettle into its own solution. Symptoms are not seen as indicators of individual pathology but rather as the byproducts of interactional sequences in relational systems that have served a purpose (if you are paying attention, you will notice I repeat this point because it is hard to grasp, taking years to fully appreciate the implications).

Neutrality

As you can imagine, when you start working with more than one person in the room, counselors are invited many, many times both verbally and nonverbally to take sides: "Counselor [wink, wink] is it healthy, natural, or normal for a person to do or feel X?" Breathlessly, everyone in the room awaits your response to see whose side you will join. Answering this or other innocent-sounding questions typically leads down a painful, slippery slope and to the erosion of a good counseling relationship. All new counselors slip and slide several times before they finally learn, but at least you have been forewarned.

Knowing this, systemic counselors advocate a *neutral* stance when working with clients (Selvini Palazzoli et al., 1978, 1980). Neutrality is practiced in two ways: with *nonpartiality*, not taking sides on particular issues, and also with *multipartiality*, the willingness to honor all perspectives.

Maneuverability

Perhaps the most adaptable and flexible in terms of forming a working alliance, systemic counselors do not use a one-size-fits-all approach to developing the counseling relationship. Systemic counselors highly value *maneuverability*, the freedom to use personal judgment in defining the counseling relationship so that it is most likely to quickly effect change (Fisch, Weakland, & Segal, 1982; Nardone & Watzlawick, 1993; Segal, 1991; Watzlawick, Weakland, & Fisch, 1974). Depending on (a) the relational rules of the particular system, and (b) the presenting problem, the counselor may play the role of an expert or take a one-down, helpless stance (see below), depending on which stance seems to help clients reach their goals more quickly, not simply adhering to what the client prefers. Furthermore, the counselor may choose to be disliked by the client or be the "bad guy" in order to achieve the desired change in the system. Thus, in the working phase, the counselor may use different relational roles with different clients to promote change.

Social Courtesy

As a rare and refreshing use of social norms in counseling relationships, Haley (1987) describes the initial stage of counseling as the *social stage*, a time when the counselor engages in casual social conversation, about the weather or traffic, as a way of making clients comfortable and reducing their sense of shame: "the model for this stage is the courtesy behavior one would use with guests in the home" (p. 15). Before moving on to discussing the problem, the counselor ensures that all members have been properly greeted. During the social stage, the counselor is assessing interactions and moods in order to know how to begin moving into discussing the problem (Haley & Richeport-Haley, 2007). Even a few moments of "normal" social conversation can help clients feel more empowered, connected, and engaged, because the counseling relationship involves something familiar.

Spontaneity

Counseling spontaneity refers to the ability to flow naturally and authentically in a variety of contexts and situations, but it does not imply a throw-caution-to-the-wind and say-what-you-please approach. Instead, systemic spontaneity is a relationally and contextually responsive expression of self that is constrained by the relational rules of the system (Minuchin & Fishman, 1981, p. 3). Much the way driving a car becomes "natural" after years of practice, systemic spontaneity is cultivated and shaped through the training process, which increases counselors' repertoire for "being natural" in a wide range of clinical situations.

Observation Team

A hallmark of systemic approaches, counselors work with an *observation team* to better observe systemic patterns (Watzlawick et al., 1974). This practice evolved from the Bateson (1972, 1979) team's early research methods where they would sit behind a one-way mirror to observe the "conductor of the session" working with the family. The team could "see" the systemic dance more rapidly and completely from there, because the person in the room very quickly falls in sync with the family system and has a more difficult time seeing the entirety of the interaction. As anyone who has spent time behind a mirror and in front of it knows, you are always "smarter" behind it. The distance created by not being part of the interactional dance of the family increases one's ability to see the steps more clearly and quickly. Arguably, the main reason family counselors still train with a mirror is to develop the ability to "see" the systemic dynamics. This is never to say that a counselor in the room *can't* see the systemic dynamics; it is just harder and takes more practice.

The Viewing: Case Conceptualization and Assessment

Systemic counselors conceptualize work with individuals, couples, and families using the following concepts:

1. Abilities and Development
    - Strengths
    - Family life cycle stage of development
2. Systemic Dynamics
    - Interactional patterns and behavioral sequences
    - Role of symptom in the relational system
3. Structure of the Relational System
    - Subsystems
    - Triangles and cross-generational coalitions
    - Boundaries
    - Hierarchy
    - Complementarity

Strengths

Systemic counselors are fundamentally *strengths-based*, keeping their focus on clients' strengths and advocating strongly against labeling families or individuals as "dysfunctional." In particular, systemic counselors focus on unique cultural and idiosyncratic strengths, such as religious beliefs or unusual hobbies, using these to design interventions (Minuchin & Fishman, 1981; Minuchin & Nichols, 1993; Watzlawick et al., 1974). Minuchin and Fishman (1981) argue powerfully against seeing the family as an enemy of its individual members, which is frequently seen in psychological literature, and instead they encourage counselors to recognize how the family provides support, protection, and a foundation for its individual members. Family strengths are used to design interventions and promote the goals of individual and family growth, as well as symptom reduction. (See Chapter 2 for a full description of assessing strengths.)

Family Life Cycle Stage of Development

Rather than as a static entity, the family is viewed as continually growing and changing in response to predictable stages of development and unexpected life events such as a death, moving, or divorce (Carter & McGoldrick, 2005; Minuchin & Fishman, 1981). Successfully navigating each stage requires changes in how the family balances interdependence and independence to meet each person's changing developmental needs. Whether working with individuals or families, systemic counselors identify their stage in the life cycle to better understand clients' developmental needs and challenges. Each stage is associated with specific developmental tasks:

1. *Leaving Home: Single Adult*: Accepting emotional and financial responsibility for self.
2. *Marriage:* Commitment to new system; realigning boundaries with family and friends.
3. *Families with Young Children:* Adjusting a marriage to make space for children; joining in child-rearing tasks; realigning boundaries with parents/grandparents.
4. *Families with Adolescent Children:* Adjusting parental boundaries to increase freedom and responsibility for adolescents; refocusing on marriage and career life.
5. *Launching Children:* Renegotiating marital subsystem; developing adult-to-adult relationships with children; coping with aging parents.
6. *Family in Later Life:* Accepting the shift of generational roles; coping with loss of abilities; middle generation taking more central role; creating space for wisdom of the elderly.

At each stage the members need to renegotiate boundaries to define levels of closeness and independence that support individual members' growth needs. Families often get stuck transitioning from one stage to another if they fail to renegotiate boundaries and hierarchy as the family develops. For example, after the birth of a child, couples need to radically reorganize how they manage independence and interdependence as they add the high-maintenance needs of a newborn into their juggling act. On the other end of the spectrum, in the case study at the end of this chapter, Billy's family is adjusting to his graduating high school and yet still living at home with his mother. The family is struggling to define and operationalize "launching" for financial reasons, and the family is not adapting well to this new stage in the family life cycle.

Interaction Patterns and Behavioral Sequences

Whether working with an individual or relational system, systemic counselors carefully assess the *interaction patterns* and *behavioral sequences* surrounding a symptom (Watzlawick, 1978; Watzlawick & Weakland, 1977). Assessing interaction patterns involves tracing the behavioral sequences in the homeostatic dance in which the symptom is embedded. The interactional sequence is traced through four general phases: (a) things being normal (homeostasis), (b) tensions escalating (early positive feedback), (c) the symptomatic feelings and behaviors (positive feedback), and, finally, (d) self-correction, with the ultimate return to normal (homeostasis). Depending on the symptom, this sequence can take several minutes or several months. Clients typically only describe the symptom, but by tracing the symptom from homeostasis to homeostasis, systemic counselors have a much better sense of how to intervene.

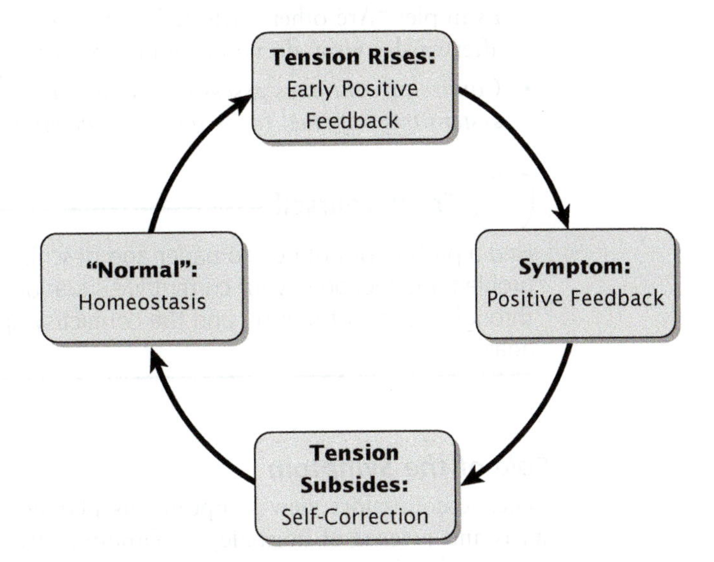

For example, if a client complains that she is anxious in public situations, a systemic counselor would explore the behaviors and interactions when the client feels "okay" or normal, then identify the behaviors, contexts, and relational interactions when the anxiety starts to rise, what she does when she feels the anxiety at its height and how others respond, and then trace the behaviors and interactions until she feels "okay" or back to normal again. Similarly, when working with a couple who argues, the counselor first asks about what types of things they are doing when things are good between the two of them, what each starts to do as tensions rise, what each says and does in response to the other during the argument, and how they get back to a sense of "normal" again.

In addition to observing actual interactions, systemic counselors *ask* a series of questions to assess the interaction sequence. For example, with the couple who is having trouble with the defiant child, in addition to observing, the counselor would ask: what is happening just before the problem incident? What is each person saying and doing? How does the child respond? How does each parent and anyone else involved respond to the defiance? How does the child respond to this?

Questions for Assessing Interactional Sequence

- *Counselor asks about "life as normal" related to the presenting issue.*
  Example: "What is going on when you feel normal (okay, good, etc.)"?
- *Counselor asks client to describe how the problem begins, inquiring about contexts and persons that seem to trigger the symptom, if these are not obvious.*
  Example: "Describe what typically happens prior to feeling anxiety. Then, how does the anxiety ultimately begin? Does it seem to happen in particular contexts or with certain people"?
- *Counselor inquires about the behavioral sequence that comprises the symptom.*
  Example: "So what do you do at the height of the anxiety? What type of dialogue is going on in your head? How do others respond to you? How do you respond to them? What happens next?" And so on.
- *Counselor continues to trace these back-and-forth interactional patterns until things return to "normal" or homeostasis.*
  Example: "How do things get back to normal? Do you have to do something? Does someone say or do something that helps? Does it generally happen the same way every time"?

(*continued*)

- *Counselor also inquires about how significant others in the system respond to the problem situation.*
  Example: "Are other's affected by this anxiety? How do they respond during or afterwards? How do you respond to them?"
- *Counselor continues assessing the interaction pattern until it is clear that the entire system has returned to its sense of "normalcy."*

Try It Yourself

Find a partner or put pen to paper and describe an interactional sequence for a problem interaction in your current life situation. Trace the interaction from "normal" through the rise of tension and the conflict/symptom and then back to "normal" again.

Role of the Symptom

Systemic counselors view symptoms as playing a role in maintaining relational homeostasis and a sense of normalcy (Colapinto, 1991). Symptoms can help maintain a sense of normalcy in a number of ways: limiting emotional intimacy, creating physical distance, forcing connection, creating distraction, or delaying developmental changes, just to name a few. Even though the symptoms are unwanted, they are often preventing or minimizing an even more distressing situation. For example, fear of going to public places (agoraphobia) often serves to force connection with a select few while creating great distance from others and avoiding numerous other responsibilities. Systemic counselors never view the *symptom bearer* or *identified patient* (IP) as the sole source of intervention, and instead the family interaction patterns are targeted for intervention. In the case study at the end of the chapter, Billy's drinking and depression are considered as part of the family homeostasis, helping to maintain his dependent status and his mother's caretaking role.

Subsystems

Using Minuchin's (1974) structural theory, systemic counselors conceptualize a family as a single system that consists of multiple *subsystems*. Certain subsystems exist in all families: couple, parental, sibling, and each individual as a separate subsystem. In addition, in some families other influential subsystems develop along gender lines, hobbies, and interests (e.g., sports, music, and so forth), and even personality (e.g., serious versus fun-loving). When assessing a client's family (see Chapter 2), the most important subsystem issues to consider are:

- Is there a clear distinction between the *parental* and *couple* subsystems?
- Is there a clear boundary between the *parental* and *child* subsystems? Alternatively stated, is there an effective *parental hierarchy*?
- Is the family divided along subsystem lines?

Many couples need help distinguishing the marital from parental subsystem when all their energy goes into caring for the children with nothing left for the relationship. Frequently parents need help distinguishing the parental and child subsystems by establishing a hierarchy (see below). Additionally, many subsystems create unhelpful dynamics that need correcting, such as coalitions across generations.

Triangles and Cross-Generational Coalitions

One type of subsystem is particularly damaging: *triangles* (Bowen, 1985), which often take the form of *cross-generational coalitions* (Minuchin & Fishman, 1991; Minuchin & Nichols, 1993). Triangles can form in any relationship where a third person is pulled in to reduce tension in a dyad, often taking the form of "confiding" in a friend or family member who takes the side of one person in the dyad against the other. Cross-generational coalitions are a *triangle* that forms between a parent and child *against* the other parent or other key caretaker. This is a common family dynamic, often involving a parent who "teams up" with one or more children against the other parent, by undermining the other parent, taking the child's side in an argument, using the child as a confidante, or simply being more invested in the parent-child relationship. In a divorce, this pattern is almost universal as parents vie to create coalitions against the other. Triangles can be *overt*, readily identifiable, or *covert*, not directly addressed or spoken about in the family but evident by secrets between the parent and child ("don't tell your mom/dad about this") or comments that compliment the child and disparage the other spouse ("I am so glad you didn't inherit your father's/mother's gene for X").

Boundaries

Boundaries refer to the relational patterns and rules for relating in a system. Each individual family has a unique set of boundaries that are closely tied to their family, cultural, socioeconomic, gender, educational, and other background variables. When initially assessing boundaries, they seem two-dimensional: too weak or too strong. But the more you work with them, the more you learn that they are far more complex than they appear at first glance. Nonetheless, let's start with the simple two-dimensional definition.

Boundaries are rules for managing physical and psychological distance between family members, defining the regulation of closeness, distance, hierarchy, and family roles (Minuchin & Fishman, 1981). Although they may sound static, they are an organic, living process. Systemic counselors identify three basic types of boundaries:

- *Clear Boundaries*: Clear boundaries refer to a range of "normal" boundaries that allow for close emotional contact with others while also allowing each person to maintain a sense of clear identity (Colapinto, 1991). Each culture defines a range of "normal" boundaries that define appropriate expressions and levels of independence versus interdependence. For example, in some cultures, more physical space is typical of clear boundaries than in others, and within a given culture families can have a wide variety of expressions of this that are considered normal. Import those same rules to another culture (e.g., from anywhere to the United States) and the once-normal boundaries may not be "normal" in the new context. Thus, immigrant and multiracial families have much more complex boundary dynamics to navigate the multiple worlds in which they live.
- *Enmeshment and Diffuse Boundaries:* If boundaries are blurry, diffuse or weak, this leads to relational *enmeshment*, which is evidenced by a lack of clear distinction between members and a strong sense of mutuality and connection at the expense of individual autonomy (Colapinto, 1991). When talking with an enmeshed family, counselors typically see family members:
    - interrupting one another and/or speaking for one another,
    - mindreading and making assumptions,
    - insisting on high levels of protectiveness and overconcern,
    - demanding loyalty at the expense of individual needs, and
    - feeling threatened when there is disagreement or difference.

  How do you sort through family and cultural differences and determine whether a particular relationship has clear or enmeshed boundaries? Simple. If there are symptoms and problems in one or more individuals and/or complaints about family interactions, then the boundaries are too diffuse for the current developmental stage and context. Thus, behaviors that constitute problematic boundaries in one cultural context may be clear in another cultural context, making it difficult for families and counselors alike to sort out relational rules in immigrant and other bicultural families because there is more than one cultural context at play (Minuchin & Fishman, 1981). Counselors must proceed slowly and mindfully to accurately assess where and how boundaries are a problem, in order to avoid imposing dominant cultural norms or psychological theory onto clients inadvertently. That said, rarely in the early stages of counseling are boundaries clear, because generally some boundary patterns need to be renegotiated to resolve the presenting complaint.

- *Disengagement and Rigid Boundaries:* Boundaries can also become highly rigid, resulting in relational *disengagement.* Families with rigid boundaries value autonomy and independence over emotional connection, creating isolation that may be more emotional than physical (Colapinto, 1991). These families have excessive tolerance for deviation, often failing to mobilize support and protection for one another. Counselors working with disengaged families notice the following:
  - A lack of reaction and repercussions, even to problems.
  - Significant freedom for most members to do as they please.
  - Few demands for or expressions of loyalty, affection, or commitment.
  - Parallel interactions (e.g., doing different activities in the same room) consistently substituting for reciprocal interactions and engagement.

  Like enmeshed boundaries, rigid boundaries cannot be accurately assessed without taking cultural and developmental variables into consideration. High levels of independence are not considered problematic unless one or more persons are experiencing symptoms.

Hierarchy

A painful, shocking reality that I was very slow to believe as a new counselor is that most child behavior issues boil down to an ineffective *parental hierarchy*—or at least greatly improve when hierarchical issues are addressed. The parental hierarchy refers to the power differential between the parent and child and the parent's ability to manage the child's behavior (Colapinto, 1991; Minuchin, 1974; Minuchin & Fishman, 1981). There are three basic forms of parental hierarchy:

- *Effective:* An effective parental hierarchy is evidenced by two things: (a) parents can effectively set boundaries and limits, while (b) still maintaining emotional connection with their children. For better or worse, children keep changing, and thus the behaviors that constitute an effective parental hierarchy at one point in time do not work at another—thus, it is hard for parents to continually shift and balance these two roles as children grow.
- *Insufficient:* A common parenting pattern, an insufficient parental hierarchy means that the parent is not able to effectively manage the child's behavior, commonly referred to as a permissive parenting style. In these families, parents cannot sufficiently influence their children's behavior to avoid problems from erupting. Often these parents hope that the counselor will "teach" their children to obey rules, be polite, and take responsibility. Alas, such a hope is in vain. Each adult must establish an effective hierarchy with a child on a one-to-one basis: this includes parents, teachers, stepparents, and, yes, counselors, too. In fact, it is commonly the case that one parent has an effective hierarchy and the other does not, thus providing evidence that the burden is on the adult rather than the child to effectively establish a hierarchy. Similar to boundaries, the outward expression of an effective versus an insufficient hierarchy can only be determined by examining the cultural context, family life stage of development, and symptomatic behavior.
- *Excessive:* The other extreme is an excessive hierarchy in which the parent maintains rules that are developmentally too strict and unrealistic and consequences that are too severe to be effective. The children typically behave well (until they decide to rebel), but at the expense of emotional closeness. These parents need assistance in developing age-appropriate rules and expectations and in developing a stronger emotional bond with their children.

Complementarity

One of the most elegant and subtle areas assessed by systemic counselors, complementarity refers to rigidly adopted patterns of opposite roles in a relational system (Colapinto, 1991). Like jigsaw puzzles, individuals develop complementary roles in their couple, family, and organizational relationships: the over-/underfunctioner, good/bad child, understanding/strict parent, logical/emotional, role model/rebel, and so on. Over time, these systemically generated roles become viewed as inherent personality characteristics that seem unchangeable within that particular relationship, even if the same dynamic is not manifested in other contexts. The more exaggerated and rigid these roles become, the more of a problem they create. After years, the individuals involved do not believe they could behave any differently, although they have ample evidence that they did in fact possess these qualities prior to being in the relationship. One of the most distinguishing features of systemic counselors is that they are able to recognize rigid complementary patterns—as part of the system dynamics, rather than focusing on individual personalities—and they can help clients move beyond them.

Targeting Change: Goal Setting

Four Steps for Setting Systemic Goals

In the MRI brief approach, counselors use a four-step process for setting goals based on the axiom that "the problem is the attempted solution," meaning that the problem is that the client has been using the wrong class or type of solution (Watzlawick et al., 1974). The counselor's task then is to identify the type of solution that *hasn't been working*, and then identify what would represent a solution that uses an alternative logic or premise. For example, if a person is trying to reduce worry by trying to control or manage it—and all those attempts have failed—the counselor would identify solutions with an alternative logic to control, such as indulging the worry by instructing the client to worry at specific times (see paradoxical interventions below).

Setting systemic goals involves four distinct steps:

Step 1: Clearly Define the Problem: *Define the problem in concrete, behavioral* terms, including the actions and reactions of all involved. When a systemic counselor hears from a client, "I worry too much," the counselor has not really heard a meaningful problem statement. The counselor's job at this point is to help the client turn this into a clear problem statement that is behavioral and concrete: "When I am assigned an important project at work, I end up thinking about it before I go to bed, during my commute, and when working on other projects; I ask my boss a thousand questions and she gets annoyed with me; I second-guess myself when talking with my partner at dinner and she keeps trying to reassure me that I am doing great, but I don't believe her because she is just saying that to make me feel better." Now *that* is a clear problem.

Step 2: Identify Prior Attempted Solutions: *Identify the attempted solutions thus far.* The counselor may ask, "How have you attempted to deal with this problem?" and listens for patterns in the various attempted solutions (e.g., I tell myself to stop worrying but can't stop; I look to others to reassure me but don't believe them either; and so on). Although a seemingly obvious thing to assess, attempted-but-failed solutions often are not spontaneously mentioned because they are typically not remembered or flagged as important because they didn't work.

Step 3: Develop a Clear Description of Preferred Change: *Develop a behavioral* description of the things to be changed. Systemic counselors take goal writing very seriously. *How* the goal is worded is a critical part of the intervention. If systemic goals are not crafted carefully using clear descriptions of *behavioral change*, failure is more likely. Watzlawick et al. (1974) identify three characteristics of helpful goals: realistic, specific, and time-limited.

- *Realistic:* Systemic counselors avoid pie-in-the-sky, utopian goals that clients hope they can achieve by seeking professional help, such as *always* be happy, *never* fight with a partner, or have a child who *always* obeys. If humans are involved, always and never are not a part of realistic goals. Instead, the counselor helps the client develop more human goals that "increase the frequency" of desired behaviors and decrease that of undesirable ones. For many clients, accepting realistic goals is a significant form of change in and of itself, often resulting in improvements just from setting a realistic goal.

- *Specific:* Goals should target clearly defined behaviors and interactions rather than vague intentions, such as "communicate better," "feel happier," or "relax more." Vague goals can set up false hopes and reduce the counselor's effectiveness. Instead, goals should be written so it is easy to determine when they have been attained: "Increase frequency of asserting needs at work" or "Increase time spent with friends."
- *Time-Limited:* Systemic counselors set clear time limits (e.g., achieve goal in four weeks or four months) to help motivate and focus both client and counselor. A written time limit helps set realistic expectations. When time limits are not met, systemic counselors view this as feedback indicating that something may be amiss and needs to be addressed, such as an unassessed dynamic, an inadequately joined counseling system, poorly designed interventions, or unrealistic initial goals.

Step 4: Develop a Systemic Treatment Plan: *Develop a plan that is based on systemic principles* to achieve change. When developing a plan, systemic counselors use two basic principles:

- The *target of change* is the *attempted solution*, meaning that a new logical premise is used (e.g., rather than forcefully trying to control a behavior, the new logic is to allow it in some form).
- The *tactic of change* is to use the *client's own language* to speak directly to the client's view of reality (e.g., if the client is athletically inclined, a sports metaphor may be used).

When designing a treatment plan, systemic counselors *never* use commonsense logic or basic psychoeducation on how to solve problems: that is the type of approach used in cognitive-behavioral or Adlerian counseling. Instead, systemic counselors alter the interaction pattern, trusting that the system will reorganize itself using its innate ability to self-correct—the counselor's role is simply to give the system a gentle nudge in the right direction, which is in the *opposite* direction of the previously attempted solution.

Systemic and Structural Goals

Systemic counselors target similar basic goals for clients that can generally be categorized as goals for (a) systemic dynamics and (b) family structure (Colapinto, 1991; Madanes, 1981, 1991; Minuchin, 1974; Watzlawick et al., 1974).

General Goals for Systemic Dynamics

- Develop relational patterns that maintain *flexible interaction and behavior patterns* without the presenting symptom(s).
  Example: Reduce pursuer-distancer pattern and increase ability to tolerate higher levels of intimacy.

General Goals for Relational Structure

- *Clear boundaries* between all subsystems that allow for *intimacy* and *individuation* appropriate within client's cultural contexts.
  Example: Reduce enmeshment between client and mother to increase client's ability to make independent decisions.
- Clear distinction between the *marital/couple subsystem* and *parental subsystem* (if children are involved).
  Example: Increase separation of parental and marital subsystems to increase emotional intimacy and solidarity in the partnership.
- *Effective parental hierarchy* and the severing of cross-generational coalitions (if children are involved).
  Example: Increase the effectiveness of the parental hierarchy and the ability of the parents to consistently set and reinforce limits.
- Relational structures that promote the *development and growth of individuals and relationships*.
  Example: Increase sense of emotional connection with father.

The Doing: Interventions

Enactments and Modifying Interactions (See "The Juice" above)

Systemic Reframing

One of the most frequently used interventions, systemic counselors use *systemic reframing* to alter interaction and behavior patterns related to the problem, by offering new frameworks for viewing the problem (Colapinto, 1991; Minuchin, 1974; Minuchin & Fishman, 1981; Watzlawick et al., 1974). Systemic counselors reframe problems in a very specific way, which distinguishes their work from other forms of counseling. Specifically, *systemic reframes illuminate how a client's symptom is part of a larger interactional pattern*. For example, if a person's worrying elicits sympathy from others by creating a sense of connection, a systemic reframe would highlight this dynamic in the reframe.

Systemic reframing focuses on reciprocal interactions, meaning that person A affects person B's response, which then affects person A's response, which affects B's response, *ad infinitum* (A ⇄ B). This process requires (1) piecing together the interaction patterns that involve the client and others involved in the problem interaction sequence, and (2) reframing it so that the broader systemic dynamic is revealed.

How to Generate Systemic Reframes

1. *Assess broader interactional patterns:* Complementary relationships, hierarchy, boundaries, and so on.
   Example: The counselor assesses a hero/damsel-in-distress pattern in which a woman's husband responds to her fear of a manic episode relapse by taking over many of her household tasks and chores; the more he does, the less capable she seemingly becomes.
2. *Redescribe the problem in a systemic frame:* Use interactional patterns to describe problem in a larger context.
   Example: The counselor can reframe the situation thusly: "Your fear and your husband's fear of relapse has resulted in him taking over many of the household tasks you dislike: cooking, cleaning, doing homework with the children, paying bills, and so on. Now you are in a situation where you have to stay worried about relapse, in order to avoid those tasks. It's a tough situation you are in. If you allow yourself to feel better, you have new problems to deal with."

Try It Yourself

Use systemic reframing for two different situations or problems in your life. Notice the effect they have on your experience of the "problem."

Circular Questions

When seeing two or more clients, circular questions should be a staple intervention. They are also invaluable when working with individuals talking about—especially complaining about—others (okay, I guess that covers virtually all clients). Developed by the Milan team, circular questioning is an elegant and highly efficient technique that simultaneously assesses interactional patterns while reframing them: thus, a winning, two-for-one assessment/intervention combination. Circular questions make overt the systemic dynamics and interactive patterns in the system, and by doing so, inherently *reframe* the problem for all participants without the counselor directly proposing a reframe (Boscolo, Cecchin, Hoffman, & Penn, 1987; Selvini Palazzoli et al., 1978; Selvini Palazzoli, Boscolo, Cecchin, & Prata, 1980). They are perhaps the most effective way means of "confronting" clients on patterns that they don't want to acknowledge without the counselor having to directly confront: instead, *the clients* are the ones who reveal the pattern by responding to questions. It's always harder to not believe oneself than to not believe another.

Specific forms of circular questions (Cecchin, 1987) include:

- *Behavioral sequences questions:* These questions trace the entire sequence of behaviors that constitute the problem, for example, "When you start to get depressed, what is your first sign? What do you do next? What do others see and how do they respond? How do you respond in turn to them? What happens next?" The counselor follows the sequence of interactions until homeostasis is restored again.
- *Behavioral difference questions:* Behavioral difference questions shatter the illusion that a particular behavior is part of a person's inherent personality. For example, if a client claims, "I am a worrier," the counselor would ask, "What do you do that makes you a worrier?" The *behavioral definition* of the problem behavior, "plan for how to handle potential problems," is then used to compare it with others: "How does your partner plan for potential problems? How did your parents plan for potential problems? Others that you know? What is similar and what is different about these approaches?"
- *Comparison and ranking questions:* Comparison and ranking questions reduce labeling and other rigid descriptions of self and others; they also help illuminate problem interaction patterns: "Who is the most anxious person you know (or in your family, office, and such)? The least anxious? How does each deal with anxiety? Who is the most upset by your anxiety? The least upset by it?"
- *Before-and-after questions:* When a particularly notable positive or negative event has occurred, counselors use before-and-after questions to assess nuances in the relational dynamics: "Before your depressive episode, did you and your partner fight more or less? Who was happier at that time? Who did more of the chores then?"
- *Hypothetical circular questions:* Hypothetical questions can be helpful in assessing how a person responds to stress and to better understand the subtle relational dynamics. For example, "If you were to suddenly lose your job, what would you do? Who would you turn to first? Who would be the first to offer help? Who would you not want to tell?"

In the case study at the end of the chapter, the counselor uses circular questions to enable Billy to see better how his depression and drinking are interrelated, how they are affected by and affect his family, and how they interrelate with his extended and tribal family.

Try It Yourself

Find a partner, have your partner identify a problem, and then ask about it using at least three types of circular questions. You can also try these by yourself by writing them out.

Directives

Frequently misunderstood because they do not follow commonsense logic, directives are a signature systemic technique (Madanes, 1991). As the name implies, directives are directions for the client to complete a specific task, usually between sessions but sometimes within the session. The key element is that the tasks are rarely "logical" or linear solutions to the problem; instead, they interrupt the system's interaction patterns in minor but meaningful ways to create new interactions (Haley, 1973, 1987). More simply stated, they are designed to "trip up" the problem, get the pattern slightly off-kilter so that clients have to rebalance. Systemic counselors trip up the problem with the *smallest change possible.* For example, if part of a client's "depression ritual" (or pattern) involves eating a pint of his favorite ice cream, a directive might involve tripping this pattern up with the least amount of change (client more likely to do it) that is still meaningful (shakes things up): such a directive might be to eat a pint of less desirable flavor, such as strawberry. Although this may sound quite ridiculous at first, for the person involved, just shifting that one element often results in a "waking up," seeing the pattern more clearly and also feeling more motivated to do something different. Because they are based in action, directives inspire a visceral form of insight because the person is in the middle of the action that needs changing, which is quite different from the more distant, cognitive insight in traditional psychodynamic theory.

Designing Directives

Step 1: Assess the Problem Sequence of Behaviors: Identify the sequence of behaviors that constitute the presenting problem: for example, the client encounters problems with a project at work, becomes intensely focused on the project, is snippy with coworkers, and ignores his family; when the work problem is solved, client is happy but has alienated people in his life.

Step 2: Target a Small Change in Behavioral Sequence: Identify one small behavioral change in the sequence that the client can reasonably make that would alter the problem sequence: for example, put on a object of clothing, hang a sign, or otherwise send a signal to others that symbolizes he is unavailable for normal human interaction until the problem is resolved.

Step 3: Motivate the Client to Follow Through: Haley (1987) emphasizes the importance of motivating the client *before* the task is issued. This is usually done by appealing to the ultimate goal: that the client and significant others wants the problem behavior to stop.

Step 4: Give Precise, Doable Instructions for the Directive: The key to directives is to be very specific: when, where, how, who, on which day of the week. The counselor should consider variations in schedules, such as vacations, illness, weekends, and so on. Furthermore, the directives should be *given* rather than casually suggested. For example, "It sounds like you would really like to do something different the next time you get pulled into a work project. So here is what I want you to do. The next time you start to feel the "pull" I want you to email your coworkers and family that you will unfortunately be absent in their lives until this problem is resolved. Feel free to add playful references to your metaphoric death, by perhaps signing it, 'Temporarily departed.'" The counselor avoids theoretical or logical explanations about "why" and "what for" and simply says, "I think this might be helpful," if the client asks.

Step 5: Review the Task in Painful Detail: Have the client describe precisely what he is to do and how he is going to do it, such as, "Just to review and make sure we understand, can you review what you are going to do this week when you feel the pull of a project?"

Step 6: Request a Task Report: The following week, the counselor asks the client "how it went." Generally, one of three things happens: the client (a) does it, (b) does not do it, or (c) partially does it (Haley, 1987). Obviously, if clients complete their tasks, they are congratulated and the counselor discusses how it went. If they have partially done the task, the counselor does not excuse them too quickly because that would send the message that undermines the counselor's authority. If they fail to attempt the task, Haley uses two responses, one nice and one not so nice. In the nice way, the counselor says, "I must have misunderstood you or your situation to ask that of you—otherwise you would have done it" (Haley, 1987, p. 71). In the not-so-nice approach, the counselor emphasizes that the client has missed an opportunity to make changes for their own good and that this is a loss for him or her (*not* that the counselor is disappointed); the counselor does not ask them to redo the task even if they say they want to. Instead, the counselor uses this experience to increase motivation for the next task.

Paradoxical Intervention and Symptom Prescription

Perhaps the most misunderstood of systemic interventions, *paradoxical intervention* and *symptom prescription* involve instructing clients to engage in the problem behavior in some fashion, such as assigning a client to worry each morning from 8:00–8:15 (Watzlawick & Weakland, 1977). Symptom prescription and other paradoxical interventions are "paradoxical" because they seem as though they will make the problem worse rather than better—or at least at first glance. I guess I should mention that, yes, indeed, they can make things worse if they are used at the wrong time or for the wrong problem—so, these interventions should only be used under careful supervision, until you understand how they work.

You will know when it is time to use one of these interventions because *when it is appropriate to use paradox it will not seem paradoxical—at least in the mind of the counselor—it will be the only logical, obvious action to take.* Generally, it takes many years of practice (and good supervision) until paradox seems like a good idea. Not a garden-variety technique that works for everybody, paradoxical interventions are appropriate for two types of problems: (a) when making any other change disrupts the client's current level of stability, or (b) when the problem seems "uncontrollable" from the client's perspective: "I can't keep myself from worrying, nagging, eating, fighting, whatever."

Paradox with Clients Resisting Change Some clients seem to resist any and all attempts at change even though they say they really, really want to change (the "really, really" part should be your first clue that things may not go as planned). No matter how great the idea and how much these clients agree to it, they never seem to follow through on anything that actually would promote change. As maddening as they can be for the counselor, these clients are not bad, hypocritical, or actively resisting. They simply need an intervention that honors the fact that this symptom is very important in maintaining homeostasis for them. Thus, they—often realistically—fear that giving it up may create *more* discomfort and chaos than they are currently experiencing; in these situations paradox can be useful (Haley, 1987). In such a situation, the counselor may restrain or caution against certain changes, such as "perhaps the couple needs to argue to keep their passion strong; if they stopped, things may get worse." Paradoxical tasks are difficult to deliver effectively because the counselor must communicate several messages at once:

- I want to help you resolve your problem.
- I am sincerely concerned about you.
- I think you can be normal, but perhaps you cannot.

When paradox is successful, change is usually spontaneous. Systemic counselors also often use paradoxical intervention in the later stages of counseling to prevent relapse by paradoxically encouraging it (Haley, 1976): "I know that you are saying that you aren't worrying any more, but now I am a bit worried about that. You might just want to let yourself worry for five to ten minutes a day a few times a week, just in case you find that it really did solve problems for you."

Paradox with "Uncontrollable" Symptoms When clients report symptoms they claim to have no control over, systemic counselors use *symptom prescription* as an intervention. Symptom prescription changes the *context* (where, when, who, what) of the problem behavior without requiring clients to stop having the symptom. If the context changes, the *meaning* of the behavior must also change. When the meaning changes, thoughts, feelings, and subsequent behaviors automatically change, too. A common example of using paradox is worrying, which is particularly difficult to intervene on because it is a thought and emotional process often with limited associated behaviors. When a client is given the directive to set an egg-timer to worry for ten minutes at a particular time in the day, it radically changes worrying from a vague, free-floating experience to a consciously chosen activity that they can voluntarily start, and most often, they quickly discover, they can also stop at will. By changing the context, the meaning and experience of worrying changes, often creating significant movement on a symptom that seemed totally out of the client's control.

Shifting Epistemologies: Expanding and Challenging the Client's Worldview

Systemic counselors carefully examine the rules, logic, and premises that clients construct their worldviews upon: what is "necessary," what is prohibited, how one shows love, what one owes to others. Most people cannot list the majority of these epistemological assumptions that inform their every action, interaction, thought, priority, and emotion. By identifying and commenting on them, systemic counselors affect the operating premises that fuel the problem (Colapinto, 1991; Minuchin, 1974; Minuchin & Fishman, 1981).

As you might have guessed this far into the chapter, systemic counselors generally don't confront these premises directly but instead use existing beliefs and *expand* and *reinterpret* them in more helpful directions. Again, this intervention involves using the symptom—not asking clients to relinquish it—and recontextualizing, stretching, and/or reordering it to resolve issues. For example, if a client tends to be a perfectionist who never stops to enjoy life, you might help them become perfect at relaxing. Alternatively, if parents were great at structuring and setting limits with young children but start to struggle with teens, they can be challenged to learn how to get the teen to structure herself and set her own behavioral standards. Like a martial artist, the systemic counselor takes a fundamental premise that has been supporting the problem and redirects its logic to support an alternative set of behaviors and interactions, allowing clients to maintain their core beliefs but use them in new ways.

Complimenting Strengths and Shaping Competence

Complimenting strengths and *shaping competence* are used to augment and reinforce the clients' natural positive interaction patterns and strengths. When systemic counselors identify client strengths, they are quick to compliment and encourage. A similar process, *shaping competence* involves noticing and complimenting small successes along the way to reaching one's goals. For example, if a client was able to stop a panic attack once during the week or keep it from getting out of control, systemic counselors compliment and encourage the client for these small successes.

Shaping competence also refers to not overfunctioning for the client, meaning doing things that the client is capable of doing and/or needs to be learning to resolve an issue. This can include setting limits with a child, jotting down an idea from a session, following up on a phone call, or making a decision about how to proceed. Depending on a client's presenting problem, all of these common in-session occurrences are opportunities for clients to shape their competence rather than have the counselor do it for them, depriving them of an opportunity to learn in a safe and supported environment. In the case study at the end of the chapter, the counselor helps shape Billy's competence by complimenting his behaviors and decisions that include taking responsibility and avoiding trouble, such as choosing to not drink and drive.

Interventions for Specific Problems

Invariant Prescription to Sever Coalitions

As the name implies, the *invariant prescription* is a directive that is not varied across families because this one task quickly severs inappropriate parent-child coalitions (Selvini Palazzoli, 1988). The prescription is essentially this: the parents are instructed to arrange to go on a date (or other outing) and they are not to tell the children where they are going or why. The desired effect is to create a *secret* between the parents, ending inappropriate coalitions by creating a clear boundary between the parents as a unified team and the symptomatic child. The child loses the status of being a special confidante of the one parent, which also lessens the emotional burden on the child, resulting in fewer problem symptoms. Although originally designed for severe pathology such as anorexia or psychosis in the child, this intervention is also effective with parents who overemphasize transparent and open communication with their children to the extent that one parent creates a coalition with the child and/or the parental hierarchy is ineffective.

Ordeals for Compulsive Behaviors

Inspired by the work of Milton Erickson (see Chapter 13), *ordeals* are often used in situations where the client feels helpless in controlling a symptom, such as overeating, smoking, nail biting, drinking, etc., and they are based on a simple premise: "If one makes it more difficult for a person to have a symptom than to give it up, the person will give up the symptom" (Haley, 1984, p. 5). Rather than try to develop linear, logical means for stopping the behavior (that would be a cognitive-behavioral approach), the strategic counselor *allows* the symptom with a twist (by now, you should recognize this theme): the client must complete another task, an "ordeal" first or afterwards.

The ordeal need not be directly related to the undesired activity but often carries a metaphoric relation to it. For example, if a person is trying to reduce their "emotional eating" to soothe difficult emotions, the ordeal would target the behavior and internal tension by logical means (e.g., write for ten minutes in a journal, jog for ten minutes, do a calorie log before the binge, etc.), metaphorically (e.g., "clean out" the refrigerator, pantry, etc.; set an elaborate table for a feast), or with a seemingly unrelated task (e.g., perform a random act of kindness for a stranger or loved one, answer three emails, etc.). In most cases, ordeals are less about creating a horrific, unappealing ordeal to stop undesired behavior and more about shaking up or perturbing the systemic pattern so that new behavioral sequences can evolve. The ordeal isn't a behavioral deterrent or punishment as much as it is adding a new—often neutral—behavior that forces clients to interrupt their patterns. As the individual or family adjusts to this rather small and innocuous twist, they *must* change to create new steps, and they are able to do so with less fear and resistance than if they were told to stop.

Boundary Making to Increase or Decrease Engagement

Boundary making is a special form of enactment that targets over- or underinvolvement to help families soften rigid boundaries or strengthen diffuse boundaries (Colapinto, 1991; Minuchin, 1974). Systemic counselors use this technique to direct who participates and how. By actively setting boundaries, counselors interrupt the habitual interaction patterns, allowing members to experience underutilized skills and abilities. Boundary making may involve several different directives:

- Asking family members to change seats.
- Asking family members to move seats farther apart or closer together or to turn toward one another.
- Having separate sessions with individuals or subsystems to strengthen subsystem boundaries.
- Asking one or more members to remain silent during an interaction.
- Asking questions that highlight a problem boundary area (e.g., "Do you always answer for your son when he is asked a question?").
- Blocking interruptions or encouraging pauses for less dominant persons to speak.

Putting It All Together: Systemic Treatment Plan Case Conceptualization and Treatment Plan Templates

Theory-Specific Case Conceptualization: Systemic

The prompts below can be used to develop a *theory-specific case conceptualization* using Adlerian theory. The cross-theoretical case conceptualizations at the end of each theory chapter provide examples for writing a conceptualization that includes key elements of this theory-specific conceptualization. Comprehensive examples of theory-specific case conceptualizations are available in *Theory and Treatment Planning in Counseling and Psychotherapy* (Gehart, 2015).

- *Strengths:* Describe individual and family strengths
- *Family Life Cycle Stage:* Describe stage of family life cycle and significant struggles related to balancing independence with interdependence:
  - Single adult
  - Marriage
  - Family with young children
  - Family with adolescent children

- Launching children
- Later life

- *Boundaries:* Describe boundaries (enmeshed, disengaged, clear) with significant persons in client's life, including:
  - *Parents*
  - *Siblings*
  - *Significant other*
  - *Children*
  - *Extended family*
  - *Friends*
- *Triangles/Coalitions:* Describe significant triangles and coalitions
- *Hierarchy:* Describe hierarchies (effective, permissive, rigid, inconsistent) with children and/or parents
- *Complementary patterns*: Describe complementary patterns in relationships, such as:
  - Pursuer/distance
  - Over-/underfunctioner
  - Emotional/logical
  - Good/bad parent
- *Intergenerational Patterns:* Describe significant intergeneration patterns:
  - Family strengths
  - Substance/alcohol abuse
  - Sexual/physical/emotional abuse
  - Parent/child relations
  - Physical/mental disorders
  - Historical incidents of presenting problem

Treatment Plan Template: Systemic

Use this Treatment Plan Template for developing a plan for clients with depressive, anxious, or compulsive types of presenting problems. Depending on the specific client, presenting problem, and clinical context, the goals and interventions in this template may need to be modified only slightly or significantly; you are encouraged to significantly revise the plan as needed. For the plan to be useful, goals and techniques should be written to target specific beliefs, behaviors, and emotions that the client is experiencing. The more specific, the more useful it will be to you.

Treatment Plan

Initial Phase of Treatment

Initial Phase Counseling Tasks

1. Develop working counseling relationship. *Diversity considerations*: Adapt style for ethnicity, gender, family dynamics, etc.
   Relationship-building approach/intervention:
   a. **Join** with client using **social courtesy** and by respecting larger systemic culture and maintaining neutral position between clients and others.
2. Assess individual, systemic, and broader cultural dynamics. *Diversity considerations: Include larger cultural systemic dynamics.*
   Assessment strategies:
   a. Obtain detailed description of **problem behavioral sequences.**
   b. Identify **boundary, subsystems, triangles, hierarchy, and complementary patterns** that contribute to the problem.

(continued)

3. Identify and obtain client agreement on treatment goals. *Diversity consideration:* Ensure goals are appropriate for individual and relational systems.
   Goal-making intervention:
   a. Develop goals that target **systemic dynamics** in **clear, doable behavioral** terms.
4. Identify needed referrals, crisis issues, and other client needs. *Diversity consideration:* Carefully assess broader systemic issues.
   a. *Crisis assessment intervention(s):* **Identify role of crisis symptom** in managing **systemic balance** and develop crisis intervention plan that accounts for these dynamics.
   b. *Referral(s):* To community resources as necessary.

Initial Phase Client Goal

1. Decrease [name specific crisis behavior] to reduce [crisis] symptoms.
   Interventions:
   a. Directives to **interrupt crisis escalation** and enable alternative means to manage crisis.
   b. **Reframing** crisis situation to reduce sense of urgency and crisis.

Working Phase of Treatment

Working Phase Counseling Tasks

1. Monitor quality of the working alliance. *Diversity considerations:* Ensure positive alliance with clients and significant others not in session.
   a. *Assessment Intervention:* Use Session Rating Scale; verbally ask client about alliance.
2. Monitor progress toward goals. *Diversity considerations:* Attend to systemic dynamics around acknowledging progress and how progress in one area can create new problems in another.
   a. *Assessment Intervention:* Use Outcome Rating Scale to measure client progress; asking about progress of out-of-session assignments week to week.

Working Phase Client Goals

1. Increase **interruptions to problem interaction cycle** to reduce depression/anxiety, etc.
   Interventions:
   a. **Directives** to do one small thing different to interrupt problem interaction pattern.
   b. **Systemic reframing** to alter response to problem pattern.
   c. **Paradoxical injunctions** to engage in symptomatic behavior in next context.
2. Increase **clear boundaries, relational structure, and communication** to reduce depression and anxiety.
   Interventions:
   a. **Enactments** to clarify boundaries, triangles, and hierarchy.
   b. **Circular questions** to make problem dynamics overt.
3. Increase developmental, relational, and cultural appropriateness of **worldview** and **rules for relating** to reduce feelings of hopelessness, anxiety, fear, etc.
   Interventions:
   a. **Circular questions** to increase awareness of relational assumptions.
   b. **Challenging worldviews and relational rules** that support and maintain the problem.

(continued)

Closing Phase of Treatment

Closing Phase Counseling Task

1. Develop aftercare plan and maintain gains. *Diversity considerations:* Reassess functioning in all areas before ending counseling to ensure problem has not shifted to another aspect of system.
   Intervention:
   a. Reinforce new **epistemology *and relational rules***; **circular questions** to apply new skills to future challenges.

Closing Phase Client Goals

1. Increase **satisfying interactions** in intimate, social, and/or work relationships (whichever were not already addressed in working phase) to reduce feelings of hopelessness, anxiety, fear, etc.
   Interventions:
   a. **Shaping competency** to transfer strengths from one area to another.
   b. **Circular questions** to capitalize on strengths and expand to new areas.
2. Increase **flexibility in worldview and relational interactions** to reduce potential for new problems to develop.
   Interventions:
   a. **Challenge rigid rules for relating and responding.**
   b. **Circular questions** to enable client to discover limits of worldview.

Bowen Intergenerational Family Approach

In a Nutshell: The Least You Need to Know

Murray Bowen's (1976, 1985) intergenerational family approach combines a psychoanalytically grounded multigenerational approach with systems theory, resulting in a distinct and fascinating approach that traces relational patterns *across generations*. Bowen's theory posits that healthy adult functioning is characterized by *differentiation*, the ability to separate thought from feeling and self from others. Differentiation is critical because of the evolutionary process that has made humans *emotionally interdependent* due to an inherent *chronic anxiety* related to survival. Each family system develops patterns for managing closeness and distance and regulating anxiety; these patterns are passed down from one generation to the next. The more the family allows for differentiation between members, the less pathology its members experience. Intergenerational counselors are quick to distinguish between *emotional cutoff* and healthy differentiation. Emotional cutoff is a sign of low levels of differentiation that require a person to stop relating to a family member because of high levels of anxiety and fusion; in contrast, healthy differentiation is marked by high levels of emotional intimacy counterbalanced with autonomy. Another problematic means of managing chronic anxiety, *triangulation* (see Triangulation above) refers to pulling in a third person to stabilize tension in a dyad, such as a mother who becomes close to a child to make up for intimacy she is not experiencing in the marriage.

The primary goals of intergenerational counseling are to (a) increase differentiation and (b) reduce emotional reactivity and chronic anxiety. Intergenerational counselors use *genograms*, a graphic representation of three or more generations that is similar to a family tree, to identify intergenerational patterns, such as emotional cutoff and triangulation. In addition, genograms can be used to identify other family patterns related to gender, death, personality, illness, mental health, substance abuse, sexual abuse, occupation, and others. In session, intergenerational counselors relate to clients using a differentiated, *nonanxious presence* that role-models differentiation, reduces triangulation, and encourages clients' differentiation. The techniques of intergenerational counseling focus on encouraging client differentiation using process questions that help clients become more aware of intergenerational patterns.

Satir's Human Growth Model

In a Nutshell: The Least You Need to Know

One of the most influential women in the field of mental health, Virginia Satir (1967, 1972, 1983, 1988) developed a comprehensive family counseling model that integrated humanism and system theory. Her theory is based on four primary assumptions:

1. People tend naturally toward positive growth (humanistic principle).
2. All people possess the resources for positive growth (humanistic principle).
3. Every person and every thing or situation impact and are impacted by everyone and everything else (systemic principle).
4. Therapy is a process, which involves interaction between counselor and client; and, in this relationship, each person is responsible for him/herself (systemic and humanistic principle). (Satir, Banmen, Gerber, & Gomori, 1991, pp. 14–15)

Similar to other experiential counselors (see Chapter 10), Satir used the person of the counselor to develop a warm, empathetic, and encouraging relationship with clients. In addition to using the systemic assessment ideas outlined above in this chapter, Satir also conceptualized family interactions in terms of the *communication* or *survival stances*. Survival stances refer to communication patterns a person adopts as a child to cope with difficult family interactions. She identified four different communication stances and one health stance.

- *Placating:* The person manages interpersonal stress by recognizing the needs of *others* and the *context* but not the *self*.
- *Blaming:* The inverse of placators, the person manages interpersonal stress by recognizing the needs of *self* and the *context* but not *others*.
- *Super-reasonable:* The person manages interpersonal stress by recognizing *contextual rules* but not more subjective needs of *self* and *others*.
- *Irrelevant:* This person manages interpersonal stress by not acknowledging *contextual demands, personal needs, or the needs of others*.
- *Congruent:* A person using a congruent stance is able to simultaneously honor the needs of self, respect the needs of others, while responding appropriately to context.

The goals of Satir's approach are twofold: (a) to communicate congruently in all relationships, and (b) to self-actualize (similar to other humanistic approaches). Satir uses an active style that includes having the family visually arrange each other to depict family dynamics using a technique called *family sculpting*. She also used communication coaching to help clients learn how to communicate congruently. Another common intervention helps clients identify the *ingredients of an interaction*, which helps them separate out the following: (a) what is heard and said, (b) what meanings are made, (c) what feelings are felt about the meanings, (d) feelings about the feelings, (e) defenses that are used to manage feelings, (f) rules for communicating about the feelings, and, finally, (g) the outward response to the situation.

Tapestry Weaving: Diversity Considerations

Ethnic, Racial, and Cultural Diversity

Because systemic and strategic family therapies do not rely on a theory-based definition of health and normalcy, they adapt relatively easily to different cultural groups and subpopulations: "Since in strategic family therapy a specific therapeutic plan is designed for each problem, there are no contraindications in terms of patient selection and suitability" (Madanes, 1991, p. 396). Furthermore, drawing on systemic and constructivist foundations, these therapies aim to work from *within* the client's worldview; when this is successfully achieved, the counselor adapts the language and interventions to the client's values and beliefs.

Hispanic and Latino Clients Of particular interest, two groups of systemic counselors have systematically adapted and used the approach with Latino/Hispanic clients. The Latino Brief Therapy Center at the MRI uses the nonnormative and nonpathologizing principles of the model to guide their work, creating unique meaning and interventions with each client, rather than relying on cultural stereotypes of the extremely diverse Latino community (Anger-Díaz, Schlanger, Rincon, & Mendoza, 2004). Similarly, Brief Strategic Family Therapy, an evidence-based approach that uses elements of systemic and structural family therapies, was developed specifically to treat Hispanic youth with high-risk behaviors and substance issues; the approach has also been found to be effective with African American youth (Robbins, Horigian, Szapocznik, & Ucha, 2010; Santisteban, Coatsworth, Perez-Vidal, Mitrani, Jean-Gilles, & Szapocznik, 1997).

In addition to these specific treatment approaches, McGoldrick, Giordano, and Garcia-Preto (2005) provide descriptions of how systemic ideas and approaches can be modified to meet the needs families from 46 different ethnicities, an invaluable resource when working with cultural groups other than one's own (and perhaps your own; read and see). Although these descriptions must be general and therefore do not capture the unique lived experience of a particular client who may be in front of you at a given moment, they can give you, the counselor, a clue about how best to understand and engage the client (and most clients appreciate your having at least a clue about their background and giving them room to share their own unique experience and beliefs).

Asian Indian Immigrants Rastogi (2007) describes how systemic family counseling can be used with Asian Indian immigrant families, the majority of whom have immigrated to the states in the past five decades. She identifies several specific cultural issues to consider when working from a systemic perspective:

- *Intergenerational family structure:* Asian Indian families are multigenerational families. Even after one generation immigrates, the family is likely to stay closely connected, both emotionally and physically, with many choosing three-generation households. Asian Indian Americans often present in counseling with intergenerational conflict, which is often exacerbated by immigration. When working with Asian Indian families, Rastogi (2007) encourages counselors to carefully consider family boundaries and role expectations from within the cultural norms. Furthermore, using a genogram to identify intergenerational patterns can also be helpful to Asian Indian families to enable them to make sense of each other's perspectives as well as identify culturally consistent possibilities for resolving concerns.
- *Collectivist value system:* Asian Indians are socialized to value family and contribute to the broader community, which also serves as a significant source of support and identity. Thus, systemic concepts such as "individual differentiation" should be used cautiously with these clients, recognizing that obligations to the community often take precedence over individual desires and that intergenerational conflict regarding these values is common.

- *Respect-based hierarchy:* Many Asian Indian families adhere to a traditional intergenerational hierarchy within the family based on age and gender. The older generations are respected, and their advice is sought by younger generations when making important life decisions. Counselors should respect this hierarchy and potentially use it to bring out the best in the elders, who are expected to be compassionate and wise leaders, and to help younger generations identify meaningful ways for them to continue this tradition.
- *Impact of modernization on Asian Indian families:* For many Asian Indian families, the effects of modernization, such as geographical mobility and egalitarian beliefs, have led to relationship crises intergenerationally. Many elders find themselves isolated and without the familial role and purpose they expected in later life, which often leads to conflict with younger generations when they embrace American values of independence. Counselors can help these clients by finding ways to honor their traditional culture while making room for the realities and demands of modern life.
- *Action Before Words:* Rastogi (2007) also notes that many Asian Indians communicate their affections and regrets through their actions rather than words. For example, after a fight, it would be more typical to reconcile by enacting the desired action that was the topic of conflict rather than saying, "I'm sorry. I won't do that again." Thus, rather than encourage clients to reconcile with words (the "natural" preference of professional counselors and contemporary American culture), counselors can help clients identify appropriate actions that would communicate the message they want to send.

Sexual Identity Diversity

Because of its nonpathologizing and nonnormative assumptions and its attention to larger systemic dynamics, systemic therapies have been widely used with clients who identify as lesbian, gay, bisexual, transgendered, or questioning (LGBTQ). Butler (2009) identifies five principles for adapting systemic therapy approaches for these clients.

1. *Understanding heterosexism:* Counselors need to be aware that gender and sexual minorities have *daily* experiences of being marginalized, judged, and ignored, and rarely see their reality reflected in advertisements, movies, and other social forums.
2. *Counselor self-reflectivity:* Heterosexual counselors need to engage in personal self-reflection of their experience of being privileged and having their sexual and gender orientations generally approved by society.
3. *Locating your position, transparency, and self-disclosure:* Based on the work of feminist counselors, Butler recommends disclosing one's gender and sexual orientation when working with LGBTQ clients. Such openness allows for frank discussions about areas of similarity and differentness, helping to address issues of power and hierarchy. However, too much self-disclosure can be nonproductive.
4. *Client as expert, and counselor as curious:* Drawing upon collaborative therapy principles (see Chapter 14), counselors should assume a curious stance, viewing the client as the expert in their life and lifestyle.
5. *Connecting to wider systems:* Finally, counselors should consider the larger social systems of which their LGBTQ clients are a part and encourage them to seek positive, supportive communities.

Butler (2009) also discusses how counselors need to adjust their approach with LGBTQ couples. First, counselors should be aware that sex, gender roles, monogamy, family of origin, family of choice, and ex-partners generally have very different meanings with these couples. Furthermore, gender roles are thought to have more impact than sexual orientation per se in these relationships, with internalized gender roles often greatly restricting same-sex relationships and being a particular issue in couples with a transgendered partner. Counselors can help couples deconstruct their gender role expectations and assumptions in ways that strengthen the partnership. Finally, counselors should keep in mind that the family life cycle looks different for most LGBTQ individuals, couples, and families (Goldenberg, 2009).

Adolescents Coming Out to Family

Another common issue that counselors address is adolescents coming out to their families (Butler, 2009). First and foremost, counselors should be aware that gay, lesbian, bisexual and transgendered youth have higher rates of suicidality, substance abuse, self-harm, depression, anxiety, and school issues; so it is important to monitor the adolescent's safety and well-being. Before coming out, most adolescents are generally able to accurately predict their parents' responses based on casual comments about sexuality over the years. Counselors can use DeVine's (1984) stage theory for the family's process of coming out to help families negotiate this transition.

- *Subliminal awareness:* The child's sexuality is suspected and sometimes provoked by inquiries about dating and same-sex friendships.
- *Impact:* The child announces his/her sexuality and suspicions are confirmed.
- *Adjustment:* The family struggles to maintain its old homeostasis while the child is expected to hide or deny his/her sexuality.
- *Resolution:* The family comes to accept the child's sexuality identity.
- *Integration:* The family shifts their values related to gender and sexual norms.

Many parents whose child comes out report a "loss" of their dreams of having a wedding or grandchildren, and much of their initial response may actually reflect the personal losses they are projecting. Counselors can help redirect parents to focus on their child's real needs at this time while also developing a more hopeful view of their future family life.

Transgendered Youth

There is little research or literature to guide counselors when working with transgendered persons, especially youth. However, unlike gay, lesbian, and bisexual youth, transgendered youth often cannot hide their difference, and thus it is more likely to be a point of family discussion whether the child wants it public or not (Coolhart, Baker, Farmer, Malaney, & Shipman, 2012). The majority of transgendered youth (59%) report negative parental reactions to their gender identity, at least initially, with those more gender-nonconforming reporting greater conflict with parents (Grossman, D'Augelli, Howell, & Hubbard, 2005). However, parental acceptance is important for transgendered individuals, since it correlates to adult life satisfaction and self-esteem (Erich, Tittsworth, Dykes, & Cabuses, 2008).

Coolhart and colleagues (2012) outline an assessment tool for counselors working with transgendered youth and their families—attending to systemic dynamics—and they recommend working with the family of transgendered youth whenever possible. The assessment tool is composed of questions that cover nine domains:

- *Early Awareness and Family Context:* These questions address the general family structure and history as well as both parents' and youth's early gender experiences. For example: "Please provide additional information about how your family's context in terms of racial, ethnic, and national communities interfaces with beliefs about variant expressions of gender and sexuality" (Coolhart et al., 2012, p. 16).
- *Parents' Attunement with Youth's Affirmed Gender:* These questions address how the parents and family have responded to the youth's transgender identity. For example: "When your child disclosed (or you discovered) their transgender identity, what was this experience like for you individually, as a couple, and as a family as a whole?" (Coolhart, 2012, p. 17).
- *Current Gender Expression:* These questions address the youth's current preference for expressing gender. For example: "Have you dressed privately in clothing typically associated with your affirmed gender? When did you first begin to dress in private? How did it feel when you first began to dress in private? Did anyone else know? If so, what was their reaction?" (Coolhart, 2012, p. 17).
- *School Context:* These questions explore the youth's experience and possible harassment at school related to gender identity. For example: "What is your current gender expression at school? Are you 'out' to any of your friends?" (Coolhart, 2012, p. 18).

- *Sexual Relationships/Development:* These questions are typically asked of the youth in private and address sexual orientation, abuse, and activity: How do you identify your sexual orientation? Have you ever experienced or witnessed sexual or physical abuse?" (Coolhart, 2012, p. 19).
- *Current Intimate Relationship(s):* If the youth is involved in a current relationship, the counselors inquires about the relationship and the partner's knowledge of the youth's gender identity and possible interest in transitioning.
- *Physical and Mental Health:* These questions assess for physical and mental health issues that may need addressing, including the potential for self-harm and substance abuse.
- *Support:* The questions aim to identify sources of support for the family and youth, including family, friends, church, neighbors, support groups, Internet connections, and so on.
- *Future Plans/Expectations:* This last set of questions explores whether the youth has plans for gender transition, hormone therapy, surgery, children, and such.

Research and the Evidence Base

Systemic therapy began as a research project: the Bateson team began by studying communication in families with members diagnosed with schizophrenia. The tradition of observational research has been integrated into the required standard training in systemic and strategic models, in the form of observation teams. Although there has been less systematic research on outcomes of specific systemic models, such as strategic, Milan, or MRI, there is consistent and growing research on the effectiveness of evidence-based systemic approaches for specific conditions, such as adolescent substance abuse, adolescent conduct issues, depression related to relationship distress, severe mental illness, and couple distress (Sprenkle, 2012). These evidence-based treatments use key theoretical concepts and techniques from systemic family therapies and apply them to a specific population.

Systemic therapies are quickly emerging as a leading force in the realm of evidence-based treatments. Numerous empirically supported treatments incorporate key elements of systemic and strategic therapies, including:

- **Brief Strategic Family Therapy** (structural ecosystemic therapy, structural ecodevelopmental preventive interventions)
- **Ecosystemic Structural Therapy** (Lindblad-Goldberg, Dore, & Stern, 1998)
- **Emotionally Focused Couples Therapy** (Johnson, 2004)
- **Functional Family Therapy** (Alexander, Waldron, Robbins, & Neeb, 2013; Sexton, 2010)
- **Multidimensional Family Therapy** (Liddle, Dakof, & Diamond, 1991)
- **Multisystemic Family Therapy** (Henggeler, Schoenwald, Borduin, Rowland, & Cunningham, 1998)

Although each of these approaches is unique, they all incorporate identifying the problem interaction sequence, and in some way interrupting or altering it by using one or more systemic or strategic techniques to address the needs of a specific population.

Questions for Personal Reflection and Class Discussion

1. Which ideas from this chapter do you find most personally relevant? Why?
2. Which ideas from this chapter do you think will be most helpful in working with clients?
3. What are the possibilities and limitations for using this approach with diverse clients? How might you address the limitations?
4. To what degree do you think a person's behavior is shaped by systemic dynamics? How?

5. Have you ever experienced a complementary dynamic, where you and another person took on opposite roles, such as good/bad kid or parent or pursuer/distance in a relationship? How did this dynamic emerge? How did it affect each person?
6. Can you describe the interactional patterns in one of your relationships? How does the tension start? What does the problem or conflict look like? How do things get back to normal?
7. What do you think about respecting and trusting the system to self-correct itself? Do you have concerns about the idea that the counselor cannot "control" how a system responds?
8. For which clients and/or presenting problems do you think this approach would be most appropriate? Least appropriate?
9. Which case conceptualization concept seems most useful for understanding a client's problem?
10. Which intervention do you think would be the most useful?
11. Do you think this approach is a good fit for you as a counselor or therapist? Why or why not?
12. In what ways would you need to grow, or what would you need to learn, to be able to use this approach well?

Online Resources

Associations and Institutes

American Association of Brief and Strategic Therapists
www.aabst.org/

American Association for Marriage and Family Therapy
www.aamft.org

Brief Strategic and Systemic World Network
www.bsst.org

Brief Strategic Family Therapy Training
www.brief-strategic-family-therapy.com

BSFT Training Manual
www.nida.nih.gov/TXManuals/bsft

Emotionally Focused Therapy: Sue Johnson, Canada
www.eft.ca

International Association of Marriage and Family Counselors
www.iamfconline.com/

Functional Family Therapy
www.fftinc.com/

Mental Research Institute
www.mri.org

Multisystemic Therapy
www.mstservices.com

Philadelphia Child and Family Therapy Training Center
www.philafamily.com

Journals

Family Process
www.familyprocess.org/

Journal of Marital and Family Therapy
www.jmft.net/

Journal of Systemic Therapies
www.guilford.com/

References

*Asterisk indicates recommended introductory readings.

Alexander, J. F., Waldron, H. B., Robbins, M. S., & Neeb, A. A. (2013). *Functional family therapy for adolescent behavior problems.* Washington, DC: American Psychological Association.

Anger-Díaz, B., Schlanger, K., Rincon, C., & Mendoza, A. (2004). Problem-solving across cultures: Our Latino experience. *Journal of Systemic Therapies, 23*(4), 11–27. doi: 10.1521/jsyt.23.4.11.57837

Aponte, H. J. (1994). *Bread and spirit: Therapy with the new poor: Diversity of race, culture, and values.* New York: Norton.

Aponte, H. J. (1996). Political bias, moral values, and spirituality in the training of psychotherapists. *Bulletin of the Menninger Clinic, 60*(4), 488–502.

*Bateson, G. (1972). *Steps to an ecology of mind; collected essays in anthropology, psychiatry, evolution, and epistemology.* San Francisco, CA: Chandler.

Bateson, G. (1979). *Mind and nature: A necessary unity.* New York: Dutton.

*Boscolo, L., Cecchin, G., Hoffman, L., & Penn, P. (1987). *Milan systemic family therapy: Conversations in theory and practice.* New York: Basic Books.

Bowen, M. (1976). Theory in practice of psychotherapy. In P. J. Guerin (Ed.), *Family therapy: Theory and practice.* New York: Gardner.

*Bowen, M. (1985). *Family therapy in clinical practice.* New York: Jason Aronson.

Butler, C. (2009). Sexual and gender minority therapy and systemic practice. *Journal of Family Therapy, 31*(4), 338–358. doi:10.1111/j.1467-6427.2009.00472.x

Carter, B., & McGoldrick, M. (Eds.). (2005). *The expanded family life cycle: Individuals, families, and social perspectives* (3rd ed.). New York: Allyn and Bacon.

*Cecchin, G. (1987). Hypothesizing, circularity, and neutrality revisited: An invitation to curiosity. *Family Process, 26*(4), 405–413.

*Colapinto, J. (1991). Structural family therapy. In A. S. Gurman & D. P. Kniskern (Eds.), *Handbook of family therapy,* (Vol. II, pp. 417–443). New York: Brunner Mazel.

Coolhart, D., Baker, A., Farmer, S., Malaney, M., & Shipman, D. (2012). Therapy with transsexual youth and their families: A clinical tool for assessing youth's readiness for gender transition. *Journal of Marital and Family Therapy* [Early View Version]. doi: 10.1111/j.1752-0606.2011.00283.x

DeVine, J. L. (1984). A systemic inspection of affectional preference orientation and the family of origin. *Journal of Social Work and Human Sexuality, 2,* 9–17.

Erich, S., Tittsworth, J., Dykes, J., & Cabuses, C. (2008). Family relationships and their correlations with transsexual well-being. *Journal of GLBT Family Studies, 4*(4), 419–432.

*Fisch, R., Weakland, J., & Segal, L. (1982). *The tactics of change: Doing therapy briefly.* New York: Jossey-Bass.

Gehart, D. (2015). *Theory and treatment planning in counseling and psychotherapy* (2nd ed.). Pacific Grove, CA: Brooks Cole.

Gehart, D. (2014). *Mastering competencies in family therapy. A practical approach to theories and clinical case documentation* (2nd ed.). Belmont, CA: Brooks/Cole.

Goldberg, A. E. (2009). Lesbian, gay, and bisexual family psychology: A systemic, life-cycle perspective. In J. H. Bray & M. Stanton (Eds.), *The Wiley-Blackwell handbook of family psychology* (pp. 576–587). Wiley-Blackwell. doi: 10.1002/9781444310238.ch40

Goldenberg, H., & Goldenberg, I. (2012). *Family therapy: An overview* (8th ed.). New York: Cengage.

Grossman, A. H., D'Augelli, A. R., Howell, T. J., & Hubbard, S. (2005). Parents' reactions to transgender youths' gender nonconforming expression and identity. *Journal of Gay and Lesbian Social Services, 18*(1), 3–16.

Haley, J. (1963). *Strategies of psychotherapy.* New York: Grune & Stratton.

Haley, J. (1973). *Uncommon therapy: The psychiatric techniques of Milton H. Erickson, M.D.* New York: Norton.

Haley, J. (1976). *Problem-solving therapy: New strategies for effective family therapy.* San Francisco, CA: Jossey-Bass.

Haley, J. (1984). *Ordeal therapy.* San Francisco, CA: Jossey-Bass.

*Haley, J. (1987). *Problem-solving therapy* (2nd ed.). San Francisco, CA: Jossey-Bass.

Haley, J., & Richeport-Haley, M. (2007). *Directive family therapy.* New York: Hawthorne.

Henggeler, S. W., Schoenwald, S. K., Borduin, C. M., Rowland, M. D., & Cunningham, P. B. (1998). *Multisystemic treatment of antisocial behavior in children and adolescents.* New York: Guilford.

Jackson, D. D. (1967). The myth of normality. *Medical Opinion and Review, 3,* 28–33.

Johnson, S. M. (2004). *The practice of emotionally focused marital therapy: Creating connection* (2nd ed.). New York: Brunner/Routledge.

Liddle, H. A., Dakof, G. A., & Diamond, G. (1991). Adolescent substance abuse: Multidimensional family therapy in action. In E. Daufman & P. Kaufman (Eds.), *Family therapy of drug and alcohol abuse* (pp. 120–171). Boston, MA: Allyn & Bacon.

Lindblad-Goldberg, M., Dore, M., & Stern, L. (1998). *Creating competence from chaos.* New York: Norton.

Madanes, C. (1981). *Strategic family therapy.* San Francisco, CA: Jossey-Bass.

Madanes, C. (1991). Strategic family therapy. In A. S. Gurman & D. P. Knishern (Eds.), *Handbook of family therapy* (pp. 396–416). New York: Brunner/Mazel.

McFarlane, W. R. (2004). *Multifamily groups in the treatment of severe psychiatric illness.* New York: Guilford.

McGoldrick, M., Giordano, J., & Garcia-Preto, N. (Eds.). (2005). *Ethnicity and family therapy* (3rd ed.). New York: Guilford.

Mental Research Institute. (2002). *On the shoulder of giants.* Palo Alto, CA: Author.

Minuchin, S. (1974). *Families and family therapy.* Cambridge, MA: Harvard University Press.

*Minuchin, S., & Fishman, H. C. (1981). *Family therapy techniques.* Cambridge, MA: Harvard University Press.

Minuchin, S., Montalvo, B., Buerney, B. G., Rosman, B., & Schumer, F. (1967). *Families of the slums: An exploration of their structure and treatment*. New York: Basic Books.
Minuchin, S., & Nichols, M. P. (1993). *Family healing: Tales of hope and renewal from family therapy*. New York: Free Press.
Minuchin, S. Nichols, M. P., Lee, W. Y. (2007). *Assessing families and couples: From symptom to system*. Bacon.
Multisystemic Therapy Services. (1998). *Multisytemic therapy*. Downloaded May 2, 2008, http://www.mstservices.com/text/treatment.html
*Nardone, G., & Watzlawick, P. (1993). *The art of change: Strategic therapy and hypnotherapy without trance*. San Francisco, CA: Jossey-Bass.
Nichols, M. P. (2012). *Family therapy: Concepts and methods* (10th ed.). Pacific Grove, CA: Pearson.
Rastogi, M. (2007). Coping with transitions in Asian Indian families: Systemic clinical interventions with immigrants. *Journal of Systemic Therapies*, *26*(2), 55–67. doi:10.1521/jsyt.2007.26.2.55
Robbins, M. S., Horigian, V., Szapocznik, J., & Ucha, J. (2010). Treating Hispanic youths using brief strategic family therapy. In J. R. Weisz & A. E. Kazdin (Eds.), *Evidence-based psychotherapies for children and adolescents* (2nd ed., pp. 375–390). New York: Guilford.
Santisteban, D. A., Coatsworth, J., Perez-Vidal, A., Mitrani, V., Jean-Gilles, M., & Szapocznik, J. (1997). Brief structural/strategic family therapy with African American and Hispanic high-risk youth. *Journal of Community Psychology*, *25*(5), 453–471. doi:10.1002/(SICI)1520-6629(199709)25:5<453::AID-JCOP6>3.0.CO;2-T
Satir, V. (1967/1983). *Conjoint family therapy* (3rd/Revised ed.). Palo Alto, CA: Science and Behavior Books.
Satir, V. (1972). *Peoplemaking*. Palo Alto, CA: Science and Behavior Books.
Satir, V. (1988). *The new peoplemaking*. Palo Alto, CA: Science and Behavior Books.
Satir, V., Banmen, J., Gerber, J., & Gomori, M. (1991). *The Satir model: Family therapy and beyond*. Palo Alto, CA: Science and Behavior Books.
Segal, L. (1991). Brief Therapy: The MRI approach. In A. A. Gurman & D. P. Knishern (Eds.), *Handbook of family therapy* (pp. 171–199). New York: Brunner/Mazel.
Selvini Palazzoli, M. (Ed.). (1988). *The work of Mara Selvini Palazzoli*. New York: Jason Aronson.
*Selvini Palazzoli, M., Boscolo, L., Cecchin, G., & Prata, G. (1980). Hypothesizing-circularity-neutrality: Three guidelines for the conductor of the session. *Family Process*, *19*(1), 3–12.
Selvini Palazzoli, M., Cecchin, G., Prata, G., & Boscolo, L. (1978). *Paradox and counterparadox: A new model in the therapy of the family in schizophrenic transaction*. New York: Jason Aronson.
Sexton, T. L. (2010). *Functional family therapy in clinical practice: An evidence-based treatment model for working with troubled adolescents*. New York: Routledge.
Sprenkle, D. H. (Ed.) (2002). *Effectiveness research in marriage and family therapy*. Alexandria, VA: American Association for Marriage and Family Therapy.
Sprenkle, D. H. (Ed.) (2011). *Effectiveness research in marriage and family therapy* (2nd ed.). Alexandria, VA: American Association for Marriage and Family Therapy.
Sprenkle, D. (Ed.). (2012). Intervention research in couple and family therapy [Special edition]. *Journal of Marital and Family Therapy*, *38*(1).
Szapocznik, J., & Williams, R. A. (2000). Brief Strategic Family Therapy: Twenty-five years of interplay among theory, research and practice in adolescent behavior problems and drug abuse. *Clinical Child and Family Psychology Review*, *3*(2), 117–134.
Walsh, F. (Ed.). (2009). *Spiritual resources in family therapy* (2nd ed.). New York: Guilford.
Watzlawick, P. (1978/1993). *The language of change: Elements of therapeutic conversation*. New York: Norton.
Watzlawick, P., Bavelas, J. B., & Jackson, D. D. (1967). *Pragmatics of human communication: A study of interactional patterns, pathologies, and paradoxes*. New York: Norton.
Watzlawick, P., & Weakland, J. H. (1977). *The interactional view: Studies at the Mental Research Institute, Palo Alto, 1965–1974*. New York: W. W. Norton & Company.
*Watzlawick, P., Weakland, J., & Fisch, R. (1974). *Change: Principles of problem formation and problem resolution*. New York: Norton.

Systemic Case Study: Substance Use and Unemployed

Billy, 23, whose mother is Sioux, comes to counseling at the urging of his sister, who notices he has started to drink excessively since he lost his busboy job three months ago. He lives with his mother and sister in a small apartment. He reports feeling hopeless because the economy is so bad, and "there aren't any good jobs in town anyway." With extra time on his hands, he has been visiting his grandmother on the reservation more frequently, where he has had some contact with the local medicine woman. When he is in town, he has a few friends from high school that he hangs out with, mostly drinking together. Billy says he no longer feels the need to sleep or eat and that there isn't anything he really enjoys doing any more. He also says that sometimes he hears the call of an eagle that he cannot see, even in town.

After an initial consultation, a systemic counselor develops the following case conceptualization.

CASE CONCEPTUALIZATION

Date: November 4, 2013 **Clinician:** Richard **Client/Case #:** 12001

I. Introduction to Client

Identify primary client and significant others

Client

Adult Male Age: 23 Native American Single heterosexual Occupation/Grade: High school graduate; unemployed busboy.

Other: Living at home with mother and sister.

Significant Others

Client's Mother Age: 53 Native American Single heterosexual Occupation/Grade: Retail

Other: ______

Other Age: 27 Native American Single heterosexual Occupation/Grade: Elementary School Teacher

Other: Client's sister

Select Person Age: ____ Select Ethnicity Select Relational Status Occupation/Grade: ______ Other: ______

Select Person Age: ____ Select Ethnicity Select Relational Status Occupation/Grade: ______ Other: ______

Others: ______

II. Presenting Concern(s)

Client Description of Problem(s): AM came to counseling primarily at his sister's urging. He was laid off from his busboy job 3 months ago and does not see any point in looking for another one since the economy in town is bad. He admits to drinking more since losing his job, but says, "What else is there to do around here?"

Significant Other/Family Description(s) of Problems: Sister: Believes her brother is depressed and drinking and headed down the wrong path, much the same as their father. She thinks he needs to get a job or go to a trade school. Mother: Less concerend about the drinking and more concerned that he is not himself: sad, hopeless, and negative. She is glad he is spending time with his grandmother, who she believes is a great influence. She believes the call of the eagle is a positive sign, that Spirit is guiding him to find his purpose as a young man.

Broader System Problem Descriptions: Description of problem from referring party, teachers, relatives, legal system, etc.:

AM Friend: One of AM's high school friends has told him that he thinks he is becoming an alcoholic like his father.

Grandmother: Sees him as needing to accept the challenge of becoming an adult young man and to use some of the ancient ways to find his path in this world. She believes the eagle he hears is a special spiritual message, calling him back to his roots.

(continued)

III. Background Information

Trauma/Abuse History (recent and past): AM denies any childhood traumas or abuse, but reports living in poverty for much of his youth.

Substance Use/Abuse (current and past; self, family of origin, significant others): AM currently drinks heavily 6–12 twelve-ounce beers per night 4–5 nights out of the week—or more if he has unrestricted access (e.g., someone else is paying). Although his father left when he was young, he has been told that he had a serious drinking problem as did his mother's father.

Precipitating Events (recent life changes, first symptoms, stressors, etc.): AM lost his busboy job that he had had since graduating high school 3 months ago; no clear cause was given.

Related Historical Background (family history, related issues, previous counseling, etc.): AM's mother lost her job several times during his youth, which were always difficult periods for AM and his sister. Although he did not party excessively in high school, he did not excel academically either, mostly for lack of effort. He enjoyed playing video games and skateboarding more than doing homework and has never had big ambitions.

IV. Client Strengths and Diversity

Client Strengths

Personal: When he had a job, AM was a diligent worker; he can be charming and fun; he is resourceful when he needs to be.

Relational/Social: He describes a deep respect for his mother, grandmother, and sister; he is proud of his Sioux heritage; he is able to maintain connections to friends from high school and the reservation.

Spiritual: Although most of his life, spirituality has not played a strong role in his life, in recent visits with his grandmother, AM has become more curious about his native spirituality. Like his grandmother and mother, he believes that the "eagle's call" is of great spiritual value.

Diversity: Resources and Limitations

Identify potential resources and limitations available to clients based on their age, gender, sexual orientation, cultural background, socioeconomic status, religion, regional community, language, family background, family configuration, abilities, etc.

Unique Resources: AM has a strong support system with his tribe, his grandmother, and the other elders living on the reservation.

Potential Limitations: Lack of a positive male role-model and mixed cultural messages toward pursuing higher education and/or a career path.

Complete All of the Following Sections for a Complete Case Conceptualization or Specific Sections for Theory-Specific Conceptualization.

(continued)

V. Psychodynamic Conceptualization

Psychodynamic Defense Mechanisms

Check 2–4 most commonly used defense mechanisms

❑ Acting Out: *Describe:*

☒ Denial: *Describe:* AM does not acknowledge troubling drinking pattern or other self-defeating behaviors.

❑ Displacement: *Describe:*

☒ Help-rejecting complaining: *Describe:* AM is quick to complain about his situation but has no motivation to do anything or accept help that is offered.

❑ Humor: *Describe:*

❑ Passive Aggression: *Describe:*

❑ Projection: *Describe:*

❑ Projective Identification: *Describe:*

❑ Rationalization: *Describe:*

❑ Reaction Formation: *Describe:*

❑ Repression: *Describe:*

❑ Splitting: *Describe:*

❑ Sublimation: *Describe:*

❑ Suppression: *Describe:*

☒ Other: Fantasy: AM retreats into a world of wishful thinking in which his problems are solved for him.

Object Relational Patterns

Describe relationship with early caregivers in past: AM was raised by his mother and grandmother. Both took a "hands-off" approach to parenting, and AM was for the most part free to do as he pleased. There were few rules or expectations.

Was the attachment with the mother (or equivalent) primarily:

☒ Generally Secure ❑ Anxious and Clingy ☒ Avoidant and Emotionally Distant ❑ Other: AM's mother was overly permissive but AM has a strong relationship with her and states he knows he can always count on her.

Was the attachment with the father (or equivalent) primarily:

❑ Generally Secure ❑ Anxious and Clingy ☒ Avoidant and Emotionally Distant ❑ Other: AM's father is an alcoholic and left the family when AM was 4 years old. They have had little contact since then.

Describe present relationship with these caregivers: AM is dependent on his mother as he is currently unemployed. She is silently supportive and enables him to drink and not search for a new job.

Describe relational patterns with partner and other current relationships: NA

Erickson's Psychosocial Developmental Stage

Describe development at each stage up to current stage

Trust vs. Mistrust (Infant Stage): AM raised by grandmother and mother

(continued)

Autonomy vs. Shame and Doubt (Toddler Stage): AM father's alcoholism grew worse during these years

Initiative vs. Guilt (Preschool Age): AM father left at age 4

Industry vs. Inferiority (School Age): AM not strongly encouraged to accel in school; he was an average-to-low-average student.

Identity vs. Role Confusion (Adolescence): During this time, he had intermittent contact with his father and limited contact with grandmother; did not develop clear sense of identity either in relation to culture or peers.

Intimacy vs. Isolation (Young Adulthood): AM has never had a serious girlfriend, only dating casually for short periods of time.

Generativity vs. Stagnation (Adulthood): ______

Ego Integrity vs. Despair (Late Adulthood): ______

Adlerian Style of Life Theme

❑ Control: ______

❑ Superiority: ______

❑ Pleasing: ______

☒ Comfort: Above all, AM has sought comfort, not wanting to study too hard, work too hard, or push himself too hard. He often feels failure is likely, so why try?

Basic Mistake Misperceptions: "Life is too hard for someone like me to be successful."

VI. Humanistic-Existential Conceptualization

Expression of Authentic Self

Problems: Are problems perceived as internal or external (caused by others, circumstance, etc.)?

❑ Predominantly internal

❑ Mixed

☒ Predominantly external

Agency and Responsibility: Is self or other discussed as agent of story? Does client take clear responsibility for situation?

❑ Strong sense of agency and responsibility

❑ Agency in some areas

☒ Little agency; frequently blames others/situation

❑ Often feels victimized

Recognition and Expression of Feelings: Are feelings readily recognized, owned, and experienced?

❑ Easily expresses feelings

❑ Identifies feelings with prompting

☒ Difficulty recognizing feelings

Here-and-Now Experiencing: Is the client able to experience full range of feelings as they are happening in the present moment?

❑ Easily experiences emotions in present moment

❑ Experiences some present emotions with assistance

☒ Difficulty with present moment experiencing

(*continued*)

Personal Constructs and Facades: Is the client able to recognize and go beyond roles? Is identity rigid or tentatively held?

❑ Tentatively held; able to critique and question

☒ Some awareness of facades and construction of identity

❑ Identity rigidly defined; seems like "fact"

Complexity and Contradictions: Are internal contradictions owned and explored? Is client able to fully engage the complexity of identity and life?

❑ Aware of and resolves contradictions

❑ Some recognition of contradictions

☒ Unaware of internal contradictions

Shoulds: Is client able to question socially imposed shoulds and oughts? Can client balance desire to please others and desire to be authentic?

❑ Able to balance authenticity with social obligation

☒ Identifies tension between social expectations and personal desires

❑ Primarily focuses on external shoulds

List shoulds: Life should be easier; AM shouldn't be able to find a job since he lost his last one

Acceptance of Others: Is client able to accept others and modify expectations of others to be more realistic?

❑ Readily accepts others as they are

❑ Recognizes expectations of others are unrealistic but still strong emotional reaction to expectations not being met

☒ Difficulty accepting others as is; always wanting others to change to meet expectations

Trust of Self: Is client able to trust self as process (rather than a stabile object)?

❑ Able to trust and express authentic self

❑ Trust of self in certain contexts

☒ Difficulty trusting self in most contexts

Existential Analysis

Sources of Life Meaning (as described or demonstrated by client): Client has done little reflecting upon the meaning of life. He values his family and is beginning to search for meaning in his cultural heritage.

General Themes of Life Meaning:

❑ Personal achievement/work

❑ Significant other

❑ Children

☒ Family of origin

❑ Social cause/contributing to others

☒ Religion/spirituality

❑ Other: ______

Satisfaction with and clarity on life direction:

❑ Clear sense of meaning that creates resilience in difficult times

❑ Current problems require making choices related to life direction

❑ Minimally satisfied with current life direction; wants more from life

☒ Has reflected little on life direction up to this point; living according to life plan defined by someone/something else

❑ Other: ______

(continued)

Gestalt Contact Boundary Disturbances

☒ *Desensitization:* Failing to notice problems
❑ *Introjection*: Take in others' views whole and unedited
❑ *Projection*: Assign undesired parts of self to others
❑ *Retroflection*: Direct action to self rather than other
❑ *Deflection*: Avoid direct contact with another or self
❑ *Egotism:* Not allowing outside to influence self
❑ *Confluence*: Agree with another to extent that boundary blurred
Describe: ______

VII. Cognitive-Behavioral Conceptualization

Baseline of Symptomatic Behavior

Symptom #1 (behavioral description): Not enjoying everyday activities; not pursuing work or school.

Frequency: Most days.

Duration: 3 months; since lost job.

Context(s): Worse at home; better with friends or when visiting grandmother on reservation.

Events Before: Getting up and having breakfast; then feels has nowhere to go or anything to do.

Events After: Continues until he drinks to "take my mind off of things."

Symptom #2 (behavioral description): Drinking alcohol

Frequency: 4–7 days per week

Duration: 3 months

Context(s): With friends from high school or on reservation.

Events Before: Feeling depressed, hopeless, bored.

Events After: Goes to bed.

A-B-C Analysis of Irrational Beliefs

Activating Event ("Problem"): Laid off from job.

Consequence (Mood, behavior, etc.): Depressed mood, feeling hopeless, drinking more, nothing to do.

Mediating Beliefs (Unhelpful beliefs about event that result in C):

1. If I can't keep a busboy job, I must be a real loser.
2. If I can't keep this job, there isn't anything else out there either.
3. ______

Beck's Schema Analysis

Identify frequently used cognitive schemas:

❑ *Arbitrary inference:*

☒ *Selective abstraction:* Focuses on difficulties/problems rather than possibilities.

❑ *Overgeneralization:* ______

☒ *Magnification/Minimization:* One setback leads him to think that cannot succeed anywhere.

☒ *Personalization:* Believes he is a loser; because there were not enough customers at his resturant.

(continued)

❑ *Absolutist/dichotomous thinking:* ________________

❑ *Mislabeling:* ________________

❑ *Mindreading:* ________________

VIII. Family Systems Conceptualization

Family Life Cycle Stage

☒ Single adult
❑ Marriage
❑ Family with Young Children
❑ Family with Adolescent Children
❑ Launching Children
❑ Later Life

Describe struggles with mastering developmental tasks in one of these stages: AM is struggling to find his place in the adult world and believes he is a "loser" because he does not have a job or a girlfriend.

Boundaries with

Parents ☒ Enmeshed ❑ Clear ❑ Disengaged ❑ NA: *Describe:* Mother is very permissive and does not set any limits for him in terms of contributing to the household or drinking.

Significant Other ❑ Enmeshed ❑ Clear ❑ Disengaged ❑ NA: *Describe:* ________________

Children ❑ Enmeshed ❑ Clear ❑ Disengaged ❑ NA: *Describe:* ________________

Extended Family ❑ Enmeshed ❑ Clear ❑ Disengaged ❑ NA: *Describe:* ________________

Other: Sister ❑ Enmeshed ☒ Clear ❑ Disengaged ❑ NA: *Describe:* AM able to talk with her about problems better than anyone.

Typical style for regulating closeness and distance with others: AM feels close to his mother, grandmother, and sister but does not talk about problems with them. Their caring is often expressed in silent presence. His mother allows him a lot of independence as the man in the family.

Triangles/Coalitions

☒ Coalition in family of origin: *Describe:* After his father left, the mother and children aligned against the father. There is very little contact with his father.

❑ Coalitions related to significant other: *Describe:* ________________

❑ Other coalitions: ________________

Hierarchy between Self and Parent/Child ❑ NA

With own children ❑ Effective ❑ Rigid ❑ Permissive

With parents (for child/young adult) ❑ Effective ❑ Rigid ☒ Permissive

Complementary Patterns with <u>Siblings</u>:

❑ Pursuer/distancer
☒ Over-/underfunctioner
❑ Emotional/logical

(*continued*)

❑ Good/bad parent
❑ Other: *Describe*

Example of complementary pattern: ______

Intergenerational Patterns

Substance/Alcohol Abuse: ❑ NA ☒ History: AM is drinking heavily; his father continues to drink; maternal grandfather also drank heavily.

Sexual/Physical/Emotional Abuse: ☒ NA ❑ History: ______

Parent/Child Relations: ❑ NA ☒ History: His father abandoned family as did his father's father.

Physical/Mental Disorders: ☒ NA ❑ History: ______

Family strengths: Describe: Strong sense of loyalty; silent suporters of one another; connection to traditional culture.

IX. Solution-Based and Cultural Discourse Conceptualization (Postmodern)

Solutions and Unique Outcomes

Attempted Solutions that DIDN'T or DON'T work:

1. Sister telling AM to stop drinking.
2. Avoiding looking for a new job and school.
3. Pretending like there is not a problem.

Exceptions and Unique Outcomes: Times, places, relationships, contexts, etc. when problem is less of a problem; behaviors that seem to make things even slightly better:

1. AM has been able to hear his grandmother and medicine woman's advice the best; he is interested in a vision quest or somehow following the cry of the eagle he has been hearing.
2. He continues to take out the trash to help his mother at home.
3. ______

Miracle Question Answer: If the problem were to be resolved overnight, what would client be doing differently the next day? (Describe in terms of doing X rather than not doing Y).

1. He would be following the eagle's cry and starting his quest toward his destiny.
2. He would would have a job he enjoys and be able to comfortably support himself.
3. He would have a serious relationship with a girlfriend.

Dominant Discourses informing definition of problem:

- *Ethnic, Class and Religious Discourses: How do key cultural discourses inform what is perceived as a problem and the possible solutions?* AM's experience of hopelessness, depression, and drinking conforms to the negative sterotype of Native Americans; AM has bought into this hopeless picture, although he argues that he has not. His interest in spiritual practices provides a hopeful avenue for AM, although the white part of him doubts that road, too. He seems to resolve these cultural tensions by taking a position in "no man's land" and avoiding taking any direction.

(*continued*)

- *Gender and Sexuality Discourses: How do the gender/sexual discourses inform what is perceived as a problem and the possible solutions?* AM is surrounded by highly capable and resilient women—mother, grandmother, and sister—and is left with a legacy of a father who deserted him and did not provide financially or emotionally. He seems to be following in his father's footsteps and might benefit from male mentorship.
- *Community, School, and Extended Family Discourses: How do other important community discourses inform what is perceived as a problem and the possible solutions?* The broader sociocultural discourse around shrinking rural towns and the poverty associated with them leads AM to conclude that there is no point in his striving to make something of himself.

Identity Narratives: How has the problem shaped each client's identity? AM seems to have concluded that since he has lost his job—his first and only job—he does not have any chance at a future until something drastic happens in town. He sees relying on his mother and sister to support him as his only option. Although he feels like a "loser," he also feels as though he does not have any other choice.

Local or Preferred Discourses: What is the client's preferred identity narrative and/or narrative about the problem? Are there local (alternative) discourses about the problem that are preferred? A part of AM is intrigued by his grandmother's belief that he is beginning a rite of passage to become a young man. The eagle's cries are part of this call to finally grow up. He is considering talking more with the medicine woman about this.

CLINICAL ASSESSMENT

Clinician: Richard	Client ID #: 12001	Primary configuration: ☒ Individual ❑ Couple ❑ Family	Primary Language: ☒ English ❑ Spanish ☒ Other: Some Lakhota

List client and significant others

Adult(s)

Adult Male Age: 23 Native American Single heterosexual Occupation: Unemployed busboy; high school graduate

Other identifier: Lives with mother and sister

Select Gender Age: _____ Select Ethnicity Select Relational Status Occupation: _____ Other identifier: ______

Child(ren)

Select Gender Age: _____ Select Ethnicity Grade: Select Grade School: _______ Other identifier: ___________

Select Gender Age: _____ Select Ethnicity Grade: Select Grade School: _______ Other identifier: ___________

Others: ______________________________

Presenting Problems

		Complete for children:
☒ Depression/hopelessness	❑ Couple concerns	❑ School failure/decline performance
❑ Anxiety/worry	❑ Parent/child conflict	❑ Truancy/runaway
❑ Anger issues	❑ Partner violence/abuse	❑ Fighting w/peers
❑ Loss/grief	❑ Divorce adjustment	❑ Hyperactivity
❑ Suicidal thoughts/attempts	❑ Remarriage adjustment	❑ Wetting/soiling clothing
❑ Sexual abuse/rape	❑ Sexuality/intimacy concerns	❑ Child abuse/neglect
☒ Alcohol/drug use	❑ Major life changes	❑ Isolation/withdrawal
❑ Eating problems/disorders	❑ Legal issues/probation	❑ Other: ___________
☒ Job problems/unemployed	❑ Other: ___________	

Mental Status Assessment for Identified Patient

Interpersonal	❑ NA	❑ Conflict ❑ Enmeshment ☒ Isolation/Avoidance ❑ Harassment ❑ Other: ___________
Mood	❑ NA	☒ Depressed/Sad ❑ Anxious ❑ Dysphoric ❑ Angry ❑ Irritable ❑ Manic ❑ Other: ___________
Affect	❑ NA	☒ Constricted ❑ Blunt ❑ Flat ❑ Labile ❑ Incongruent ❑ Other: ___________

(continued)

Sleep	❑ NA	❑ Hypersomnia ☒ Insomnia ❑ Disrupted ❑ Nightmares ❑ Other: ______
Eating	❑ NA	❑ Increase ☒ Decrease ❑ Anorectic restriction ❑ Binging ❑ Purging ❑ Other: ______
Anxiety	☒ NA	❑ Chronic worry ❑ Panic ❑ Phobias ❑ Obsessions ❑ Compulsions ❑ Other: ______
Trauma Symptoms	☒ NA	❑ Hypervigilance ❑ Flashbacks/Intrusive memories ❑ Dissociation ❑ Numbing ❑ Avoidance efforts ❑ Other: ______
Psychotic Symptoms	❑ NA	❑ Hallucinations ❑ Delusions ❑ Paranoia ❑ Loose associations ☒ Other: ______
Motor activity/ Speech	❑ NA	☒ Low energy ❑ Hyperactive ❑ Agitated ❑ Inattentive ☒ Impulsive ❑ Pressured speech ❑ Slow speech ❑ Other: ______
Thought	❑ NA	☒ Poor concentration ☒ Denial ❑ Self-blame ☒ Other-blame ❑ Ruminative ❑ Tangential ❑ Concrete ☒ Poor insight ☒ Impaired decision making ❑ Disoriented ❑ Other: ______
Socio-Legal	☒ NA	❑ Disregards rules ❑ Defiant ❑ Stealing ❑ Lying ❑ Tantrums ❑ Arrest/ incarceration ❑ Initiates fights ❑ Other: ______
Other Symptoms	☒ NA	______

Diagnosis for Identified Patient

Contextual Factors considered in making diagnosis: ☒ Age ☒ Gender ☒ Family dynamics ☒ Culture ☒ Language ☒ Religion ☒ Economic ❑ Immigration ❑ Sexual/Gender orientation ❑ Trauma ❑ Dual diagnosis/comorbid ☒ Addiction ❑ Cognitive ability ❑ Other: ______

Describe impact of identified factors on diagnosis and assessment process: Hallucinations considered within cultural/religious traditions in which this particular hallucination (hearing an eagle cry) is not unusual; no other psychotic symptoms, thus the client will only be monitored for additional indications of psychotic symptoms before diagnosing such issues. Family pattern of addiction used to provide context for diagnosing alcohol abuse issues.

DSM-5 Code	Diagnosis with Specifier *Include V/Z/T-Codes for Psychosocial Stressors/Issues*
1. F32.1	1. Major Depression, Single Episode, Moderate
2. F10.20	2. Alcohol Use Disorder, Moderate
3. ______	3. ______
4. ______	4. ______
5. ______	5. ______

(*continued*)

Medical Considerations

Has patient been referred for psychiatric evaluation? ☒ Yes ❑ No

Has patient agreed with referral? ❑ Yes ☒ No ❑ NA

Psychometric instruments used for assessment: ❑ None ☒ Cross-cutting symptom inventories ❑ Other: ________

Client response to diagnosis: ❑ Agree ☒ Somewhat agree ❑ Disagree ❑ Not informed for following reason:

Agree with depression; disagree with alcohol abuse diagnosis.

Current Medications (psychiatric & medical) ☒ **NA**

1. ______; dose ______ mg; start date: ______
2. ______; dose ______ mg; start date: ______
3. ______; dose ______ mg; start date: ______
4. ______; dose ______ mg; start date: ______

Medical Necessity: *Check all that apply*

☒ Significant impairment ❑ Probability of significant impairment ❑ Probable developmental arrest

Areas of impairment:

☒ Daily activities ☒ Social relationships ❑ Health ☒ Work/School ❑ Living arrangement ❑ Other: ________

Risk and Safety Assessment for Identified Patient

Suicidality	Homicidality	Alcohol Abuse
☒ No indication/Denies	☒ No indication/Denies	❑ No indication/denies
❑ Active ideation	❑ Active ideation	❑ Past abuse
❑ Passive ideation	❑ Passive ideation	☒ Current; Freq/Amt: 6–12 per day
❑ Intent without plan	❑ Intent without means	**Drug Use/Abuse**
❑ Intent with means	❑ Intent with means	☒ No indication/denies
❑ Ideation in past year	❑ Ideation in past year	❑ Past use
❑ Attempt in past year	❑ Violence past year	❑ Current drugs: ________
❑ Family or peer history of completed suicide	❑ History of assaulting others	Freq/Amt: ________
	❑ Cruelty to animals	❑ Family/sig.other use

Sexual & Physical Abuse and Other Risk Factors

❑ Childhood abuse history: ❑ Sexual ❑ Physical ❑ Emotional ❑ Neglect

❑ Adult with abuse/assault in adulthood: ❑ Sexual ❑ Physical ❑ Current

❑ History of perpetrating abuse: ❑ Sexual ❑ Physical ❑ Emotional

❑ Elder/dependent adult abuse/neglect

❑ History of or current issues with restrictive eating, binging, and/or purging

❑ Cutting or other self-harm: ❑ Current ❑ Past: Method: ________

❑ Criminal/legal history: ________

❑ Other trauma history: ________

☒ None reported

(continued)

Indicators of Safety

❑ NA

☒ At least one outside support person

☒ Able to cite specific reasons to live or not harm

❑ Hopeful

❑ Willing to dispose of dangerous items

❑ Has future goals

❑ Willingness to reduce contact with people who make situation worse

❑ Willing to implement safety plan, safety interventions

❑ Developing set of alternatives to self/other harm

❑ Sustained period of safety:

☒ Other: Agrees to harm reduction goals, including not drivdriving while drunk.

Elements of Safety Plan

❑ NA

❑ Verbal no harm contract

❑ Written no harm contract

☒ Emergency contact card

☒ Emergency therapist/agency number

❑ Medication management

❑ Plan for contacting friends/support persons during crisis

☒ Specific plan of where to go during crisis

☒ Specific self-calming tasks to reduce risk before reach crisis level (e.g., journaling, exercising, etc.)

❑ Specific daily/weekly activities to reduce stressors

❑ Other: ____________

Legal/Ethical Action Taken: ☒ NA ❑ Action: ____________

Case Management

Collateral Contacts

- Has contact been made with treating *physicians or other professionals*: ❑ NA ☒ Yes ❑ In process.
  Name/Notes: Consult with physican regarding alcohol use
- If client is involved in mental health *treatment elsewhere*, has contact been made? ❑ NA ❑ Yes ☒ In process.
  Name/Notes: Client refuses to attend specific program for alochol use
- Has contact been made with *social worker*: ☒ NA ❑ Yes ❑ In process. Name/Notes: ____________

Referrals

- Has client been referred for *medical assessment*: ☒ Yes ❑ No evidence for need
- Has client been referred for *social services*: ❑ NA ☒ Job/training ☒ Welfare/Food/Housing ❑ Victim services ❑ Legal aid ❑ Medical ❑ Other: ____________
- Has client been referred for *group* or other support services: ☒ Yes: AA and/or other alcohol program; client has not agreed to attend ❑ In process ❑ None recommended
- Are there anticipated *forensic/legal processes* related to treatment: ☒ No ❑ Yes; describe: ____________

Support Network

- Client social support network includes: ☒ Supportive family ❑ Supportive partner ☒ Friends ☒ Religious/spiritual organization ❑ Supportive work/social group ❑ Other: ____________

(continued)

- Describe anticipated effects treatment will have on others in support system (Children, partner, etc.): As he takes greater responsibility for his life, his mother may feel loss of "little boy."
- Is there anything else client will need to be successful? Connection with tribal family and support

Expected Outcome and Prognosis

☒ Return to normal functioning ❑ Anticipate less than normal functioning ❑ Prevent deterioration

Client Sense of Hope: 2

Evaluation of Assessment/Client Perspective

How were assessment methods adapted to client needs, including age, culture, and other diversity issues? Diagnosis of hallucinations not made based on religious/cultural tradition.

Describe actual or potential areas of client-clinician agreement/disagreement related to the above assessment: AM does not agree with alcohol abuse label but did agree to harm reduction plan.

______________________, ______________ ______________

Clinician Signature License/Intern Status Date

______________________, ______________ ______________

Supervisor Signature License Date

TREATMENT PLAN

Date: November 7, 2013 Case/Client #: 12001

Clinician Name: Richard Theory: Systemic Counseling

Modalities planned: ☒ Individual Adult ❑ Individual Child ❑ Couple ☒ Family ❑ Group: ______

Recommended session frequency: ☒ Weekly ❑ Every two weeks ❑ Other: ______

Expected length of treatment: 6 months

Initial Phase of Treatment

Initial Phase Counseling Tasks

1. Develop working counseling relationship. *Diversity considerations:* Proceeded slowly and with respect for cultural and spiritual traditions. Avoid intense, direct eye contact. Educate self on native spiritual traditions and tribal norms. Use stories when appropriate.

   Relationship building approach/intervention:

   a. Joined with AM by adapting to his slower pace, quiet mannerisms, etc.

2. Assess individual, systemic, and broader cultural dynamics. *Diversity considerations:* Invited mother, sister, grandmother, and tribal elders to an assessment session.

   Assessment strategies:

   a. Assess sequence of AM behaviors and interactions around depression and drinking.

   b. Assess worldview, rules for relating, boundaries, hierarchy, and complementarity patterns in his family, social network, and tribal family.

3. Identify and obtain client agreement on treatment goals. *Diversity note:* Use harm reduction since client does not agree to abstinence goal at this time.

   Goal-making intervention:

   a. Develop systemically framed doable, behaviorally defined goals for both depression and alcohol use.

4. Identify needed referrals, crisis issues, and other client needs. *Diversity note:* Contact physican about drinking safety plan.

   a. *Crisis assessment intervention(s):* Use harm reduction model to stop drunk driving and minimize harm from alcohol use; ensure no suicidal thoughts.

   b. *Referral(s):* Refer AM to job placement program and/or junior college; support group for drinking (if he will go); encourage AM to connect with medicine woman he has had contact with.

Initial Phase Client Goal

1. Decrease alcohol use to reduce drunk driving.

   Interventions:

   a. Family session with mother, sister, and grandmother; use circular questions to gently reframe their concerns and motivate responsible drinking.

(continued)

b. Shaping competency by highlighting past responsible decisions and apply to drinking and Ordeal Therapy to reduce compulsive behaviors related to drinking.

Working Phase of Treatment

Working Phase Counseling Tasks

1. Monitor quality of the working alliance. *Diversity considerations:* Periodically ask clients about comfort level in session as well as monitor nonverbal cues in session and between session (e.g., no-shows, etc.)
   a. *Assessment Intervention:* Check in verbally on each week's task; check in with AM/family members.

2. Monitor progress toward goals. *Diversity considerations:* Include family/tribal feedback on progress
   a. *Assessment Intervention:* Weekly check-in on homework/directives. In family sessions, ask for feedback on progress.

Working Phase Client Goals

1. Decrease enmeshment with mother to increase responsibility for self to reduce depression and helplessness.
   Interventions:
   a. Circular questioning to highlight how he has chosen to remain a child rather than become a man.
   b. Directives to provide opportunities to experiment with greater personal responsibility.

2. Increase interruptions in drinking cycle to reduce alcohol abuse.
   Interventions:
   a. Family sessions with circular questions and reframing to motivate AM to not follow path of father.
   b. Directives that playfully interrupt his drinking pattern/rituals.

3. Increase identity as young man who is on a quest and responsible for his destiny to reduce depression.
   Interventions:
   a. Reinforce cultural stories and resources about spiritual journey and transition to manhood; work with grandmother and medicine woman to facilitate this journey.
   b. Paradoxical directives that encourage him to be a loser every other day.

Closing Phase of Treatment

Closing Phase Counseling Task

1. Develop aftercare plan and maintain gains. *Diversity considerations:* Involve mother, grandmother, sister, and tribal elders/members.
   Intervention:
   a. Circular questions to reinforce new worldview and view of self.

(*continued*)

Closing Phase Client Goals

1. Increase ability to support self in meaningful employment/education to reduce depression.

   Interventions:

   a. Circular questions to motivate AM to identify his goals and ways to pursue them.

   b. Directives to enable AM to change his self-defeating patterns.

2. Increase and strengthen sense of personal agency and responsibility while also part of larger family/tribal system to reduce depression and drinking.

   Interventions:

   a. Systemic reframing and circular questions related to his role in family, tribe, larger society.

   b. Challenge rigid rules for relating and defining himself as a half-Native American man.

PROGRESS NOTE FOR CLIENT #12001

Date: November 14, 2013 **Time:** 1:00 ❑ am/☒pm **Session Length:** ☒ 45 min. ❑ 60 min. ❑ Other: ____ minutes

Present: ☒ Adult Male ❑ Adult Female ❑ Child Male ❑ Child Female ❑ Other: ____

Billing Code: ❑ 90791 (eval) ☒ 90834 (45 min. therapy) ❑ 90837 (60 min. therapy) ❑ 90847 (family)

❑ Other: ____

Symptom(s)	Duration and Frequency Since Last Visit	Progress
1: Drinking	5 days/6–12 sixteen ounce drinks per day (reported)	**Maintained**
2: Depressed Mood	Moderate, most days	**Maintained**
3: Loss of interest	Significantly reduced with parents; tension remains	**No Progress**

Explanatory Notes on Symptoms: AM reports not driving while intoxicated during past week; using friend to drive him home or staying overnight. Reports continued depression on most days; he did follow through on directive related to conversation with medicine woman and says it helped a little.

In-Session Interventions and Assigned Homework

Follow-up on prior week's homework; circular questions to help AM generate new frames for understanding his situation based on directive assignment and perspectives of mother, sister, grandmother, father, and tribe. Reframing to motivate AM to take more adult position related to his mother. Delivered new directive to have AM alternate loser days with adult days.

Client Response/Feedback

AM seems to enjoy the challenge of directives; struggles some with circular questioning but seems to get the point by the end.

Plan

☒ Continue with treatment plan: plan for next session: Follow up on directive intervention.

❑ Modify plan: ____

Next session: Date: November 21, 2015 Time: 1:00 ❑ am/☒pm

Crisis Issues: ☒ No indication of crisis/client denies ☒ Crisis assessed/addressed: describe below

Reports adhering to harm reduction plan; not drinking and driving.

____, ____ ____

Clinician's Signature License/Intern Status Date

Case Consultation/Supervision ❑ Not Applicable

Notes: Encouraged exploration of drinking within cultural frame; harnassing spiritual beliefs to support sobriety/reduced harm goals.

Collateral Contact ❑ Not Applicable

Name: Amy Biehl Date of Contact: November 14, 2013 Time: 10:15 ☒am/❑pm

(continued)

☒ Written release on file: ☒ Sent/❑ Received ❑ In court docs ❑ Other: ______

Notes: Contacted local job placement program to see if AM qualifies for program; unfortunately, he does not because supported by mother.

______, ______ ______
Clinician's Signature License/Intern Status Date

______, ______ ______
Supervisor's Signature License Date

CHAPTER 13

Solution-Based Counseling

"One of the most important aspects of SFBT is the general tenor and stance that is taken by the therapist. The overall attitude is positive, respectful, and hopeful. There is a general assumption that people have within them strong resiliencies, and can utilize these to make changes. Further, there is a core belief that most people have the strength, wisdom, and experiences to effect change.

—de Shazer et al. (2007, p. 4)

Lay of the Land

The quintessential strength-based approach, solution-based counseling is a positive, future-focused, and active approach that helps clients take small, consistent steps toward enacting their solutions. Broadly speaking, there are two strands of practice, which share more similarities than differences:

- *Solution-Focused Brief Therapy (SFBT)*, developed by Steve de Shazer (1985, 1988, 1994) and Insoo Berg at the Milwaukee Brief Family Therapy Center, emphasizes a future focus with minimal discussion of the presenting problem or the past; interventions target small steps in the direction of the solution.
- *Solution-Oriented Therapy* (O'Hanlon & Weiner-Davis, 1989) and the related approach *Possibility Therapy* (O'Hanlon & Beadle, 1999), developed by Bill O'Hanlon and colleagues, shares many tenants and practices with SFBT, adding more language-based techniques as well as more interventions that draw from the past and present to identify potential solutions.

Due to the numerous commonalities, I will present brief solution-focused and solution-oriented approaches together in this chapter.

Solution-Based Counseling

In a Nutshell: The Least You Need to Know

Solution-based counseling evolved from systemic family counseling (see Chapter 12) and the work of the Mental Research Institute (MRI) as well as Milton Erickson's brief therapy and trance work (de Shazer, 1985, 1988, 1994; O'Hanlon & Weiner-Davis, 1989). In contrast to the problem-focused approach at the MRI institute, de Shazer and Berg based their work on solutions, boldly proclaiming that the *solution is not necessarily related to the problem* (de Shazer, 1988). They developed their model around the miracle question, which invites clients to describe what they would notice happening differently (not what would *not* be happening) if the problem were miraculously solved overnight without their knowledge. This concrete, behavioral description of the solution is then used to develop interventions to help clients take small, consistent steps toward change. In addition to the miracle questions, solution-based counselors use exception questions to identify times without the problems and scaling questions to break the solution down into small, easily achievable steps. Rather than being "solution-givers," solution-based counselors collaborate with the client to envision potential solutions based on the client's experience and values. If ever the process seems to get stuck, the counselor does not blame the client's lack of effort, but instead works with the client to identify more appropriate and viable routes to change. As this approach is goal-focused and emphasizes measurable change, it tends to be brief, making it a favorite approach in managed care environments, schools, and other time-limited contexts.

The Juice: Significant Contributions to the Field

If you remember one thing from this chapter, it should be ...

Scaling Questions and the Miracle Scale

If you were challenged to use only one technique, and one technique only, to work with clients from start to finish, scaling questions would have to top the list of possibilities, because they are arguably one of the most versatile and comprehensive interventions. Counselors can use scaling questions to (a) assess strengths and solutions, (b) set goals, (c) design homework tasks, (d) measure progress, and (e) manage crises with safety plans (see Scaling for Safety in Chapter 3). They can be used in the first session and can be reused weekly until the last. Like many modern-day miracle, all-in-one products—such as shampoo-conditioners, moisturizer-sunscreen-foundations, and car wash-and-waxes—this technique is likely to be one of your go-to techniques for years to come.

As the name indicates, *scaling questions* involve asking clients to define their goals and rate their progress toward them using a scale, most often a ten-point scale but sometimes percentages, or shorter, nonnumeric versions are often used with children (Bertolino, 2010; de Shazer, 1994; O'Hanlon & Weiner-Davis, 1989; Selekman, 1997). de Shazer, Dolan, Korman, Trepper, McCollum, and Berg (2007) recommend having 0 represent "*when you decided to seek help*" rather than when things are "at their worst." When scaling 0 to mean "at their worst," this can refer to decades earlier or have different meanings to different people. Instead, scaling from "when you decided to seek help" allows for a clearer system for measuring progress from the beginning to end of counseling; counselors refer to these as "*miracle scales*" and use these scales to follow up with the miracle question (see Case Conceptualization below). Others use 0 or 1 to represent things at their *worst* (Bertolino, 2010).

Two Approaches to Scaling

Miracle Scale: Measures Progress from Beginning of Counseling

When you decided to seek help — *Miracle Situation*

0---------1---------2---------3---------4---------5---------6---------7---------8---------9---------10

Worst-to-Solution Scale: Measures Progress in General

Things at their worst — *Solution*

0---------1---------2---------3---------4---------5---------6---------7---------8---------9---------10

Scaling questions can be used early in the counseling process to help identify meaningful long-term goals, much the way the miracle question is used (see below):

Scaling Question for Long-Term Goal Setting (Assessing solutions and setting goals)

If you were to put your situation on a scale from 1–10, with 0 being where you were when you decided to seek help (or at their worst) and 10 being where you'd like them to be, can you describe to me what you would be doing (**not** what you would **not** be doing) if things were at a 10? Where are you today? What was happening and what were you doing at a 0?

As the client responds, the counselor listens for clear, specific descriptions of what life would be like at a 10, helping the client to paint a clear, behavioral picture: what is the client doing, what are others doing, how does the day go? Once a clear description of the 10 scenario is developed, the counselor can then ask where things are today and obtain a behavioral description of the current situation. A concrete description of when things were at the point the client decided to seek help or at their worst (0 or 1) can also be useful assessment information. Once the big picture is assessed, the same scale can be used to identify *what works*.

Scaling Question for Assessing What Works

If 0 is where you were when you decided to seek help and 10 is where you would be if the problem you came here for was resolved, where are you today? [If above a 0] What are you doing or what is happening that tells us you are at a 3 and not 0? How did you get from a 0 to here?

This next set of questions helps identify what works, exceptions, and potential solutions that need to be assessed before more specific interventions can be developed. If the client gets stuck answering any of these questions, it can be helpful to ask what significant others might rate them on the scale. After exploring where a client is this week, where he/she was when deciding to seek counseling, and where he/she would like to be, then it is time to use scaling to identify the next step.

Scaling Question for Designing Week-to-Week Interventions and Tasks

On a scale from 0–10 with 10 being your desired goal, where are you this week? [Client responds and rates: e.g., 3]. If you are at a 3 this week, what things would need to be different in your life for you to come in and say you were at a 4, one step higher (or *half* a step higher if client tends toward pessimism or needs to keep goal smaller)?

Try It Yourself

Find a partner, identify a problem, and use scaling to identify small action steps your partner is willing to take for the next week to improve things one point on the scale.

This is not an easy question to answer. Often clients rush ahead and describe an 8, 9, or 10 when the next step is really a 4. In such cases, the counselor needs to help clients identify more realistic expectations. In other cases, clients say, "I don't know";

when this happens, counselors need to practice patience, silence, and encouragement to help clients identify mini-steps toward their goal, which is a critical part of the process. The client—not the counselor—is the only person who can answer this question in any meaningful way. Remember, the counselor is *not* a solution-giver.

Once a clear description of the next step is developed, this information is used to identify specific, small tasks the client can undertake during the next week to move one step higher on the scale. It generally takes an entire session to fully flesh out concrete steps that are (a) realistic and meaningful, and (b) something that the client is motivated to try. For the intervention to work, the counselor and client need to develop micro-steps that take into account the client's motivation, willingness, schedule, variations in the schedule, reactions of others, and so forth. The counselor asks questions to identify and listen for potential barriers and pitfalls, in addition to helpful resources, working with the client to find ways to negotiate these. Together, the clients and counselors work together to develop specific homework tasks that clients believe will help move them toward their goals.

For example, if the client's initial response is that "At a 4, I would feel less anxious," the counselor needs to ask follow-up questions such as "How would you know you were less anxious?" "What would you be doing differently" "How would your days be different?" "What changes would other people notice in you?" These questions help the client identify one to two specific, small steps to be taken over the week, such as "invite a friend over," "go to the mall alone," "watch a funny movie," for example. The steps need to be small enough that the client thinks the steps are easily attainable, especially early in the process.

Scaling Question for Measuring Progress

Last week you said you were at a 3, where would you say you are this week and why? [If things got better] What did *you do* that helped move you up the scale? [If things stayed the same or got worse] What happened that kept things the same (or made them worse)?

The counselor follows up the next week to see if the homework tasks helped move clients closer to their goals. If so, they explore what helped and how to do more of it. If clients don't report progress or they report that things got worse [with or without doing the homework], the counselor does not despair, but simply goes back to more carefully assess whether (a) the solution has been meaningfully assessed and concretely identified, and (b) whether the task was small enough, concrete enough, and motivating enough. This scale can be used to measure progress from the beginning to end of the counseling process. In the case study at the end of this chapter, scaling questions are used throughout treatment to help Sarah best manage her response to her parents' refusal to support her choice of whom to marry; in the early stages, scaling questions are used to help manage her drinking, and in the later phases to help her make a decision and take action to resolve her dilemma.

Big Picture: Overview of Counseling Process

Solution Building

The process of solution-based counseling is described as *solution building* rather than problem solving, highlighting that the problem is not necessarily related to the solution (De Jong & Berg, 2002). By design, the solution-building process is brief and forward-focused. "Brief" can mean as few as one to ten sessions a year or more, depending on the severity of the problem, client resources, and numerous other factors (O'Hanlon & Weiner-Davis, 1989). The process focuses on identifying where the client wants to go (the solution) rather than trying to analyze and troubleshoot the problem. For example, rather than identify the cause of depression, the focus is on identifying what life would look like without depression and start taking steps to move in that direction.

After a relatively brief assessment phase, solution-based counselors quickly move to helping clients take *small action steps* between sessions to help clients move toward their identified solutions. These steps are practical and small enough to be achievable between sessions, such as call a friend to go to lunch, exercise three days a week, or go on a date night with a partner. Thus, most weeks, clients leave with some sort of homework assignment or task that involves taking action toward the identified solutions. An important part of the counselor's role is to help motivate the client to take these action steps, which requires working closely with the client to develop meaningful goals and tasks. A less obvious part of this process is that, in session, counselors ask questions and offer observations that shift *how* clients think about their situation so that they move from a problem focus to a perspective that emphasizes resources, strengths, abilities, possibilities, and the future. In general, counselors maintain an upbeat, hopeful attitude in session. In the closing phase of the counseling process, counselors work with clients to identify strategies for managing future problems using the newly acquired resources and strategies.

Making Connection: Counseling Relationship

Optimism and Hope

A signature characteristic, optimism and hope are immediately and undeniably palpable in solution-based counseling (Miller, Duncan, & Hubble, 1996, 1997). Solution-based counselors assume that change is inevitable and that improvement—in some form—is always possible, and they clearly communicate this verbally and nonverbally to clients (O'Hanlon & Weiner-Davis, 1989). Their optimism and hope do not stem from naïveté but rather are grounded in their ontology and epistemology: their theory of what it means to be human and how people learn. Because change is always happening—moods, relationships, emotions, and behaviors are in constant flux—*change is inevitable* (Walter & Peller, 1992). They have hope that the change will be positive because the client is in therapy to make an improvement and because over 90% of clients report positive outcomes in psychotherapy (Miller et al., 1997). Hope is cultivated early in therapy to develop motivation and momentum (Bertolino & O'Hanlon, 2002).

Carl Rogers with a Twist: Channeling Language

O'Hanlon and Beadle (1999) describe how they build counseling relationships by reflecting feelings, similar to Carl Rogers, but with a twist. The solution-oriented twist is that their reflections *delimit* the difficult feeling, behavior, or thought by reflecting on a time, context, or relational limit. Such reflections generally use one or more of three strategies for delimiting the problem:

1. **Past Tense:** Rather than describe a person's mood as a chronic state or characteristic, reflect statements back to clients in the *past tense,* for example, "You were feeling down *yesterday.*"
2. **Partial:** Rather than using global descriptions of people, situations, or things, describe these as *partial* or *periodic*, for example, "*A part of you* thinks things will never get better."
3. **Perception:** When the client makes an unhelpful global truth statement (e.g., "Life will never get better"), reflect back the sentiment as a *perception,* for example, "Right now *it seems to you* that things will never get better."

For example, a client-centered reflection with a client who is telling a story about how her boyfriend got angry at her for "no reason" would be something like "you aren't feeling understood" (present-focused statement about client's unexpressed emotion), whereas the solution-focus twist to delimit would be "you were not feeling understood *by your boyfriend last Saturday.*" The solution-oriented twist emphasizes the limited time and relational context in order to (a) define the problem in more solvable ways, and (b) engender hope. O'Hanlon and Beadle (1999) refer to this process as "channeling language." By channeling a client's language while listening to the client's story, both the client and counselor transition more easily to identifying desired outcomes. Channeling language is actually a very difficult skill to develop because it requires a paradigm shift in how the counselor listens for problems and strengths, but with practice it becomes habit. In the case study at the end of the chapter, the counselor uses channeling language to reduce Sarah's sense of hopelessness and feeling that "life is over" because her parents do not approve of her marrying her boyfriend.

Beginner's Mind

O'Hanlon and Weiner-Davis (1989) use *beginner's mind* when forming a relationship, referring to the classic Zen saying: "In the beginner's mind there are many possibilities; in the expert's mind there are few" (p. 8). Assuming a position of beginner's mind involves listening to each client's story as if you are listening for the first time, not filling in blanks with personal or professional knowledge. Most counselors underestimate how hard this is to do. When a client starts talking about "feeling depressed," most clinicians believe they have useful diagnostic information, unthinkingly assuming that clients have read diagnostic manuals and use the term as a professional would. In contrast, solution-oriented counselors bring a beginner's mind to the conversation and are curious about *how this person experiences his/her unique depression.* If you get in the habit of asking, you will find that every depression is surprisingly "one of a kind." Thus, solution-oriented counselors make no assumptions when they are listening, asking to hear more about clients' unique experiences and understandings.

Echoing Client's Key Words

Solution-based counselors carefully attend to *client word choice* and echo their key words whenever possible (De Jong & Berg, 2002). For example, rather than teaching clients to use psychiatric terms such as depression or hallucinations to describe their experience, the counselor prefers to use the client's own language, such as "feeling blue" or "schizos." Using client language often makes the problem more "solvable" and engenders greater hope. For many, "ending the blahs" or "getting back to my old self" is a more attainable goal than treating a psychiatrically defined problem of "296.22 Major Depressive Disorder, Single Episode, Moderate."

The Viewing: Case Conceptualization

Introduction to Solution-Based Case Conceptualization

Unlike most forms of counseling, solution-based counseling primarily involves conceptualizing *where to go from here* (a.k.a., the solution) rather than where the client has been (a.k.a., the problem). A basic tenant of solution-based counseling is that *the solution is not necessarily related to the problem*, and thus, the solution—where to go—is the focus of assessment (de Shazer et al., 2007). This does not mean that the past is ignored; instead, it is only discussed as long as is necessary to better understand the potential solution. Outside of exceptions (see below), the past is not the focus of the assessment and case conceptualization process.

The Miracle and Other Solution-Generating Questions

The original solution-generating question, the *miracle question* serves to both (a) conceptualize and assess, and (b) set goals in solution-based counseling. Legend (and good authority) has it that Insoo Kim Berg developed the miracle question based on a client's desperate and exasperated claim to Insoo that "maybe only a miracle will help." So, Insoo, using the clients' language and worldview, played with the idea and had the client describe how life would be if there were a miracle (de Shazer, 1988; de Shazer et al., 2007). The intervention was so successful that it was crafted into a hallmark intervention that is frequently used early in treatment, in order to identify the focus of treatment. Since then several variations have been developed, including the crystal ball technique (de Shazer, 1985), magic wand questions (Selekman, 1997), and time machine (Bertolino & O'Hanlon, 2002). When successfully delivered, these questions help clients envision a future without the problem, thus generating hope, motivation, and goals.

- *Miracle Question:* Imagine that you go home tonight and during the middle of the night a miracle happens: all the problems you came here to resolve are miraculously resolved. However, when you wake up, you have no idea a miracle has occurred. What are some of the first things you would notice that would be different? How would you know that the problems that brought you here were resolved?
- *Crystal Ball Question:* Imagine I had a crystal ball that allowed us to look into the future to a time when the problems you came here for are already resolved. I hold it up to you, and you look in. What do you see?
- *Magic Wand Question:* Imagine we had a magic wand (or imagine that this magic wand I have here actually works), and you could wave it and all of the problems you came here for are miraculously resolved. What would be different?
- *Time Machine:* Imagine I had a time machine that could propel you into the future to a point in time when the problems you came to see me for are totally resolved. Imagine you stepped in: Where do you end up? Who is with you? What is happening? How is your life different? How did your problems go away?

Successfully delivering one of these solution-generating questions is far more difficult than it appears. As you can imagine, if done poorly, these hit the floor like a lead balloon. To avoid such humiliation, solution-focused experts have several suggestions for successfully delivering the miracle question (Bertolino, 2010; Bertolino & O'Hanlon, 2002: De Jong & Berg, 2002; de Shazer, 1988; de Shazer et al., 2007). Additionally, I suggest you think of asking of the miracle question as having three specific phases:

- Phase 1: Setup for the Miracle
- Phase 2: Delivery of the Miracle Question
- Phase 3: Facilitation of the Answer

Phase 1: Setup for the Miracle: 3 Steps with 3 Nods

- *Phase 1-Step 1: Obtain Client Agreement and Wait for Nod #1:* The first and most critical step is to prepare clients by changing their state of mind so that they are willing to engage in an atypical conversation. By asking, "May I ask an unusual question?" or "Would you be willing to play along if I ask a somewhat odd question?" The counselor signals clients to change their frame of mind so that they are better able to enter a more fanciful, creative conversation. The counselor waits for the client to say "okay" or nod in agreement.
- *Phase 1-Step 2: Custom-Tailor Initial Setup and Wait for Nod #2:* After the client agrees to the odd question, begin delivering the question but customize it to include numerous little details from the client's everyday life to get him or her fully engaged in the story and enable him or her to better visualize the miracle. For example, you might say, "Let's imagine that after we are done talking here, you get in your car and drive home; you make dinner for the family like you usually do; you clean up dishes like you usually do; and check the kids' homework like you usually do." *Continue describing the typical day and evening until the client starts to nod.*
- *Phase 1-Step 3: Setup for Miracle and Wait for Nod #3:* Once the client nods, continue with, "Then you get the kids to bed, maybe do some minor chores or watch television, and then you finally get to bed and fall asleep." Up to this point, you have only asked the client to imagine a regular day, but this is very important. The goal is to have the client psychologically leave the session and vividly envision being at home where the miracle is to occur. *Pause and wait for the nod or verbal affirmation before moving on to the miracle; don't move on to the miracle without such confirmation.*

Phase 2: Deliver the Miracle Question: 4 Steps and 3 Pauses and a Snap

- *Phase 2-Step 1: Introduce the Miracle with Pause #1:* "Then, during the night ... while you are sleeping ... a miracle happens" (de Shazer et al., 2007, p. 42). Pause and wait for a reaction that signals surprise or that they are thinking: a smirk,

laugh, tilting of the head, raised eyebrow, or funny look. Insoo reportedly looks intently at the client and smiled; Steve warned that if you pause for too long, the client is likely to respond with, "I don't believe in miracles"; so keep moving.
- *Phase 2: Step 2: Specifically Define the Terms of the Miracle with Optional Snap:* "And it's not just any miracle. This miracle makes the problems that brought you here today disappear ... just like *that*" (de Shazer et al., 2007, p. 43; emphasis). Snapping your fingers at this point is optional but adds flair (might need extra practice with that part). If you forget to include the "problems that brought you here" part of the question, you most likely will get a wish list appropriate for a genie in a lantern, which is not the answer we want for this question. Without this limit on the miracle, clients will spend a lot of time exploring vague and unrelated goals, and the counselor will spend more time with follow-up questions to get a useful answer.
- *Phase 2-Step 3: Add Mystery with Pause #2:* "However, because you were sleeping, you don't know that *the miracle has happened*" (De Jong & Berg, 2002, p. 85). If delivered well, most clients start bobbing their heads at this point, stare off into space, or otherwise begin to behave as if they were thinking about the proposition.
- *Phase 2-Step 4: Ask What Is Different with Pause #3:* "So, you wake up the morning after the miracle happens during the night. All the problems that brought you here are gone—poof—just like that. What is the very first thing you notice after you wake up? What are the little changes you start to notice that tell you the problem is gone?" (de Shazer et al., 2007, p. 43). At this point, many clients need some time to think about their answer, often becoming quiet, still, and pensive. This is generally a sign that the client is generating new ideas, so it is important that the counselor patiently *wait* for the response. Rushing clients at this point will likely generate more-of-the-same thinking.

Phase 3: Facilitating the Description of the Miracle: 2 Steps with 1 List

- *Phase 3-Step 1: Focus Client on Behavior Changes in Positive Language:* Those new to this intervention often imagine their work is done once the question has been asked. For the miracle question to be useful in case conceptualization, the counselor needs to skillfully facilitate the description of the miracle—not just any miracle will do. Once the client begins to describe what is different, the counselor helps focus the answer by asking about *observable behavioral changes* in the client and others. In typical solution-focused style, the counselor is interested not in what the client is *not* doing but instead in what the client *is doing*. For example, if the client says, "I will not be depressed any more," the counselor responds with, "What will you be doing instead?"
- *Phase 3-Step 2: Continue Until You Have Enough to Identify Clear Goals:* Once the client identifies one new behavior, the counselor asks for more: "What else would be different?" The counselor continues until several (three or more) concrete miracle behaviors are identified that can be useful for developing goals and clear direction for change. In the case study at the end of this chapter, the counselor uses the miracle question with Sarah to better understand her goals, values, and priorities regarding her relationship with her parents and boyfriend.

Exceptions, Previous Solutions, and "What Works"

Successful solution-based counseling requires developing an uncanny, sleuth-like ability to detect even the minutest exceptions to problems (this is generally an endearing quality in personal relations, by the way; so it is worth cultivating). Solution-based counselors assess for *exceptions*, *previous* (helpful) *solutions*, and examples of *what works* in three different ways: 1) as part of the follow-up to the miracle question, 2) listening for spontaneous descriptions of exceptions, and 3) directly asking about exceptions (de Shazer, 1985, 1988; de Shazer et al., 2007; O'Hanlon & Weiner-Davis, 1989). First, if the miracle or other solution-generating question has been used, exceptions can be identified by asking, "What elements of the miracle are happening now, even just a little?" This prompt often results in a heartening description for both client and counselor of what elements of the miracle are already there; most are thrilled to think that half (or a quarter) of the work is already done. Alternatively, the finely tuned solution-focused ear attends to clients' spontaneously offered descriptions of exceptions and examples of what works: "Except for when I am on my boat, I am always depressed" or "The only time I don't worry is when I am playing with my kids" or "Suzy is the only one who cares about me." These seemingly minor exceptions provide clues as to what works, and therefore what clients need to do more frequently. Additionally, solution-based counselors directly ask about exceptions to gather more information about what works:

Examples of Exception Questions

- Are there any times when the problem is less likely to occur or be less severe?
- Can you think of a time when you expected the problem to occur but didn't?
- Are there any people who seem to make things easier?
- Are there places or times when the problem is not as bad?

Try It Yourself

Find a partner, identify a problem, and use exception questions to assess potentials for solutions.

The vast majority of clients will be able to identify exceptions with questions such as these; note that the assumption underlying most of these questions is that the problem varies in *intensity*; the times when the problem is *less severe* is considered a type of exception and generally provides clues as to what works (de Shazer, 1985; O'Hanlon & Weiner-Davis, 1989). Especially true with diagnoses such as depression that are experienced most of the time most days, counselors need to focus on the varying of intensity, rather than on the absence of, the symptom, in order to identify exceptions.

Pre-Session Change

Solution-based counselors pay careful attention to *pre-session change*: change that occurs *after* the initial phone call to make an appointment and *before* the first session (de Shazer et al., 2007). Counselors can assess this by asking, "Since we spoke on the phone (or you made the appointment), what changes have you noticed that have happened or started to happen?" In early research surveys, Weiner-Davis, de Shazer, and Gingerich (1987) reported that the majority of clients reported *some* positive changes *before* the first changes, leading them to hypothesize that simply the anticipation of change and making a commitment to change (i.e., an appointment with a professional) mobilizes clients resources and begins the change process. This question is asked *very early* in the first session to assess for what works, strengths, and resources.

Assessing Client Strengths

Assessing client strengths is one of the key areas of assessment in solution-based counseling (Bertolino & O'Hanlon, 2002; De Jong & Berg, 2002; O'Hanlon & Weiner-Davis, 1989). Strengths include resources in a person's life, personally, relationally, financially, socially, or spiritually, and may include family support, positive relationships, and religious faith. Most counselors *underestimate* the difficulty of identifying strengths. In fact, identifying client strengths is often *harder* than diagnosing pathology because clients come in with a long list of problems they want to be fixed and are thus prepared to discuss pathology. Surprisingly, many clients, especially those with depressive or anxious tendencies (the majority of outpatient cases), have great difficulty identifying areas without problems in their lives. Similarly, many couples who have been distressed and arguing for long periods of time have difficulty identifying positive characteristics in their partners, happy times in the marriage, and, in the most desperate of cases, the reasons they got together in the first place. Therefore, counselors often have to ask more subtle questions and attend to vague clues in order to assess strengths well.

Solution-based counselors assess strengths in two ways: (a) by directly asking about strengths, hobbies, and areas of life that are going well, and (b) by listening carefully for *exceptions* to problems and for areas of unnoticed strength (Bertolino & O'Hanlon, 2002; De Jong & Berg, 2002). Furthermore, I have found that any strength in one context has the potential to be a liability in another context and that the inverse is also true: any weakness in one area is generally a *strength* in another area (see Assessing Strengths section in Chapter 2). Therefore, if a client has difficulty identifying strengths and more readily discusses weaknesses and problems, a fine-tuned solution-focused ear will be able to identify potential areas in which the "weakness" is a strength. For example, a person who is critical, anxious, and/or negative in a relational context typically excels at detailed or meticulous work and tasks. This insight can be useful in identifying ways for clients to move toward their goals.

Solution-based counselors have been on the vanguard of a larger movement within mental health that emphasizes identifying and utilizing client strengths to promote better clinical outcomes (Bertolino & O'Hanlon, 2002). Increasingly, county mental health and insurance companies are requiring assessment of strengths as part of initial intake assessments. The key to successfully assessing strengths is the unshakable belief that *all* clients have significant and meaningful strengths no matter how dire and severe their situations appear in the moment. It is helpful for counselors to remember that we see people typically in their worst moments; therefore, even if we are not seeing strengths in the moment, they are undoubtedly there. Solution-based counselors maintain that all people have strengths and resources and make it their job to help identify and utilize them toward achieving client goals.

Client Motivation: Visitor, Complainant, and Customers

Steve de Shazer (1988) assessed client motivation for change using three categories: visitors, complainant, and customers. These categories are used to understand the type of *relationship* the counselor has with the client rather than to label the client (De Jong & Berg, 2002).

- *Visitor-Type Relationship:* In this relationship, the client does not have a complaint, but generally others have a complaint against him or her. These clients are typically brought to therapy by an outside other, such as courts, parents, or spouse. They are often most motivated to get the third party "off their back"; thus, the counselor should honor this and quickly identify the specific goals that would achieve this end.
- *Complainant-Type Relationship:* In this type of relationship, the client identifies a problem but expects the counselor or some other person to be the primary source of change. Rather than try to convince these clients to change their perspectives, the solution-focused counselor works with these clients to identify small ways they can positively affect the situation.
- *Customer-Type Relationship:* In this type of relationship, the client and counselor jointly define a problem and solution picture, and the client is motivated to take action toward the solution.

	Visitor-Type	Complainant-Type	Customer-Type
Motivation	Low	Moderate to High	High
Source of Problem or Solution	Outside other (spouse, parent, court) thinks client has a problem.	Problem generally related to outside cause or person; expect counselor or another to be source of solution.	Self as part of problem and active agent in solution.

(continued)

View of who needs to change	Outside other needs to see there is no problem.	Outside other needs to change and/or fix it.	Self needs to take action to fix things.
Building Therapeutic Alliance	Identify areas where client sees problem willing to work on to make them a customer for change.	Honoring client's view of the situation while identifying specific instances where client can make a difference.	Join with client by complimenting readiness for change.
Focus of Interventions	Building alliance; understanding client perspective; framing outside request for change as the problem.	Observation-oriented tasks (e.g., identifying exceptions over week; Selekman, 1997, 2010).	Reframing; identifying what does not work; action-oriented tasks.
Readiness for Action	Not ready for making active changes in life until client believes there is a problem and is motivated for change.	Not ready for action until open to the idea that their actions can make a difference.	Ready to take action to make changes.

Assessing clients' motivation is helpful in knowing how to build relationships with the client as well as how to proceed. Many new counselors assume that all clients are customers for change: ready to take action to improve their situation simply because they showed up for a therapy session. However, this is often not the case. People come to therapy with mixed emotions and varying levels of motivation. Generally, most mandated clients are "visitors," and counselors need to find a way to connect with their agenda while still working with the referring party's agenda. This same dynamic is often the case with children, teens, and even one half of a couple. In complainant relationships, counselors need to either find ways that the client can contribute to making a difference or help shift the viewing of the problem to increase client willingness to take action. In the case study at the end of the chapter, Sarah is a complainant, feeling helpless since her parents' refusal to allow her to marry her boyfriend. The counselor helps her redefine the problem—finding ways to honor her Iranian heritage and parents' wishes while also integrating American values and personal desires—so that she can direct her energy in fruitful directions.

Details, Details, Details

Throughout the assessment and case conceptualization process, solution-focused counselors are continually asking about the *details:* who, what, where, why, and when. Effective "solution building requires getting details, details, and more details" (De Jong & Berg, 2002, p. 24). By learning more about when symptoms are better or worse, who is around when things are better or worse, what happens step by step when things get a little better, counselors become well provisioned for helping to build solutions. For example, when a client reports that the depressed feelings are reduced at work or when busy (very common), the counselor asks about the details of what happens in these contexts to identify potential elements of solutions, such as being around people or away from people, have a purpose, being outside, avoiding thinking about another problem, and so on.

Targeting Change: Goal Setting

Goal Language: Positive and Concrete

Solution-based counselors state their goals in positive, observable terms (De Jong & Berg, 2002). Positive goal descriptions emphasize what the client is *going to be doing* rather than focusing on symptom reduction, which is typical in pathology-focused counseling approaches. Observable descriptions include clear, specific behavioral indicators of the desired change.

Positive, Observable Goal Example	Negative (Symptom Reducing), Nonobservable Goal Examples
Increase periods of engaging in hobbies and enjoyable activities	Reduce depression
Increase sense of confidence and calm in social situations	Reduce panic attacks
Increase frequency of choosing healthy foods and healthy portions	Reduce binging and purging

You may have noticed that simply reading the left column generates more hope and provides greater direction for clinical intervention than the right column. Positive, observable goals provide a constant reminder to the counselor and client of the goal and they reinforce a solution-focused and solution-oriented perspective. Many solution-based techniques, such as scaling questions (see above), invite the client to measure goal progress weekly; thus, carefully crafted goal language is particularly critical to success in solution-based counseling.

Additional qualities of solution-based goals include (Bertolino & O'Hanlon, 2002; De Jong & Berg, 2002):

- *Meaningful to client:* Goals must be *personally* important to the client, not just a "good idea."
- *Interactional:* Rather than reflect a general feeling (e.g., "feeling better"), the goals should describe how interactions with others will change.
- *Situational:* Rather than global terms, goals are stated in situational terms (e.g., improved mood at work).
- *Small steps:* Goals should be short-term and with identifiable small steps.
- *Clear role for client:* Goals should identify a clear role for the client rather than for others.
- *Realistic:* Goals need to be realistic for this client at this time.
- *Legal and Ethical:* Goals should be legal and adhere to client, counselor, and professional ethics.

One Thing Different

In the beginning, goals should focus on doing one small thing differently rather than target broad, lofty goals (e.g., call a friend this week rather than visit with someone every day; de Shazer, 1985, 1988; O'Hanlon, 2000; O'Hanlon & Weiner-Davis, 1989). Similarly, a goal such as "get up and exercise one day this week," rather than "every day this week," is more likely to generate change and motivation for further action. In most cases, making this *one small change* starts a cascade of change events that are inspired from the client's *own* motivation rather than the prescription of the counselor (or even co-created solution with the counselor). Ideas generated in therapy are not viewed as the "best," "only," or "correct" solution but rather activities that will spark clients to identify what works for them.

The Doing: Interventions

Solution-Focused Tenants for Intervention

de Shazer et al. (2007, p. 2) identify basic tenants of solution-focused intervention that counselors can use to guide their work.

1. *If it isn't broken, don't fix it:* Don't use therapeutic theory to determine areas of intervention.
2. *If it works, do more of it:* Amplify and build upon things that are currently working.
3. *If it's not working, do something different:* Even if it's a good idea, if it's not working, find another solution.
4. *Small steps can lead to big changes:* Begin with small doable changes; these typically happen and quickly lead to more change.
5. *The solution is not necessarily related to the problem:* Focus on moving forward, not on understanding why there is a problem.
6. *The language for solution development is different from that needed to describe a problem:* Problem-talk is negative and past-focused; solution-talk is hopeful, positive, and future-focused.
7. *No problem happens all the time; there are always exceptions that can be utilized:* Even the smallest exception is useful for identifying potential solutions.
8. *The future is both created and negotiable:* Clients have a significant role in designing their future.

Scaling and Miracle Questions

Described in "The Juice" above, scaling and miracle questions are the bread-and-butter techniques for week-to-week interventions. They can be used to (a) assess whether the last week's tasks were helpful or not, (b) identify potential areas for change, and (c) develop specific homework tasks for the following week.

Formula First Session Task

As the name implies, the *formula first session task* (de Shazer, 1985) is typically used in the first session with all clients, regardless of the issue, to increase client hope in the therapy process and motivation for change.

> *Formula First Session Task:* Between now and the next time we meet, we [I] would like you to observe, so that you can describe to us [me] next time, what happens in your [pick one: family, life, marriage, relationship] that you want to continue to have happen" (de Shazer, 1985, p. 137).
>
> *Formula First Session Task (paraphrased with introduction):* "As we are starting therapy, many things are going to change. However, I am sure that there are many things in your life and relationships that you do *not* want to have change. Over the next week, I want you to generate a list of the things in your life and relationships that you *do not* want to have changed by therapy. Notice small things as well as big things that are working right now."
>
> 
>
> **Try It Yourself**
>
> Take a moment to generate a list of things that you do **not** want to change in your life and/or relationships right now. Notice how you feel afterwards.

This directive stimulates clients to notice what is working, identify their strengths and resources, and it helps generates hope and agency.

Presuppositional Questions and Assuming Future Solution

Presuppositional questions and talk that assume future change help clients envision a future without the problem, generating hope and motivation (O'Hanlon & Beadle, 1999; O'Hanlon & Weiner-Davis, 1989). Solution-focused counselors assume change based on the observation that all things change: a client's situation *cannot* change. Knowing that change is inevitable and that most clients benefit from therapy, counselors can be confident when they ask presuppositional questions such as:

- What will you be doing differently once we resolve these issues?
- Do you think there are other concerns you will want to address once we resolve these issues?
- When the problem is resolved, what is one of the first things you will do to celebrate?

Questions such as these can be very helpful in cases where clients feel hopeless or have difficulty imagining a future without the problem.

Videotalk

Videotalk is a technique that distinguishes between two basic levels of experience: (a) *facts*, and (b) *stories and experience* (Hudson & O'Hanlon, 1991). The *facts* are a behavioral description of what was done and said, what would be recorded on videotape (hence the name). The *story* is the interpretation and meaning that a person associates with the behaviors and words, while the *experience* is a person's internal thoughts and feelings. The overarching goal of videotalk is to separate out facts (what behavior happened) from interpretation (stories and subjective experience in response to what happened). By separating what happened to how clients interpret the events, counselors and clients can closely examine how meanings were made and responses created, allowing new understandings and responses.

Anatomy of Videotalk: Facts versus Interpretation

- *Facts:* What is captured by video camera; *behavioral description* of what was said and done.

Examples:

"If I had a video camera, what would I see you do or say when you are feeling depressed?"

"If I had a video camera, what would I see you do or hear you say the day of your miracle?"

- *Interpretations:* Description of the *stories* (interpretations) and subjective *experiences* (what was thought and felt)

Examples:

"When you are lying in bed not wanting to get up, what are you thinking and feeling? What type of meaning do you make of this situation and who you are because of it?"

"When you are getting up before the alarm rings and going for a run, what are you thinking and feeling? What type of meanings are you making about yourself and your choice to get up and run before the alarm goes off? How do you feel about yourself?"

When a client reports vague feelings or goals, counselors can help them bring greater clarity and to descriptions of the problem and solution by using videotalk. These descriptions are used to define the problem behaviorally and identify potential solutions using small weekly behavioral tasks. In addition, solution-oriented counselors prefer to use the descriptive language of videotalk to describe problems and solutions (e.g., "wanting to sleep in" or "when you are running in the mornings again") rather than vague interpretation or experience labels, such as "depressed" or "feeling better." When counselors consistently use videotalk to separate the *behaviors* from *interpretation of the behaviors*, clients are better able to identify where and how to make changes. For example, in the case study at the end of this chapter, the counselor uses videotalk to help Sarah redefine her problem as one of deciding how she can best integrate her Iranian and American cultures and values, and to help her realize how these values affect her sense of self and who she wants to become.

Utilization

Based on the hypnotic work of Milton Erickson, de Shazer (1988) employed *utilization* techniques to help clients identify and enact solutions. Utilization refers to finding a way to use and leverage whatever the client presents as a strength, interest, proclivity, or habit to develop meaningful actions and plans that will lead in the direction of solutions. For example, if a client has difficulty making friends and close relations but has numerous pets, the counselor would utilize the client's interest in animals to develop more human connections, perhaps by taking a dog for a walk in public places, joining a dog agility class, or volunteering at a pet shelter.

Coping Questions

Coping questions generate hope, agency, and motivation, especially when clients are feeling overwhelmed (De Jong & Berg, 2002; de Shazer & Dolan, 2007). They are used when the client is not reporting progress, is describing an acute crisis, or is otherwise feeling hopeless. Coping questions direct clients to identify how they have been coping through a current or past difficult situation:

- "This sounds hard—how have you managed to cope with this to the degree that you have?" (de Shazer & Dolan, 2007, p. 10)
- "How have you managed to prevent the situation from getting worse?" (p. 10)

Compliments and Encouragement

Solution-based counselors use compliments and encouragement to motivate clients and highlight strengths (De Jong & Berg, 2002). The key with compliments is to compliment *only* when clients are making steps toward goals *that they have set* or compliment *specific strengths that relate to the problem.* This is so important I am going to say it again and put it in a special box so you don't forget:

Compliment only when clients are making steps toward goals that they have set or compliment specific strengths that relate to the problem; compliment their progress, not their personhood.

Basic therapeutic compliment:

- "Wow. You made real progress toward your goal this week."

Even better therapeutic compliment:

- "I am impressed; you not only followed through on the chart idea we developed last week but you came up with your own additional strategies—setting up a weekend outing with his friend—to improve your relationship with your son." [compliment specific behavior toward goal].

Not-so therapeutic compliment:

- "I really admire what you have done with your life" (too personal and does not clearly relate to the problem; sounds like you are "buttering up" client).
- "You really are a great mom" (nonspecific; evaluating mothering skills globally; not allowing client to reflect upon and evaluate her own behavior).

When you compliment on anything else, you are setting up a situation where you are rendering judgment, albeit a positive one, on the clients and/or their life. Compliments should not be used to be "nice" to clients (De Jong & Berg, 2002). Instead, compliments should be used to reinforce progress toward goals that clients have set for themselves, and should be stated in such a way that the compliments encourage clients to validate themselves instead of relying on an outside authority figure to do so. When clients can set goals and make progress toward them, they develop a greater sense of *self-efficacy*, which is a greater predictor of happiness than self-esteem (Seligman, 2004).

Homework and Experiments

Just in case it hasn't been obvious, most every week solution-based counselors assign a homework assignment or task that requires the clients to take small, concrete steps toward their desired goals. These tasks are collaboratively identified during session using any number of techniques listed above. The counselor's role is to help concretely define the task so that the client (a) knows exactly what to do, (b) is motivated to do it, and (c) is likely to succeed. To ensure success, counselors should also identify potential obstacles, including weekends, holidays, visitors, schedule changes, or anything that might keep clients from attaining their goals.

Interventions for Specific Problems

Sexual Abuse

Yvonne Dolan (1991) and Bill O'Hanlon and Bob Bertolino (2002) use solution-based counseling with child and adult survivors of childhood sexual abuse. Solution-based approaches stand out from traditional approaches to sexual abuse treatment in their optimistic and hopeful stance that emphasizes the resiliencies of survivors. Given that survivors of sexual abuse have *survived* such a difficult trauma, solution-oriented counselors harness those strengths in new ways to help them resolve current issues. Some of the distinctive qualities of solution-oriented approaches to treating sexual abuse include:

Honoring the Agency of Survivors More so than traditional approaches, solution-based counselors honor the agency of survivors, allowing them to decide whether to tell their abuse stories and determine the pacing of their treatment (Dolan, 1991; O'Hanlon & Bertolino, 2002). Although many counselors insist that a survivor cannot heal without sharing the details of their abuse to their counselors, solution-based counselors would not readily agree. Instead, solution-based counselors work with clients to identify if, when, how, and to whom it is best to tell their stories. By fully honoring their agency, counselors create a relationship in which survivors reclaim full authority over the private aspects of their lives, reclaiming autonomy that was lost through the abuse. Counselors who play a more directive role in working with a survivor may unintentionally replicate the abuse pattern by forcing clients to reveal parts of their sexual life in the name of "treatment" before the client is ready, leaving the client feeling violated and retraumatized.

The Recovery Scale: Focusing on Strengths and Abilities Dolan (1991, p. 32) uses the *Solution-Focused Recovery Scale* to identify what areas of the client's life were not affected by the abuse, reducing the sense that the client's whole life and self has been affected. The success strategies in these areas are used to address areas that are affected by the abuse. Questions from this scale are rated "not at all," "just a little," "pretty much," and "very much" and include:

- Able to think/talk about the trauma
- Feels part of family
- Goes to work
- Cares for pets, plants
- Holds hands with loved one
- Able to relax without drugs or alcohol
- Accepts praise well
- Shows healthy appetite

3-D Model: Dissociate, Disown, and Devalue O'Hanlon and Bertolino (2002) conceptualize the aftereffects of abuse and trauma using the *3-D Model*, which postulates that abuse leads people to *dissociate, disown, and devalue* aspects of the self. The goal of counseling is to reconnect people with these disowned parts, parts that tend to either inhibit experience (e.g., lack of sexual response, lack of memories, lack of anger) or create intrusive experiences (e.g., flashbacks, sexual compulsions, or rage). O'Hanlon and Bertolino (2002) note that many of the symptoms related to sexual abuse are experienced as a sort of *negative trance*, feeling as though the experience is uncontrollable and involving only a part of the self. Solution-oriented counselors use *permission* (i.e., allowing clients to express and feel undesirable feelings), *validating* (i.e., helping clients acknowledge difficult or unwanted feelings), and *inclusive language* (i.e., creating space for contradictory parts or feelings to be simultaneously recognized) to encourage clients to revalue and include the devalued aspects of self that were disowned through the abuse.

Constructive Questions Dolan (1991) uses constructive questions to construct solutions by identifying the specifics of clients' unique solutions:

- What will be the first (smallest) sign that things are getting better, that this (the sexual abuse) is having less of an impact on your current life?
- What will you be doing differently when this (sexual abuse trauma) is less of a current problem in your life?
- What will you be doing differently with your time?
- What will you be thinking about (doing) *instead* of thinking about the past?
- Are there times when the above is already happening to some (even a small) extent? What is different about those times? What is helpful about those differences?
- What differences will the above healing changes make when they have been present in your life over an extended time (days, weeks, months, years)?
- What do you think your (significant other) would say would be the first sign that things are getting better? What do you think your significant other will notice first?
- What do you think your (friends, boss, significant other, etc.) will notice about you as you heal even more?
- What differences will these healing changes you've identified make in future generations of your family? (pp. 37–38)

Videotalk (Action Terms) with Abuse and Trauma Survivors

Due to the intense emotions that characterize abuse and trauma, survivors often have difficulty identifying the current effects of abuse in their present life. O'Hanlon and Bertolino (2002) use *videotalk* (see above) with survivors to help identify specific actions and patterns of behavior that recreate the traumatic experience, including the sequence of events, antecedents, consequences, invariant actions, repetitive actions, and body responses. Once these recurrent patterns are identified, counselors help clients either change one part of the context to interrupt the cycle and create space for new responses, or, if the client feels a certain degree of control over the symptoms, identify new, alternative solution-generating actions. For example, if a client gets flashbacks when watching sexual scenes in movies, the counselor helps identify the behaviors before and after the flashbacks as well as the thoughts, feelings, and interpretations of these events. Using this information—such as the client's anxiety building as the suspense builds in the movie, the counselor can help the client identify ways to interrupt the cycle by hitting the mute button, turning on the lights, or going for a bathroom break.

Putting It All Together: Solution-Based Treatment Plan Case Conceptualization and Treatment Plan Templates

Theory-Specific Case Conceptualization: Solution-Based

The prompts below can be used to develop a *theory-specific case conceptualization* using Adlerian theory. The cross-theoretical case conceptualizations at the end of each theory chapter provide examples for writing a conceptualization that includes key elements of this theory-specific conceptualization. Comprehensive examples of theory-specific case conceptualizations are available in *Theory and Treatment Planning in Counseling and Psychotherapy* (Gehart, 2015).

- *Strengths:* Describe unique client strengths, including:
  - Personal strengths and abilities
  - Relational and social strengths and resources
  - Spiritual resources
- *Exceptions, Previous Solutions, and What Works:* Describe times, places, relationships, contexts, and such, when the problem is less of a problem or when things are even slightly better.
- *Miracle question answer:* Identify what client will be doing differently when the problem is resolved.
- *Client Motivation:* Describe client's level of motivation: visitor, complainant, or customer for change.
- *Solution-Focused Description of Problem and/or Solution:* Describe problem using solution-focused language that avoids pathologizing language and negative labels and instead highlights concrete behaviors that need to be changed and/or new behaviors to be adopted. The solution-focused language should be detailed and should inspire hope and/or a positive vision of change.

Treatment Plan Template: Solution-Based

Use this Treatment Plan Template for developing a plan for clients with depressive, anxious, or compulsive types of presenting problems. Depending on the specific client, presenting problem, and clinical context, the goals and interventions in this template may need to be modified only slightly or significantly; you are encouraged to significantly revise the plan as needed. For the plan to be useful, goals and techniques should be written to target specific beliefs, behaviors, and emotions that the client is experiencing. The more specific, the more useful it will be to you.

Treatment Plan

Initial Phase of Treatment

Initial Phase Counseling Tasks

1. Develop working counseling relationship. *Diversity considerations:* Attend to relevant diversity issues.
   Relationship-building approach/intervention:
   a. Build rapport by identifying **strengths, resources, and channeling language to delimit problem**, identify areas of **functioning**, and generate **hope.**
2. Assess individual, systemic, and broader cultural dynamics. *Diversity considerations:* Identify resources related to diversity.
   Assessment Strategies:
   a. **Miracle question** to obtain behavioral description of solutions and motivate clients.
   b. **Identify exceptions, previous solutions, "what works," pre-session change, and strengths.**
3. Identify and obtain client agreement on treatment goals. *Diversity considerations:*
   Goal-making Intervention:
   a. Develop **concrete, attainable, step-by-step goals** stated in **positive terms** based on **miracle questions**.

(continued)

4. Identify needed referrals, crisis issues, and other client needs. *Diversity considerations:*
   a. *Crisis-assessment Intervention(s):* Use **scaling for safety** to manage crisis issues.
   b. *Referral(s):* Refer to solution-based groups; connect with community resources, including activities, hobbies, and classes related to elements identified in miracle question.

Initial Phase Client Goal

1. Increase safety and ability to **use resources** to prevent crisis situations to reduce [crisis-related behavior].
   Interventions:
   a. Motivate client to use **scaling for safety** to generate **step-by-step safety plan**.
   b. Identify personal, relational, and community **resources** to provide immediate support for client.
   c. **Formula first session task** to identify what IS working well right now and to generate hope.

Working Phase of Treatment

Working Phase Counseling Tasks

1. Monitor quality of the working alliance. *Diversity considerations*: Address diversity issues.
   a. *Assessment Intervention*: Use Session Rating Scale; adjust alliance based on client level of **motivation** (visitor, complainant, or customer); if intervention does not work, **do something different**.
2. Monitor progress toward goals. *Diversity considerations*: Select measures with consideration for diversity.
   a. *Assessment Intervention*: Outcome Rating Scale; **weekly scaling questions** to monitor progress.

Working Phase Client Goals

1. Increase* [behaviors derived from "**exceptions**," "**what works**," and/or "**previous solutions**"] (personal/relational dynamic) to reduce depressed mood, anxiety, problem behaviors, etc.
   Interventions:
   a. **Scaling questions** to identify specific behavioral tasks each week to generate incremental improvement.
   b. **Coping questions** to augment areas of strength and resource utilization.
2. Increase [one set of behaviors identified **in miracle question**] (personal/relational dynamic) to reduce depressed mood, anxiety, problem behaviors, etc.
   Interventions:
   a. **Scaling questions** to identify specific behavioral tasks each week to generate incremental improvement.
   b. **Videotalk** to identify specific behaviors and how they inform client's personal and relational identities.
3. Increase [another set of behaviors identified in **miracle question**] (personal/relational dynamic) to reduce depressed mood, anxiety, problem behaviors, etc.
   Interventions:
   a. **Scaling questions** to identify specific behavioral tasks each week to generate incremental improvement.
   b. **Pre-suppositional questions** to help client envision solution and build hope.

*Note: Solution-based treatment plans will *only* have goals that begin with "increase" since they use positively stated goals.

(continued)

Closing Phase of Treatment

Closing Phase Counseling Task

1. Develop aftercare plan and maintain gains. *Diversity considerations*: Include individual, family, and community resources to support client.
   Intervention:
   a. Adapt **miracle question** to have client envision future problem and how they used resources learned in counseling to handle it.

Closing Phase Client Goals

1. Increase confidence and solidify **new identity** related to living the solution (personal/relational dynamic) to reduce depressed mood, anxiety, problem behaviors, etc.
   Interventions:
   a. **Compliments and encouragement** to build new identity based on solution behaviors, choices, etc.
   b. **Scaling questions** to reflect on progress and what worked; discuss how to maintain.
2. Increase use of new skills to **build solutions** in personal, family, interpersonal, and occupational situations (personal/relational dynamic) to reduce depressed mood, anxiety, problem behaviors, etc.
   Interventions:
   a. **Compliments and encouragement** of new skills and ability to adapt them to new situations.
   b. **Scaling into the future** to anticipate ups and downs and how to manage.

Tapestry Weaving: Working with Diverse Populations

Ethnic, Racial, and Cultural Diversity

Because it does not use a theory of health to predefine client goals (O'Hanlon & Weiner-Davis, 1989), solution-focused therapy can be adapted to a wide range of populations and value systems. This therapy is widely used with diverse populations in North America, South America, Europe, the Middle East, Asia, and Australia (Gingerich & Patterson, 2007). It has also been studied with a range of clients, including immigrants, African Americans, Hispanics, Saudi Arabians, Chinese, and Koreans; and in a wide range of contexts, such as schools, prisons, hospitals, businesses, and colleges (Gingerich & Patterson, 2007). When working with diverse clients, solution-focused therapists access their unique emotional, cognitive, and social resources, which often relate to issues of diversity.

Corcoran (2000) identifies several reasons why solution-focused therapy is generally a good fit for diverse populations:

- *Behavior considered in context:* The solution-based viewing of behaviors in context allows for a more fair understanding of problem behaviors of marginalized populations.
- *Client-generated, behavioral goals:* The goal-setting process of solution-based therapies is a good fit for many ethnic groups because the goals are set in client language, they are concrete and behavioral, and they are generally short-term.
- *Behavioral rather than emotional focus:* The focus on behavior rather than emotion is more comfortable and value-consistent for many ethnic minority groups.
- *Future orientation:* The focus on solving problems in the future rather than understanding the past makes sense to many ethnic minorities.

Asian Americans Several therapists have explored using solution-based therapies with Asians and Asian Americans. Hsu and Wang (2011) describe solution-focused counseling as being highly compatible for Asian clients because of its positive reframing (client avoids losing face), relation-based perspective, and its focus on pragmatic solutions. Considerations for working with Asian clients include:

- *Filial Piety:* Several therapists have used solution-focused therapy to help clients navigate issues of filial piety, a common Asian value in which elders are obeyed and honored (Hsu & Wang, 2011; Lee & Mjelde-Mossey, 2004). Solution-focused approaches help reframe each generation's perspective in positive terms, so the good intentions of each are better understood.
- *Form and content:* Many Asian societies value the *form—how* something is done—as much as the *content—what* is done (Berg & Jaya, 1993). This can translate to family members being more concerned about how someone approached a problem than they are about what was done to solve it.
- *Practical solutions:* Asian cultures generally discourage dramatic displays of emotion, and this often translates to a preference for therapeutic approaches that focus on pragmatic solutions rather than explore feelings and causes (Berg & Jaya, 1993).
- *Saving face:* Solution-focused therapy is unique in that its focus on "what to do from here" rather than identifying root causes more easily allows for Asian clients to save face. Asian cultures are *shame*—not guilt—based, and thus positive reframes and compliments work particularly well with these populations (Berg & Jaya, 1993).
- *Brief treatment:* As therapy is usually a last resort for Asian families who prefer privacy, the brief approach of solution-focused therapy is an excellent fit (Berg & Jaya, 1993).

Middle Eastern and South Asian and Muslim Americans Chaudhry and Li (2011) have identified solution-focused counseling as a theoretical approach that can be culturally sensitive and appropriate for working with Middle Eastern and South Asian Muslim Americans. They believe that the general approach to having a future focus, concrete goals, and limited self-disclosure is a good cultural fit. In addition, Muslim Americans typically have strong family and community ties, resources that solution-focused counselors are typically quick to acknowledge and utilize. Furthermore, as Middle Eastern and South Asian Muslim Americans tend to first seek support through family, community, and their religious clergy, they tend to seek professional counseling for only specific problems; thus, the "don't fix what isn't broken" philosophy of solution-focused counseling will respect this cultural boundary.

Specifically, Chaudhry and Li (2011) cite the following elements of solution-focused counseling as particularly applicable for working with Middle Eastern and South Asian Muslim Americans:

- *Problem-Free Talk:* Problem-free talk allows for a greater sense of privacy and reduces a sense of shame, which is important for Muslim Americans who have encountered a significant increase in discrimination in past decades in the United States.
- *Pre-Session Change:* Identifying pre-session change similarly reduces embarrassment and can honor and acknowledge resources in the client's existing family and community.
- *Goal Setting:* The positive framework for goal setting in solution-focused counseling, combined with the focus on client goals rather than counselor-defined goals, can help Muslim American clients become engaged and trusting of the counseling process.
- *Competence Seeking:* By taking time to identify competence, the counselor has an opportunity to acknowledge numerous culture-based strengths and resources, conveying a sincere sense of respect and understanding of the client's culture.
- *Miracle Question:* Using the miracle question early in the process can improve engagement of Muslim Americans by creating a clear vision and purpose for the counseling process and enhancing their sense of safety, because hopeful, uplifting emotions are invoked.

Sexual Identity Diversity

Because it does not have a predefined theory of health and it focuses on client-defined goals, solution-based therapies can be appropriate when working with gay, lesbian, bisexual or transgendered clients. However, to be sensitive to these issues, therapists should inquire with "beginner's mind" about their possible role in the client's presenting problem rather than assume that, because it is not mentioned, it is not part of the problem or solution. Little has specifically been written on solution-based therapies and these populations. However, this approach has been used to facilitate adjustment to one's spouse coming out. Treyger, Ehlers, Zajicek, and Trepper (2008) found solution-based therapy appropriate for a case in which a woman's spouse announced he was gay. The approach was used to help the client identify her own solutions to the situation in a supportive, nonpathologizing context. They used Buxton's (2004) seven-stage model for partner adjustment to news that their spouse is homosexual or bisexual; the stages include: disorientation/disbelief, facing and acknowledging reality, accepting, letting go, healing, reconfiguring and refocusing, and transforming. The client in Treyger et al. (2008) reported that what helped the most from the approach was talking without being judged, not being given advice (which her family and friends offered plenty of), positive feedback and compliments, and scaling questions to concretely measure progress.

Research and the Evidence Base

Solution-based therapies have a steadily growing foundation of empirical support. Two recent meta-analyses of well-controlled, clinical trial studies (Stams, Dekovic, Buist, & De Vries, 2006; Kim, 2008) found that the solution-focused brief therapy has modest effect sizes and typically has equivalent outcomes to other approaches but typically does so in less time and therefore at less cost (Gingerich, Kim, Stams, & MacDonald, 2012). As further evidence of its growing evidence base, the Office of Juvenile Justice and Delinquency Prevention has recognized it as a promising practice, setting the stage for recognition as an evidence-based practice (Kim, Smock, Trepper, McCollum, & Franklin, 2010).

The majority of research has been conducted on solution-focused brief therapy, which was first described in the literature in 1986, had its first controlled study 1993, and has had a total of 48 published studies and two meta-analytic reviews (Gingerich et al., 2012). The quality of studies is steadily improving, including randomized samples, treatment fidelity measures, and standardized outcome measures. Researchers have studied the effectiveness of solution-focused brief therapy with a wide range of clinical populations and problems, including domestic violence offenders, couples, schizophrenics, child abuse, troubled youth, school settings, parenting, alcohol, and foster care (Franklin, Trepper, Gingerich, & McCollum, 2012). Research on the process of solution-focused brief therapy suggests that presuppositional questions, the miracle question, the first-session task, scaling questions, and solution-talk have been found to accomplish their intended therapeutic effect and that the model in general engenders hope and optimism in clients (McKeel, 2012).

Currently, quantitative research in solution-focused brief therapy has focused on refining and improving clinical trial studies through the expansion of a standardized treatment manual (Trepper et al, 2012) and development of improved adherence and fidelity measures (Lehman & Patton, 2012). In addition, process research is being done on in-session therapeutic alliance and client progress as both an outcome measure and a collaborative intervention (Duncan, Miller, & Sparks, 2004; Gillaspy & Murphy, 2012). Finally, of great current in psychotherapy research is the examination of the mechanisms of change, which underlie an evidenced-based clinical approach such as solution-focused brief therapy. Laboratory experiments have provided evidence for some of the major underlying theoretical assumptions of solution-focused brief therapy—for example, that collaboration and co-construction led significantly better outcomes in the laboratory

(Bavelas, 2012). Also, microanalysis research has shown that solution-focused therapists are overwhelmingly positive in their formulations and questions as compared with client-centered and cognitive-behavioral therapists, whose formulations and questions were primarily negative (Korman et al., 2012; Smock et al., 2012; Tomori & Bavelas, 2007). It was also shown that this "positive talk" led to more positive talk, and negative talk led to more negative talk (Smock, et al, 2012). Thus "... a therapist's use of positive content seems to contribute to the co-construction of an overall positive session, whereas negative content would do the reverse." (Bavelas, 2012; p. 159). This area of research may someday refine our understanding of the exact mechanisms of change in solution-focused brief therapy and of how this approach differs from other clinical models.

Questions for Personal Reflection and Class Discussion

1. Which ideas from this chapter do you find most personally relevant? Why?
2. Which ideas from this chapter do you think will be most helpful in working with clients?
3. What are the possibilities and limitations for using this approach with diverse clients? How might you address the limitations?
4. Are you optimistic that all clients can change and possess strengths? Why or why not?
5. Do you think solution-focused interventions are too optimistic or simple to work? Why or why not?
6. Do you think it would be hard for you to stay focused on solutions, exceptions, and possibilities with clients? Why or why not?
7. What are your thoughts about focusing on problems versus solutions? Do you think understanding why the problem exists is critical to resolving it? In which cases might that be more true than others?
8. For which clients and/or presenting problems do you think this approach would be most appropriate? Least appropriate?
9. Which case conceptualization concept seems most useful for understanding a client's problem?
10. Which intervention do you think would be the most useful?
11. Do you think this approach is a good fit for you as a counselor or therapist? Why or why not?
12. In what ways would you need to grow, or what would you need to learn, to be able to use this approach well?

Online Resources

Milton H. Erickson Foundation
www.erickson-foundation.org

Solution-Focused Brief Therapy Association
www.sfbta.org

Solution-Oriented, Possibility Therapy
www.billohanlon.com

Divorce Busting
www.divorcebusting.com

European Brief Therapy Association
www.ebta.nu

Review of Solution-Focused Therapy Research
http://gingerich.net/SFBT/2007_review.htm

References

*Asterisk indicates recommended introductory readings.

Bavelas, J. B. (2012). Connecting the lab to the therapy room: Microanalysis, co-construction, and solution-focused brief therapy. In C. Franklin, T. S. Trepper, W. J. Gingerich, & E. E. McCollum (Eds.), *Solution-focused brief therapy: A handbook of evidence-based practice* (pp. 144–164). London: Oxford University Press.

Berg, I. K., & Jaya, A. (1993). Different and same: Family therapy with Asian-American families. *Journal of Marital and Family Therapy, 19*, 31–38.

Bertolino, B. (2010). *Strength-based engagement and practice: Creating effective helping relationships*. New York: Allyn and Bacon.

Bertolino, B., & O'Hanlon, B. (1998). *Therapy with troubled teenagers: Rewriting young lives in progress*. New York: Wiley.

*Bertolino, B., & O'Hanlon, B. (2002). *Collaborative, competency-based counseling and therapy*. New York: Allyn & Bacon.

Buxton, A. P. (2004). Paths and pitfalls: How heterosexual spouses cope when their husbands or wives come out. *Journal of Couple and Relationship Therapy, 3*(2–3), 95–109.

Chaudhry, S., & Li, C. (2011). Is solution-focused brief therapy culturally appropriate for Muslim American counselees? *Journal of Contemporary Psychotherapy, 41*(2), 109–113. doi:10.1007/s10879-010-9153-1

Corcoran, J. (2000). Solution-focused family therapy with ethnic minority clients. *Crisis Intervention & Time-Limited Treatment, 6*(1), 5–12.

*De Jong, P., & Berg, I. K. (2002). *Interviewing for solutions* (2nd ed.). New York: Brooks/Cole.

*de Shazer, S. (1985). *Keys to solution in brief therapy*. New York: Norton.

*de Shazer, S. (1988). *Clues: Investigating solutions in brief therapy*. New York: Norton.

de Shazer, S. (1994). *Words were originally magic*. New York: Norton.

*de Shazer, S., Dolan, Y., Korman, H., Trepper, T., McCollum, E., & Berg, I. K. (2007). *More than miracles: The state of the art of solution-focused brief therapy*. New York: Haworth.

*Dolan, Y. (1991). *Resolving sexual abuse: Solution-focused therapy and Ericksonian hypnosis for survivors*. New York: Norton.

Duncan, B., Miller, S. D., & Sparks, J. A. (2004). *The heroic client: A revolutionary way to improve effectiveness through client-directed, outcome-informed therapy*. New York: Jossey-Bass.

Franklin, C., Trepper, T. S., Gingerich, W. J., & McCollum, E. E. (Eds.). (2012). *Solution-focused brief therapy: A handbook of evidence-based practice*. New York: Oxford University Press.

Gehart, D. (2015). *Theory and treatment planning in counseling and psychotherapy* (2nd ed.). Pacific Grove, CA: Brooks Cole.

Gillaspy, A., & Murphy, J. J. (2012). Incorporating outcome and session rating scales in solution-focused brief therapy. In C. Franklin, T. S. Trepper, W. J. Gingerich, & E. E. McCollum (Eds.), *Solution-focused brief therapy: A handbook of evidence-based practice* (pp. 73–94). New York: Oxford University Press.

Gingerich, W. J., & Eisengart, S. (2000). Solution-focused brief therapy: A review of the outcome studies. *Family Process, 39*, 477–498.

Gingerich, W. J., Kim, J. S., Stams, G. J. J. M., & MacDonald, A. J. (2012). Solution-focused brief therapy outcome research. In C. Franklin, T. S. Trepper, W. J. Gingerich, & E. E. McCollum (Eds.), *Solution-focused brief therapy: A handbook of evidence-based practice* (pp. 95–111). New York: Oxford University Press.

Gingerich, W. J., & Patterson, L. (2007). The 2007 SFBT effectiveness project. Retrieved March 20, 2008 from http://gingerich.net/SFBT/2007_review.htm

Hsu, W., & Wang, C. C. (2011). Integrating Asian clients' filial piety beliefs into solution-focused brief therapy. *International Journal for the Advancement of Counselling, 33*(4), 322–334. doi:10.1007/s10447-011-9133-5

Hudson, P. O., & O'Hanlon, W. H. (1991). *Rewriting love stories: Brief marital therapy*. New York: Norton.

Kim, J. S. (2008). Examining the effectiveness of solution-focused brief therapy: A meta-analysis. *Research on Social Work Practice, 18*(2), 107–116. doi:10.1177/1049731507307807

Kim, J. S., Smock, S., Trepper, T. S., McCollum, E. E., & Franklin, C. (2010). Is solution-focused brief therapy evidence based? *Families in Society, 91*, 300–306. doi:10.1606/1044-3894.4009

Korman, H., Bavelas, J. B., & De Jong, P. (2012). Microanalysis of formulations, Part II: Comparing Solution-Focused Brief Therapy, Cognitive-Behavioral Therapy, and Motivational Interviewing. (In Press)

Lee, M., & Mjelde-Mossey, L. (2004). Cultural dissonance among generations: A solution-focused approach with East Asian elders and their families. *Journal of Marital and Family Therapy, 30*(4), 497–513.

Lehmann, P., & Patton, J. D. (2012). The development of a solution-focused fidelity instrument: A pilot study. In C. Franklin, T. S. Trepper, W. J. Gingerich, & E. E. McCollum (Eds.), *Solution-focused brief therapy: A handbook of evidence-based practice* (pp. 39–54). New York: Oxford University Press.

McCollum, E. (2007). Introduction to special issue. *Journal of Family Psychotherapy, 18*(3), 1–9.

McKeel, J. (2012). What works in solution-focused brief therapy: A review of change process research 2012. In C. Franklin, T. S. Trepper, W. J. Gingerich, & E. E. McCollum (Eds.), *Solution-focused brief therapy: A handbook of evidence-based practice* (pp. 130–143). New York: Oxford University Press.

Miller, S. D., Duncan, B. L., & Hubble, M. (Eds.). (1996). *Handbook of solution-focused brief therapy*. San Francisco, CA: Jossey-Bass.

Miller, S. D., Duncan, B. L., & Hubble, M. A. (1997). *Escape from Babel: Towards a unifying language for psychotherapy practice*. New York: Norton.

O'Hanlon, B. (2000). *Do one thing different: Ten simple ways to change your life*. New York: Harper.

*O'Hanlon, B., & Beadle, S. (1999). *A guide to possibilityland: Possibility therapy methods*. Omaha, NE: Possibility Press.

O'Hanlon, B., & Bertolino, B. (2002). *Even from a broken web: Brief and respectful solution-oriented therapy for resolving sexual abuse*. New York: Norton.

*O'Hanlon, W. H., & Weiner-Davis, M. (1989). *In search of solutions: A new direction in psychotherapy*. New York: Norton.

Parsons, R. (2009). *Thinking and acting like a solution-focused school counselor*. Thousand Oaks, CA: Corwin Press.

Selekman, M. D. (1997). *Solution-focused therapy with children: Harnessing family strengths for systemic change*. New York: Guilford.

*Selekman, M. D. (2010). *Collaborative brief therapy with children*. New York: Guilford.

Seligman, M. (2004). *Authentic happiness*. New York: Free Press.

Smock, S., Froerer, A., & Bavelas, J. B. (2012). Microanalysis of positive and negative content in Solution-Focused Brief Therapy and Cognitive-Behavioral Therapy Expert Sessions. Manuscript submitted for publication.

Stams, G., Deković, M., Buist, K., & de Vries, L. (2006). Effectiviteit van oplossingsgerichte korte therapie: Ein meta-analyse. *Gedragstherapie*, *39*(2), 81–94.

Tomori, C., & Bavelas, J. B. (2007). Using microanalysis of communication of communication to compare solution-focused and client-centered therapies. *Journal of Family Psychotherapy*, *18*, 25–43.

Trepper, T. S., McCollum, E. E., de Jong, P., Korman, H., Gingerich, W. J., & Franklin, C. (2012). Solution-focused brief therapy treatment manual. In C. Franklin, T. S. Trepper, W. J. Gingerich, & E. E. McCollum (Eds.), *Solution-focused brief therapy: A handbook of evidence-based practice* (pp. 20–38). New York: Oxford University Press.

Treyger, S., Ehlers, N., Zajicek, L., & Trepper, T. (2008). Helping spouses cope with partners coming out: A solution-focused approach. *American Journal of Family Therapy*, *36*(1), 30–47. doi:10.1080/01926180601057549

Walter, J. L., & Peller, J. E. (1992). *Becoming solution-focused in brief therapy*. New York: Brunner/Mazel.

Weiner-Davis, M., de Shazer, S., & Gingerich, W. J. (1987), Building on pretreatment change to construct the therapeutic solution: An exploratory study. *Journal of Marital and Family Therapy*, *13*, 359–363. doi:10.1111/j.1752-0606.1987.tb00717.x.

Solution-Based Counseling Case Study: Family Conflict Over Biracial Relationship

A 24-year-old registered nurse, Sarah is the daughter of Iranian immigrants who had always done well in school and never got in trouble. Recently, when she announced she was planning on marrying her African American boyfriend, Alan, who works in retail, her parents informed her that this was not acceptable on numerous counts. They insist that she marry someone with a professional background and from within their culture who speaks their language. Never having had much tension with her family, Sarah feels betrayed, hurt, and angry, but is not sure how she will resolve the issue—caught between her family and the man she loves. Her boyfriend is surprised by how she lets her family influence her in this way, leaving her feeling distant from him, too. This tension began a month before coming to counseling, during which time she has begun to drink more frequently to manage the stress. She states: "I have only been doing it since I was told they would disown me if I marry him; once this all blows over, I won't need it. I just have to figure out what to do." After an initial consultation, a solution-based counselor develops the following case conceptualization.

CASE CONCEPTUALIZATION

Date: April 23, 2013 **Clinician:** Demetria **Client/Case #:** 13009

I. Introduction to Client

Identify primary client and significant others

Client

Adult Female Age: 24 Middle Eastern American Partnered heterosexual Occupation/Grade: Registered Nurse

Other: Living with parents and siblings; dating 26-year-old African American man

Significant Others

Client's Male Partner Age: 26 African American Partnered heterosexual Occupation/Grade: Assistant Store Manager Other:_______

Client's Mother Age: 54 Middle Eastern American Married heterosexual Occupation/Grade: Homemaker; officer in local woman's club. Other:

Client's Father Age: 65 Middle Eastern American Married heterosexual Occupation/Grade: Engineer Other:____

Select Person Age: ______ Select Ethnicity Select Relational Status Occupation/Grade: Other: ______

Others: AF has one younger female sibling (19) and an older male sibling (26). Both are currently in college. Her brother is studying to be an engineer like their father, and her sister is studying to be a physician.

II. Presenting Concern(s)

Client Description of Problem(s): Client views parents' refusal to allow her to marry man of her choosing as her primary problem. She reports feeling trapped between having to choose between her family and the man she loves. She says she has always been loyal to the family and now feels betrayed by them. She does not believe her recent increase in drinking is a long-term issue: "I have only been doing it since I was told they would disown me if I marry him; once this all blows over, I won't need it."

Significant Other/Family Description(s) of Problems: AF54 and AM65, AF24's parents, believe their daughter is not thinking about her future and is too young to make a good decision without their help. They view their refusal as their responsibility as loving parents to ensure that their daughter ends up in a healthy marriage and is well cared for. They are unaware of her recent drinking but are very concerned about her withdrawal from them and the family, avoiding family meals, not saying more than "hi" and "bye." They feel they are being reasonable by allowing her to still see and talk with AM26.

(continued)

Broader System Problem Descriptions: Description of problem from referring party, teachers, relatives, legal system, etc.:

AM26: believes AF should not allow her parents to control her and her life decisions for her. He sees her as being manipulated by them. He thinks her drinking is becoming a problem.

Siblings: Her 19-year-old sister thinks everyone is being overly dramatic, yet does not clearly take a side and is currently the closest to AF at this time. The 26-year-old brother clearly sides with the parents.

III. Background Information

Trauma/Abuse History (recent and past): AF's parents left Iran after the revolution ended in 1984, having seen much of violence in person. AF says that her parents avoid talking about the war, but she knows her mother in particular seems scared by it.

Substance Use/Abuse (current and past; self, family of origin, significant others): AF has been drinking 2–4 drinks per night for the past month; prior to this she reported periodically partying with her friends (2–4 drinks on 2 nights out of the month), but otherwise nothing in between. She denies use of other recreational and prescription drugs. She does not report a family history of alcohol abuse but she also says that many of her family never left Iran.

Precipitating Events (recent life changes, first symptoms, stressors, etc.): AF began dating AM two years ago, and they recently began to discuss marriage. When she mentioned this to her parents, she expected resistance from them, but not their threat to disown her if she did. They want her to marry someone who is from a more similar ethnic group and who has a professional career. They state that they only have her long-term and best interests at heart. AF's physician sent her to counseling when she learned about her family stress and drinking.

Related Historical Background (family history, related issues, previous counseling, etc.): AF parents come from the upper-middle class in Iran, her parents leaving as soon as they could after the revolution. Her father was an engineer and easily found work upon arriving in the states. They have since supported father's parents and several of his siblings in Iran. The family is Muslim but not strictly observant, the family often integrating American values and practices. They raised AF and her siblings (one older brother and one younger sister) to be respectful and to excel in scholastics. Her brother is studying to be an engineer like his father, and her sister is in college studying medicine.

IV. Client Strengths and Diversity

Client Strengths

Personal: AF is intelligent, self-disciplined, and socially skilled. She has developed sensitivity as a nurse and enjoys helping others. She avoided typical teenage and college troubles and has generally gotten along well with her family.

(*continued*)

Relational/Social: AF's family is generally close, all still living together in the family house. Her family values education and status, and her parents have done well trying to balance Iranian tradition with modern American lifestyle.

Spiritual: AF was raised Muslim but as a young adult has not found great solace from it. She reports that the politics of being Muslim in America have probably been a factor in her feeling less connected. She states that she really is not sure there is a god.

Diversity: Resources and Limitations

Identify potential resources and limitations available to clients based on their age, gender, sexual orientation, cultural background, socioeconomic status, religion, regional community, language, family background, family configuration, abilities, etc.

Unique Resources: AF has a strong social support system and friends from other cultures who offer her a different perspective. While her sister is often busy with school, she is also a strong source of support for her and has also dated men from other cultures. She can relate to what AF24 is going through.

Potential Limitations: AF's traditional Iranian background as well as the local Iranian American community have certain standards and expectations that are in conflict with AF's desire to marry AM26.

Complete All of the Following Sections for a Complete Case Conceptualization or Specific Sections for Theory-Specific Conceptualization.

V. Psychodynamic Conceptualization

Psychodynamic Defense Mechanisms

Check 2–4 most commonly used defense mechanisms

❑ Acting Out: *Describe:* ____

❑ Denial: *Describe:* ____

❑ Displacement: *Describe:* ____

❑ Help-rejecting complaining: *Describe:* ____

❑ Humor: *Describe:* ____

☒ Passive Aggression: *Describe:* When dealing with her parents and boyfriend, AF reports using passive-aggressive means to get what she wants.

❑ Projection: *Describe:* ____

❑ Projective Identification: *Describe:* ____

☒ Rationalization: *Describe:* When dealing with her parents and boyfriend, AF reports using passive-aggressive means to get what she wants.

❑ Reaction Formation: *Describe:* ____

❑ Repression: *Describe:* ____

❑ Splitting: *Describe:* ____

❑ Sublimation: *Describe:* ____

❑ Suppression: *Describe:* ____

❑ Other: ____

(continued)

Object Relational Patterns

Describe relationship with early caregivers in past: AF's mother was a stay-at-home mom and the primary caretaker for the family. Her father worked long hours to support their family as well as his extended family. Both parents placed a high value on education and hovered over the children's schoolwork. As a young child and teenager AF always complied with her parents' wishes and was dependent upon them to make most of her decisions.

Was the attachment with the mother (or equivalent) primarily:

❑ Generally Secure ☒ Anxious and Clingy ❑ Avoidant and Emotionally Distant ❑ Other:______

Was the attachment with the father (or equivalent) primarily:

❑ Generally Secure ❑ Anxious and Clingy ☒ Avoidant and Emotionally Distant ❑ Other: ______

Describe present relationship with these caregivers: AF's parents have strong opinions about the way in which AF24 should live her life. They are frequently involved in her life decisions and feel as though she is not mature enough to make her own decisions, especially in choosing a romantic partner. This has caused a strain in AF's present relationship with her parents as she is realizing that this way of relating is not adaptive for her.

Describe relational patterns with partner and other current relationships: The relationship between AF24 and AM26 is strained due to AM26 not being accepted by her family as a suitable life partner for AF24. AF26 has been patient with AF24 and is genuinely willing to do whatever he can to help alleviate some of her stress and to win over her family.

Erickson's Psychosocial Developmental Stage

Describe development at each stage up to current stage

Trust vs. Mistrust (Infant Stage): AF describes normal infancy with mother at home with children.

Autonomy vs. Shame and Doubt (Toddler Stage): AF reports that her parents used shame to get her and her siblings to behave.

Initiative vs. Guilt (Preschool Age): Shame and guilt often used to manage children's behavior in family.

Industry vs. Inferiority (School Age): AF remembers being strongly encouraged to excel in school.

Identity vs. Role Confusion (Adolescence): Teen years were marked by struggling to integrate Iranian heritage and values with American values. AF feels "American" outside the home and "Iranian" when around her family.

Intimacy vs. Isolation (Young Adulthood): AF is currently having to decide between her boyfriend and her family—or at least so it seems to her. This struggle will be central in defining her cultural identity and the type of relationship/family she will have.

Generativity vs. Stagnation (Adulthood): ______

Ego Integrity vs. Despair (Late Adulthood): ______

(continued)

Adlerian Style of Life Theme

☒ Control: Although on the outside AF appears to devote much energy to pleasing others, inside she is highly concerned with who is in charge and who is not; her current struggle with her parents heightens her sense of being out of control, which is terrifying for her.

❏ Superiority: ____________________

❏ Pleasing: ____________________

❏ Comfort: ____________________

Basic Mistake Misperceptions: I must be in control to make life safe.

VI. Humanistic-Existential Conceptualization

Expression of Authentic Self

Problems: Are problems perceived as internal or external (caused by others, circumstance, etc.)?

❏ Predominantly internal

❏ Mixed

☒ Predominantly external

Agency and Responsibility: Is self or other discussed as agent of story? Does client take clear responsibility for situation?

❏ Strong sense of agency and responsibility

☒ Agency in some areas

❏ Little agency; frequently blames others/situation

☒ Often feels victimized

Recognition and Expression of Feelings: Are feelings readily recognized, owned, and experienced?

❏ Easily expresses feelings

❏ Identifies feelings with prompting

☒ Difficulty recognizing feelings

Here-and-Now Experiencing: Is the client able to experience full range of feelings as they are happening in the present moment?

❏ Easily experiences emotions in present moment

❏ Experiences some present emotions with assistance

☒ Difficulty with present moment experiencing

Personal Constructs and Facades: Is the client able to recognize and go beyond roles? Is identity rigid or tentatively held?

❏ Tentatively held; able to critique and question

☒ Some awareness of facades and construction of identity

❏ Identity rigidly defined; seems like "fact"

Complexity and Contradictions: Are internal contradictions owned and explored? Is client able to fully engage the complexity of identity and life?

❏ Aware of and resolves contradictions

☒ Some recognition of contradictions

❏ Unaware of internal contradictions

(*continued*)

Shoulds: Is client able to question socially imposed shoulds and oughts? Can client balance desire to please others and desire to be authentic?
❑ Able to balance authenticity with social obligation
☒ Identifies tension between social expectations and personal desires
❑ Primarily focuses on external shoulds

List shoulds:

Acceptance of Others: Is client able to accept others and modify expectations of others to be more realistic?
❑ Readily accepts others as they are
☒ Recognizes expectations of others are unrealistic but still strong emotional reaction to expectations not being met
❑ Difficulty accepting others as is; always wanting others to change to meet expectations

Trust of Self: Is client able to trust self as process (rather than a stabile object)?
❑ Able to trust and express authentic self
☒ Trust of self in certain contexts
❑ Difficulty trusting self in most contexts

Existential Analysis

Sources of Life Meaning (as described or demonstrated by client): AF24 takes a great deal of pride in her work as a nurse and believes that her purpose in life is to help others. She also places a great deal of value on family, and it is very important to her to start a family of her own with a man that she truly loves.

General Themes of Life Meaning:
☒ Personal achievement/work
❑ Significant other
❑ Children
☒ Family of origin
❑ Social cause/contributing to others
❑ Religion/spirituality
❑ Other:

Satisfaction with and clarity on life direction:
❑ Clear sense of meaning that creates resilience in difficult times
❑ Current problems require making choices related to life direction
☒ Minimally satisfied with current life direction; wants more from life
❑ Has reflected little on life direction up to this point; living according to life plan defined by someone/something else
❑ Other:

Gestalt Contact Boundary Disturbances
❑ *Desensitization:* Failing to notice problems
☒ *Introjection*: Take in others' views whole and unedited
❑ *Projection*: Assign undesired parts of self to others
❑ *Retroflection*: Direct action to self rather than other
❑ *Deflection*: Avoid direct contact with another or self
❑ *Egotism:* Not allowing outside to influence self
❑ *Confluence*: Agree with another to extent that boundary blurred

Describe: AF24 believes she must choose between the man that she loves and her family. She is unable to see any other possible solutions.

(*continued*)

VII. Cognitive-Behavioral Conceptualization

Baseline of Symptomatic Behavior

Symptom #1 (behavioral description): Anger and sense of powerlessness in response to parents saying they will not allow her to marry boyfriend.

Frequency: Reports daily feelings of anger and powerlessness.

Duration: 1 month

Context(s): Anytime she is not working.

Events Before: Seeing family, being around family.

Events After: Tries to leave house to get away.

Symptom #2 (behavioral description): Drinking

Frequency: 6-7 days of every week

Duration: 4 weeks

Context(s): With boyfriend or friends; at home in room.

Events Before: Fight with parents over boyfriend.

Events After: Goes to sleep.

A-B-C Analysis of Irrational Beliefs

Activating Event ("Problem"): Parents told her they do not approve of her marrying boyfriend.

Consequence (Mood, behavior, etc.): Feeling angry; betrayed; confused; trapped; drinking to manage conflicting emotions.

Mediating Beliefs (Unhelpful beliefs about event that result in C):

1. I can't give up connection to my family but I can can't live without my boyfriend.
2. My parents can't make this decision for me.
3. ______

Beck's Schema Analysis

Identify frequently used cognitive schemas:

❑ *Arbitrary inference:* ______

❑ *Selective abstraction:* ______

❑ *Overgeneralization:* ______

☒ *Magnification/Minimization:* My life is over if I cannot be with AM; if I don't marry AM now, I'll never be happy again.

☒ *Personalization:* My parents are doing this to me because I am a girl.

☒ *Absolutist/dichotomous thinking:* I am now forced to choose between parents and boyfriend.

❑ *Mislabeling:* ______

☒ *Mindreading:* ______

(continued)

VIII. Family Systems Conceptualization

Family Life Cycle Stage

☒ Single adult
❑ Marriage
❑ Family with Young Children
❑ Family with Adolescent Children
❑ Launching Children
❑ Later Life

Describe struggles with mastering developmental tasks in one of these stages: AF24 is struggling to create boundaries with her family of origin and exercise her autonomy as an adult. She would like to start a family with the man that she loves but fears rejection from her family and the need to choose one or the other.

Boundaries with

Parents ☒ Enmeshed ❑ Clear ❑ Disengaged ❑ *NA: Describe:* Although unable to directly communicate about conflict with her father, AF's identity is closely tied to her parents' approval and support. She has difficulty accepting when her thoughts and feelings are different from theirs, as do they.

Significant Other ☒ Enmeshed ❑ Clear ❑ Disengaged ❑ *NA: Describe:* AF has difficulty standing up for herself in relationship to AM, not having had direct communication with her father.

Children ❑ Enmeshed ❑ Clear ❑ Disengaged ❑ *NA: Describe:* ______

Extended Family ☒ Enmeshed ❑ Clear ☒ Disengaged ❑ NA: *Describe:* The extended family is very involved in the family's affairs, offering strong opinions.

Other: Siblings ❑ Enmeshed ☒ Clear ❑ Disengaged ❑ NA: *Describe:* AF has a more distant but respectful relationship with her brother; she and her sister are close but not dependent on each other.

Typical style for regulating closeness and distance with others: The father is recognized as the head of the family and no one openly challenges him; the mother has always quietly mediated conflict between the children and the father/parents by talking to one and then the other in private, always trying to strike a realistic middle ground. The eldest brother has special status in the family, receiving extra attention and praise from the parents. The sisters are close but each is busy with school and career. The family finds closeness in encouraging each other in professional pursuits and in their cultural heritage.

Triangles/Coalitions

☒ Coalition in family of origin: *Describe:* AF's mother typically triangulated with the children against the father's traditional rules; this current conflict is atypical, thus AF feels betrayed by her mother.

❑ Coalitions related to significant other: *Describe:* ______

❑ Other coalitions: ______

Hierarchy between Self and Parent/Child ❑ NA

With own children ❑ Effective ☒ Rigid ❑ Permissive
With parents (for child/young adult) ❑ Effective ❑ Rigid ❑ Permissive

(continued)

Complementary Patterns with Siblings:

❑ Pursuer/distancer
❑ Over-/underfunctioner
❑ Emotional/logical
❑ Good/bad parent
☒ Other: *Good/bad child*

Example of complementary pattern: AF's sister has typically been the rebel and AF was the "good girl." Their roles are shifting with AF's decision to date and marry AM.

Intergenerational Patterns

Substance/Alcohol Abuse: ☒ NA ❑ History: AF currently; no other reported family history.

Sexual/Physical/Emotional Abuse: ☒ NA ❑ History: AF reports very strict father with minimal spanking.

Parent/Child Relations: ❑ NA ☒ History: As is typical in Iranian culture, parents and children are very close, especially mothers and their children; sons are closest to the parents.

Physical/Mental Disorders: ❑ NA ❑ History: Family experienced extensive trauma, loss of brothers and young men during the revolution.

Family strengths: *Describe:* Value education; strong sense of cultural heritage; have adapted well as immigrants.

IX. Solution-Based and Cultural Discourse Conceptualization (Postmodern)

Solutions and Unique Outcomes

Attempted Solutions that DIDN'T or DON'T work:

1. Arguing with parents (mostly mother)
2. Trying to get extended family members and siblings to take her side against parents.
3.

Exceptions and Unique Outcomes: Times, places, relationships, contexts, etc., when problem is less of a problem; behaviors that seem to make things even slightly better:

1. Staying away from the house.
2. Talking with sister and friends.
3. Going to work and focusing on something else.

Miracle Question Answer: If the problem were to be resolved overnight, what would client be doing differently the next day? (Describe in terms of doing X rather than not doing Y).

1. AF would be more assertive in expressing her needs and feelings to her family about her desire to marry AF26.
2. AF would decrease her weekly intake of alcohol.
3. Family would accept AM26.

(continued)

Dominant Discourses informing definition of problem:

- *Ethnic, Class and Religious Discourses: How do key cultural discourses inform what is perceived as a problem and the possible solutions?* AF's Iranian heritage informs marital choices that provide a stable, happy lifestyle more than romantic love. Her parents are most concerned about her quality of life married to AM, more than about her personal happiness. This is somewhat at odds with the American culture in which romantic love is highly valued and viewed as the primary reason to marry.
- *Gender and Sexuality Discourses: How do the gender/sexual discourses inform what is perceived as a problem and the possible solutions?* As a young Iranian woman, AF has little power within the family, and is expected to be compliant and helpful. AF has always done this without question. Her current situation now has her questioning this role in the family.
- *Community, School, and Extended Family Discourses: How do other important community discourses inform what is perceived as a problem and the possible solutions?* AF's family values education and status, and AF has generally adopted these values. She recognizes that her current boyfriend is not an equal to her in these ways, but says she loves him anyway.

Identity Narratives: *How has the problem shaped each client's identity?* AF feels more alone than she ever has before and is terrified of losing her family. Up to this point, she felt that they had done a good job balancing their Iranian heritage with modern American values. This current dilemma has her feeling trapped and without her mother's or extended family support, which she was used to. She has also never felt love like she feels for AM and is afraid to lose it. This dilemma has her feeling frozen, unsure what to do, as she has tried to do her normal working from behind the scenes, but having it fail.

Local or Preferred Discourses: What is the client's preferred identity narrative and/or narrative about the problem? Are there local (alternative) discourses about the problem that are preferred? The client wants to be able to marry whomever she choose AND continue to have her parents' approval. She has always had a pull toward the freedom of American culture yet feels comfort in her Iranian heritage.

CLINICAL ASSESSMENT

Clinician: Demetria	Client ID #: 13009	Primary configuration: ☒ Individual ❑ Couple ❑ Family	Primary Language: ☒ English ❑ Spanish ❑ Other: _______

List client and significant others

Adult(s)

Adult Female Age: 24 Middle Eastern American Partnered heterosexual Occupation: Nurse; Roosevelt Hospital Other identifier: _______

Adult Male Age: 26 African American Partnered heterosexual Occupation: Assistant Store Manager Other identifier: _______

Child(ren)

Select Gender Age: _______ Select Ethnicity Grade: Select Grade School: _______ Other identifier: _______

Select Gender Age: _______ Select Ethnicity Grade: Select Grade School: _______ Other identifier: _______

Others: _______

Presenting Problems

☒ Depression/hopelessness
☒ Anxiety/worry
❑ Anger issues
❑ Loss/grief
❑ Suicidal thoughts/attempts
❑ Sexual abuse/rape
☒ Alcohol/drug use
❑ Eating problems/disorders
❑ Job problems/unemployed

❑ Couple concerns
☒ Parent/child conflict
❑ Partner violence/abuse
❑ Divorce adjustment
❑ Remarriage adjustment
❑ Sexuality/intimacy concerns
❑ Major life changes
❑ Legal issues/probation
❑ Other: _______

Complete for children:

❑ School failure/decline performance
❑ Truancy/runaway
❑ Fighting w/peers
❑ Hyperactivity
❑ Wetting/soiling clothing
❑ Child abuse/neglect
❑ Isolation/withdrawal
❑ Other: _______

Mental Status Assessment for Identified Patient

Interpersonal	❑ NA	☒ Conflict ☒ Enmeshment ☒ Isolation/avoidance ❑ Harassment ❑ Other: _______
Mood	❑ NA	❑ Depressed/Sad ☒ Anxious ☒ Dysphoric ❑ Angry ❑ Irritable ❑ Manic ❑ Other: _______
Affect	❑ NA	☒ Constricted ❑ Blunt ❑ Flat ❑ Labile ❑ Incongruent ❑ Other: _______
Sleep	❑ NA	❑ Hypersomnia ❑ Insomnia ☒ Disrupted ❑ Nightmares ❑ Other: _______

(continued)

Eating	❑ NA	❑ Increase ☒ Decrease ❑ Anorectic restriction ❑ Binging ❑ Purging ❑ Other: ____
Anxiety	❑ NA	❑ Chronic worry ❑ Panic ❑ Phobias ❑ Obsessions ❑ Compulsions ❑ Other: ____
Trauma Symptoms	☒ NA	❑ Hypervigilance ❑ Flashbacks/Intrusive memories ❑ Dissociation ❑ Numbing ❑ Avoidance efforts ❑ Other: ____
Psychotic Symptoms	☒ NA	❑ Hallucinations ❑ Delusions ❑ Paranoia ❑ Loose associations ❑ Other: ____
Motor activity/ Speech	❑ NA	❑ Low energy ☒ Hyperactive ❑ Agitated ❑ Inattentive ❑ Impulsive ❑ Pressured speech ❑ Slow speech ❑ Other: ____
Thought	❑ NA	☒ Poor concentration ☒ Denial ❑ Self-blame ☒ Other-blame ❑ Ruminative ❑ Tangential ❑ Concrete ❑ Poor insight ☒ Impaired decision making ❑ Disoriented ❑ Other: ____
Socio-Legal	☒ NA	❑ Disregards rules ❑ Defiant ❑ Stealing ❑ Lying ❑ Tantrums ❑ Arrest/incarceration ❑ Initiates fights ❑ Other: ____
Other Symptoms	❑ NA	____

Diagnosis for Identified Patient

Contextual Factors considered in making diagnosis: ☒ Age ☒ Gender ☒ Family dynamics ☒ Culture ☒ Language ☒ Religion ☒ Economic ☒ Immigration ❑ Sexual/gender orientation ❑ Trauma ❑ Dual diagnosis/comorbid ❑ Addiction ❑ Cognitive ability ❑ Other: ____

Describe impact of identified factors on diagnosis and assessment process: Immigration/cultural/class issues considered in assessing severity of response to conflict with parents to qualify as "excessive distress"; coping strategies considered in relation to gender norms within Iranian culture for unmarried women. Fluent in English; did not want translation.

DSM-5 Code	Diagnosis with Specifier *Include V/Z/T-Codes for Psychosocial Stressors/Issues*
1. F43.23	1. Adjustment Disorder, Mixed anxiety and depression
2. F10.10	2. Rule out Alcohol Use Disorder, Mild
3. V61.20	3. Parent-child relational problem
4. ____	4. ____
5. ____	5. ____

Medical Considerations

Has patient been referred for psychiatric evaluation? ☒ Yes ❑ No

Has patient agreed with referral? ❑ Yes ☒ No ❑ NA

(*continued*)

Psychometric instruments used for assessment: ❑ None ☒ Cross-cutting symptom inventories ❑ Other:_______

Client response to diagnosis: ❑ Agree ☒ Somewhat agree ❑ Disagree ❑ Not informed for following reason: _______

Current Medications (psychiatric & medical) ☒ NA

1. _______; dose mg _______; start date: _______
2. _______; dose mg _______; start date: _______
3. _______; dose mg _______; start date: _______
4. _______; dose mg _______; start date: _______

Medical Necessity: *Check all that apply*

☒ Significant impairment ☒ Probability of significant impairment ❑ Probable developmental arrest

Areas of impairment:

☒ Daily activities ☒ Social relationships ☒ Health ☒ Work/School ☒ Living arrangement ❑ Other: _______

Risk and Safety Assessment for Identified Patient

Suicidality	Homicidality	Alcohol Abuse
☒ No indication/Denies	☒ No indication/Denies	☒ No indication/denies
❑ Active ideation	❑ Active ideation	❑ Past abuse
❑ Passive ideation	❑ Passive ideation	☒ Current; Freq/Amt: 2-4 drinks per day
❑ Intent without plan	❑ Intent without means	**Drug Use/Abuse**
❑ Intent with means	❑ Intent with means	☒ No indication/denies
❑ Ideation in past year	❑ Ideation in past year	❑ Past use
❑ Attempt in past year	❑ Violence past year	❑ Current drugs: _______
❑ Family or peer history of completed suicide	❑ History of assaulting others	Freq/Amt: _______
	❑ Cruelty to animals	❑ Family/sig.other use

Sexual & Physical Abuse and Other Risk Factors

❑ Childhood abuse history: ❑ Sexual ❑ Physical ❑ Emotional ❑ Neglect

❑ Adult with abuse/assault in adulthood: ❑ Sexual ❑ Physical ❑ Current

❑ History of perpetrating abuse: ❑ Sexual ❑ Physical ❑ Emotional

❑ Elder/dependent adult abuse/neglect

❑ History of or current issues with restrictive eating, binging, and/or purging

❑ Cutting or other self harm: ❑ Current ❑ Past: Method: _______

❑ Criminal/legal history: _______

☒ Other trauma history: Significant family history of war-related trauma and loss

❑ None reported

(continued)

Indicators of Safety

❑ NA

❑ At least one outside support person
❑ Able to cite specific reasons to live or not harm
❑ Hopeful
❑ Willing to dispose of dangerous items
❑ Has future goals
❑ Willingness to reduce contact with people who make situation worse
☒ Willing to implement safety plan, safety interventions
☒ Developing set of alternatives to self-/other harm
❑ Sustained period of safety: ______
☒ Other: Agreed to harm reduction plan for drinking

Elements of Safety Plan

❑ NA

❑ Verbal no harm contract
❑ Written no harm contract
☒ Emergency contact card
☒ Emergency therapist/agency number
❑ Medication management
❑ Plan for contacting friends/support persons during crisis
❑ Specific plan of where to go during crisis
☒ Specific self-calming tasks to reduce risk before reach crisis level (e.g., journaling, exercising, etc.)
❑ Specific daily/weekly activities to reduce stressors
❑ Other: ______

Legal/Ethical Action Taken: ☒ NA ❑ Action: ______

Case Management

Collateral Contacts

- Has contact been made with treating *physicians or other professionals*: ☒ NA ❑ Yes ❑ In process. Name/ Notes: ______
- If client is involved in mental health *treatment elsewhere*, has contact been made? ☒ NA ❑ Yes ❑ In process. Name/Notes: ______
- Has contact been made with *social worker*: ☒ NA ❑ Yes ❑ In process. Name/Notes: ______

Referrals

- Has client been referred for *medical assessment*: ☒ Yes ❑ No evidence for need
- Has client been referred for *social services*: ☒ NA ❑ Job/training ❑ Welfare/Food/Housing ❑ Victim services ❑ Legal aid ❑ Medical ❑ Other: ______
- Has client been referred for *group* or other support services: ❑ Yes: ____ ❑ In process ☒ None recommended
- Are there anticipated *forensic/legal processes* related to treatment: ☒ No ❑ Yes; describe: ______

Support Network

- Client social support network includes: ❑ Supportive family ☒ Supportive partner ☒ Friends ❑ Religious/ spiritual organization ☒ Supportive work/social group ❑ Other: ______
- Describe anticipated effects treatment will have on others in support system (Children, partner, etc.): Treatment, specifically how counselor approaches culturally based conflict regarding boyfriend, will significantly impact family of origin and boyfriend.

(*continued*)

Is there anything else client will need to be successful? Thoughtful awareness of how resolving this issue will impact future relationship with family, religion, and culture.

Expected Outcome and Prognosis

☒ Return to normal functioning ❑ Anticipate less than normal functioning ❑ Prevent deterioration

Client Sense of Hope: 2

Evaluation of Assessment/Client Perspective

How were assessment methods adapted to client needs, including age, culture, and other diversity issues? Assessment of "excessive response" to stressor for adjustment disorder considered within her cultural/family context; bilingual services offered and refused; couple and family sessions will be offered, but AF does not believe her parents would ever come in. Counselor must be particularly careful to allow client to define and use her values to decide whether to follow her cultural versus the dominant U.S. cultural norms regarding her decision to marry.

Describe actual or potential areas of client-clinician agreement/disagreement related to the above assessment: AF does not believe her drinking situation will develop into a long-term problem; counselor using harm reduction model to plan for safey while drinking and reduce overall use.

_______________________, ______________ ____________

Clinician Signature License/Intern Status Date

_______________________, ______________ ____________

Supervisor Signature License Date

TREATMENT PLAN

Date: May 13, 2013

Case/Client #: 13009

Clinician Name: Demetria

Theory: Solution-Focused

Modalities planned: ☒ Individual Adult ❑ Individual Child ❑ Couple ❑ Family ❑ Group: ______

Recommended session frequency: ☒ Weekly ❑ Every two weeks ❑ Other: ______

Expected length of treatment: 4 months

Initial Phase of Treatment

Initial Phase Counseling Tasks

1. Develop working counseling relationship. *Diversity considerations:* Adapt relationship to respond to cultural expectations of an "expert" while still maintaining collaborative stance by providing information when asked but not solutions.

   Relationship-building approach/intervention:

   a. Identify AF strengths, resources, especially as they relate to cultural and religious background; channel language to focus on relatively short duration of problem.

2. Assess individual, systemic, and broader cultural dynamics. *Diversity considerations:* Obtain immigration history; carefully assess each member of the family's approach to acculturation, especially as it relates to presenting problems.

   Assessment strategies:

   a. Adapt miracle question: "when you wake up, you know what you need to do to resolve this problem between you, your parents, and your boyfriend."

   b. Identify "what works," exceptions, and systemic dynamics of extended family/cultural systems to identify resources and possibilities for communication.

3. Identify and obtain client agreement on treatment goals. *Diversity note:* Be extremely careful to not inadvertantly support one set of cultural values or another; instead, allow AF (in dialogue with family) to decide which cultural norms she chooses to value in her life and how to do so; instead, help her to thoughtfully exam each set and potential implications in her life. Harm reduction for safety plan for drinking.

   Goal-making intervention:

   a. Based on adapted miracle question, develop goals that will enable her to define a satisfying process for resolving these issues.

4. Identify needed referrals, crisis issues, and other client needs. *Diversity note:* Consult with referring physician

   a. *Crisis assessment intervention(s):* Harm reduction and scaling for safety to manage increase in drinking.

(*continued*)

b. *Referral(s):* Discussed option of psychiatric medications as alternative to alcohol to manage stress; client refused for now but will consider if things get worse; agreed to harm reduction related to drinking.

Initial Phase Client Goal

1. Increase connection with "neutral" friends and family to reduce drinking, isolation, and hopelessness.

   Interventions:

   a. Use harm reduction model to identify ways AF is willing to reduce harmful effects of drinking.

   b. Use exceptions and scaling to help AF identify small steps and more effective strategies to cope by connecting with neutral friends and family to reduce sense of isolation and hopelessness.

Working Phase of Treatment

Working Phase Counseling Tasks

1. Monitor quality of the working alliance. *Diversity considerations:* Follow up with Outcome Rating Scale with discussion to ensure interpreted in culturally sensitive way.

   a. *Assessment Intervention:* Outcome Rating Scale.

2. Monitor progress toward goals. *Diversity considerations:* Follow up with discussion to ensure interpreted correctly for culture and gender.

   a. *Assessment Intervention:* Session Rating Scale; checking in verbally; watching nonverbal cues.

Working Phase Client Goals

1. Increase client's sense of agency in making a decision and defining bicultural identity to reduce hopelessness.

   Interventions:

   a. Define problem in solution-oriented terms: The problem is that you are in a position to choose and define how you will integrate your Iranian heritage with American culture, especially as it relates to future relationships and family life.

   b. Use formula first session task, echoing key words, and beginner's mind to help client articulate values, hopes, and dreams to help client identify what matters most to her.

2. Increase authentic connection with family and cultural traditions to reduce isolation.

   Interventions:

   a. Scaling questions to identify small steps of feeling authentically and meaningfully connected to family and community, connections that are not based solely on duty.

   b. Videotalk to identify the positive and negative effects of various family and community relationships on her sense of self.

(*continued*)

3. Increase direct, open communication with boyfriend to reduce isolation and passive-aggressive communication patterns.

   Interventions:

   a. Scaling questions to identify small steps toward more open, proactive communication, which may include couple sessions.

   b. Videotalk to identify how various communication efforts (positive and negative) affect her sense of identitiy and intimacy.

Closing Phase of Treatment

Closing Phase Counseling Task

1. Develop aftercare plan and maintain gains. *Diversity considerations:* Include connections in Iranian and Muslim community as desired by client.

   Intervention:

   a. Adapt miracle question to help identify how she will handle future problems, addressing family and community dynamics and resources; ensure drinking has returned to pre-crisis levels.

Closing Phase Client Goals

1. Increase integrated, bicultural sense of identity to reduce sense of feeling torn between two cultures.

   Interventions:

   a. Miracle quesiton to identify behaviors and activities that characterize how AF wants to define herself as an Iranian American woman.

   b. Scaling questions with specific behavioral tasks for resolving current dilemma regarding boyfriend and family.

2. Increase relationships in which AF is able to appropriate assert needs while respecting those of others to reduce isolation and hopelessness.

   Interventions:

   a. Scaling questions to identify where and how she can appropriately have needs met in relationships, both familial, romantic, and friendship.

   b. Compliments and encouragements to support AF in maintaining relationships that support her.

PROGRESS NOTE FOR CLIENT #13009

Date: May 4, 2013 **Time:** 2:00 ❑ am/☒ pm **Session Length:** ☒ 45 min. ❑ 60 min. ❑ Other: ______ minutes

Present: ❑ Adult Male ☒ Adult Female ❑ Child Male ❑ Child Female ❑ Other: ______

Billing Code: ❑ 90791 (eval) ☒ 90834 (45 min. therapy) ❑ 90837 (60 min. therapy) ❑ 90847 (family)

❑ Other: ______

Symptom(s)	Duration and Frequency Since Last Visit	Progress
1: Drinking	4 days/2-3 drinks per day	Progressing
2: Hopelessness	Mild; 5-6 days	Progressing
3: Conflict	Significantly reduced with parents; tension remains	Maintained

Explanatory Notes on Symptoms: AF reports adhering to harm reduction drinking agreement; denies drinking and driving; reports generally more hopeful and less depressed; reports not arguing with parents, able to have dinner with them again, hiding more information regarding AM from them to reduce tension.

In-Session Interventions and Assigned Homework

Follow-up on prior week's homework; AF reported on how she had conversation with AM about his vision of marriage and career; used scaling questions to identify tasks for next week: have conversation with aunt and spend time with sister. Went over drinking pattern and AF asserted that she felt comfortable with current usage.

Client Response/Feedback

AF finds small tasks helpful in thinking through "big" question of what to do; wants to keep connected to better understand family members.

Plan

☒ Continue with treatment plan: plan for next session: ______

❑ Modify plan: ______

Next session: Date: May 11, 2015 Time: 2:00 ❑ am/☒ pm

Crisis Issues: ☒ No indication of crisis/client denies ❑ Crisis assessed/addressed: describe below

Reports adhering to harm reduction plan; not drinking and driving.

______, ______ ______

Clinician's Signature License/Intern Status Date

Case Consultation/Supervision ❑ Not Applicable

Notes: Supervisor reviewed substance use and encouraged getting third-party reports of progress, too; recommend giving AF permission to take time in exploring issue.

(continued)

Collateral Contact ❑ Not Applicable

Name: Dr. Ahmid Date of Contact: May 4, 2013 Time: 1:15 ❑ am/☒pm

☒ Written release on file: ☒ Sent/❑ Received ❑ In court docs ❑ Other: ______

Notes: Consulted with MD on harm reduction plan; MD okay with plan; willing to prescribe antidepressant if client wants them.

______, ______ ______

Clinician's Signature License/Intern Status Date

______, ______ ______

Supervisor's Signature License Date

Digital Download Download from CengageBrain.com

CHAPTER

14

Postmodern and Feminist Counseling Approaches

Lay of the Land

The newest kids on the block, postmodern and feminist counseling approaches are grounded in social constructionist theories that examine how societal discourses (e.g., "talk of the town," media images, movie plots, and so on) about gender, culture, race, religion, and economic status affect a person's sense of personhood and the development of problems. Much like systemic approaches, these theories place an emphasis on interpersonal relationships and how they shape a person's understanding and experience of self. In fact, they radically posit that one's sense of self is constructed in and through relationships rather than being independently thought up in one's head. These approaches can be broadly divided into three streams of practice:

- **Narrative Counseling:** Based on the work of Australia- and New Zealand-based practitioners Michael White and David Epston (1990), narrative counselors help separate people from their problems by exploring the sociocultural influences and language habits that maintain problems.
- **Feminist and Multicultural Approaches:** Evolved from the work of numerous feminist thinkers and practitioners, including Carol Gilligan (1982/1993), Jean Baker Miller (1976/1986), and Judith Jordan (2010; Jordan, Kaplan, Miller, Stiver & Surrey, 1991), feminist approaches have been expanded over the years to include working with various forms of diversity.
- **Collaborative Approaches:** Developed by Harlene Anderson and Harry Goolishian (1988, 1992) in Texas and Tom Andersen in Norway (1991), collaborative approaches focus on facilitating dialogical conversations that "dissolve" problems with conversations and relationships that allow for the co-creation of new meaning related to problems. This approach is covered in an online module available from cengagebrain.com as part of this text.

Digital Download Download from CengageBrain.com

Similar to solution-based counselors (Chapter 13), postmodernists optimistically focus on client strengths and abilities. Despite many philosophical similarities (Gergen, 1999), these approaches differ in significant ways, most notably their philosophical foundations, the stance of the counselor, the role of interventions, and the emphasis on political issues.

	Feminist	Narrative	Collaborative
Primary Philosophical Foundations	Feminist, multicultural, and sexual orientation theories; social constructionism	Foucault's philosophical writings; critical theory; social constructionism	Postmodernism, social constructionism; hermeneutics (the study of interpretation)
Counseling Relationship	Mutuality; egalitarian; growth-fostering relationships	Active role as "coeditor" or "coauthor"	Facilitative role; democratic; "client is the expert"
Counseling Process	Focuses on identifying societal oppression	Uses structured interventions; focus on various forms of oppression.	Avoid formal interventions; counselor focuses on facilitating dialogical process
Politics and Social Justice	Social justice issues regularly included in counseling conversations and techniques	Social justice issues regularly included in counseling conversations	Political issues raised tentatively for client consideration

Narrative Approaches

In a Nutshell: The Least You Need to Know

Developed by Michael White and David Epston in Australia and New Zealand, narrative counseling is based on the premise that we "story" and create meaning of life events using available *dominant discourses*—broad societal stories, sociocultural practices, assumptions, expectations about how we should live. People experience "problems" when their personal life does not fit with these dominant societal discourses and expectations. The process of narrative counseling involves *separating the person from their problem* by critically examining the assumptions that inform how the person evaluates him or herself and his/her life. Through this process, clients identify alternative ways to view, act, and interact in daily life. Narrative counselors assume all people are resourceful and have strengths, and they do not see "people" as having problems but rather seeing people as being imposed upon by unhelpful or harmful societal cultural practices.

The Juice: Significant Contributions to the Field

If you remember one thing from this chapter, it should be ...

Understanding Oppression: Dominant versus Local Discourses

Like feminist approaches, narrative counseling is one of the few theories that integrates societal and cultural issues into its core conceptualization of how problems form and are resolved. Narrative counselors maintain that problems do not exist separate from their sociocultural contexts, which are broadly constituted in what philosopher Michel Foucault referred to as *dominant discourses* (Foucault, 1972, 1979, 1980; White & Epston, 1990). *Dominant discourses* are culturally generated stories about how life should go that are used to coordinate social behavior, such as how married people should act, what happiness looks like, and how to be successful. These dominant discourses organize social groups at all levels: large cultural groups down to individual couple and family stories about how life should go. These discourses are described as *dominant* because they are foundational to how each of us behaves and evaluates our lives and yet we are rarely conscious of their impact or origins.

Foucault contrasts *dominant discourses* with *local discourses*, which occur in our heads, our closer relationships, and marginalized (not mainstream) communities. Local discourses have different "goods" and "shoulds" than dominant discourses. A classic example is women's valuing of relationship compared to men's valuing of outcome in typical work environments (see Feminist Theories). Both discourses have a value they are working toward; however, men's is generally privileged over women's, thus it is considered a dominant discourse and women's is local. Narrative counselors closely attend to the fluid interactions of local and dominant discourses and how these different stories of what is "good" and valued collide in our web of social relationships, creating problems and difficulties. By attending to this level of social interaction, narrative counselors help clients become aware of how these different discourses are impacting their lives; this awareness serves to increase clients' sense of agency in their struggles, allowing them to find ways to more successfully resolve their issues.

Big Picture: Overview of Counseling Process

The process of narrative counseling involves helping clients find new ways to view, interact with, and respond to problems in their lives by redefining the role of problems in their lives (White, 2007). From a narrative perspective, "persons are not the problem; problems are the problem." Although there is variety among practitioners, narrative counseling broadly involves the following phases (Freedman & Combs, 1996; White & Epson, 1990):

- *Meeting the Person:* Getting to know people separate from their problems by learning about hobbies, values, and everyday aspects of their lives.
- *Listening:* Listening for the effects of dominant discourses and identifying times without the problems.
- *Separating Persons from Problems:* Externalizing and separating people from their problems to create space for new identities and life stories to emerge.
- *Enacting Preferred Narratives:* Identifying new ways to relate to problems that reduce their negative effects on the lives of all involved and to "thicken" their identity and problem stories (see Thickening Descriptions).
- *Solidifying:* Strengthening preferred stories and identities by having them witnessed by significant others in a person's life.

Thickening Descriptions

Narrative counseling process is a *thickening* and enriching of the person's identity and life accounts rather than a "story-ectomy," the replacing of a problem story with a problem-free one. Instead, narrative counselors *add* new strands of identity to the problem-saturated descriptions with which clients enter counseling. In a given day, there are an infinite number of events that can be storied into our accounts of the day and who we are. When people begin to experience problems, they tend to notice *only* those events that fit with the problem narrative. For example, if a person is feeling hopeless, they tend to notice when things do not go their way during the day and do not give much weight to the good things that happened. Similarly, when couples start a period of fighting, they start to notice only what the other person is doing that confirms their position in the fight and ignore and/or forget other events. In narrative counseling, the counselor helps clients create more *balanced* descriptions of the events of their lives to enable clients to build more accurate and appreciative descriptions of themselves and others, which helps clients build successful and enjoyable lives.

Making Connection: Counseling Relationship

Meeting the Person Apart from the Problem

Narrative counselors generally begin their first session with clients by *meeting the person apart from the problem*: meeting clients as everyday people before learning about the problem (Freedman & Combs, 1996). When meeting a client apart from the problem, narrative counselors ask questions such as the following to familiarize themselves with clients' everyday lives:

Questions for Meeting the Person Apart from the Problem

- What do you do for fun? Do you have hobbies?
- What do you like about living here? What don't you like?
- Tell me about your friends and family.
- What is important to you in life?
- What is a typical weekday like? Weekend?

The answers to these questions enable narrative counselors to know and view their clients much in the same way that clients view themselves, as an everyday person. This brief and seemingly mundane intervention can have profound effects in terms of developing an effective counseling relationship and informing meaningful interventions. In the case study at the end of the chapter, the counselor makes a concerted effort to meet Jose apart from his problems of substance use and attention deficit hyperactivity disorder (ADHD), both of which have strong, negative social stereotypes, thus helping Jose to feel accepted and valued as a person from the beginning of their relationship.

Separating People from Problems: The Problem Is the Problem

In narrative counseling, the motto is: "The problem is the problem. The person is not the problem" (Winslade & Monk, 1999, p. 2). Once counselors have come to know the client apart from the problem and have a clear sense of who the client is as a person, they begin to "meet" the problem in much the same way, keeping their identities separate. The problem—whether depression, anxiety, marital conflict, ADHD, defiance, loneliness, or a breakup—is viewed as a separate entity or situation that is *not* inherent to the person of the client. The attitude is again one of a polite, social "getting to know you" feel.

Questions for "Meeting" the Problem

- When did the problem first enter your life?
- What was going on with you then?
- What were your first impressions of the problem? How have they changed?
- How has your relationship with the problem evolved over time?
- Who else has been affected by the problem?

Narrative counselors can take an adversarial stance (wanting to outwit, outsmart, or evict the problem; White, 2007) or a more compassionate stance (wanting to understand its message and concerns; Gehart & McCollum, 2007) toward the problem.

Optimism and Hope

Because narrative counselors view problems as problems and people as people, they have a deep, abiding optimism and hope for their clients (Monk et al., 1997; Winslade & Monk, 1999). Their hope and optimism are not a sugarcoated, naïve wish but instead are derived from their understanding of how problems are formed—through language, relationship, and social discourse—having confidence that their approach can make a difference. Furthermore, by separating people from their problems, they quickly connect with the "best" in the client, which reinforces a sense of hope and optimism.

Coauthor/Coeditor

The role of the counselor is often described as a *coauthor* or *coeditor*, emphasizing that the counselor and client engage in a joint process of constructing meaning (Freedman & Combs, 1996; Monk et al., 1997; White & Epston, 1990). Rather than attempting to offer a "better story," the counselor works alongside the client to generate a more useful narrative. The degree and quality of input on the part of the counselor varies greatly among narrative counselors, and there is a tendency to focus on the sociopolitical aspects of a client's life. In fact, some narrative counselors maintain that counselors should take a stance on broader sociocultural issues of injustice with all clients (Zimmerman & Dickerson, 1996), although this agenda is not shared by all narrative counselors (Monk & Gehart, 2003).

The Viewing: Case Conceptualization

Problem-Saturated Stories

As clients are talking, narrative counselors listen for the *problem-saturated story* (Freedman & Combs, 1996; White & Epston, 1990), the story in which the "problem" plays the leading role and the client plays a secondary role, generally that of victim. The counselor attends to the ways the problem affects the client at an *individual level* (health, emotions, thoughts, beliefs, identity, relationship with the divine) and how it affects them at a *relational level* (significant other, parents, friends, coworkers, teachers, and others) as well as how it affects each of these significant others at a personal level. While listening to a client's problem-saturated story, the counselor listens closely for alternative endings and subplots in which the problem is less of a problem and the person is an effective agent in the story; these are referred to as *unique outcomes*.

Unique Outcomes and Sparkling Events

Unique outcomes (White & Epston, 1990) or *sparkling events* (Freedman & Combs, 1996) refer to stories or subplots in which the problem-saturated story does not play out in its typical way: the child cheerfully complies with a parent's request; a couple is able to stop a potential argument from erupting with a soft touch; a teenager decides to call a friend rather than allow herself to cut. These stories often go unnoticed because they have no dramatic ending or particularly notable outcome that warrants attention, and therefore they are not "storied" in clients' or others' minds. These unique outcomes are used to help clients create the lives they prefer and to develop a more full and accurate account of their and others' identities.

Dominant Cultural and Gender Discourses (also see "The Juice" above)

Narrative counselors listen for dominant cultural and gender themes that have informed the development and perception of a problem (Monk et al., 1997; White & Epston, 1990). The purpose of all discourses is to identify the set of "goods" and "values" that organize social interaction in a particular culture. All cultures are essentially a set of dominant discourses—social rules and values that make it possible for a group of people to meaningfully interact.

Dominant discourses are the societal stories of how life "should" go: for example, to be a "happy" and "good" person, you should get married, get a stable, high-paying job, have kids, get a nice car, buy a house, volunteer at your child's school, and build a white-picket fence. Whether you comply with this vision of happiness, rebel against it, or simply are not even in the game due to social or physical limitations that prevent it, problems can arise in relation to it. In working with clients, narrative counselors listen closely for the dominant discourses that are most directly informing the perception of a problem. In response, they inquire about *local* or *alternative discourses*.

Local and Alternative Discourses: Attending to Client Language and Meaning

Local and *alternative discourses* are those that do not conform to the dominant discourse (White & Epston, 1990): couples who choose not to have children; same-sex relationships; immigrant families wanting to preserve their roots; speaking English as a second language; teen subculture in any society, among others. The local discourses offer a different set of "goods," "shoulds," and ethical "values" from what is portrayed in the dominant discourse. If we take the case of teens and adults in the same culture, the teens have created a subculture with a different set of "goods," beauty standards, sexual norms, vocabulary, friendship rules, and so on. The teen culture represents an alternative discourse that counselors can tap into to understand the teen's worldview and values, and explore with the teen how this alternative discourse can successfully coexist with the dominant discourse. Thus, the local discourse provides a resource for generating new ways of viewing the self and talking and interacting with others around the problem.

Targeting Change: Goal Setting

Preferred Realities and Identities

As a postmodern approach, narrative counseling does not include a set of predefined goals that can be used with all clients. Instead, goal setting in narrative counseling is unique to each client. In the broadest sense, the goal of narrative counseling is to help clients enact their *preferred realities and identities* (Freedman & Combs, 1996). In most cases, enacting preferred narratives involves increasing clients' sense of *agency*, the sense that they have influence in the direction of their lives. When identifying preferred realities, counselors work with clients to develop thoughtfully reflected goals that consider local knowledges, rather than simply adopting the values of the dominant culture. During the process of counseling, clients often redefine their preferred reality to incorporate local knowledges and thus lessen the influence of dominant discourses. For example, many gay men find that they prefer the gay subculture in one city to another, highlighting that even within local cultures there can be multiple variations of local knowledge that a person can choose to connect with. Thus, the key is defining the "preferred" reality and identity thoughtfully and with intention, after considering the impact of dominant and local discourses. This process is often a gradual shift from "make this problem go away" to "I want to create something beautiful/meaningful/great with my/our life(ves)."

Examples of Middle Phase: Targeting Immediate Symptoms and Presenting Problem

- Reduce frequency of allowing Depression to talk client into avoiding pleasurable activities.
- Increase opportunities to interact with friends using "confident, social" self.
- Increase instances of defiance in response to Anorexia's directions to not eat.

Examples of Late Phase: Targeting Personal Identity, Relational Identity, and Expanded Community

- *Personal Identity:* Solidify a sense of personal identity that derives self-worth from meaningful activities, relationships, and values other than body size.
- *Relational Identity:* Develop a family identity narrative that allows for greater expression of differences while maintaining the family's sense of closeness and loyalty.
- *Expanded Community:* Expand preferred "outgoing" identity to social relationships and contexts.

The Doing: Interventions

Externalizing: Separating the Problem from the Person

The signature technique of narrative counseling, *externalizing* involves conceptually and linguistically separating the person from the problem (Freedman & Combs, 1996; White & Epston, 1990). To be successful, externalization requires a sincere belief that people are separate from their problems; thus, the *attitude* of externalization is key to its effectiveness (Freedman & Combs, 1996). More than a single-session intervention, externalization is an organic and evolving process—a process of shifting the client's perception of their relationship to the problem—from "having" it, to seeing it outside the self. Counselors can externalize by naming the problem as an external other, switching a descriptive adjective into a noun: for example, from a client being depressed to having a relationship with Depression. Other times, clients respond better talking about "sides" of themselves or a relationship, for example, "the little girl in me who is afraid" or "the competitive side of our relationship."

For externalization to work, it cannot be forced onto the client, but rather it needs to emerge from the dialogue or be introduced as a possibility for how to think about the situation. In most cases, using techniques such as *mapping the influence of the problem and persons* (see below), invites a natural, comfortable process for externalizing the problem. Periodically, clients already have a name for the problem and conceptualize the problem as a sort of external entity or very discrete part of themselves, and in such cases counselors need only to build upon the externalization process the client has started.

Relative Influence Questioning: Mapping the Influence of the Problem and Persons

Relative influence questioning was the first detailed method for externalization (White & Epston, 1990). Used early in counseling, relative influence questioning serves as an assessment and intervention simultaneously and is composed of two parts: (a) mapping the influence of the problem, and (b) mapping the influence of persons.

Mapping the Influence of Problems When mapping the influence of problems, counselors inquire about the ways the problem has affected the life of the client and significant others in the client's life, often *expanding* the reach of the problem beyond how the client generally thinks of it; thus, it is critical that this is followed up by *mapping the influence of person* questions to ensure that the client does not feel worse afterwards. Mapping the influence of problems involves asking about how the problem has affected:

Questions for Mapping the Influence of the Problem

How did the problem affect:

- The client at a physical, emotional, and psychological level?
- The client's identity story and what they tell themselves about their worth and who they are?
- The client's closest relationships: partner, children, parents?
- Other relationships in the client's life: friendships, social groups, work/school colleagues, and others?
- The health, identity, emotions, and other relationships of significant people in the client's life (e.g., how parents may pull away from friends because they are embarrassed about a child's problem)?

Mapping the Influence of Persons Mapping the influence of persons begins the externalization process more explicitly. This phase of questioning, which should immediately follow *mapping the influence of problems*, involves identifying how the person has affected the life of the problem, reversing the logic of the first series of questions:

Questions for Mapping the Influence of Persons

- When have the persons involved kept the problem from affecting their mood or how they value themselves as people?
- When have the persons involved kept the problem from allowing them to enjoy special and/or casual relationships in their lives?
- When have the persons involved kept the problem from interrupting their work or school lives?

(*continued*)

- When have the persons involved been able to keep the problem from taking over when it was starting?

Try It Yourself

Find a partner, ask your partner to identify a problem, and map the influence of the problem in the person's life. Then map the influence of persons. Notice how you both feel afterwards.

Externalizing Conversations: The Statement of Position Map

White (2007) describes his more recently developed process for facilitating externalizing conversations, *the statement of position map*. This map includes four categories of inquiry, which are used multiple times throughout a session and across sessions to shift the client's relationship with the problem and open new possibilities for action:

Inquiry Category 1: Negotiating a particular, experience-near definition of the problem White begins by defining the problem using the client's language (experience-near) rather than professional or global terms (e.g., a diagnosis). Thus, "feeling blue" is preferred to "depressed."

Inquiry Category 2: Mapping the effects of the problem Similar to his early work (White and Epston, 1990), mapping the effects of problems involves identifying how the problem has affected the various domains of the client's life: home, work, school, and social contexts; relationships with family, friends, and oneself; one's identity and future possibilities.

Inquiry Category 3: Evaluating the effects of the problem's activities After identifying the effects of the problem, the counselors asks the client to evaluate these effects (White, 2007, p. 44):

- Are these activities okay with you?
- How do you feel about these developments?
- Where do you stand on these outcomes?
- Is the development positive or negative—or both, or neither, or something in between?

Inquiry Category 4: Justifying the evaluation In the final phase, the counselor asks about how and why clients have evaluated the situation the way they did (White, 2007, p. 48):

- Why is/isn't this okay for you?
- Why do you feel this way about this development?
- Why are you taking this stand/position on this development?

These "why" questions must be offered in a spirit of allowing clients to give voice to what is important to them, rather than creating a sense of moral judgment. These questions should open up conversations about what is important to clients, what motivates them, and how they want to shape their identities and futures.

Metaphors When externalizing using the four above categories, White (2007, p. 32) employs various metaphors for relating to problems:

- Walking out on the problem
- Going on strike against the problem
- Defying the problem's requirements
- Disempowering the problem
- Educating the problem
- Escaping the problem
- Recovering or reclaiming territory from the problem
- Refusing invitations from the problem
- Disproving the problem's claims
- Resigning from the problem's service
- Stealing their lives from the problem
- Taming the problem
- Harnessing the problem
- Undermining the problem

Avoid Totalizing and Dualistic Thinking White (2007) avoids totalizing descriptions of the problem—the problem being all-bad—because such descriptions promote dualistic, either/or thinking, which can be invalidating to the client and/or obscure the problem's broader context. In the case study at the end of the chapter, the counselor uses statement of position maps to enable Jose to clearly define a healthy and desired relationship to drugs and alcohol, rather than directly confronting him on these issues.

Externalizing Questions

Narrative counselors use *externalizing questions* to help clients build different relationships with their problems (Freedman & Combs, 1996). In most cases, externalizing questions involve changing *adjectives* (e.g, depressed, anxious, angry, etc.) to *nouns* (e.g, Depression, Anxiety, Anger, etc.; capitalization is used to emphasize that the problem is viewed as a separate entity). Externalizing questions *presume* that the person is separate from the problem and that the person has a two-way relationship with the problem: it affects them, and they affect it.

To experience the liberating effects of externalizing, Freedman and Combs (1996, pp. 49–50) have developed the following two sets of questions: one representing conventional counseling questions and the other externalizing. To do this exercise, choose a quality or trait that you or others find problematic, usually an adjective; substitute this for X in the questions below. Then find a noun form of that trait; substitute this for Y in the questions below. Examples include: X = depressed/Y = Depression; X = critical/Y = Criticism; X = angry/Y = Anger.

Conventional Questions (Insert problem description as adjective for X)	Externalizing Questions (Insert problem as noun for Y)
When did you first become X?	What made you vulnerable to the Y so that it was able to dominate your life?
What are you most X about?	In what contexts is the Y most likely to take over?
What kinds of things happen that typically lead to your being X?	What kinds of things happen that typically lead to the Y taking over?
When you are X, what do you do that you wouldn't do if you weren't X?	What has the Y gotten you to do that is against your better judgment?
What are the consequences for your life and relationships of being X?	What effects does the Y have on your life and relationships?
How is your self-image different when you are X?	How has the Y led you into the difficulties you are now experiencing?
If by some miracle you woke up some morning and were not X anymore, how, specifically, would your life be different?	Does the Y blind you from noticing your resources, or can you see them through it?
	Have there been times when you have been able to get the best of the Y? Times when the Y could have taken over but you kept it out of the picture?

Try It Yourself

First answer the list of convention questions, then go back and answer the list of externalizing questions. Notice how your feel after each set.

Problem Deconstruction: Deconstructive Listening and Questions

Based on the philosophical work of Jacques Derrida, narrative counselors use deconstructive listening and questions to help clients trace the effects of dominant discourses and to empower clients to make more conscious choices about which discourses they allow to affect their life (Freedman & Combs, 1996). *Deconstructive listening* involves the counselor listening for "gaps" in clients' understanding and asking them to fill in the details or have them explain the ambiguities in their stories. For example, if a client reports feeling rejected because friends did not call when they said they would, the counselor would listen for the meanings that led to the sense of feeling "rejected."

Deconstructive questions help clients to further "unpack" their stories to see how they have been constructed, identifying the influence of dominant and local discourses. Typically used in externalizing conversations, these questions target problematic beliefs, practices, feelings, and attitudes by asking clients to identify:

- The *history of their relationship* with the problematic belief, practice, feeling, or attitude ("When and where did you first encounter the problem?")
- *The contextual influences* on the problematic belief, practice, feeling, or attitude ("When is it most likely to be present?")
- *The effects or results* of the problematic belief, practice, feeling, or attitude ("What effects has this had on you and your relationships?")
- *The interrelationship with other* beliefs, practices, feelings, or attitudes ("Are there other problems that feed this problem?")
- *Tactics and strategies* used by the problem belief, practice, feeling, or attitude ("How does it go about influencing you?")

Mapping in Landscapes of Action and Identity/Consciousness

Based on the narrative theory of Jerome Bruner (1986), *mapping the problem in the landscape of action and identity* (White, 2007) or *consciousness* (Freedman & Combs, 1996) refers to a specific technique for harnessing unique outcomes to promote desired change. Mapping in the landscapes of action and identity generally involves the following steps:

1. *Identify a Unique Outcome:* Listen for and ask about times when the problem could have been a problem but it was not.
2. *Ensure the Unique Outcome is Preferred:* Rather than assume, ask clients about whether the unique outcome is a preferred outcome: Is this something you want to do or have happen more often?
3. *Mapping in the Landscape of Action:* First, the counselor begins by mapping the unique outcome in the landscape of action, identifying what actions were taken by whom in which order. The counselor does this by asking specific details: What did you do first? How did the other person respond? What did you do next? The counselor carefully plots the events until there is a step-by-step picture of the actions of the client and involved others, gathering details about:
    - Critical events
    - Circumstances surrounding events
    - Sequence of events
    - Timing of events
    - Overall plot
4. *Mapping in the Landscape of Identity/Consciousness:* After obtaining a clear picture of what happened during the unique outcome, the counselor begins a process of mapping in the landscape of identity. This phase of mapping *thickens the plot* associated with the successful outcome, thus directly strengthening the connection of the preferred outcome with the client's personal identity. Mapping in the landscape of identity focuses on the psychological and relational implications of the unique outcomes. Areas of impact include:
    - What do you believe this says about you as a person? About your relationship?
    - What were your intentions behind these actions?
    - What do you value most about your actions here?

- What, if anything, did you learn or realize from this?
- Does this change how you see life/God/your purpose/your life goals?
- Does this affect how you see the problem?

Scaffolding Conversations

White (2007) uses *scaffolding conversations* to move clients from that which is familiar to that which is novel, using developmental psychologist Vygotsky's concept of *zones of proximal development.* Vygotsky emphasized that learning is inherently relational, requiring adults to structure the child's learning in ways that make it possible for them to interact with new information. The *zone of proximal development* is the distance between what the child can do independently and what the child can do in collaboration with others. *Scaffolding* is a term White developed to describe five incremental and progress movements across this zone of learning with clients.

- *Low-level distancing tasks: Characterizing a unique outcome:* Tasks that are at a low-level distance and very close to what is familiar to the client, encouraging the attribution of meanings to events that have gone unnoticed.
- *Medium-level distancing tasks: Unique outcomes taken into a chain of association:* Tasks that introduce greater "newness," encouraging greater comparison and categorization of difference and similarity.
- *Medium-high-level distancing tasks: Reflection on chain of associations:* Tasks that encourage clients to reflect on, evaluate, and learn from the differences and similarities.
- *High-level distancing tasks: Abstract learning and realizations:* Tasks that require clients to assume a high level of distance from their immediate experience, promoting increased abstract conceptualization of life and identity.
- *Very high-level distancing tasks*: *Plans for action:* Tasks that promote a high-level distancing from immediate experience to enable clients to identify ways of enacting their newly developed concepts about life and identity.

Over the course of a conversation, counselors move back and forth between various levels of distancing tasks, progressively moving to higher levels of action planning. In the case study at the end of the chapter, scaffolding questions are used to gently move Jose from noticing one exception of avoiding substances to developing concrete and motivating action plans for managing his substance use.

Permission Questions

Narrative counselors use permission questions to emphasize the democratic nature of the counseling relationship and to encourage clients to maintain a strong and clear sense of agency when talking with the counselor. Quite simply, permission questions are questions counselors use to ask permission to ask a question. This goes against the prevailing assumptions that counselors can ask any question they want to gather information they purportedly need to be helpful to the client. Socially, counselors are exempt from the prevailing social norms of polite conversation topics and are free to bring up taboo subjects such as sex, past abuse, relationship problems, death, fears, and weaknesses. Many clients feel compelled to answer these questions even if they are not comfortable doing so. Narrative counselors are sensitive to the power dynamic related to taboo and difficult subjects and therefore *ask for the client's permission* before asking questions that are generally taboo or that the counselor anticipates will make this particular client feel uncomfortable. For example, "Would it be okay if I ask you some questions about your sex life?"

In addition, permission questions are used throughout the interview related to *what* is being discussed and *how* to ensure that the conversation is meaningful and comfortable for the client. For example, often when starting a session the counselor may briefly outline his ideas for how to use the time, asking for client input and permission to continue with a particular topic or line of questioning. Similarly, in a situation such as a family session, where the counselor finds herself asking one person more questions than the others, she would pause to ask permission to continue to ensure everyone was okay with what was going on.

Situating Comments

Similar to permission questions, *situating comments* are used to maintain a more democratic counseling relationship and reinforce client agency by ensuring that comments from the counselor are not taken as a "higher" or "more valid" truth than the client's (Zimmerman & Dickerson, 1996). Drawing on the distinction between dominant and local discourses, narrative counselors are keenly aware that any comment made by the counselor is often considered more "valid" than anything the client might say. Thus, counselors *situate* their comments by revealing the source of the perspective they are offering, emphasizing that it is only one perspective among others. By revealing the source and context of a comment, a client is less likely to overprivilege counselor comments.

Counselor Comment Without Situating	Situating Counselor Comment
I am noticing that you tend to....	Having grown up on a farm, my attention is of course drawn to....
Research indicates that....	There is one counselor who has developed a theory/done a study that suggests.... Does this sound like something that would be true for you?
I suggest that you....	Since you are asking me for a suggestion, I can only tell you what I think as someone who believes action is more productive than talk....

Leagues

As a means of solidifying the new narrative and identities, narrative counselors have created *leagues* (or clubs, associations, teams, and such), membership to which signifies an accomplishment in a particular area. In most cases, leagues are virtual communities of concern (e.g., giving a child a membership certificate to the Temper Tamer's Club), although some meet face to face or interact via the Internet (Anti-Anorexia/Anti-Bulimia League; see www.narrativetherapy.com).

Letters and Certificates

Narrative letters are used to develop and solidify preferred narratives and identities (White & Epston, 1990). Counselors can write *letters* after sessions detailing a client's emerging story, in lieu of doing case notes (unless you work in a practice environment that requires a specific format). Narrative letters use the same techniques that are used in session to reinforce the emerging narrative and are characterized by the following:

- **Emphasizing Client Agency:** Highlighting client agency in their lives, including small steps in becoming proactive.
- **Taking Observer Position:** The counselor clearly takes the role of *observing* the changes the client is making, citing specific, concrete examples whenever possible.
- **Highlighting Temporality:** The time dimension is used to plot the emerging story: where clients began, where they are now, where they are likely to go.
- **Encouraging Polysemy:** Rather than proposing singular interpretations, multiple meanings are entertained and encouraged.

Letters can be used early in counseling to engage clients, during counseling to reinforce the emerging narrative and reinforce new preferred behaviors, or at the end of counseling to consolidate gains by narrating the change process.

Sample Letter White and Epston (1990) offer numerous sample letters, such as the following:

Dear Rick and Harriet,

I'm sure that you are familiar with the fact that the best ideas have the habit of presenting themselves after the event. So it will come as no surprise to you that I often think of the most important questions after the end of an interview.... Anyway, I thought I would share a couple of important questions that came to me after you left our last meeting: Rick, how did you decline Helen's [the daughter] invitation to you to do the reasoning for her? And how do you think this could have the effect of inviting her to reason with herself? Do you think this could help her to become more responsible? Harriet, how did you decline Helen's invitations to you to be dependable for her? And how do you think this could have the effect of inviting her to depend upon herself more? Do you think that this could have the effect of helping her to take better care of her life? What does this increased vulnerability to Helen's invitations to have life for her reflect in you both as people? By the way, what ideas occurred to you after our last meeting? M.W. (pp. 109–110).

Certificates

Certificates are used often with children to recognize the changes they have made and to reinforce their new "reputation" as a "temper tamer," "cooperative child," or such.

Certified Temper Tamer

This is to certify that

____

has proven himself as a skilled Tamer of Tempers,

having gone two months without temper problems at home or school

using the following taming techniques that he developed for himself:

1. Asking for help when confused
2. Taking three deep breathes when the scent of Temper appears
3. Using soft words to talk about anger and frustration

Date of award: ________________________

Witnessed by: ________________________(counselor)

________________________(parents)

________________________(teacher)

Putting It All Together: Narrative Treatment Plan Case Conceptualization and Treatment Plan Templates

Theory-Specific Case Conceptualization: Narrative

The prompts below can be used to develop a *theory-specific case conceptualization* using Adlerian theory. The cross-theoretical case conceptualizations at the end of each theory chapter provide examples for writing a conceptualization that includes key elements of this theory-specific conceptualization. Comprehensive examples of theory-specific case conceptualizations are available in *Theory and Treatment Planning in Counseling and Psychotherapy* (Gehart, 2015).

- *Meeting Person Apart from the Problem:* Describe who the persons/people are apart from the problem: hobbies, interests, career, and such.
- *Problem-Saturated Narrative:* Describe how the problem is affecting the persons involved at all levels:
  - Personal level: emotional, behavioral, identity narrative, and so on
  - Relational level: conflicts or distance in significant relationships
  - Broader life circumstances: work, school, hobbies, and so on
- *Unique Outcomes/Sparkling Events:* Describe:
  - Times, contexts, relationships, and so on, when the problem is less of a problem or not a problem.
  - The effect of persons on the problem: what things do people do that make the problem less of a problem?
- *Dominant Discourses*
  - *Cultural, ethnic, SES, religious, and such*: How do key cultural discourses inform what is perceived as a problem and the possible solutions?
  - *Gender, sexual orientation, and such:* How do the gender/sexual discourses inform what is perceived as a problem and the possible solutions?
  - *Contextual, family, community, school, and other social discourses:* How do other important discourses inform what is perceived as a problem and the possible solutions?
- *Local/Alternative Narratives*
  - Identity/Self Narratives: How has the problem shaped each family member's identity?
- *Local or Preferred Discourses:* What is the client's preferred identity narrative and/or narrative about the problem? Are there local (alternative) discourses about the problem that are preferred?

Treatment Plan Template: Narrative

Use this Treatment Plan Template for developing a plan for clients with depressive, anxious, or compulsive types of presenting problems. Depending on the specific client, presenting problem, and clinical context, the goals and interventions in this template may need to be modified only slightly or significantly; you are encouraged to significantly revise the plan as needed. For the plan to be useful, goals and techniques should be written to target specific beliefs, behaviors, and emotions that the client is experiencing. The more specific, the more useful it will be to you.

Treatment Plan

Initial Phase of Treatment

Initial Phase Counseling Tasks

1. Develop working counseling relationship. *Diversity considerations:* Describe how you will specifically adjust to respect cultured, gendered, and other styles of relationship building and emotional expression.
   Relationship-building approach/intervention:
   a. Meet the **person apart from the problem** to generate **hope**.
2. Assess individual, systemic, and broader cultural dynamics. *Diversity considerations:* *Describe how you will specifically adjust assessment based on cultural, socioeconomic, sexual orientation, gender, and other relevant norms. Consider inviting significant friends and family for assessment session(s).*

(continued)

Assessment strategies:

a. **Relative influence questioning** and **deconstructive questions** to identify effects of problem and effects of persons, noting key **dominant and local discourses**.

b. Identify **unique outcomes and sparkling moments** that do not conform to problem-saturated narrative.

3. Identify and obtain client agreement on treatment goals. *Diversity considerations: Describe how you will specifically modify goals to correspond with values from the client's cultural, religious, and other value systems.*

   Goal-making intervention:

   a. Identify **preferred realities** using **unique outcomes**; **map** these in the **landscapes of action and consciousness** to generate thick descriptions of goals.

4. Identify needed referrals, crisis issues, and other client needs. *Diversity considerations: Describe diversity issues related to specific crisis issues and referral options.*

   Crisis assessment intervention(s): Use **relative influence questioning** to identify the "problem's strategies for creating crisis" as well as the person's strategies for managing it.

   Referral(s): To face-to-face, "**narrative leagues**," and/or online communities that support the person in relating differently to the problem.

Initial Phase Client Goal

1. Increase the client's ability **resist invitations** to engage in [crisis behavior] to reduce [crisis symptom(s)].

   Interventions:

   a. **Relative influence questioning** to identify how client is "enticed" to engage in crisis behavior as well as times when the client resists these invitations.

   b. **Statement of position map** to identify client's desired "position" in relation to crisis behaviors; identify strategies, persons, and contexts that support the desired position.

Working Phase of Treatment

Working Phase Counseling Tasks

1. Monitor quality of the working alliance. *Diversity considerations: Describe how you will specifically adapt expectations for age, gender, cultural, sexual orientation, socioeconomic status, and other norms for relating.*

   a. *Assessment Intervention:* Use **situating comments** and **permission questions** to situate counselor as **coeditor/investigative reporter**; regularly check in with client about alliance; use Session Rating Scale.

2. Monitor progress toward goals. *Diversity considerations: Describe how you will specifically adapt the monitoring of progress for age, ethnicity, educational level, language, etc. Involve client in deciding how best to measure progress.*

   a. *Assessment Intervention:* Regularly ask about frequency of elements of **preferred reality** that are occurring; use Outcome Rating Scale to measure client progress.

Working Phase Client Goals

1. Increase client's sense of **separation from** and **agency in relation to [the problem]** to reduce [specific symptoms: depression, anxiety, etc.].

   Interventions:

   a. **Externalizing questions** to separate client's identity from problem-saturated story.

   b. **Statement of position map** and **relative influence questioning** to externalize problem.

(continued)

2. Increase frequency of [specific behavior] that supports the client's **preferred reality** to reduce [specific symptoms: depression, anxiety, etc.].
   Interventions:
   a. **Mapping in the landscapes of action and consciousness** to identify specific behaviors that support change.
   b. **Scaffolding questions** to help client move toward a new relationship with the problem.
3. Increase frequency of [specific behavior] that supports the client's **preferred reality** to reduce [specific symptoms: depression, anxiety, etc.].
   Interventions:
   a. **Mapping in the landscapes of action and consciousness** to identify specific behaviors that support change.
   b. **Scaffolding questions** to help client move toward a new relationship with the problem.

Closing Phase of Treatment

Closing Phase Counseling Task

1. Develop aftercare plan and maintain gains. *Diversity considerations: Describe specific diversity considerations and unique resources for the ending treatment and sustaining gains posttreatment.*
   Intervention:
   a. Use **mapping in the landscape of action and consciousness** questions to help clients identify how they can resist invitations from the presenting problem and similar problems in the future.

Closing Phase Client Goals

1. Increase and **thicken the plot** around the client's **new sense of identity** and **agency** in relation to the problem to reduce [specific symptoms: depression, anxiety, etc.].
   Interventions:
   a. **Scaffolding questions** to develop action plans to bolster and sustain new identity.
   b. **Landscape of action and consciousness questions** to thicken new narratives that capture the outer and inner experience of client's preferred reality.
2. Increase **involvement of significant persons** in client's life to **witness and support new identity narrative** and new relationship to the problem to reduce [specific symptoms: depression, anxiety, etc.].
   Interventions:
   a. **Invite significant persons, leagues, and/or reflecting teams to session** to witness changes and identify ways to support client.
   b. **Certificates, letters, and other written documents** to solidify new identity and preferred narrative.

Digital Download Download from CengageBrain.com

Feminist and Cultural Theories

In a Nutshell: The Least You Need to Know

Feminist counseling theories focus on how the effects of gender, cultural, heterosexual, and other stereotypes affect an individual's identity and relationships and how these lead to the types of problems for which a person seeks counseling. Informed by cultural theory, feminist approaches are based on the premise that *humans seek, grow through, and move toward connection* with others across the life span (Jordan, 1997, 2010; Jordan et al., 1991). A sense of connection and community is fundamental to an individual's sense of well-being. *Disconnection*, then, is the root cause of most forms of emotional distress, and this becomes the focus of treatment. The counseling process is characterized by egalitarianism, empathy, and mutuality; the relationship is an authentic and human encounter for both client and counselor. Through this relationship, clients learn to engage in *growth-fostering relationships*, relationships that enhance both parties' sense of well-being. The counseling process also involves analyzing the effects of oppression and social power on the client and their impact on the presenting concern. The process of counseling increases clients' awareness of sociopolitical issues in individual lives and empowers clients to make meaningful change in their personal lives, relationships, and larger community.

The Juice: Significant Contributions to the Field

If there is one thing you remember from this chapter, it should be:

Growth-Fostering Relationships, and the Five Good Things

Feminists maintain that humans are primarily *relational*, that they seek, grow through, and move toward connection with others (Jordan, 2010; Jordan et al., 1991). The desire for connection is the primary motivating force, in contrast to more traditional human development models that emphasize individuation. Feminists view the idea of a separate self as a myth that is based on a spatial metaphor of separateness, with psychodynamic theories generally positing that the more separate the self, the better it functions (Jordan, 2010; Jordan et al., 1991). In contrast, feminists use a model of human development that recognizes the inherent interdependence of humans for survival, both physical and psychological (Comstock, 2005). Rather than a stage-based model of human development, feminists describe development as a complex, multifaceted process in which people increase their abilities to be differentiated *within* relationships and increase their capacity for *mutuality*.

However, all relationships are not created equal. The types of relationships that we seek, that are good for us, and that help us to grow are different from others, because they allow us to fully experience and safely explore our sense of self. Relational cultural counselors refer to these as *growth-fostering relationships*, which are characterized by the *five good things* (Jordan, 2010; Miller & Stiver, 1997).

- Increased zest and energy
- Increased sense of self-worth
- Increased knowledge and clarity about one's own experience, the other person, and the relationship
- Increased creativity and productivity
- Increased desire for more connection without feeling helpless or needy

Feminist counselors build growth-fostering relationships with clients to (a) foster personal growth and (b) increase clients' capacity to authentically be in relationship outside of session. When assessing clients, feminist counselors listen carefully for growth-fostering relationships in clients' lives that are characterized by the five good things. Counselors help clients nurture the growth-fostering relationships that they already have, transform other relationships to be growth-fostering, and/or develop new ones.

Big Picture: Overview of Counseling Process

The feminist counseling process evolved around two primary themes: (a) an egalitarian counseling relationship and (b) recognition of sources of oppression. The process of counseling involves the following:

1. *Developing an egalitarian relationship:* The initial goals of the counseling process are to develop (a) a relationship in which clients feel safe and understood and (b) a sense of having a voice in shaping the process.

2. *Exploring Sources of Marginalization and Disconnection:* Next the counselor works with the client to identify sources of relational disconnection and social marginalization that relate to and fuel the presenting problem.
3. *Fostering Authenticity and Empowerment:* Using the counseling relationship as a place to experience empathy and authenticity, counselors empower clients to transfer learning in session to address areas of concern in their everyday life.
4. *Building Better Relationships and Communities:* In the later stages of the counseling process, clients are encouraged to promote social change to reduce forms of oppression for themselves and others as a means of increasing their sense of being part of growth-fostering relationships and communities.

Making Connection: Counseling Relationship

Egalitarian

Since social power is a central focus in feminist counseling, the counselor strives to make the counseling relationship *egalitarian* by closely attending to the inherent power imbalance in the relationship (Brown, 1996, 2010; Enns, 2004). How exactly do they achieve this seeming paradox? Feminist counselors have open discussions about the power dynamics and politics of counseling, such as the diagnosis process, communications with other professionals, and the counseling theories chosen. In these conversations, the counselor *demystifies* the counseling process and invites clients to share their opinions, ask questions, and do their own research, all of which is considered equally alongside the counselor's thoughts and theory (Worell & Remer, 1992). Much like in collaborative therapy, the feminist counseling process is a *mutual exploration* of how best to resolve clients' issues, an exploration in which counselors recognize clients' expertise in their own lives.

In addition, feminist counselors use *self-disclosure* to increase the sense of equality in the relationship and help clients develop hope and courage in their own lives. Counselors' egalitarian self-disclosure also involves admitting when they are wrong, being open to correction, and acknowledging personal defensiveness, rather than assuming that relational disruptions are solely clients' faults. Instead, the counseling relationship is—in good times and bad—a two-way street where the counselor is equally responsible for bumpy roads and misunderstandings.

Mutual Empathy and Growth

A unique feminist concept, *mutual empathy* refers to two-way empathy in which each person—counselor and client—is able to see, know, and feel the inner experience of the other and experience *responsiveness* from the other. Mutual empathy involves *both persons impacting the other*, caring for the other, and responding to the other. This experience of mutuality repairs empathetic failures in early, formative childhood relationships; in addition, recent research indicates that there is active brain resonance between people experiencing empathy and that this alters the functioning of the brain in positive ways (Schore, 1994). The counselor allows clients to see that what they say touches and moves the counselor in a personal and human way. These exchanges help clients feel more connected, reducing their sense of isolation from others and increasing their capacity for relationships that foster growth (see Growth Fostering Relationships in "The Juice" above). In addition, the counselor is authentically and personally touched in the process, enhancing the counselor's growth, too.

Counseling relationships built upon mutuality should not be misunderstood as sappy, saccharin-sweet relationships in which there is no conflict, disagreement, or confrontation. In fact, these relationships demand high levels of honesty and authenticity, which inherently bring differences and conflicts to the surface. However, because of the relational context, these differences can lead to "good conflict," in which each person's unique experiences, beliefs, and feelings are heard and *responded to*, allowing for each member to learn and grow (Jordan, 2010). In good conflict, even though there is a difference, each person fundamentally feels safe and trusts that the relationship is not threatened. Thus, the counselor cannot retreat into a position of power, but instead maintains an egalitarian, human presence and respectfully works through the differences with clients. In fact, moments of conflict and disconnection provide the most fertile opportunities for growth, for it is precisely in these moments when counselors can stay present and responsive and help clients have a *corrective relational experience*, enabling clients to develop new relational patterns (Jordan, 2010). Clients first learn to do this with the counselor and then transfer this to relationships outside the counseling process.

Authenticity

Feminist counselors cultivate *authenticity* in their relationships with clients. Authenticity in the counseling context does not mean that the counselor expresses just *any* old emotion, thought, or reaction that spontaneously arises, but instead implies a genuine *responsiveness* that keeps the well-being and needs of the client in mind. Clinical judgment and ethics always guide the counselors' expressions of authenticity (Jordan, 2010; Jordan et al., 1991). In determining which authentic expressions are appropriate with a given client, feminists ask themselves, "*Will this* [information, action, expression, etc.] *facilitate the client's growth? Will this further healing? Will this strengthen the relationship?*" Errors can occur, and when they do, the counselor needs to be ready to apologize and correct the relational disconnection, remaining responsive and open to hearing the client's response.

Feminist Code of Ethics

Feminists at the Feminist Therapy Institute (2000) have developed a *Feminist Code of Ethics*, which counselors use to guide their work and relationships with clients *in addition to* other professional codes. This ethical code describes a commitment to recognizing the impact of dominant cultural norms, acknowledging power differentials in relationships, managing overlapping relationships to avoid abuse, establishing counselor accountability, and promoting social change:

> ... feminists believe the personal is political. Basic tenets of feminism include a belief in the equal worth of all human beings, a recognition that each individual's personal experiences and situations are reflective of and an influence on society's institutionalized attitudes and values, and a commitment to political and social change that equalizes power among people. Feminists are committed to recognizing and reducing the pervasive influences and insidious effects of oppressive societal attitudes and society. (p. 1)

Men and Feminist Counseling

Can men be feminist counselors? Do feminist counselors work with men? Yes and yes. Although many of the seminal ideas originated in feminist literature, the applications and values behind them are universal. Contemporary feminist approaches, such as relational-cultural therapy, emphasize diversity and relational responsiveness more than simply women's issues. The values that define feminist approaches—ending oppression, equality, and mutuality—have validity for men and women, and have the potential to help both sexes live more authentically and with greater social connection.

Ironically, in the future, feminist approaches may have increased relevance for men. Twenty-first century economic, political, and social changes are rapidly redefining the role of men in society, and men have had—as a group—more difficulty with adapting to these changes than women had in the 20th century as their social roles were redefined (Rosin, 2010). For example, in 2010, for the first time, more American women worked then men. At the same time, 60% of college graduates were female. Many men are struggling to define themselves in a postindustrial economy, where flexibility, relationships, and collaboration matter more than physical strength and size. Additionally, male socialization pushes many men into disconnection from themselves and emotions in boyhood, leaving them searching for ways to connect in adulthood (Shepherd, 2005). In the years ahead, feminist counselors may find they are surprisingly well equipped to help men struggling to find meaning, identity, and connection as their social roles are dramatically and rapidly redefined.

The Viewing: Case Conceptualization

The Personal Is Political; The Political Is Personal

One of the foundational assumptions of feminist counseling is that *the personal is political*, meaning that a person's internal reality—and therefore pathology—is inherently interconnected with political issues from the broader social context (Brown, 2006; Remer, 2008). This is true for men as well as women; heterosexuals as well as those with alternative sexual orientations; and persons of all cultural and ethnic backgrounds. The reverse is also true: the political is also personal (Brown, 2006), meaning that what happens at the societal level affects people in a very personal way. Thus, when developing a case conceptualization, feminist counselors help clients separate internal and external sources of problems by *raising awareness* of oppression, privilege, and societal impact on individual experience. For example, a professional Hispanic mother who is feeling depressed would be encouraged to look at the numerous and contradictory expectations society maintains for the roles of "mother" and "professional," as well as the American stereotypes of Hispanic women and the Hispanic community's expectations of her. Similarly, a working-class, African American father struggling with substance abuse would be encouraged to examine social roles associated with his class, race, and gender in relation to his problems. In the case study at the end of this chapter, the counselor helps Jose examine the political effects of being gay, Mexican American, working-class, and diagnosed with ADHD and substance abuse, and consequently considering multiple, interlocking layers of marginalization.

The Politics of DSM Diagnosis

Like other postmodernists in this chapter, feminists have long challenged the practice of DSM diagnosis as an oppressive practice. Long from over, this critique is more alive than ever:

> I would submit that feminist critiques of the diagnostic process exemplified by the *DSM* remain fresh and will be even more necessary in the future as increasing numbers of people receive one of these labels during the course of their lives. What does it mean that almost half of the U.S. population qualifies for a formal diagnosis, according to recent news reports? Feminist critique demands a complex analysis and synthesis of the emerging data about the biology of various forms of distress, on the one hand calling into question assumptions about the hard-wired, evolutionarily immutable nature of some phenomena, and on the other calling attention to the profound changes made to neuro-anatomy by exposure to traumatic stress. Feminist theory requires that we conceptualize our clients' distress... [using] a range of factors that include the parameters of distress and dysfunction as currently subjectively experienced by our clients. (Brown, 2006, p. 19)

As you may have surmised, feminist counselors are in no rush to find a diagnostic label to slap on clients. Instead, they carefully develop a thoughtful case conceptualization that includes the impact of social norms, cultural differences, gender politics, trauma, and clients' subjective experience and understanding of their situations (Brown, 2010). Most feminists would agree that in some cases, a diagnostic label can be helpful and even liberating. For example, women who have been sexually abused often feel quite relieved to hear that flashbacks, nightmares, and hypervigilance are quite normal responses to trauma. In every case, feminist counselors are keenly aware of the political impact that diagnosis has in relationships (e.g., how friends, partners, and family see the person), in medical treatment (e.g., services and fees by insurance companies), and, most important, on how clients see and understand themselves.

Gender Roles

One of the primary areas of assessment, feminist counselors carefully explore clients' *gender role expectations* and how these relate to the presenting problem and clients' lives more broadly (Miller, 1986). Feminists note that "gender is commonly the first identity that people experience, coming before other identity markers such as culture, ethnicity, or social class, because gender, as a sex-derived social construct, is frequently the variable of greatest importance to the human world into which a child is born" (Brown, 2010, p. 52). Counselors explore how the client has internalized social messages about gender and how an individual's social class, cultural background, profession, and sexual orientation shape the clients' understanding of gender roles. For example, many women who report feeling depressed strongly maintain gendered expectations that women put the needs of others before their own, physically, emotionally, and professionally. Not surprisingly, the National Institutes of Mental Health report that women are more likely than men to be diagnosed with Major Depressive Disorder as well as any mental health disorder (NIMH, 2010). The social pressure for women to be nice, not make waves, and care for others takes a personal toll and sets the stage for depression (Kaplan, 1991). Feminist counselors explore the interaction of gender role and the development of psychological distress.

Self-in-Relation

One of the original theories at the Stone Center, *self-in-relation* theory refers to an alternative model for conceptualizing women's development (Surrey, 1991). In contrast to traditional developmental theories, "self-in-relation involves the recognition that, for women, the primary experience of self is relational, that is, the self is organized and developed in the context of important relationships" (p. 52). Thus, rather than follow the Ericksonian developmental model that emphasizes autonomy, self-reliance, self-actualization, and other forms of separation (see Chapter 8), feminists describe women as developing their sense of self *in and through relationships*. Accordingly, when developing case conceptualizations with clients, the counselor views women's development through a relational lens, exploring the evolution and development of self through significant relationships in the woman's life.

Marginalization and Oppression

Contemporary "feminist" counselors have far more than women's issues on their agenda. They are aware that in addition to gender, people can be marginalized due to culture, race, sexual orientation, age, ability, economic class, religion, and numerous other factors. All of these contribute to a person feeling *disconnected* and marginalized from the dominant group, rejected for one's "otherness." Chronically having to hide parts of the self to be accepted leads to psychological symptoms and pathology (Jordan, 2010). Thus, feminist counselors consider *social oppression* and isolation the root cause of clients' problems (Brown, 2010). By identifying these sources of marginalization in the case conceptualization process, counselors identify where and how to help clients build the connections they need to live full, authentic lives.

Relational Images

Relational-cultural counselors assess clients' *relational images*, internal constructs and expectations of relationship based on early life experience, and carefully trace how these affect present-day relationships (Jordan, 2010). People who experience chronic disconnection and relational trauma develop negative relational images that diminish their ability to fully participate in growth-fostering relationships and restrict their ability to experience authenticity. Such negative images are projected onto to other relationships, repeating a painful life pattern. Thus, the case conceptualization process involves identifying these patterns, which are both verbally described and often reenacted in the counseling relationship. In particular, counselors pay attention to *controlling images* that result in *shame* and *disempowerment*, defining what is acceptable and who the client is. These controlling images are often experienced as immutable by clients, resulting in *internal oppression*, where the client rejects parts of the self, thus becoming disconnected from the self as well as others. The counseling relationship is used as a forum for clients to modify their relational images so that they can experience more satisfying relationships, referred to as *correctional relational experiences* (similar to *corrective emotional experiences* described in Chapter 8).

Relational Resilience and Courage

A critical quality for healing, *relational resilience* refers to the ability to move back into relationship following disconnection and empathetic failures, as well as the ability to ask for help when needed (Jordan, 2010). Counselors don't force or push clients to work through disconnections, either in session or in their personal lives, but instead they create a context in which it is safe to do so, modeling that the well-being of the relationship has priority over making a point and being right. Developing relational resilience requires courage, but not in the form of heroic legend, which glorifies individual accomplishment and typically domination of another. Instead, *relational courage* is far quieter and scarier: it requires vulnerability and the willingness to open up to another. The counselor's role is to help "en-courage" clients so that they are willing to take the risks that intimacy and relationship demand.

"Mattering" and Connection

When assessing, feminist counselors pay particular attention to the growth-fostering relationships and other contexts in which clients feel that they "matter," that they are valued and cherished by another (Jordan, 2010). This sense of "mattering" to someone—either in a personal relationship or in broader social communities—is considered vital to mental and relational health and well-being; recent research has shown that this is particularly important for persons diagnosed with severe mental illness (Davidson, Tondora, Lawless, O'Connell, & Rowe, 2008). Counselors listen for both (a) areas of strength—relationships where clients feel they matter to someone—and (b) areas where a sense of connection needs to be built, and they use these areas to identify goals and build upon strengths.

Disconnection Strategies and the Central Relational Paradox

In addition to identifying sources of connection, feminist counselors also identify the strategies that clients use to disconnect from others when they feel vulnerable. Counselors use several questions to guide their assessment of disconnection:

Assessment of Disconnection

1. What strategies are used to disconnect from others: family, partner, friends, colleagues, children, and such?
2. Where were these methods first learned and used?
3. Does shame or disempowerment fuel the need for disconnection?
4. How useful are these strategies in current relationships?
5. Does the client know how and when to reconnect?

Try It Yourself

Find a partner and answer each of these questions. You can also do this alone in written form.

One way that people cope with repeated disconnection is to alter the self to fit the wishes of others, at the expense of personal authenticity; this is referred to as the *central relational paradox*, because it describes how, in response to disconnection, a person seeks connection by avoiding authentic connection. This paradoxical attempt to connect without connecting must change in order for clients to experience growth-fostering relationships that promote wellness.

Targeting Change: Goal Setting

Sociopolitical Awareness and Empowerment

Feminist counselors strive to increase a person's *sociopolitical awareness* of how their individual identity is interconnected with one's broader place in society and to *empower* clients to define themselves by alternative standards. Feminists strive to have all clients become more aware of how their *gender, ethnicity, social class, sexual orientation, physical characteristics, and physical abilities* significantly affect a person's identity and sense of self-worth (Worell & Johnson, 2001). Thus, one of the goals is to help clients develop greater awareness of how these sociocultural variables inform their identity, critically evaluate their effects, and ultimately develop their identity by crafting their sense of identity with full awareness, using personal values and the values from communities that have personal significance.

Connection

The overarching goal of feminist counseling, specifically relational-cultural counseling, is to build *connection*, specifically *growth-fostering relationships* (Jordan, 2010). When clients are able to establish such relationships, they create contexts in which they can authentically experience themselves while feeling a zest for life, valuing the self, being productive, and learning more about who they are: quite simply, a recipe for a lifelong process of evolving into one's best self.

The Doing: Interventions

Introduction to Feminist Techniques

The emphasis of feminist counseling is on the "viewing," case conceptualization, and quality of the counseling relationship, more so than on intervening. In fact, intervention from other approaches may be used *if adapted* in a gender and culturally sensitive manner (Enns, 1995; Worell & Remer, 1992). The techniques below are some of the unique ones used in feminist counseling.

Gender Role Analysis

A hallmark and defining intervention, *gender role analysis* involves encouraging clients to exam how cultural rules about male and female behavior affect the client's current distress, including multiple cultural rules from the different contexts of a client's life, such as religious, work, family, and ethnic traditions (Enns, 2000; Worell & Remer, 1992). Used with both men and women, gender role analysis helps clients better identify the often unacknowledged pressures and beliefs that support the problem. In the case study at the end of the chapter, the counselor helps Jose increase his awareness of how his gender role interacts with being gay, working-class, Mexican American, and from a Catholic family, and how this contributes to his ADHD diagnosis and substance misuse.

Questions to Facilitate Gender Role Analysis

- What beliefs do you have about being a "good woman" (or man) that might be related to the presenting problem?
- In what ways do you see gender stereotyping affecting you at work, at home, in your family, with friends, with your children, in your religious community, in your ethnic community, or somewhere else?
- What did you learn from your parents about what it means to be a girl/boy or man/woman? Which of these concepts still affect you today?
- What do you believe is a woman's (or man's) role in work? In a relationship? In a family? Regarding finances? Regarding health?
- What are your relationships like with men, women, heterosexuals, and persons who identify as gay/lesbian/bisexuals/transgendered?
- [If in a heterosexual relationship] How do you see gender roles playing out in your relationship? Do you like these effects?
- [If in a same-sex relationship] How do you see gender stereotypes and gay/lesbian stereotypes playing out in your relationships?
- What is your philosophy on gender relations and cultural issues?
- How have gender, culture, sexual orientation, class, ability, and other diversity variables affected how you see yourself?

Try It Yourself

Find a partner and use these questions to explore the experience of gender and how it affects his/her life.

Assertiveness Training

A classic cognitive-behavioral technique, feminists adapt *assertiveness training* to help empower clients, most notably women, who have been socialized to put the needs of others before their own (Worell & Remer, 1992). Assertiveness training involves teaching clients the difference between assertive, passive, and aggressive behaviors:

- *Assertive:* Able to balance the needs of self and others.
- *Passive:* Attends only to the needs of others.
- *Aggressive:* Attends only to the needs of self.

Using a psychoeducational approach, clients are taught in role-plays and real-world experiments how to advocate for their needs while honoring the needs of others in difficult interpersonal situations.

Self-Esteem Training

Proposed as an alternative to assertiveness training for women with very low self-esteem and/or who are constricted by rigid gender role stereotypes, self-esteem training emphasizes increasing a client's self-awareness and confidence, which ultimately enables her to assert her needs in interpersonal relationships (Stere, 1985). Self-esteem training involves developing four areas of personal skills:

1. *Accepting Feelings as Rational and Valid:* Validating feelings of guilt and resentment related to sociocultural inequities; trusting feeling reactions; expressing feelings.
2. *Being Able to Please Self:* Knowing what one wants; feeling worthy; taking action and making requests on one's own behalf.
3. *Identifying Personal Strengths:* Valuing feminine qualities; feeling courage to be successful; making positive self statements.
4. *Being Gentle with Self and Accepting Personal "Imperfections":* Developing realistic expectations for self; feeling calm when criticized; stating what shortcomings are.

Corrective Relational Experiences

Relational-cultural theory describes how the mutuality of the counseling relationship provides numerous opportunities for *corrective emotional experiences*, experiences in which old relational images are reworked by the counselor—providing an alternative, connecting response in a situation where the client had only experienced disconnect in other relationships (Jordan, 2010). For example, clients who had highly critical parents often experience extreme, painful disconnection with even the slightest negative comment. When counselors are able to stay connected and empathetic with clients who feel criticized or as if they have failed in some way, the counselor provides a *corrective relational experience* by not disengaging when clients have come to expect the other to abandon them. By maintaining an empathetic and mutually engaged relationship, counselors help clients work through various corrective emotional experiences, first in session and ultimately in relationships outside of the counseling context.

Self-Empathy

Relational-cultural approaches emphasize the importance of developing *self-empathy* in clients, the ability to bring empathetic awareness and a gentle presence to one's own experience (Jordan, 2010). Rather than judging or rejecting, clients learn how to stay with their feelings and experience empathy for how they came about. Clients first experience empathy from without, from the counselor, but are then encouraged to use this same kind of empathy in their inner dialogues. Counselors promote self-empathy by questioning their negative self statements, such as, "I shouldn't feel this way" or "I was a fool to do X." Such statements are countered with questions, such as "You are so accepting of others, but you do not accept the same qualities (actions, feelings, etc.) in yourself." If a client is particularly self-loathing, the counselor may ask the client to imagine it was a friend who was experiencing the situation and to have the client identify how she would see the situation in that case.

Social Activism and Social Justice

Feminist counseling is not a solitary process. Clients cannot meaningfully redefine their gender and personal identity stories or seek connection in a vacuum, or even in the dyad of the counseling relationship. By definition, changing one's gender identity and building connection happens in relationship and community. Thus, for clients to change, their relationships and social connections must also change. One way this is commonly achieved is through *social activism* and *social justice work* of various forms, activities that clients often spontaneously seek in the closing phase of treatment. This can involve something as stereotypical as becoming involved in activist groups, but more often it takes far subtler forms, such as getting a group of mothers or fathers together from work, or taking a stand on body issues in a circle of friends. Sometimes clients ask counselors where they can make a difference in the community with certain groups, such as children who have been sexually abused or immigrants needing assistance, and counselors should be ready and able to help them connect with appropriate community resources. Often, helping others who have experienced similar painful situations can be a transformative experience in which a client shifts from feeling like a victim to full recovery.

In addition, feminist counselors themselves are committed to social justice causes, using both professional and personal venues to effect societal change. This may take the form of advocating for clients by obtaining mental health or other services, in court situations, or in other contexts related to the client. Additionally, feminist counselors typically are involved in broader social movements, women's movements, clients' rights groups, children's advocacy, political campaigns, and similar efforts to promote social change.

Putting It All Together: Feminist Treatment Plan Case Conceptualization and Treatment Plan Templates

Theory-Specific Case Conceptualization: Feminist

The prompts below can be used to develop a *theory-specific case conceptualization* using Adlerian theory. The cross-theoretical case conceptualizations at the end of each theory chapter provide examples for writing a conceptualization that includes key elements of this theory-specific conceptualization. Comprehensive examples of theory-specific case conceptualizations are available in *Theory and Treatment Planning in Counseling and Psychotherapy* (Gehart, 2015).

- *Personal as Political/Political as Personal:* Describe how the client's presenting problem relates to broader political and social contexts and how the political affects the client's personal life.
- *Politics of Diagnosis:* Describe political and social considerations related to the client's DSM diagnosis.
- *Gender Roles:* Describe how gender role expectations are affecting the client, related to the presenting problems.
- *Self-in-Relation:* Describe how significant relationships have shaped the client's sense of self.
- *Marginalization and Oppression:* Describe the ways the client may be experiencing a sense of marginalization and oppression. These experiences may be due to race, culture, gender, sexual/gender orientation, economic class, religion, ability, age, and so on. These experiences may vary from context to context: work, home, community, for example.
- *Relational Images:* Describe significant relational constructs and expectations based on early life relationships. In particular, are there controlling images that evoke shame or disempowerment?
- *Relational Resilience and Courage:* Is client able to reconnect following disconnection and empathic failures in significant relationships?
- *"Mattering" and Connection:* Does client feel as though he/she matters to significant others, and is there a sufficient sense of connection with others?

- *Disconnection Strategies and the Central Relational Paradox:* Describe strategies for disconnecting, for others when feeling vulnerable. Is shame or disempowerment related to the pattern of disconnection? Does the client know how to safely reconnect?

Treatment Plan Template: Feminist

Use this Treatment Plan Template for developing a plan for clients with depressive, anxious, or compulsive types of presenting problems. Depending on the specific client, presenting problem, and clinical context, the goals and interventions in this template may need to be modified only slightly or significantly; you are encouraged to significantly revise the plan as needed. For the plan to be useful, goals and techniques should be written to target specific beliefs, behaviors, and emotions that the client is experiencing. The more specific, the more useful it will be to you.

Treatment Plan

Initial Phase of Treatment

Initial Phase Counseling Tasks

1. Develop working counseling relationship. *Diversity considerations:* *Describe how you will specifically adjust to respect cultured, gendered, and other styles of relationship building and emotional expression.*
   Relationship-building approach/intervention:
   a. Develop **growth-fostering relationship** using **mutual empathy** and **authenticity**.
2. Assess individual, systemic, and broader cultural dynamics. *Diversity considerations:* *Describe how you will specifically adjust assessment based on cultural, socioeconomic, sexual orientation, gender, and other relevant norms.*
   Assessment strategies:
   a. Identify **gender role expectations** and the effects of the **political on the personal**, including sources of **marginalization** and **oppression**.
   b. Assess sources of "**mattering,**" **relational resilience**, and **disconnection strategies**.
3. Identify and obtain client agreement on treatment goals. *Diversity considerations:* Ensure client's authentic agreement with goals.
   Goal-making intervention:
   a. **Mutually** determine goals, attending to **sociopolitical and gender** influences and impact.
4. Identify needed referrals, crisis issues, and other client needs. *Diversity considerations:* *Describe diversity issues related to specific crisis issues and referral options.*
   a. *Crisis assessment intervention(s):* Explore how **marginalization** and **relational disconnection** relate to sense of crisis; mobilize **relational resilience** and sense of connection to create safety plan.
   b. *Referral(s):* Connect with communities that will **empower** client and reduce sense of marginalization.

Initial Phase Client Goal

1. Increase **empowerment** and feelings of "**mattering**" to reduce [specific crisis symptoms].
   Interventions:
   a. Identify sources of **marginalization, oppression, and disconnection** that fuel sense of crisis.
   b. Identify **relationships and communities** that provide support and connection when needed to manage feelings that lead to crisis.

(continued)

Working Phase of Treatment

Working Phase Counseling Tasks

1. Monitor quality of the working alliance. *Diversity considerations:* Attend to issues of power and client's sense of **empowerment** to provide honest feedback to counselor.
   a. *Assessment Intervention:* Look for evidence of and ask about client experiencing "**five good things**" in counseling relationship; use Session Rating Scale.
2. Monitor progress toward goals. *Diversity considerations:* Attend to issues of **power and politics** if using standardized measurements.
   a. *Assessment Intervention:* Inquire with client about sense of progress while attending to **power** dynamics in counseling relationship; use Outcome Rating Scale to measure client progress.

Working Phase Client Goals

1. Increase awareness of the effects of **politics-as-personal, gender roles, and marginalization** to reduce [specific symptoms: depression, anxiety, etc.].
   Interventions:
   a. **Gender role analysis** and **analysis of sociopolitical influences** and how they affect the problem.
   b. Connect with friends, groups, and causes that create a sense of **empowerment** in relation to the problem issue.
2. Increase ability to relate to people and situations from **an assertive** position of respect for self and other to reduce [specific symptoms: depression, anxiety, etc.].
   Interventions:
   a. **Assertiveness training** to learn how to balance asserting one's needs while respecting those of others.
   b. **Self-esteem training** to develop a greater sense of self-acceptance.
3. Increase number and quality of **mutual growth-fostering relationships** to reduce [specific symptoms: depression, anxiety, etc.].
   Interventions:
   a. **Corrective emotional experiences** to learn how to relate more authentically.
   b. Learn to identify **disconnection strategies** and ways to repair the disconnection.

Closing Phase of Treatment

Closing Phase Counseling Task

1. Develop aftercare plan and maintain gains. *Diversity considerations:* Include unique relational and community resources to support client after counseling ends.
   Intervention:
   a. Identify **relational** and **sociopolitical** forces that are likely to generate problems in the future, prevention, and potential assertive responses.

Closing Phase Client Goals

1. Increase client's sense of **relational resilience, "mattering,"** and **empowerment** to reduce feelings of disconnection [OR anxiety, fear, etc.].
   Interventions:
   a. Apply learning from **corrective emotional experiences** in session to relationships outside.
   b. Empower client to advocate for **relational resilience** and **marginalized others** in relationships.

(continued)

2. Increase **advocacy** and **social justice** efforts for self and/or marginalized others to reduce sense of disempowerment [OR depressive, anxious, compulsive behaviors, etc.].
   Interventions:
   a. Identify contexts and relationships for **advocacy efforts** that enhance client's sense of self-esteem.
   b. Identity relationships and organizations that foster client's ongoing **growth** and **resilience**.

Tapestry Weaving: Working with Diverse Populations

Cultural and Ethnic Diversity

If you have not already noticed, more than any other approach covered in this book, postmodern and feminist approaches integrate consideration of cultural issues at the most fundamental level of their method. Therefore, many would consider them the quintessential approach for diverse populations. The broader questions of diversity and of how society, its norms, and the use of language affect individuals are the guiding premises in postmodern philosophical literature, making these therapies particularly suitable for clients from marginalized groups (for an in-depth discussion, see Monk et al., 2008). Unlike most mental health therapies, feminist and narrative theories place societal issues of oppression at the heart of their therapeutic interventions, and many narrative counselors are active agents of social justice (Jordan, 1997, 2010; Zimmerman & Dickerson, 1996). Collaborative therapy attends more to local discourses, working closely with the client and significant others to determine what the problem is (for the moment, knowing its definition will continually evolve) and how best to resolve it. This focus on local knowledges ensures that the client's cultural values and beliefs are a central part of the therapy process. Postmodern approaches have international roots and are practiced in numerous countries around the world.

Applications with Native American, First Nations, and Aboriginals

Narrative therapy approaches have been widely used and researched with native cultures in Canada, Australia, New Zealand, and the United States. In one study, counselors who worked with Native Americans in Wyoming identified communication and therapy practices, all of which were descriptive of narrative therapy practices, that seemed best suited for this culture, (Lee, 1997). Some of the observations from these counselors include:

- *Subtle eye contact:* Native Americans generally do not maintain sustained eye contact, and counselors should follow the client's lead.
- *Active listening:* Counselors should use nonverbal and verbal feedback to signal that the client's meanings are understood.
- *Subtle emotional expression:* Native Americans are not prone to strong, demonstrative expressions of emotions, and counselors must respect this by not pushing hard for emotional expression.
- *Spirituality:* Spirituality is generally highly valued by Native Americans, and counselors need to respectfully address and find ways to integrate these practices into therapeutic work.
- *Self-in-relation:* Native Americans are likely to construct their identity within relationships, seeing much of their identity as tied to family or the tribe.
- *Home visits:* The counselor making home visits is generally appreciated by Native Americans, helpful in terms of comfort, familiarity, and time flexibility.
- *Gentle, reflective stance:* Counselors described a therapeutic stance that was calm, reflective, nonconfrontational, and nonconflictual.
- *Art, Storytelling, and Metaphor:* The use of art, drawing, storytelling, and metaphor were found to be particularly helpful interventions.

In another study set in Manitoba, Canada, native healers and their clients were interviewed and asked to identify what they believed to be helpful in changing emotions, cognitions, and behaviors (McCabe, 2007). This study included many of the above practices, in addition to the following:

- *Ceremonies and rituals:* Ceremony and rituals are powerful allies in the healing process and are used throughout.
- *Spiritual guidance:* Native Americans with traditional spiritual beliefs generally believe in a Creator spirit that provides guidance in the healing process.
- *Self-acceptance:* For many, themes of self-acceptance of one's identity, especially within the larger context of marginalization.
- *Lessons of daily living:* Using opportunities in daily living to apply learning.
- *Empathy:* Expressions of empathy from the healer help in the healing process.
- *Role modeling:* The healer serves as a role model for the client in terms of lifestyle, behaviors, and attitudes.

Narrative counselors readily use native rituals, ceremonies, spiritual beliefs, and cultural stories to create therapeutic contexts that are respectful and responsive to the needs of native and aboriginal clients, often inviting tribal elders, leaders, and healers into the broader therapeutic dialogue. In particular, separating the person from the problem and meeting the person apart from the problem can be particularly useful. In addition, counselors can use situating and permission comments to increase the client's sense of voice and autonomy in the therapeutic relationship, and to help create a more respectful healing context.

Hispanic Youth

Narrative counseling has also been used with Hispanic children and adolescents with depression, high-risk behaviors, and/or substance abuse (Malgady & Costantino, 2010). Some of their unique applications with this population include:

- *Cuento therapy:* Puerto Rican folktales, *cuentos*, were used to convey themes and morals, providing models for adaptive responses to problems such as acting out, self-esteem, and anxiety. They adapted the tales to incorporate traditional Puerto Rican values as well as Anglo cultural values.
- *Hero/Heroine therapy:* Since many children were in single-parent households, the counselors had children identify male and female Puerto Rican heroes and heroines to help bridge bicultural and intergenerational gaps, and to identify conflicts commonly experienced in adolescence.
- *Temas storytelling therapy:* Counselors selected pictures from the Thematic Apperception Tests that represented Hispanic cultural elements: traditional food, games, family scenes, and neighborhoods. Then the group of children was asked to develop a story with the cards. Then each group member was invited to share personal experiences that relate to the story the group created. The counselor reinforced adaptive, preferred narratives and helped find alternatives to maladaptive responses. Finally, the group did a dramatization of the story in class to practice preferred behaviors and responses.

Sexual Identity Diversity

Postmodern therapies are often the theory of choice for working with lesbian, gay, bisexual, transgendered, and questioning (LGBTQ) clients, because these therapies help deconstruct the heterosexist discourses that often are the source of greatest suffering in LGBTQ clients (Simon & Whitfield, 2000). Deconstructionist practices can help clients critically examine how their understanding of their sexuality emerged, the consequences of these descriptions, and options for alternative understandings (Simon & Whitfield, 2000). When working with LGBTQ clients, some counselors recommend an advocacy stance with expertise in the subject matter, rather than a strict not-knowing stance (Aducci & Baptist, 2011; Perez, 1996). In addition, many LGBTQ clients benefit form therapeutic conversations that help them construct positive labels and identity narratives for themselves and their relationships (Perez, 1996). Furthermore, it is important for counselors to identify how much of the presenting problem is due directly to a client's sexual identity, versus more general life or relationship circumstances (Aducci & Baptist, 2011).

Narrative counselors have developed a specific approach that can be used with LGBTQ clients struggling with dissonance between heterosexual dominant discourses and their own lived experience. Yarhouse (2008) describes *narrative sexual identity therapy* as a middle ground to *gay-affirmative therapy* on one hand, which affirms the inherent goodness of identifying as LGBT, and *reorientation therapy* on the other, a highly controversial approach (so much so that it is under legislative scrutiny in California at the moment) designed to help clients change their sexual orientation to heterosexual. In contrast, narrative sexual identity therapy, which is based on narrative therapy principles, helps clients seek to live their lives in *congruence* between their personal beliefs and behaviors, a process that focuses on deconstructing dominant discourses that constrain and confuse clients' sexual identity. Designed to help clients struggling with their sexual identity, this approach is particularly relevant for clients from religious and cultural backgrounds that have strong anti-gay messages.

Drawing from standard narrative therapy practices, the counselor helps clients identify the problem narrative and then identify potential counternarrative that is more congruent with the client's lived experience and values. In this approach, the client determines what values and intentions they want to define their lives. The approach has six general steps or phases, which are of course fluid but which can nonetheless be helpful to counselors in conceptualizing treatment.

1. *Client Presents Sexual Identity Concern*
   Initially, a client presents with concerns about sexual identity. These concerns may be related to external (e.g., religious, cultural, or family) or internal voices (e.g., personal values) that believe their lived experience of sexual attraction is somehow wrong, immoral, or otherwise problematic.
2. *Map Dominant Narratives*
   The next step is to explore the dominant discourse, its origin, and specific nuanced meanings. Questions counselors can ask to map the dominant discourse include:
   - What were some of the messages you received growing up about identifying as gay? (Yarhouse, 2008, p. 205)
   - How was the message communicated to you that feelings toward someone from the same sex meant you were gay? (Yarhouse, 2008, p. 205)
   - How did you respond to these views of same-sex attraction?
3. *Identify Preferred Narratives*
   In the next phase, clients reflect on their own personal lived experience of same-sex attraction. Most often the metaphor used to describe this is "*discovery*": discovering a preexisting fact about their true selves. In other cases, the metaphor is more one of "integration": integrating their experience of same-sex attraction with other aspects of their identity. The metaphor of integration is more common when a person chooses not to assume a gay identity but instead chooses to only integrate certain elements.
4. *Recognize Exceptions/Emerging Counternarrative*
   Next, the counselor helps clients identify exceptions to the dominant discourses, to create space for a counternarrative to emerge. Questions counselors can use to facilitate this process include:
   - In what ways are you understanding your sexual identity differently from when you first thought of yourself? (Yarhouse, 2008, p. 206)
   - Have you had experiences that call into question the meaning of same-sex attraction that you learned when you were young?
   - In what ways have your personal experiences of same-sex attraction contrasted with messages you have heard about what gay people are like?
5. *Highlight Identity-Congruent Attributes, Activities, and Resources*
   As the counternarrative emerges, the counselor listens for and highlights personal attributes, activities, and resources that are congruent with the client's preferred identity.

- In what ways would you like to challenge some of the messages you received about your sexual identity? (Yarhouse, 2008, p. 207)
- In what ways are you already living in accordance—even in small measure—with your preferred values and identity?
- What type of relationships, activities, or communities might further provide support for your preferred identity and values?

6. *Resolution/Congruence*
   Finally, clients are able to live according to their preferred sexual identity, one that is congruent with their lived experience, spiritual beliefs, and cultural values. Questions counselors can use to facilitate this process include:
   - In the course of the next few months or so, what do you see as the relationship between your sexual identity and your religious or spiritual identity? (Yarhouse, 2008, p. 208).
   - Can you share a little of the way you would like to describe your sexual identity in the year to come? (Yarhouse, 2008, p. 208).

Research and the Evidence Base

Consistent with their philosophical underpinnings, feminist, narrative and collaborative counselors have conducted more qualitative than quantitative investigations about their approaches to therapy (Anderson, 1997; Gehart et al., 2007). Qualitative research on postmodern therapies has focused on clients' lived experience of therapy and its effects on their lives, emphasizing the clients' experience over researcher-defined measures of successful therapy (Andersen, 1997; Gehart & Lyle, 1999; Levitt & Rennie, 2004; London, Ruiz, & Gargollo, 1998). A notable exception, Finnish psychiatrist Jaakko Seikkula (2002) and his team (Haarakangas et al., 2007) have used qualitative and quantitative methods to study their open-dialogue approach to working with psychosis and other severe diagnoses for over 20 years, generating significant evidence for their model's effectiveness (see Clinical Spotlight discussion). They report that they have effectively eradicated chronic cases of psychosis, with most clients returning to normal functioning within two years; their work is an exemplary, evidence-based approach for recovery-oriented approaches to treating severe mental health issues (see Recovery in Mental Health Movement in Chapter 3).

Outcome research on narrative therapy has increased in recent years. For example, one study from Australia examined the effectiveness of narrative therapy for treating major depressive disorders and found its effects were comparable to other approaches, with 74% of clients achieving reliable improvement (Vromans & Schweitzer, 2011). In another Australian study, women with eating disorders and depressive issues engaged in a ten-week narrative therapy group that resulted in reduced self-criticism and changes in daily practices/activities. Process research on narrative therapy indicates that unique outcomes that specifically enable clients to reconceptualize their problems and foster new experiences are correlated with positive outcomes (Matos, Santos, Gonçalves, & Martins, 2009).

The assumptions and premises of postmodern therapy are also receiving support from an unexpected arena: psychiatry, more specifically interpersonal neurobiology (Beaudoin & Zimmerman, 2011; Gehart, 2012; Siegel, 2012). Like postmodern counselors, Siegel proposes that storytelling is how humans make sense of life:

> We are storytelling creatures, and stories are the social glue that binds us to one another. Understanding the structure and function of narrative is therefore a part of understanding what it means to be human. (pp. 31–32)

Siegel describes how in childhood, humans are born into story, take on cultural meaning, and then in adolescence and adulthood continue to reshape these meanings, thus evolving human culture. These narratives constrain or expand a person's options for responding to life. Siegel suggests that *reflection*—a detached examination of these narratives—enable clients to liberate themselves from these limiting stories of who they are and what their life is; this same process is emphasized in postmodern therapies.

In describing how people change, Siegel (2012) emphasizes the importance of *bottom-up processing*, which is compared to *top-down processing*. Bottom-up processing refers to processing experiences using the bottom three layers of the prefrontal cortex to generate new understandings, categories, and stories for what is happening. In contrast, top-down processing involves using the top three layers of the prefrontal cortex to categorize lived experience with preexisting categories. Both forms of processing are important, but most people who feel "stuck" related to a problem are stuck in top-down processing, unable to change how they see their situation or the possibilities for changing it. The *not-knowing* position of postmodern counselors is an excellent approach for facilitating bottom-up processing: in fact, the entire collaborative therapy process can be viewed as an approach for expanding bottom-up processing (Gehart, 2012).

Additionally, Siegel (2012) describes trauma resolution as a process of creating an integrative narrative, similar to thickening the plot in narrative therapy. Traumatic experiences overwhelm the hippocampus and explicit (narrative) memory not encoded with implicit memory, as happens in nontraumatic situations. Thus, traumatic memories are encoded primarily as implicit memories, which do not have a sensation of being from the past and are often experienced as fragmented auditory, visual, and sensual experiences that are occurring in the here-and-now (i.e., flashbacks). These fragmented memories create chaotic and rigid patterns that impair the brain's ability to enter into healthy, integrated neural states. Siegel suggests that the treatment from trauma essentially involves pulling the implicit memories together into a coherent narrative, which is most easily achieved by entering into "interpersonal attunement" with a counselor. He proposes that when two minds become entrained, in sync, the client can "borrow" the counselor's neural integrated state to help cope with the traumatic memories long enough to put them into a coherent narrative. Through this process of recreating an integrated explicit narrative of the trauma, the client is then able to recall the trauma while remaining in an integrated neural state (i.e., not have symptoms when recalling the trauma).

Finally, Beaudoin and Zimmerman (2011) note that the postmodern techniques that help clients "give voice" to their lived experience and put into words things that have never been said before also help move clients from their anxiety-focused limbic system to the more calm and reason-focused prefrontal cortex. By labeling and giving voice to their stress-based experiences, clients are able to reduce the firing of the limbic system, allowing the client to make more conscious choices and responses. Furthermore, therapeutic conversations about preferred realities strengthen neural connections that support clients' preferred identities and associated behaviors. In particular, *affect-infused descriptions* of preferred realities help to solidify new identity narratives, which are predominantly associated with the right-brain hemisphere; such affect-infused descriptions include not only emotion but also sensory experiences, such as imagery, scent, and tactile experiences.

Questions for Personal Reflection and Class Discussion

1. Which ideas from this chapter do you find most personally relevant? Why?
2. Which ideas from this chapter do you think will be most helpful in working with clients?
3. What are the possibilities and limitations for using this approach with diverse clients? How might you address the limitations?
4. Which dominant discourses are most significant in your life? Gender, culture, success, beauty, wealth, health, family, and so on.
5. Describe the growth-fostering relationships in your life. How have they been most impactful?
6. Describe your experiences of marginalization. How did you respond to others? How did these experiences shape your identity and behavior? What helped you cope or overcome these experiences?
7. Describe your experience of gender [or other diversity factor] and how it has shaped your identity, the possibilities you see in your life, your relationship, and your professional life.

8. For which clients and/or presenting problems do you think this approach would be most appropriate? Least appropriate?
9. Which case conceptualization concept seems most useful for understanding a client's problem?
10. Which intervention do you think would be the most useful?
11. Do you think this approach is a good fit for you as a counselor or therapist? Why or why not?
12. In what ways would you need to grow, or what would you need to learn, to be able to use this approach well?

Online Resources

Harlene Anderson
www.harleneanderson.org

Anti-Anorexia/Anti-Bulimia League
www.narrativeapproaches.com/antianorexia%20folder/anti_anorexia_index.htm

Dulwich Centre: Michael White's Narrative Therapy
www.dulwichcenter.com

Evanston Family Therapy Center: Freedman and Combs' Narrative Therapy
www.narrativetherapychicago.com

Feminist Therapy Institute
www.feminist-therapy-institute.org/

Feminist Therapy Code of Ethics
www.feminist-therapy-institute.org/ethics.htm

Houston Galveston Institute: Collaborative language systems
www.talkhgi.com

Narrative Approaches
www.narrativeapproaches.com

Taos Institute: Collaborative Practices in Therapy, Consultation, Education, Business
www.taosinstitute.net

Yaletown Family Therapy: Narrative Therapy, Canada
www.yaletownfamilytherapy.com

References

*Asterisk indicates recommended introductory readings.

Aducci, C. J., & Baptist, J. A. (2011). A collaborative-affirmative approach to supervisory practice. *Journal of Feminist Family Therapy: An International Forum, 23*(2), 88–102. doi:10.1080/08952833.2011.574536

*Andersen, T. (1991). *The reflecting team: Dialogues and dialogues about the dialogues.* New York: Norton.

Andersen, T. (1995). Reflecting processes; acts of informing and forming: You can borrow my eyes, but you must not take them away from me! In S. Friedman (Ed.), *The reflecting team in action: Collaborative practice in family therapy* (pp. 11–37). New York: Guilford.

*Andersen, T. (2007). Human participating: Human "being" is the step for human "becoming" in the next step. In H. Anderson & D. Gehart (Eds.), *Collaborative therapy: Relationships and conversations that make a difference* (pp. 81–97). New York: Brunner-Routledge.

Anderson, H. (1993). On a roller coaster: A collaborative language systems approach to therapy. In S. Friedman (Ed.), *The new language of change* (pp. 323–344). New York: Guilford.

Anderson, H. (1995). Collaborative language systems: Toward a postmodern therapy. In R. Mikesell, D. D. Lusterman, & S. McDaniel (Eds.), *Family psychology and systems therapy* (pp. 27–44). Washington, DC: American Psychological Association Press.

*Anderson, H. (1997). *Conversations, language, and possibilities: A postmodern approach to therapy.* New York: Basic Books.

Anderson, H. (2005). Myths about "not knowing". *Family Process, 44*, 497–504.

Anderson, H. (2007). Historical influences. In H. Anderson & D. Gehart (Eds.), *Collaborative therapy: Relationships and conversations that make a difference* (pp. 21–31). New York: Brunner-Routledge.

*Anderson, H., & Gehart, D. (2007). *Collaborative therapy: Relationships and conversations that make a difference.* New York: Brunner-Routledge.

Anderson, H., & Goolishian, H. (1988). Human systems as linguistic systems: Preliminary and evolving ideas about the implications for clinical theory. *Family Process, 27,* 157–163.

*Anderson, H., & Goolishian, H. (1992). The client is the expert: A not-knowing approach to therapy. In S. McNamee & K. J. Gergen (Eds.), *Therapy as social construction* (pp. 25–39). Newbury Park, CA: Sage.

Beaudoin, M., & Zimmerman, J. (2011). Narrative therapy and interpersonal neurobiology: Revisiting classic practices, developing new emphases. *Journal of Systemic Therapies, 30*(1), 1–13. doi:10.1521/jsyt.2011.30.1.1.

Brown, L. (1994). *Subversive dialogues: Theory in feminist therapy.* New York: Basic Books.

Brown, L. (2006). Still subversive after all these years: The relevance of feminist therapy in the age of evidence-based practice. *Psychology of Women Quarterly, 30*(1), 15–24. doi:10.1111/j.1471-6402.2006.00258.x

Brown, L. (2010). *Feminist therapy.* Washington, DC: American Psychological Association.

Bruner, J. (1986). *Actual minds, possible worlds.* Cambridge, MA: Harvard University Press.

Comstock, D. (Ed.). (2005). *Diversity and development: Critical contexts that shape our lives and relationships.* Pacific Grove, CA: Brooks Cole.

Davidson, L., Tondora, J., Lawless, M. S., O'Connell, M. J., & Rowe, M. (2008). *A practical guide to recovery-oriented practice: Tools for transforming mental health care.* New York: Oxford University Press.

Enns, C. Z. (1995). Toward integrating feminist psychotherapy and feminist philosophy. *Professional Psychology: Research and Practice, 24,* 453–466.

Enns, C. Z. (2000). Gender issues in counseling. In S. D. Brown & R. W. Rice (Eds.), *Handbook of counseling psychology* (3rd ed., pp. 601–669). New York: Wiley.

Enns, C. Z. (2004). *Feminist theories and feminist psychotherapies: Origins, themes, and diversity* (2nd ed.). New York: Haworth Press.

Feminist Therapy Institute. (2000). *Feminist code of ethics.* Georgetown, ME: Author.

Foucault, M. (1972). *The archeology of knowledge* (A. Sheridan-Smith, trans.). New York: Harper & Row.

Foucault, M. (1979). *Discipline and punish: The birth of the prison.* Middlesex: Peregrine Books.

Foucault, M. (1980). *Power/knowledge: Selected interviews and other writings.* New York: Pantheon Books.

*Freedman, J., & Combs, G. (1996). *Narrative therapy: The social construction of preferred realities.* New York: Norton.

Gehart, D. (2012). *Mindfulness and acceptance in couple and family therapy: The art and science of learning to be present in relationships and life.* New York: Springer.

Gehart, D. (2015). *Theory and treatment planning in counseling and psychotherapy* (2nd ed.). Pacific Grove, CA: Brooks Cole.

Gehart, D., & McCollum, E. (2007). Engaging suffering: Towards a mindful re-visioning of marriage and family therapy practice. *Journal of Marital and Family Therapy, 33*(2), 214–226.

Gehart, D. R., & Lyle, R. R. (1999). Client and therapist perspectives of change in collaborative language systems: An interpretive ethnography. *Journal of Systemic Therapy, 18*(4), 78–97.

Gehart, D., Tarragona, M., & Bava, S. (2007). A collaborative approach to inquiry. In H. Anderson & D. Gehart (Eds.), *Collaborative therapy: Relationships and conversations that make a difference* (pp. 367–390). Brunner-Routledge.

*Gergen, K. (1999). *An invitation to social construction.* Newbury Park, CA: Sage.

Gilligan, C. (1982/1993). *In a different voice: Psychological theory and women's development.* Cambridge, MA: Harvard University Press.

Haarakangas, K., Seikkula, J., Alakare, B., & Aaltonen, J. (2007). Open dialogue: An approach to psychotherapuetic treatment of psychosis in Northern Finland. In H. Anderson & D. Gehart (Eds.), *Collaborative therapy: Relationships and conversations that make a difference* (pp. 221–233). New York: Brunner-Routledge.

Jordan, J. (1997). *Women's growth in diversity.* New York: Guilford.

Jordan, J. (2010). *Relational-cultural therapy.* Washington, DC: American Psychological Association.

Jordan, J., Kaplan, A., Miller, J., Stiver, I., & Surrey, J. (1991). *Women's growth in connection: Writings from the Stone Center.* New York: Guilford.

Kaplan, A. G. (1991). The self-in-relation: A theory of women's development. In J. Jordan, A. G. Kaplan, J. B. Miller, I. P. Stiver, & J. L. Surrey (Eds.), *Women's growth in connection: Writings from the Stone Center* (pp. 206–222). New York: Guilford.

Levitt, H., & Rennie, D. L. (2004). Narrative activity: Clients' and therapists' intentions in the process of narration. In L. Angus & J. McLeod (Eds.), *The handbook of narrative and psychotherapy: Practice, theory, and research* (pp. 299–313). Thousand Oaks, CA: Sage.

London, S., Ruiz, G., & Gargollo, M. C. (1998). Client's voices: A collection of client's accounts. *Journal of Systemic Therapies, 17*(4), 61–71.

Malgady, R. G., & Costantino, G. (2010). Treating Hispanic children and adolescents using narrative therapy. In J. R. Weisz & A. E. Kazdin (Eds.), *Evidence-based psychotherapies for children and adolescents* (2nd ed., pp. 391–400). New York: Guilford.

Matos, M., Santos, A., Gonçalves, M., & Martins, C. (2009). Innovative moments and change in narrative therapy. *Psychotherapy Research, 19*(1), 68–80. doi:10.1080/10503300802430657.

McCabe, G. H. (2007). The healing path: A culture and community-derived indigenous therapy model. *Psychotherapy: Theory, Research, Practice, Training, 44*(2), 148–160. doi:10.1037/0033-3204.44.2.148

Miller, J. B. (1976/1986). *Toward a new psychology of women* (2nd ed.). Boston, MA: Beacon.

Miller, J. B., & Stiver, I. (1997). *The healing connection: How women form relationships in therapy and in life.* Boston, MA: Beacon.

Monk, G., & Gehart, D. R. (2003). Conversational partner or socio-political activist: Distinguishing the position of the therapist in collaborative and narrative therapies. *Family Process, 42,* 19–30.

Monk, G., Winslade, J., Crocket, K., & Epston, D. (1997). *Narrative therapy in practice: The archaeology of hope.* San Francisco: Jossey-Bass.
Monk, G., Winslade, J., & Sinclair, S. (2008). New horizons in multicultural counseling. Thousand Oaks, CA: Sage.
National Institutes of Mental Health (NIMH). (2010). The numbers count: Mental disorders in America. Downloaded June, 30, 2010 http://www.nimh.nih.gov/health/publications/the-numbers-count-mental-disorders-in-america/index.shtml#MajorDepressive
Perez, P. J. (1996). Tailoring a collaborative, constructionist approach for the treatment of same-sex couples. *The Family Journal, 4*(1), 73–81. doi:10.1177/1066480796041016
Remer, P. (2008). *Feminist therapy.* In J. Frew & M. D. Spiegler (Eds.), *Contemporary psychotherapies for a diverse world* (pp. 397–441). Boston, MA: Lahaska.
Rosin, H. (2010). The end of men. *The Atlantic, July/August.* Downloaded June, 20, 2010. http://www.theatlantic.com/magazine/archive/2010/07/the-end-of-men/8135/
Schore, A. (1994). *Affect regulation and the origins of the self: The neurobiology of emotional development.* Hillsdale, NJ: Erlbaum.
Seikkula, J. (2002). Open dialogues with good and poor outcomes for psychotic crises: Examples from families with violence. *Journal of Marital and Family Therapy, 28*(3), 263–274.
Shepherd, D. (2005). Male development and the journey toward disconnection. In D. Comstock (Ed.), *Diversity and development: Critical contexts that shape our lives and relationships* (pp. 133–157). Pacific Grove, CA: Brooks Cole.
Siegel, D. J. (2012). *The developing mind: How relationships and the brain interact to shape who we are* (2nd ed.). New York: Guilford.
Simon, G., & Whitfield, G. (2000). Social constructionist and systemic therapy. In D. Davies & C. Neal (Eds.), *Therapeutic perspectives on working with lesbian, gay and bisexual clients* (pp. 144–162). Maidenhead, England: Open University Press.
Surrey, J. L. (1991). The self-in-relation: A theory of women's development. In J. Jordan, A. G. Kaplan, J. B. Miller, I. P. Stiver, & J. L. Surrey (Eds.), *Women's growth in connection: Writings from the Stone Center* (pp. 51–66). New York: Guilford.
Vromans, L. P., & Schweitzer, R. D. (2011). Narrative therapy for adults with major depressive disorder: Improved symptom and interpersonal outcomes. *Psychotherapy Research, 21*(1), 4–15. doi:10.1080/10503301003591792.
Winslade, J., & Monk, G. (1999) *Narrative counseling in schools: Powerful and brief* (1st ed.). Thousand Oaks, CA: Corwin Press.
*White, M. (2007). *Maps of narrative practice.* New York: Norton.
*White, M., & Epston, D. (1990). *Narrative means to therapeutic ends.* New York: Norton.
Worell, J., & Johnson, D. (2001). Therapy with women: Feminist frameworks. In R. K. Unger (Ed.), *Handbook of the psychology of women and gender* (pp. 317–329). New York: John Wiley.
Worell, J., & Remer, P. (1992). *Feminist perspectives in therapy: An empowerment model for women.* New York: Wiley.
Yarhouse, M. A. (2008). Narrative sexual identity therapy. *American Journal of Family Therapy, 36*(3), 196–210. doi:10.1080/01926180701236498.
Zimmerman, J. L., & Dickerson, V. C. (1996). *If problems talked: Narrative therapy in action.* New York: Guilford.

Postmodern Case Study: ADHD, Substance Use, Coming Out

Jose, a 43-year-old Mexican American male, enters counseling at the urging of his partner, Robert, with whom he has been in a committed relationship for ten years. Robert believes that Jose's "partying" has been out of control for the past three years, going from drinking and smoking pot a few nights per month to smoking pot most days of the week and partying with "whatever he has access to" on the weekends, including ecstasy, meth, and cocaine. A construction worker, Jose has always had an irregular schedule, but is working less and less because he is "out of commission" more often. As a child, Jose was diagnosed with ADHD but never took any medication for it. When sober, Jose admits to feeling like nothing is interesting any more and periodically having thoughts of suicide. He says that although his family tries to be supportive, he does not feel they fully accept him the way he is.

CASE CONCEPTUALIZATION

Date: Sept 14, 2013 **Clinician:** Michael **Client/Case #:** 14002

I. Introduction to Client

Identify primary client and significant others

Client

Adult Male Age: 43 Hispanic/Latino Partnered Gay/Lesbian/Bisexual Occupation/Grade: Construction worker/ carpenter Other: Mexican American (second generation; fluent in English and Spanish; prefers sesssions in English)

Significant Others

Client's Male Partner Age: 44 Caucasian Partnered Gay/Lesbian/Bisexual Occupation/Grade: CPA Other: ____

Select Person Age: ______ Select Ethnicity Select Relational Status Occupation/Grade: ______ Other: ______

Select Person Age: ______ Select Ethnicity Select Relational Status Occupation/Grade: ______ Other: ______

Select Person Age: ______ Select Ethnicity Select Relational Status Occupation/Grade: ______ Other: ______

Others: ______

II. Presenting Concern(s)

Client Description of Problem(s): AM believes he is "self-medicating" his ADHD and admits his partying has gotten out of hand. He is particularly motivated to change in order to keep his partner happy. He believes that if he felt more accepted by his family, he might be less "stressed out."

Significant Other/Family Description(s) of Problems: Partner: Thinks that AM43 is depressed and self-medicating with drugs and alcohol. He wants to see AM43 get back to his "happy self" again. He believes AM43 is hanging with a young party crowd and that he is trying to extend his college years.

Broader System Problem Descriptions: Description of problem from referring party, teachers, relatives, legal system, etc.:

Parents: Describe AM as always being a "trouble maker" and "rebellious one." They do not "believe in" ADHD and always tried to impart better discipline. They "respect" AM43's choice of partner, but admit that they are disappointed that he will never have kids and that he has abandoned his Catholic faith.

______: ______

III. Background Information

Trauma/Abuse History (recent and past): AM43 reports that he was frequently spanked as a child for his unruly behavior. He also reports one incident of sexual abuse at 8 years old by a 16-year-old male cousin at a family event.

(*continued*)

Substance Use/Abuse (current and past; self, family of origin, significant others): Current substance and alcohol abuse; began abusing 3 years ago. Brothers and father also have pattern of heavy drinking and brothers also smoke marijuana.

Precipitating Events (recent life changes, first symptoms, stressors, etc.): Three years ago, AM43 turned 40, which highlighted for him that he was getting older and, for his family, that he would never have kids and a family. He began hanging out with younger group of coworkers from one of his work sites who partied "harder" than he and his partner had in past. Also during that time, his partner was working longer hours as a CPA.

Related Historical Background (family history, related issues, previous counseling, etc.): AM's father was always a heavy drinker but never used other drugs. He has never been in counseling before. AM is the first openly gay man in his family.

IV. Client Strengths and Diversity

Client Strengths

Personal: Good sense of humor; wants to improve his life; open to suggestions and help; social and meets friends easily.

Relational/Social: AM and partner are committed to each other and relationship; family tries to support him as best as they can; AM belongs to several friendship networks.

Spiritual: Raised Catholic but no longer practicing, AM believes in God and that things happen for a reason.

Diversity: Resources and Limitations

Identify potential resources and limitations available to clients based on their age, gender, sexual orientation, cultural background, socioeconomic status, religion, regional community, language, family background, family configuration, abilities, etc.

Unique Resources: Strong connection to and support system within the Latino gay community; easily connects with others.

Potential Limitations: Some of AM's extended family are not so supportive of his sexuality, especially his grandparents. He also feels rejected by the Catholic Church that he was raised in.

Complete All of the Following Sections for a Complete Case Conceptualization or Specific Sections for Theory-Specific Conceptualization.

V. Psychodynamic Conceptualization

Psychodynamic Defense Mechanisms

Check 2-4 most commonly used defense mechanisms

☒ Acting Out: *Describe:* Historically AM has acted out and rebelled in response to inner conflict.

☒ Denial: *Describe:* AM has been in denial about his substance abuse issues for the past 3 years.

❑ Displacement: *Describe:* ________

❑ Help-rejecting complaining: *Describe:* ________

(*continued*)

☒ Humor: *Describe:* AM often uses humor to reduce intimacy.

❑ Passive Aggression: *Describe:*

❑ Projection: *Describe:*

❑ Projective Identification: *Describe:*

❑ Rationalization: *Describe:*

❑ Reaction Formation: *Describe:*

❑ Repression: *Describe:*

❑ Splitting: *Describe:*

❑ Sublimation: *Describe:*

❑ Suppression: *Describe:*

☒ Other: In anticipation of being judged, AM finds reasons to preemptively criticize and judge others.

Object Relational Patterns

Describe relationship with early caregivers in past: AM's mother was the primary caretaker when he was a child since his father often worked long hours. AM was very close with both his mother and father as a child although was generally more of a "mama's boy." His father was strict and AM rebelled against his father throughout his teenage years.

Was the attachment with the mother (or equivalent) primarily:

☒ Generally Secure ❑ Anxious and Clingy ❑ Avoidant and Emotionally Distant ❑ Other: AM's mother has been overly involved for most of his life. She babies him and believes that her son can "do no wrong." They have a strong bond and have a generally secure attachment.

Was the attachment with the father (or equivalent) primarily:

❑ Generally Secure ❑ Anxious and Clingy ☒ Avoidant and Emotionally Distant ❑ Other: AM's father was the disciplinarian in the household. He was strict with his children and showed little affection; however, he took pride in AM43 as he was the only son.

Describe present relationship with these caregivers: AM is close with both of his parents. His father is uncomfortable with AM's sexuality; however, both he and AM's mother are respectful of their son's choices.

Describe relational patterns with partner and other current relationships: AM43 is overdependent on his partner and is very sensitive to what his partner thinks about his behavior. He wants to make him happy and feels very distressed when they argue.

Erickson's Psychosocial Developmental Stage

Describe development at each stage up to current stage

Trust vs. Mistrust (Infant Stage): Report normal early attachment

Autonomy vs. Shame and Doubt (Toddler Stage): Reports "always in trouble"; often spanked.

Initiative vs. Guilt (Preschool Age): Often in trouble for "acting up"; reports often feeling like "bad child"

(*continued*)

Industry vs. Inferiority (School Age): Sexually abused by teenaged cousin

Identity vs. Role Confusion (Adolescence): Struggled against attraction to other men; tried dating women; continued to not succeed in school; "trouble maker" reputation.

Intimacy vs. Isolation (Young Adulthood): Accepted sexual orientation in late teens; came out in early 20s to family.

Generativity vs. Stagnation (Adulthood): "Slow to be an adult"; doesn't want to grow old; does not like responsibility, time schedules, "boring life."

Ego Integrity vs. Despair (Late Adulthood): ______

Adlerian Style of Life Theme

❑ Control: ______

❑ Superiority: ______

❑ Pleasing: ______

☒ Comfort: AM has always sought fun, adventure, and comfort above all else.

Basic Mistake Misperceptions: I am a "bad" person because I don't like to work; because I am different.

VI. Humanistic-Existential Conceptualization

Expression of Authentic Self

Problems: Are problems perceived as internal or external (caused by others, circumstance, etc.)?

❑ Predominantly internal

☒ Mixed

❑ Predominantly external

Agency and Responsibility: Is self or other discussed as agent of story? Does client take clear responsibility for situation?

❑ Strong sense of agency and responsibility

❑ Agency in some areas

☒ Little agency; frequently blames others/situation

☒ Often feels victimized

Recognition and Expression of Feelings: Are feelings readily recognized, owned, and experienced?

❑ Easily expresses feelings

☒ Identifies feelings with prompting

❑ Difficulty recognizing feelings

Here-and-Now Experiencing: Is the client able to experience full range of feelings as they are happening in the present moment?

❑ Easily experiences emotions in present moment

❑ Experiences some present emotions with assistance

☒ Difficulty with present moment experiencing

Personal Constructs and Facades: Is the client able to recognize and go beyond roles? Is identity rigid or tentatively held?

❑ Tentatively held; able to critique and question

☒ Some awareness of facades and construction of identity

❑ Identity rigidly defined; seems like "fact"

(continued)

Complexity and Contradictions: Are internal contradictions owned and explored? Is client able to fully engage the complexity of identity and life?

❑ Aware of and resolves contradictions

☒ Some recognition of contradictions

❑ Unaware of internal contradictions

Shoulds: Is client able to question socially imposed shoulds and oughts? Can client balance desire to please others and desire to be authentic?

❑ Able to balance authenticity with social obligation

☒ Identifies tension between social expectations and personal desires

❑ Primarily focuses on external shoulds

List shoulds: I should be more invested in work and career. I should have started a family and have kids of my own by now.

Acceptance of Others: Is client able to accept others and modify expectations of others to be more realistic?

❑ Readily accepts others as they are

☒ Recognizes expectations of others are unrealistic but still strong emotional reaction to expectations not being met

❑ Difficulty accepting others as is; always wanting others to change to meet expectations

Trust of Self: Is client able to trust self as process (rather than a stabile object)?

❑ Able to trust and express authentic self

❑ Trust of self in certain contexts

☒ Difficulty trusting self in most contexts

Existential Analysis

Sources of Life Meaning (as described or demonstrated by client): AM finds meaning through his social relationships and family. He believes that the purpose of life is to have fun and be happy. He is very involved in the Latino gay community and has become an advocate for gay rights within his community. He is particularly passionate about creating a wider acceptance within the Catholic Church for LGBT individuals.

General Themes of Life Meaning:

❑ Personal achievement/work

☒ Significant other

❑ Children

☒ Family of origin

☒ Social cause/contributing to others

❑ Religion/spirituality

❑ Other: ______

Satisfaction with and clarity on life direction:

❑ Clear sense of meaning that creates resilience in difficult times

❑ Current problems require making choices related to life direction

☒ Minimally satisfied with current life direction; wants more from life

❑ Has reflected little on life direction up to this point; living according to life plan defined by someone/something else

❑ Other: ______

Gestalt Contact Boundary Disturbances

❑ *Desensitization:* Failing to notice problems

❑ *Introjection*: Take in others' views whole and unedited

(continued)

❑ *Projection*: Assign undesired parts of self to others
❑ *Retroflection*: Direct action to self rather than other
☒ *Deflection*: Avoid direct contact with another or self
❑ *Egotism:* Not allowing outside to influence self
❑ *Confluence*: Agree with another to extent that boundary blurred
Describe: AM avoids many of his feelings and problems through drinking and partying.

VII. Cognitive-Behavioral Conceptualization

Baseline of Symptomatic Behavior

Symptom #1 (behavioral description): Uses substances to point of intoxication

Frequency: Most days of the week

Duration: 4-6 hours

Context(s): At home during the week; at friend's house or club on Fri-Sun

Events Before: Have fun with friends; watching TV; come home from work

Events After: Go to sleep; pass out

Symptom #2 (behavioral description): Loss of interest in hobbies, relationship, and other normal activities

Frequency: Most days

Duration: 1-2 hours

Context(s): When not using substances; after using substances is worst

Events Before: Drinking alcohol or using substances

Events After: Watches television; goes to sleep

A-B-C Analysis of Irrational Beliefs

Activating Event ("Problem"): Having nothing "exciting" to do

Consequence (Mood, behavior, etc.): Using substances; feeling like nothing in life is worth it; feeling as though life is too hard.

Mediating Beliefs (Unhelpful beliefs about event that result in C):

1. Lack of excitement means something is wrong.
2. If he is not happy and having fun then it is not worth it.
3. __________

Beck's Schema Analysis

Identify frequently used cognitive schemas:

❑ *Arbitrary inference:* __________
☒ *Selective abstraction:* Focus on negative: "glass half empty"
❑ *Overgeneralization:* __________
☒ *Magnification/Minimization:* Exaggerates minor criticisms from others.
❑ *Personalization:* __________

(*continued*)

☒ *Absolutist/dichotomous thinking:* Either life is great or it is the pits.

❑ *Mislabeling:* ____

❑ *Mindreading:* ____

VIII. Family Systems Conceptualization

Family Life Cycle Stage

❑ Single adult
☒ Marriage/Partnered
❑ Family with Young Children
❑ Family with Adolescent Children
❑ Launching Children
❑ Later Life

Describe struggles with mastering developmental tasks in one of these stages: AM struggles with the responsibilities of being an adult and prefers to "have fun" and live carefree. This is hindering the growth of many of his relationships including that with his partner and family.

Boundaries with

Parents	☒ Enmeshed	❑ Clear	❑ Disengaged	❑ NA: *Describe:* Esp. with mother
Significant Other	☒ Enmeshed	❑ Clear	❑ Disengaged	❑ NA: *Describe:* Complementary roles of under-/overfunctioner.
Children	❑ Enmeshed	❑ Clear	❑ Disengaged	☒ NA: *Describe:*
Extended Family	❑ Enmeshed	❑ Clear	☒ Disengaged	☒ NA: *Describe:* Maternal grandparents very distant after he came out.
Other: Sister	☒ Enmeshed	❑ Clear	❑ Disengaged	❑ NA: *Describe:*

Typical style for regulating closeness and distance with others: Family often becomes overinvolved in each others' lives, feeling rejected or offended if a person even slightly disagrees.

Triangles/Coalitions

☒ Coalition in family of origin: *Describe:* Mother's favorite; she protected him against father's rules.

❑ Coalitions related to significant other: *Describe:* ____

❑ Other coalitions: ____

Hierarchy between Self and Parent/Child ☒ NA

With own children	❑ Effective ❑ Rigid ❑ Permissive
With parents (for child/young adult)	❑ Effective ❑ Rigid ❑ Permissive

Complementary Patterns with Significant Other:

❑ Pursuer/distancer
☒ Over/under-functioner
❑ Emotional/logical
❑ Good/bad parent
❑ Other: *Describe*

(continued)

Example of complementary pattern: AM's partner takes care of the responsibilities that AM does not view as "fun" or worthwhile. This allows AM43 to avoid responsibilities of adulthood and spend more time partying.

Intergenerational Patterns

Substance/Alcohol Abuse: ❑ NA ☒ History: Father heavy drinker; brothers also heavy drinkers and use substances.

Sexual/Physical/Emotional Abuse: ❑ NA ☒ History: Sexually abused by teenaged cousin; frequently spanked when young.

Parent/Child Relations: ❑ NA ☒ History: Generations are generally close with mothers especially connected with children.

Physical/Mental Disorders: ☒ NA ❑ History: ______

Family strengths: *Describe:* Family has been generally supportive of sexual orientation, although he has lost status as "favorite." Family generally supportive of one another and get together often.

IX. Solution-Based and Cultural Discourse Conceptualization (Postmodern)

Solutions and Unique Outcomes

Attempted Solutions that DIDN'T or DON'T work:

1. Using more substances.
2. Partner ignoring partying.
3. Avoiding work and family.

Exceptions and Unique Outcomes: Times, places, relationships, contexts, etc. when problem is less of a problem; behaviors that seem to make things even slightly better:

1. When partner demands AM "shape up," he usually reduces his substance and alcohol use for a week or two.
2. AM tends to control drinking somewhat better around family because they do not allow as much drinking as friends when partying (e.g., does not get "wasted").
3. When AM hangs out with partner, partner's circle of friends, and AM's old circle of friends, he does better.

Miracle Question Answer: If the problem were to be resolved overnight, what would client be doing differently the next day? (Describe in terms of doing X rather than not doing Y).

1. He would be socializing with people more close to his age.
2. He would be spending more time with his partner and family.
3. He would be working in a meaningful job that he enjoys going to.

Dominant Discourses informing definition of problem:

- *Ethnic, Class and Religious Discourses: How do key cultural discourses inform what is perceived as a problem and the possible solutions?* AM is a second-generation Mexican American living in the Southwest and

(*continued*)

earning a working wage. He generally feels proud of his heritage and is connected to the local Latino gay scene as well as "straight" Latino community. He feels less "at home" in his partner's social circles, which include more professionally trained white gay males. He feels most alienated in relation to the Catholic Church, where he feels accepted on the surface but then is painfully reminded that he is not.

- *Gender and Sexuality Discourses: How do the gender/sexual discourses inform what is perceived as a problem and the possible solutions?* In some ways, AM feels "outmanned" by his professional partner, especially when he is unable to work and contribute equally in terms of finances. Although he generally feels supported by his family, he also reports a lingering sense that he is a bit of disappointment to his parents because he is gay and does not have children. Thus, both with his partner and family, he has a nagging sense of not being man enough and also feeling like there is no way to change it.
- *Community, School, and Extended Family Discourses: How do other important community discourses inform what is perceived as a problem and the possible solutions?* As one of the "older" workers at most of his work sites, AM has been feeling increasing pressure to fit in with the younger crowd, which has been his access to increasingly more substances. Spending time with these friends triggers a feeling of "where is my life going?" and "how did I end here?"

Identity Narratives: How has the problem shaped each client's identity? AM's partying is driving a wedge between him and his partner; as AM becomes less functional, his partner becomes more functional, both in the relationship and at work. The roller coaster of substance use appears to be augmenting AM's sense that nothing in life has interest for him.

Local or Preferred Discourses: What is the client's preferred identity narrative and/or narrative about the problem? Are there local (alternative) discourses about the problem that are preferred? Although a part of AM feels that partying helps give him a sense of "having a life," another part of him (and certainly his partner) believes it leads to avoiding and not accepting the life he has and keeps him from creating an appropriate and meaningful life for a 43-year-old man.

CLINICAL ASSESSMENT

Clinician: Michael	Client ID #: 14002	Primary configuration: ☒ Individual ❑ Couple ❑ Family	Primary Language: ☒ English ❑ Spanish ❑ Other: ______

List client and significant others

Adult(s)

Adult Male Age: 43 Hispanic/Latino Partnered Gay/Lesbian/Bisexual Occupation: Construction Worker/ Carpenter Other identifier: ______

Adult Male: Partner Age: 44 Caucasian Partnered Gay/Lesbian/Bisexual Occupation: CPA Other identifier: Partner for 10 years

Child(ren)

Select Gender Age: ______ Select Ethnicity Grade: Select Grade School: ______ Other identifier: ______

Select Gender Age: ______ Select Ethnicity Grade: Select Grade School: ______ Other identifier: ______

Others: ______

Presenting Problems

☒ Depression/hopelessness
❑ Anxiety/worry
❑ Anger issues
❑ Loss/grief
☒ Suicidal thoughts/attempts
❑ Sexual abuse/rape
☒ Alcohol/drug use
❑ Eating problems/disorders
☒ Job problems/unemployed

☒ Couple concerns
❑ Parent/child conflict
❑ Partner violence/abuse
❑ Divorce adjustment
❑ Remarriage adjustment
❑ Sexuality/intimacy concerns
❑ Major life changes
❑ Legal issues/probation
❑ Other: ______

Complete for children:
❑ School failure/decline performance
❑ Truancy/runaway
❑ Fighting w/peers
❑ Hyperactivity
❑ Wetting/soiling clothing
❑ Child abuse/neglect
❑ Isolation/withdrawal
❑ Other: ______

Mental Status Assessment for Identified Patient

Interpersonal	❑ NA	❑ Conflict ☒ Enmeshment ❑ Isolation/Avoidance ❑ Harassment ☒ Other: Couple Problems
Mood	❑ NA	☒ Depressed/Sad ☒ Anxious ❑ Dysphoric ❑ Angry ❑ Irritable ❑ Manic ❑ Other: ______
Affect	❑ NA	☒ Constricted ❑ Blunt ❑ Flat ❑ Labile ❑ Incongruent ❑ Other: ______

(continued)

Sleep	❑ NA	☒ Hypersomnia ❑ Insomnia ❑ Disrupted ❑ Nightmares ❑ Other: ______
Eating	❑ NA	☒ Increase ❑ Decrease ❑ Anorectic restriction ❑ Binging ❑ Purging ❑ Other: ______
Anxiety	☒ NA	❑ Chronic worry ❑ Panic ❑ Phobias ❑ Obsessions ❑ Compulsions ❑ Other: ______
Trauma Symptoms	☒ NA	❑ Hypervigilance ❑ Flashbacks/Intrusive memories ❑ Dissociation ❑ Numbing ❑ Avoidance efforts ❑ Other: ______
Psychotic Symptoms	☒ NA	❑ Hallucinations ❑ Delusions ❑ Paranoia ❑ Loose associations ❑ Other: ______
Motor activity/ Speech	❑ NA	❑ Low energy ❑ Hyperactive ❑ Agitated ☒ Inattentive ☒ Impulsive ❑ Pressured speech ❑ Slow speech ❑ Other: ______
Thought	❑ NA	☒ Poor concentration ☒ Denial ❑ Self-blame ❑ Other-blame ❑ Ruminative ❑ Tangential ☒ Concrete ☒ Poor insight ❑ Impaired decision making ❑ Disoriented ❑ Other: ______
Socio-Legal	❑ NA	☒ Disregards rules ❑ Defiant ❑ Stealing ❑ Lying ❑ Tantrums ❑ Arrest/incarceration ❑ Initiates fights ❑ Other: ______
Other Symptoms	☒ NA	______

Diagnosis for Identified Patient

Contextual Factors considered in making diagnosis: ☒ Age ☒ Gender ☒ Family dynamics ☒ Culture ❑ Language ☒ Religion ☒ Economic ❑ Immigration ☒ Sexual/Gender orientation ☒ Trauma ☒ Dual diagnosis/Comorbid ☒ Addiction ❑ Cognitive ability ❑ Other: ______

Describe impact of identified factors on diagnosis and assessment process: ______

DSM-5 Code	Diagnosis with Specifier *Include V/Z/T-Codes for Psychosocial Stressors/Issues*
1. F10.20	1. Alcohol Use Disorder; Moderate
2. F90.2	2. ADHD; Combined Type
3. Z63.0	3. Relationship distress with spouse or intimate partner
4. Z56.9	4. Other problem related to employment
5. ______	5. ______

Medical Considerations

Has patient been referred for psychiatric evaluation? ☒ Yes ❑ No

Has patient agreed with referral? ☒ Yes ❑ No ❑ NA

(continued)

Psychometric instruments used for assessment: ❑ None ❑ Cross-cutting symptom inventories

❑ Other: Michigan Alcoholic Screening Test; Outcome questionnaire

Client response to diagnosis: ❑ Agree ☒ Somewhat agree ❑ Disagree ❑ Not informed for following reason: _______

Current Medications (psychiatric & medical) ❑ NA

1. Adderal; dose 40 mg; start date: September 10, 2010
2. _______; dose _______ mg; start date: _________
3. _______; dose _______ mg; start date: _________
4. _______; dose _______ mg; start date: _________

Medical Necessity: *Check all that apply*

☒ Significant impairment ❑ Probability of significant impairment ❑ Probable developmental arrest

Areas of impairment: ☒ Daily activities ☒ Social relationships ❑ Health ☒ Work/School ❑ Living arrangement

❑ Other: ___________________________

Risk and Safety Assessment for Identified Patient

Suicidality	Homicidality	Alcohol Abuse
☒ No indication/Denies	☒ No indication/Denies	❑ No indication/denies
❑ Active ideation	❑ Active ideation	❑ Past abuse
☒ Passive ideation	❑ Passive ideation	☒ Current; Freq/Amt: Most days/4-12
❑ Intent without plan	❑ Intent without means	**Drug Use/Abuse**
❑ Intent with means	❑ Intent with means	❑ No indication/denies
❑ Ideation in past year	❑ Ideation in past year	❑ Past use
❑ Attempt in past year	❑ Violence past year	☒ Current drugs: MJ; esctasy; cocaine
❑ Family or peer history of completed suicide	❑ History of assaulting others	Freq/Amt: 1–2 × week; varies
	❑ Cruelty to animals	❑ Family/sig.other use

Sexual & Physical Abuse and Other Risk Factors

☒ Childhood abuse history: ☒ Sexual ☒ Physical ❑ Emotional ❑ Neglect

❑ Adult with abuse/assault in adulthood: ❑ Sexual ❑ Physical ❑ Current

❑ History of perpetrating abuse: ❑ Sexual ❑ Physical ❑ Emotional

❑ Elder/dependent adult abuse/neglect

❑ History of or current issues with restrictive eating, binging, and/or purging

❑ Cutting or other self harm: ❑ Current ❑ Past: Method: ___________________

❑ Criminal/legal history: ___________________________

❑ Other trauma history: ___________________________

❑ None reported

(continued)

Indicators of Safety

❑ NA

☒ Willingness to reduce contact with people who make situation worse

☒ At least one outside support person

☒ Willing to implement safety plan, safety interventions

☒ Able to cite specific reasons to live or not harm

☒ Developing set of alternatives to self/other harm

❑ Hopeful

☒ Sustained period of safety: Has never acted on passive ideation

☒ Willing to dispose of dangerous items

❑ Other: ______

❑ Has future goals

Elements of Safety Plan

❑ NA

☒ Plan for contacting friends/support persons during crisis

☒ Verbal no harm contract

❑ Specific plan of where to go during crisis

❑ Written no harm contract

☒ Specific self-calming tasks to reduce risk before reach crisis level (e.g., journaling, exercising, etc.)

☒ Emergency contact card

❑ Specific daily/weekly activities to reduce stressors

☒ Emergency therapist/agency number

❑ Other: ______

☒ Medication management

Legal/Ethical Action Taken: ☒ NA ❑ Action: ______

Case Management

Collateral Contacts

- Has contact been made with treating *physicians or other professionals*: ❑ NA ☒ Yes ❑ In process. Name/Notes: Dr. Gonzalez; Consulted briefly with MD on harm reduction plan; MD okay with progress.
- If client is involved in mental health *treatment elsewhere*, has contact been made? ☒ NA ❑ Yes ❑ In process. Name/Notes: ______
- Has contact been made with *social worker*: ☒ NA ❑ Yes ❑ In process. Name/Notes: ______

Referrals

- Has client been referred for *medical assessment*: ☒ Yes ❑ No evidence for need
- Has client been referred for *social services*: ☒ NA ❑ Job/training ❑ Welfare/Food/Housing ❑ Victim services ❑ Legal aid ❑ Medical ❑ Other: ______
- Has client been referred for *group* or other support services: ☒ Yes: ______ ❑ In process ❑ None recommended
- Are there anticipated *forensic/legal processes* related to treatment: ☒ No ❑ Yes; describe: ______

(continued)

Support Network

- Client social support network includes: ☒ Supportive family ☒ Supportive partner ☒ Friends ❑ Religious/spiritual organization ❑ Supportive work/social group ❑ Other: ______
- Describe anticipated effects treatment will have on others in support system (children, partner, etc.): Partner supportive; family of origin may have difficulty with AM deciding to reduce or stop drinking.
- Is there anything else client will need to be successful? Dual treatment of substances and ADHD

Expected Outcome and Prognosis

☒ Return to normal functioning ❑ Anticipate less than normal functioning ❑ Prevent deterioration

Client Sense of Hope: 3

Evaluation of Assessment/Client Perspective

How were assessment methods adapted to client needs, including age, culture, and other diversity issues? Carefully considered family and cultural drinking and socialization norms; gay Latino socializing patterns.

Describe actual or potential areas of client-clinician agreement/disagreement related to the above assessment: AM does not see self as alcoholic or substance abuser; agrees with ADHD and willing to try medication as an adult.

______, ______ ______

Clinician Signature License/Intern Status Date

______, ______ ______

Supervisor Signature License Date

TREAMENT PLAN

Date: September 14, 2013 Case/Client #: 14002

Clinician Name: Michael Theory: Postmodern (integrate feminist, narrative, collaborative)

Modalities planned: ☒ Individual Adult ❑ Individual Child ☒ Couple ❑ Family ❑ Group: ______

Recommended session frequency: ☒ Weekly ❑ Every two weeks ❑ Other: ______

Expected length of treatment: 9 months

Initial Phase of Treatment

Initial Phase Counseling Tasks

1. Develop working counseling relationship. *Diversity considerations:* Involve partner, family of origin, and key friends. Consider dynamics of working with a straight male therapist and carefully attend to creating a strong sense of safey and respect for AM. As a professional male, counselor must consider how the counseling relationship may replicate the white-collar/blue-collar tension he has with his partner and must identify ways to use this to increase his awareness and sense of safety at home.

   Relationship building approach/intervention:

   a. Meet client apart from "Partying"/ADHD and provide opportunities to share experience as gay, working-class male from immigrant Latino, Catholic family.

2. Assess individual, systemic, and broader cultural dynamics. *Diversity considerations:* Attend to substance use patterns across systems, considering cultural norms for drinking. Assess AM role in and effects of gay community, Latino community, and white-collar/blue-collar social groups.

   Assessment strategies:

   a. Deconstructive questions and relative influence questions to explore effect of "Partying"/ADHD on all involved and effect of persons (strengths and resources) on the life of the "Partying"/ADHD and to explore effects of the political on the personal.

   b. Hear from all parties affected by and discussing the "Partying"/ADHD to understand their definitions of the problem and ideas on how best to deal with it.

3. Identify and obtain client agreement on treatment goals. *Diversity note:* Ensure client agreement with dual dx goals.

   Goal-making intervention:

   a. Be public with counselor goals and utilize client expertise to develop goals to address both substance use and ADHD.

4. Identify needed referrals, crisis issues, and other client needs. *Diversity note:* Work with MD and psychiatrist on possible need for detox and/or medication management.

(continued)

a. *Crisis assessment intervention(s):* Develop safety plan regarding passive suicidal ideation.

b. *Referral(s):* Work with MD on plan for reducing/ending substance use and monitor detox complications; refer to dual dx group where AM feels accepted and comfortable.

Initial Phase Client Goal

1. Increase identification with his "responsible" (preferred) self to reduce alcohol and substance use.

Interventions:

a. Statement of position map to enable AM to develop a clear and strong position on his relationship to alcohol and drugs, including his use of Adderall to manage ADHD, as well as articulate his values and identity apart from substance use; involve partner and family in discussions.

b. Mutual puzzling, not knowing, and curiosity to help AM develop stategies and solutions to managing his substance use, that he is committed to employ.

Working Phase of Treatment

Working Phase Counseling Tasks

1. Monitor quality of the working alliance. *Diversity considerations:* Continually monitor for client sense of feeling accepted and not being judged by counselor related to sexual orientation, socioeconomic status, or substance use.

   a. *Assessment Intervention:* Publicly discuss counseling alliance, esp. as it relates to feeling pushed by counselor on substance use issues and to ensure AM openly shares thoughts and experiences and maintains sense of agency and investment in change.

2. Monitor progress toward goals. *Diversity considerations:* Use reports of partner and family as well as client to monitor progress, esp. with substance use.

   a. *Assessment Intervention:* Regularly check with partner and family as well as client on progress; use Outcome Rating Scale.

Working Phase Client Goals

1. Increase identification with preferred self and preferred behaviors to reduce impulsivity and irresponsible choices.

   Interventions:

   a. Deconstructive questions and statement of position map to identify affects of ADHD behaviors, and label from childhood through adulthood, considering political impact of other labels: gay, male, Latino, working-class, adult with ADHD, etc.; develop position in relation to ADHD.

   b. Scaffolding conversations to thicken identity narrative around being a "mature adult" who is able to balance fun, work, and personal obligations.

2. Increase sense of personal empowerment and "mattering" to others to reduce loss of interest and connection.

(continued)

Interventions:

a. Identify sources of marginalization and oppression and how they have affected his choices to "party" and his ADHD behaviors over the years; link to motivation to make better choices with drugs and alcohol.

b. Build relationships and connect with communities in which he feels he matters and feels empowered to make good decisions for his life.

3. Increase number of growth-fostering relationships to reduce substance use.

Interventions:

a. Mutual puzzling in couple sessions with AM44 to increase intimacy and equal functioning in the relationship.

b. Scaffolding questions to explore how to deepen relationship with family of origin and to choose how to relate to each group of friends to promote best self.

Closing Phase of Treatment

Closing Phase Counseling Task

1. Develop aftercare plan and maintain gains. *Diversity considerations:* Include resources and supportive others in gay and Latino communities.

Intervention:

a. Map in landscapes of action and consciousness as to how to respond to invitations to misuse substances again or to act on ADHD habits.

Closing Phase Client Goals

1. Increase personal investment in identity as "an adult who makes mature, responsible decisions and can still have fun" to reduce misuse of substances and failure to respond to ADHD symptoms.

Interventions:

a. Statement of position map and relative influence questioning to have AM redefine relationship to substances and ADHD; involve AM44 in positioning conversations.

b. Involve AM in social advocacy activities in which he serves as role model to others (e.g., Latino teens) on how to make responsible decisions.

2. Increase social connections that support AM's "mature but fun" identity to reduce relapse potential.

Interventions:

a. Invite partner, family, and friends to share their experiences of AM's new choices and behaviors; map each person's perspective in landscapes of action and consciousness.

b. Have AM create written or artistic documentation of his counseling journey, to solidify new narrative and identity; write a final closing letter that documents journey from counselor perspective.

PROGRESS NOTE FOR CLIENT #14002

Date: Sept 21, 2013 **Time:** 5:00 ❑ am/☒ pm **Session Length:** ☒ 45 min. ❑ 60 min. ❑ Other: ______ minutes

Present: ☒ Adult Male ❑ Adult Female ❑ Child Male ❑ Child Female ☒ Other: AM44 (Partner)

Billing Code: ❑ 90791 (eval) ❑ 90834 (45 min. therapy) ❑ 90837 (60 min. therapy) ☒ 90847 (family)

❑ Other: ______

Symptom(s)	Duration and Frequency Since Last Visit	Progress
1: Drinking	3 days/4-6 drinks per day	**Progressing**
2: Impulsivity	Mild; 2 days	**Progressing**
3: Responsible choices	Significantly improved; on time to work 5 days; more proactive at work.	**Significantly Improved**

Explanatory Notes on Symptoms: Reports no substance use besides alcohol on weekend; AM44 verified report; AM43 reports that having AM44 there helps keep him accountable. AM43 reports renewed commitment to work and AM44 feels increased energy and hope.

In-Session Interventions and Assigned Homework

Map positive developments in landscapes of action and consciousness to increase both men's awareness of how positive choices affect both parties' sense of well-being, "mattering," and positive identity. Discuss both partners' position in relation to alcohol, substances, and social networks who use substances. Identified best social scenes to bring out "mature fun." Identified how to continue with positive choices for next week.

Client Response/Feedback

AM43 energized by landscape of consciousness conversations where he "sees" how choices affect how he feels. AM44 eager to be part of process.

Plan

☒ Continue with treatment plan: plan for next session: Follow up on homework with socializing in supportive networks.

❑ Modify plan: ______

Next session: Date: Sept 28, 2016 Time: 5:00 ❑ am/☒ pm

Crisis Issues: ☒ No indication of crisis/client denies ❑ Crisis assessed/addressed: describe below

Reports adhering to harm reduction plan; not drinking and driving; partner and he report no substance use other than alcohol.

______, ______ ______

Clinician's Signature License/Intern Status Date

Case Consultation/Supervision ❑ Not Applicable

Notes: Reviewed substance use and safety issues with supervisor, who continued to encourage contact with partner to get accurate monitoring of substance use.

(continued)

Collateral Contact ❑ Not Applicable

Name: Dr. Gonzalez Date of Contact: September 15, 2013 Time: 10:45 ☒am/❑pm

☒ Written release on file: ☒ Sent/❑ Received ❑ In court docs ❑ Other: ______

Notes: Consulted briefly with MD on harm reduction plan; MD okay with progress.

______,	______	______
Clinician's Signature	License/Intern Status	Date
______,	______	______
Supervisor's Signature	License	Date

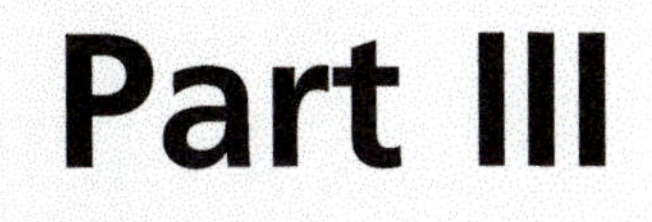

Part III

The Competent Supervisee

CHAPTER

15

The Competent Supervisee

What I Wish I'd Known Before I Saw My First Client

I began seeing clients at a domestic violence center in the Southwest when I was 23 years old. I had taken only two graduate classes—counseling theories and ethics—during the introductory summer session before having to enroll in my first fieldwork class that required seeing clients (yes, they changed their course sequencing the next year). Excited and terrified, I greeted my first client in the waiting room and awkwardly walked her to the counseling room. My client was a petite and delicate woman, slightly older than myself. Her hair was black, which was striking against her alabaster skin; I would later learn that she was a quarter Cherokee, a heritage in which she took pride.

After I inelegantly introduced her to the confidentiality clauses, mandated reporting, and agency policies, she began to speak. After describing her current violent relationship, I happened to ask about any prior abuse, which prompted her to describe three separate incidents of childhood sexual abuse perpetrated by U.S. military personnel (her mother was attracted to men in uniform) and another emotionally abusive dating relationship as an adult that included stalking. I listened intently, but periodically my mind would flash with the thought: "This woman needs a *real* counselor—not me. I can't possibly help her—she has *real* problems. I don't know enough. I won't be good enough to help her for years. Certainly not without a license or doctoral degree in hand. Even then, she needs a specialist. Some who is *really*, *really* good. Not me." Needless to say, my first session was a bit overwhelming.

At the end of the session, the woman paused and stared at me intently. There were several seconds (seemed like millennia) of dead silence in the room as I waited for her to say what was clearly on the tip of her tongue. As I quietly waited, I expected (and almost hoped) she would say something like, "Clearly, you are totally incapable of helping me. Can I please be assigned a competent counselor?" Instead, she calmly said with a sense of certainty, "I think I can work with you. I have had several other counselors in the past who didn't seem to get me. But, I think I can work with you." And we did. She taught me a lot over the two-plus years we worked together making sense of her difficult past and creating a safe and joyful future together. The dream catcher she made me still hangs in my office as a reminder of what is important in counseling—being fully present as a compassionate witness for another person's suffering. It's an attitude, a way of being. I didn't have to be perfect to be helpful to someone in pain. I just had to be there—*really* there.

Obviously, I had significant help from my supervisor, who spent over an hour after the intake session trying to get the information she needed to help me manage the various crises, abuse, and reporting issues; had I known what to tell her, it would have taken less than fifteen minutes. With that first client, I also learned that being an effective supervisee is different from learning to be an effective counselor—two separate skill sets.

As you now know, I stumbled initially, learning to be a counselor and supervisee. I began with the incorrect assumption that what I said mattered more than who I was in the room. I also incorrectly believed that my supervisor would have to do most of the thinking work because I didn't know enough. This chapter is designed to help you more gracefully enter the profession.

In this chapter, I discuss much of what I wish I'd known before I met my first client, knowledge about how to be a competent supervisee. Some might argue that a supervisee cannot be competent by definition. However, over the years I have come to realize there are specific skills, attitudes, and behaviors that are unique to being a successful *supervisee*. Traditionally, most counselors learn these rarely spoken expectations through trial and error and experience, the great teacher. But, I believe many people are capable of learning these things in a more gentle way: simple explanation. Thus, in this chapter, I will cover the seldom-discussed essentials skills of being a competent counselor supervisee:

- Managing Initial Anxiety
- Understanding Your Role as Supervisee
- Setting Realistic Expectations of the Supervisor's Role
- Managing Professional Paperwork
- Getting the Most from Supervision
- Handling Problems in Supervision
- Finding a Training Site

Managing Initial Anxiety

After a few weeks of seeing clients, many of the students in my fieldwork classes at the university exclaim: "Why did you let us go into the field? We aren't ready! We need more classes, role-plays, videos, knowledge, experience!" In response, I unapologetically share an uncomfortable truth: they could enroll in 100 classes and watch 1,000 hours of videos of the world's best counselors and therapists but would never feel truly "ready" to see clients—or if they did, they wouldn't for long. Learning to counsel is much like learning how to swim: you can watch hours of YouTube videos and read a tower of how-to books, but you still have to get wet to figure it out. Even with the best classroom training, you *will* struggle at first—there is no avoiding it. After a fair amount of practice, there will still be days when it feels like you have been dumped into the deep end of the pool without a swim lesson (or role-play). In these moments, your ability to manage your anxiety will determine whether you sink or swim. So, let's make sure you swim.

One of the more surprising secrets to becoming a competent supervisee is that in the first years of training it isn't how much you know that determines your competence but rather your ability to simply *recall* what you have learned thus far. In many cases, the primary impediment to competency in this early period is anxiety—not lack of knowledge. In general, optimal performance is associated with optimal levels of anxiety: not too much or too little (Eysenck, 2013). For new counselors, the struggle is typically feeling overwhelmed by too much performance anxiety when they start seeing clients (Lawrence, Cassell, Beattie, Woodman, Khan, Hardy, & Gottwald, 2013; Tsai, 2012). This anxiety triggers the stress response, a physiological response designed to help us outrun bears and fight saber-toothed tigers. However, this hyperphysical state typically diminishes a person's access to the prefrontal cortex, where language, higher reasoning, and everything learned in class are stored (Siegel, 2010). Thus, many new counselors often report "going blank" when first talking to clients. After years of watching even the brightest and most articulate students go silent in session with the deer-in-the-headlight response, I have found the most expedient means to competent counseling in the first year of training is to help new trainees manage their stress response—so they can access what they know.

Supervisees have many options for learning how to manage their anxiety. Most of the theories in this book offer options, most notably the cognitive-behavioral methods. Other possibilities include exercise, meditation, spiritual practices, breathing exercises, and practice with anxiety (Lawrence et al., 2013). Of these, my colleague Eric McCollum and I have found mindfulness—and contemplative practices more broadly—surprisingly effective and easy to implement with our students in their first year of training (Gehart & McCollum, 2007, 2008; McCollum & Gehart, 2010). I find it second only to live supervision, in terms of helping new counselors develop competence in the first year.

Mindfulness (discussed more fully in Chapter 11) is a meditation technique that involves simply observing a single phenomenon as it occurs in the moment (such as watching yourself breathe) while quieting the mind's inner chatter. Each time the mind wanders off, the practitioner compassionately returns to the point of focus without berating the self or otherwise giving oneself a hard time. This practice—when done regularly—increases a person's physiological and psychological ability to manage the stress response (Siegel, 2010); translated to the life of a supervisee, that means when you begin to become anxious in session with a client, you will be able to quickly calm yourself so that you can access all of the wonderful information you have learned in class and in the volumes of books you have read.

To examine whether mindfulness really makes a difference, my colleague and I did a study to analyze the changes students noticed after practicing mindfulness (McCollum & Gehart, 2010). We asked our students to practice five to ten minutes per day, five to seven days per week, and virtually all reported that they noticed significant changes both in and out of the therapy session. Specifically, supervisees reported being better able to be emotionally present with clients, less anxious in session, and better able to respond in difficult moments. Most report that their overall level of stress decreased noticeably within two weeks of practicing five days a week for two to ten minutes; they also report better relationships and a greater sense of inner peace. Not bad for a 10–50-minute-per-week investment. So you might want to give it a try.

Starting Your Personal Mindfulness Practice

1. **Find a Regular Time:** The most difficult part of doing mindfulness is finding time—two to ten minutes—several days a week. My colleague Eric and I have our students do five days per week. It is best to "attach" mindfulness practice to some part of your regular routine, such as before or after breakfast, working out, brushing your teeth, seeing clients, coming home, or going to bed (if you are not too tired).
2. **Find a Partner or Group (Optional):** If possible, find a partner or meditation group with whom you can practice on a regular basis. The camaraderie will help keep you motivated.
3. **Find a Timer (Highly Advisable):** Using a timer helps structure the mindfulness session, and many find it helps them focus better because they don't wonder if time is up. Most mobile phones have alarms and timers that work well; you can also purchase meditation apps with Tibetan chimes for iPhones and other smartphones. Digital egg-timers work well, too—avoid the ones that tick. You may also try a recorded meditation like the ones listed below.
4. **Sit Comfortably:** When you are ready, find a comfortable chair to sit in. Ideally, you should not rest your back against the chair, but rather sit toward the front so that your spine is erect. If this is too uncomfortable, sit normally with your spine straight—but not rigid.
5. **Breathe:** Set your timer for two minutes initially and then watch yourself breathe while quieting the thoughts and any other chatter in your mind.

   - Don't try to change your breathing; just notice its qualities, not judging it as good or bad.
   - Know that your mind will wander off numerous times—both to inner and outer distractions—each time it does gently notice it without judging—perhaps

(*continued*)

imagine it disappearing like a cloud drifting off, soap bubbles popping, or say "ah, that too"—and then gently return your focus to watching your breath.

- Accept your mind how it is each time you practice; some days it is easier to focus than others. The key is to practice acceptance of "what is," rather than fall into the common pattern of being frustrated with what is not happening.
- The goal is *not* to have extended periods without thinking but rather to practice nonjudgmental acceptance and cultivate a better sense of how the mind works.

6. **Notice:** When the bell rings, notice how you feel. The same, more relaxed, more stressed? Try only to notice without judging. You may or may not feel much difference; the most helpful effects are cumulative rather than immediate. If you happen to notice that you wish the bell did not ring so soon, go ahead and add a minute or two the next time you practice. Slowly, you will add minutes until you find a length of time that works well for you. Don't extend the time until you feel a desire to do so.
7. **Repeat:** Our students report the best outcomes with shorter, regular practices rather than longer but infrequent practices. Thus, doing five two-minute practices is likely to produce better outcomes than one ten-minute session each week.

Resources to Support Your Practice

- *Free Meditation Podcasts:* You can download free guided mindfulness meditations and other free resources to support your practice from my website www.dianegehart.com and from UCLA's Mindfulness Awareness Research Center website www.marc.ucla.edu.
- *Workbooks: The Mindfulness-Based Stress Reduction Workbook* (Stahl & Goldstein, 2010) and *Get Out of Your Mind and into Your Life: The New Acceptance and Commitment Therapy* (Hayes & Smith, 2005) are excellent workbooks to teach you practical techniques.

If mindfulness is not your thing, that is fine. There are numerous other practices, tools, and self-care techniques that can help you manage anxiety and to reduce the sense of "going blank" or feeling overwhelmed in session. I promise, although any anxiety-management approach takes time, it will be worth it, and you will find yourself feeling "competent" far sooner.

Your Role as Supervisee: Proactive Learner

Training programs cover a lot of material before sending new supervisees out to do counseling for the first time: empathetic responding, crisis management, theory, diagnosis, techniques, laws, and ethics. But something is missing. Because, upon arriving at their first clinical experience, supervisees are placed in a supervision group and then "expected" to magically know what to do. Most supervisors assume their supervisees will know how to effectively "receive" supervision; but that is probably because they forgot how little they knew as first-year trainees and how lost they felt. Additionally, as we have more diverse supervisees and supervisors, the assumption that each instinctively knows or can quickly decipher the expectations of his/her role is problematic. Being an effective supervisee is a unique skill that must be learned as part of becoming a competent counselor.

The Hallmarks of a Professional

When I was in graduate school, I was hired to do career assessment and counseling for a large military grant my professor oversaw. Upon hiring me, my professor clarified what he meant by "professional behavior" and "punctuality": "I don't care if you are in the morgue with a toe tag, someone better be here to meet your clients in the morning—and they better be on time." He was dead serious. At first, I was taken aback by his expectations—almost offended. But over the years, those words and the dedication they imply have stayed with me, echoing in my head. In addition to always having a plan in case of my untimely demise, these words impressed upon me that being a professional entails obligations that do not come with other types of jobs. Being a professional requires a deep sense of dedication, discipline, and selflessness that is hard to learn from a book (even though I am trying with this one).

My appreciation for what it means to be a professional was further shaped by the calls I have received from potential employers of my former students and supervisees. When I first started answering such calls, I was surprised to learn that they were more interested in the professional habits of my students than in their counseling skills. They focused their reference questions on character and habits:

- Is the applicant typically on time and reliable?
- Is the applicant easy to supervise?
- Does the applicant follow through on instructions?
- Does the applicant know when to ask for help and when to handle things independently?
- Does the applicant get along well with others?
- Can the applicant write?
- Can the applicant solve problems independently?
- Can the applicant manage paperwork and keep up with deadlines?
- Can the applicant work with a variety of personalities and ages?
- Does the applicant work well in diverse settings?

Although prospective employers also asked about actual counseling skills—forming relationships with clients and intervening—their greatest concern is virtually always about professional skills. Over the years, it has dawned on me that the reason they focus on this is that these professional habits and personal qualities are much harder to teach than actual counseling skills. Otherwise stated, supervisors are trained and ready to teach a person how to become a better counselor; that typically happens relatively easily. But the habits that define professionalism—punctuality, reliability, discernment, and judgment—are much more difficult to impart to a new counselor. Thus, these are important skills to cultivate early in one's career.

Proactive Learner

Although there are many models of supervision (Aasheim, 2012; Bernard & Goodyear, 2009; Bradley & Ladany, 2010; Campbell, 2000; Harris & Brockbank, 2011; Stoltenberg, McNeill, & Delworth, 2010), they all share the goal of developing supervisee autonomy. Thus, it is fair to say—although few supervisors say it this plainly—that being a proactive learner is the foundation to being successful. More so than in the classroom, where a passive learning style is typically rewarded, learning how to be a counselor requires far more initiation and self-guided learning (Tsai, 2012; Weimer, 2002). Supervisees hoping for a supervisor to tell them what to do, think, or say will not thrive—even when a supervisor is willing to oblige such expectations. Instead, a more preferred stance for a supervisee is to actively be in charge of identifying what they need to learn and determining how best to learn it.

Each supervisee—even those at the same agency—has a unique learning agenda based on the particular clients/cases assigned and each supervisee's personal set of strengths and areas for growth. There is no single learning agenda that fits all supervisees, even though there are some common competencies that all must learn (Lee & Nelson, 2014; Rust, Raskin, & Hill, 2013). Quite honestly, unless your supervisor is observing most of your cases, there is no way for your supervisor to psychically or magically know what your learning agenda needs to be, either. If relying primarily on a case report (your description of what happened in session), your supervisor is seriously handicapped in terms of knowing precisely what it is you need and how to help you best.

Thus, requesting as much live supervision as possible is critical in the first year of training. After that, it is up to you to critically examine what is and is not happening in your sessions, and to identify what you need most help with.

For many students, the role of proactive learner is awkward if not foreign. Let's face it: most graduate students have achieved their success because they have excelled at and mastered the essential skills of higher learning: sit quietly, listen, read, take notes, follow instructions, and remember what you were told. Unfortunately, initiative is not the first skill rewarded in modern education, although there are movements to change this (Weimer, 2002). For successful counselor trainees, the shift to practicum and fieldwork is the shift to proactive learning.

Proactive learning as a supervisee generally entails the following:

- *Answering Your Own Questions:* Whether about an agency policy, state regulatory board rule, or clinical issue, it is best to assume that you should try to answer your questions first through your own research and resources rather than running to your supervisor with every single little question (and there will be a ton of them). Even if your supervisor is happy to answer these for you, you will become competent faster if you at least do a little searching before you raise a white flag.
- *Asking Great Questions:* When you do ask questions, ask them well. I address specifically how to do this later in the chapter; we need to cover more ground covering this important topic.
- *Identify What Needs to Happen:* You should have a good road map of what needs to happen (a) for you to get the hours you need, (b) for a client to be seen at your agency, and (c) for a session to go well. Study the agency's policy manual if you need to, but it is important to have a very clear picture of all the steps that need to happen so that you can intelligently identify what you need to be doing.
- *Identify Where You Need Help:* At the end of each session, it is important to reflect on what went well and what may not have gone so well. Rather than berate yourself or consider a change of career, spend some time figuring out what you need to know and trying to educate yourself so that you can then get the most out of your supervisee experience.

For many, the greatest impediment to being a proactive learner is confidence—lacking confidence that they can succeed in this field (Fernando, 2013; Tsai, 2012). The truth is: No new supervisee is totally ready and prepared to effectively and easily carry out the many and varied tasks associated with being a competent counselor. And that is okay. It really is. But having the right attitude, one in which you take full responsibility for learning what you need to know is the key to competence.

Receiving Feedback

For many, one of the greatest challenges of being a supervisee is being able to receive feedback (Reifer, 2001; Tsai, 2012). Especially if you have already been accomplished in another field, learning to take the position of a novice who receives constant correction can be difficult. Some start out with the secret hope that learning to do professional counseling and psychotherapy will be easy: that somehow, "I will be the exception." Similarly, even though most states require a process that spans a minimum of five years to practice independently, many still have the unspoken hope that most of what they are going to hear from a supervisor will be a continuous series of positive affirmations similar to what they received in school: "good job," "A+," "best I've ever seen," "amazing work." Although this is often the case toward the end of those five years, in the beginning virtually all new counselors will receive a constant stream of constructive feedback and/or—the more dreaded term—criticism.

Perhaps because the counseling process touches on such vulnerable emotions and the stakes often feel high (that is, supervisees sincerely want to be helpful to those they work with), many supervisees have great difficulty hearing constructive criticism and feedback from their supervisors, even when the feedback is well intended (Reifer, 2001; Tsai, 2012). It is true that some supervisors will be "harsher" than others, but over the years I have found that the best supervisors (a) are generally surprisingly direct and

(b) provide lots of constructive criticism and suggestions for improvement. Much as we may enjoy their positive, nonthreatening attitudes, supervisors who are saccharine-sweet cheerleaders and give you the sense that you are a gifted-genius-prodigy of a counselor often are the ones from which you learn the least. Much like the teachers who are "hard" and "intimidating" in the classroom, you often learn the most from those supervisors who are able to show you where and how to improve.

Typically, early in the process of being supervised, you will want reassurance from your supervisor about whether you are doing a "good" job (Reifer, 2001; Tsai, 2012). First of all, I encourage you to set your standard at doing a "good enough" job: you really do not need to be perfect to be helpful to your clients. If, early on, you need reassurance that you are good enough and your supervisor is not freely giving it, simply ask your supervisor directly rather than anxiously wonder and second-guess yourself or your supervisor. Sometimes supervisors need the nudge. Otherwise, if your supervisor is quick to make suggestions, put your pride aside if you need to and then take notes, and learn. It is such a precious time in your professional life that you have someone sit down with you and help you think through your work with clients. It is a rare and special gift, even if your ego stings a little bit. Once it is no longer there, you will miss it.

The Developing Supervisee

Another way to understand your journey as a supervisee is to consider it from a developmental perspective. Stoltenberg et al. (2010) conceptualize the development of counselors and therapists in three phases:

- *Level 1: The New Supervisee:* Entry-level counselors typically are highly motivated yet also highly anxious. Because these counselors are still learning what to focus on, observation by a supervisor is particularly helpful at this stage.
- *Level 2: Mid-Level Supervisee:* As supervisees gain experience, they begin to develop a sense of confidence, which can fluctuate significantly based on a given experience with clients. During Level 2, supervisees are more willing to explore new approaches and become comfortable with a wider range of skills. At this level, supervisees also become better able to identify and process their own personal issues that may be affecting the counseling process.
- *Level 3: Advanced Supervisee:* As supervisees become more experienced and autonomous, they develop a more secure and stable sense of confidence and motivation. At this stage, supervisees are able to better balance (a) being empathetic and emotionally attuned, with (b) challenging clients to grow. They are also better able to use the "self of the counselor" to promote change with clients.

Your Supervisor's Role: Realistic Expectations

Neither Omniscient nor Omnipotent

When most of us meet our first supervisor, it is common to assume that all supervisors are competent in all areas of counseling and psychotherapy practice. Supervisors have passed the licensing exam, after all—and, certainly if they did it 30 years ago, then they are really, really competent. Since supervisors already finished all the classes in their master's programs—or even doctoral programs—and have been practicing for years, then they should be very knowledgeable. Perhaps. Often that is the case. But not always. Although such an assumption is sound and logical, it does not capture the complexity of real-world practice.

A more realistic assumption is that any given supervisor has special areas of competence and expertise. One may be an excellent diagnostician, another a theoretician, and yet a third well grounded in law, ethics, and case documentation. Ideally, all supervisors are basically competent in all these areas. More realistically, most are competent in a few. Too often, my students describe supervision experiences in which a supervisor is not up to par in one or more areas.

What is a supervisee to do? Having realistic expectations of your future or current supervisor can significantly reduce potential frustrations. Here are some realistic expectations:

- Supervisor is competent in seeing the average client in your clinical setting.
- Supervisor will know the most commonly used legal and ethical guidelines in his/her work context.
- Supervisor—if an employee of the site—will have a general sense of policies and procedures of the site. If not, the clinical supervisor may expect you to master these with the help of a site coordinator.
- Supervisor may identify his/her preferred therapeutic model, but may not have extensive training or expertise with the model.
- Supervisor may not have any specific therapeutic model and may work from an "eclectic" approach.
- Supervisor will have decent skills in managing common crisis issues.
- Supervisor will be able to tell you what he/she would do in a given situation (but his/her supervision model may not allow them to do it directly).

Unrealistic expectations of a supervisor:

- Supervisor is a master of all knowledge in the field (e.g., since he/she already got a degree, he/she has memorized all information presented in master's program and/or for license).
- Supervisor is able to supervise in any "standard" theory in the field.
- Supervisor is interested in supporting you in developing your personal theory of choice; some will, but others will require you to use their perspective, because that is what they have skill and competence to teach (valid arguments for either approach).
- Supervisor wants to hear about struggles in your personal life; some will insist on it and even focus on it; some won't want to hear about any of it. Each supervisor model has a different approach to self-of-the-counselor/therapist issues.
- Supervisor will always support you.
- Supervisor will always have something useful to say about each case and situation.
- Supervisor has been trained to do supervision and/or any good therapist can be a good supervisor. Supervision is a unique and separate skill from doing therapy; although being a good therapist is generally a prerequisite for being a good supervisor, the two skills don't always correlate.
- Supervisors supervise in the same way. It is natural to assume that supervisors will be more alike than different; however, there is a surprising, if not startling, variety of ways to do supervision. Be prepared to work with vastly different approaches.
- I must like my supervisor, and the supervisor must like me. Although either party will enjoy the process less if there is not mutual fondness, it is possible to still learn quite a bit from a supervisor with whom you don't have great chemistry. Often, such a supervisor requires one to become more independent, reflect on one's own interactions with others, and generally recognize areas from growth, even if it is just in the area of tolerance and acceptance of human differences.

The World from Your Supervisor's Perspective

As a supervisee, it is often hard to imagine the world from the supervisor's perspective. At the other end of the professional spectrum, they have an entirely different set of concerns and issues. To begin, in most states, supervisees work under the license of their supervisors, not under the auspices of the agency. So, the supervisors' licenses are on the line—and they are held responsible for any harm that comes to your clients. If your supervisors have done due diligence and gone to trainings that cover the ethical and legal implications of supervising, they probably have been given a long and scary list of the ways they can be sued for a supervisee's mistake. Thus, a major concern of all supervisors is their exposure to significant liability due to actions of supervisees whom they cannot fully control.

Next, many organizations that are large enough to train new counselors generally have significant paperwork and a complex bureaucracy. In such a system, the supervisor is expected to ensure that their supervisees follow all of the detailed rules and complete copious amounts of paperwork. In most cases, these same supervisors maintain a caseload of their own and also handle numerous client crisis issues and various unsavory administrative tasks. Most are given the workload for two and expected to complete it flawlessly in a 40-hour workweek without overtime. Thus, they are very interested in having trainees learn the paperwork and organizational systems as quickly as possible.

Finally, most supervisors want you to succeed. They chose to become a supervisor because they find the extra work and liability are worth the reward of helping a new counselor develop and flourish. For most, it is a gratifying process because they are helping another person learn to help countless others. They are excited to serve in this capacity and to help you achieve your goals. However, how they do that is often a matter of *style*.

Styles of Supervision

Another surprising discovery for new supervisees is that there are many different styles of supervision. In fact, the degree of variety can be shocking, and in some cases painfully so. Some of the differences are related directly to the theoretical model of supervision employed, and other differences have more to do with relational style.

Theoretical Differences in Supervision Style

Most schools of counseling and psychotherapy have a correlated supervision approach that relies on the philosophy and methods of the approach. For most readers, it is a bit early to go over theories of supervision, but below are some highlights that new supervisees might find useful to know.

- *Psychodynamic:* The ultimate goal of psychodynamically oriented supervision is to refine the "analytic instrument," which is the counselor or therapist (Watkins, 2013). Thus, these supervisors spend quite a bit of time talking about *you, the supervisee*—not the client. Often, this is discussed in terms of your internal reaction to the client, or countertransference (see Chapter 8). In some cases, you may wonder if this is a therapy session or supervision. Also common within this tradition is for the supervisor (parallel to the counselor-client relationship) to share minimal personal information about himself or herself in supervision. This may come across as distant or aloof, but it is an intentional part of the process.
- *Adlerian:* Adlerian supervisors embody Adlerian counseling attitudes more generally and typically combine an educational component within an encouraging supervisory relationship. A supervision group may be used to provide support and also to provide reflection about how others experience you relationally (McMahon & Fall, 2006). Most notably, you will be challenged on your private logic and how it affects your clinical work.
- *Humanistic-Existential:* Like their psychodynamic peers, humanistic supervisors tend to focus on the personal experiences and self-awareness of the supervisee (Farber, 2012). However, you will likely experience a greater sense of personal connection with the supervisor, because humanistic-existential supervisors use the self of the supervisor to model how you can use your authentic self to meaningfully engage clients (Farber, 2012). When discussing clients and counseling skills, the supervisor will focus on your abilities to facilitate the exploration and expression of emotion with clients.
- *Cognitive-Behavioral:* Cognitive-behavioral supervisors tend to have a more businesslike approach to supervision, often beginning with a clear agenda and ending with clear follow-up tasks or homework (Reiser & Milne, 2012). The sessions will generally focus on the case conceptualization and intervention, using direct instruction or Socratic questions (see Chapter 11) to help the supervisee learn to think through clinical issues independently. Of all supervisors, they are the most likely to use a supervision contract (see Supervision Contract below).

- *Systemic:* Systemically oriented supervisors focus on the relational and cultural dynamics (a) in the client's life, (b) between you and the client, and, if they are good, (c) between the supervisor and you (Lee & Nelson, 2014). Much of their attention will be on how to "view" the client and then skillfully intervene with the systemic dynamics. They are also likely to be interested in "live supervision," such as watching you with a client either behind a one-way mirror or using video.
- *Solution-Focused:* With a distinct strengths-orientation, solution-focused supervisors are likely to focus on what you are doing well and on helping you do more of that (Hsu, 2009). They also help you identify exceptions to problems in clients' lives and your own development as a counselor. They will typically provide supportive feedback and education to help you develop your case conceptualization and learn specific skills (Hsu, 2009).
- *Postmodern/Feminist:* Postmodern and feminist supervisors are likely to focus on cultural and gender politics of the supervision relationship and those relating to the client, the client's problem, and the relationship between you and the client (Ungar, 2006). They tend to have a collaborative style, using nonassuming questions to help you reflect on the counseling process with your clients (Anderson, 1997). Often, postmodern supervisors will use reflecting teams (see Chapter 14) and related processes, both in supervision and as part of live supervision with clients.

Relational Style

The other issue to consider is the relational style of your supervisor, which is often directly related to their supervisory model, the supervisee's level of development, the demands of the clinical context, and the client in question. More subtly, a supervisors' relational style may flow from their natural or personality style of relating, and, to a certain extent, from the "chemistry" between supervisor and supervisee. Supervisory relational style can take on many forms, and typically, one supervisor will embody several of the following roles when working with a single supervisee (Lee & Nelson, 2014; Morgan & Sprenkle, 2007):

- *Coach:* Supervisors use coaching when they focus on teaching supervisees specific in-session competencies or skills, such as reframing or setting boundaries. Coaching may involve role-plays or talking through an intervention in detail.
- *Teacher:* Supervisors can also take on the role of teacher, instructing supervisees on various therapy approaches and how to employ them. The teacher relational style is distinguished from coaching in that it is more conceptual and general, whereas the coach is focusing on specific clinical interventions.
- *Administrator:* Increasingly, supervisors must also take on an administrative role with supervisees, overseeing the completion and quality of documentation and ensuring that supervisees follow agency policies and procedures (Tromski-Klingshirn, 2007). The administrative role also involves helping supervisees track their supervision and clinical hours.
- *Mentor:* More common later in a supervisee's prelicensing training period, mentoring from a supervisor involves helping supervisees reflect on and consider the larger picture of professional development, including guidance through licensure, development of a specialization, and identifying a career path.
- *Advocate:* Sometimes your supervisor will serve as your advocate within an agency to help ensure that you receive adequate resources for your training. Be sure to show your appreciation.
- *Gatekeeper:* One role all supervisors must accept at one level is gatekeeper of the profession, ensuring that no clients are harmed by supervisees. Thus, there is an expectation that they evaluate and monitor the work of supervisees and do what is necessary to protect both supervisees and clients.

Learning to Work with All Supervisory Styles and Personalities

Although you may be tempted to wish for a particular relational style or good chemistry in general with all of your supervisors, I no longer believe that is actually desirable (but as a trainee I thought it was). The reason for this is that it is essential for mental health professionals to work well with all sorts of people, especially "different" and "difficult" people. Ultimately, that is our job. I believe we all have valuable professional and life lessons to learn from all sorts of people in our lives, not just the ones we like. Quite frankly, we need those lessons—whether we want to learn them or not—to be able to help the people who seek our counsel. Looking back over my training and career, I can confidently say that I have learned the most from people with whom I struggled to work. Generally, our clients are coming to us with concerns about those difficult relationships; and when we have worked through these successfully in our own lives, we are of more use to them. Therefore, I encourage you to be open to learning from all of your supervisors, no matter their style or approach—with the very rare exceptions discussed in the "When to Leave" section below.

Supervision Contract

Given that there is such a variety of supervision styles, it is generally considered a best practice for supervisors to provide supervisees with a supervision contract that clearly spells out their expectations and style of working (Aasheim, 2012; Bradley & Ladany, 2010; Lee & Nelson, 2014; Thomas, 2007). Yet, you may find that a minority of supervisors actually uses a written contract, and some do a verbal contract only minimally. To be fair, it is a bit of work on their part. If you happen to be working with a supervisor who does not provide you with a written supervision contract, you may want to ask them some of the following questions so that you clearly understand his/her expectations from the beginning (Lee & Nelson, 2014; Thomas, 2007):

- *Supervision Approach, Style, and Format:* Can you describe your approach to supervision? Do you have a specific model or theory you use? To what degree to you focus on (a) theoretical orientation, (b) diagnostic assessment, (c) case conceptualization, and (d) specific interventions? To what degree am I free to choose my theoretical model or orientation? Which supervision formats do you use: case report, live, video-/audiotaped, co-therapy, group, or others? Do you have expectations about reading or additional training?
- *Self-of-the-Counselor:* Do you tend to focus on self-of-the-counselor issues and if so, how? How much self-disclosure and personal information do you expect? What format do you prefer for such conversations?
- *Privacy and Confidentiality:* How do you handle privacy issues in supervision, both related to what I discuss personally and with client information?
- *Preparation for Supervision and Case Presentation:* How would you like for me to present my cases and prepare for supervision? Is there a specific format you would like for me to use and/or a specific ordering of cases?
- *Crisis Protocols:* What are the protocols for handling crisis? Who should I contact if you are not available? At what point in my assessment (at what level of risk) should I contact you? If you are not on-site at the time, how best should I contact you?
- *Documentation:* How will you be overseeing my clinical documentation? How do you typically handle hour logs and documentation for licensure?
- *Supervisee Status:* What are your guidelines for my explaining my status with clients and other stakeholders?
- *Illness, Vacation, and Leave:* What are the policies and procedures for handling time off for illness, vacation, and/or leave by supervisee *and* supervisor? If the supervisor is ill or out of town, how is the missed supervision handled? Is there a backup supervisor? Who is expected to notify clients if the counselor is ill for a day?
- *Evaluation:* What are the procedures for evaluating my skills and performance?
- *Handling Difficult Issues:* If you have concerns about my performance in any way, how would you typically raise these? If for any reason I have a difficult issue I need to raise, how would you prefer I handle it? Is there an established protocol for handling such situations?
- *Site-Specific Concerns:* What is the most common problem you see trainees have at this site/with this population?
- *Duration and Termination:* What is the expected duration of and process for terminating the supervision arrangement?

What to Know and Do Before You Start Seeing Clients

Training Agreements

After rejoicing upon being accepted to your first trainee site, you should quickly get your paperwork in order—but not *too* quickly. You want to take time to actually read and understand what you are agreeing to. If you are still in school, your university will typically have a three-way training agreement between you, them, and the field site. Your site may also have another agreement they want you to sign. These contracts or agreements are not casual matters. You are committing yourself to certain things, and the site is committing certain things to you. Thus, you will be expected to uphold your end of the bargain, and you want to make sure that you understand and like the deal.

Although these are boilerplate to some degree, the most common problems arise from the following issues, which I encourage you to carefully think about before signing:

- *Start and End Dates:* You want to carefully approach the start and end dates on the agreement. You need to make sure you will be enrolled in a class in which you are allowed to see clients (based on state licensing laws and university rules) and that you will commit to an end date. Most sites are not happy if you ask to leave early, which could have negative repercussions for you in multiple ways. That said, you might not be able to extend your contract, depending on how the site enters and exits trainees. Thus, I suggest working closely with the supervisor to identify realistic dates that comfortably allow you get the hours you need and are within university and site timelines.
- *Total Weekly Time Commitment:* You should ask enough questions to get a clear picture of the full time commitment. First, you should ask about the initial training period, which can be substantial, and how long it will take to build up a full load of clients. In addition, you want to get specific information about the days per week and hours per week. In some cases, you will not be able to negotiate certain times, such as staff meetings or supervision, and these may conflict with other school or work obligations. Finally, you want a realistic expectation for hours spent on paperwork, administrative tasks, crisis counseling, overload clients, staffing the phone, driving, and perhaps other tasks; these "extra" hours are often the ones that surprise you and throw a monkey wrench in your otherwise balanced schedule. It is best to clarify the hour expectations in detail before signing on the dotted line.
- *Hours Required by University/Licensing Board:* Although most trainees don't feel competent about much, most supervisors expect you to be the expert on knowing how many of which type of hours you need for graduation and licensing requirements. Licensing requirements change frequently and are different from discipline to discipline. So, even if your supervisor has your same license, the supervisor likely earned hours under a different set of requirements. Therefore, it really is the supervisee's job to clearly communicate the type of hours needed for licensure. In addition, each university has a set of unique requirements, so even if the site already has an agreement with a given university, this does not mean that the supervisor remembers or understands those requirements. That is the trainee's responsibility.
- *Vacation:* Discuss and put into writing the expectations around vacations and other forms of leave. Most sites will rarely allow for more than two weeks of vacation over a one-year period of training, because your consistent engagement is important for clients and your training.
- *Mileage:* If you will be doing home visits or otherwise traveling frequently for the organization, it is customary to receive mileage reimbursement. Don't forget to ask for it!
- *Training Fees:* Some training sites do require students to pay for certain expenses, often an initial training fee and in some cases a monthly training fee. You should ask about such requirements in your early negotiations with a site.

Licensing Requirements

As mentioned above, supervisees are responsible for understanding the requirements for licensure in their state. This includes understanding the following:

- *Sites:* Appropriate sites for training; most states limit the type of businesses and organizations a trainee can work in.
- *Supervisor:* Each state has unique laws for who can supervise a trainee; trainees should confirm a supervisor's license is current and in good standing (if not, no hours will count). This information is available on the website of the licensing body in each state. Check it out; one day soon, your license may be there. In addition, supervisees are responsible for confirming whether the supervisor has obtained the necessary training to be a supervisor for your license in your state. It is not rude or inappropriate to ask for the evidence (e.g., CEU certificate or certificate of supervisor status).
- *Hours:* Each state has unique hour requirements for supervisees pursuing licensure. Although it would seem logical that either your clinical supervisor or university professor would be an expert at this and responsible for guiding you, that is not required by any state law of which I am aware. Also, it would seem logical that more-senior supervisees would be a good source of information about these requirements; trust me, this is not always the case. Ultimately, it is your job not only to educate yourself on the current requirements for licensure in your state but also to stay up-to-date about any changes. It is more than likely that some significant requirement will change at least once before you get licensed. Although supervisors, university faculty, and more-senior peers often do understand and accurately communicate the requirements, it is foolhardy to rely on such information alone. If you want to be competent, you need to roll up your sleeves, take a deep breath, and read the painfully detailed rules and regulations for licensing. The benefits of such efforts will pay dividends because you will be more confident and will understand how to best document your experience to get a license significantly sooner than those who rely on hearsay.
- *Documentation:* While you are befriending your state licensing board, don't forget to study and master their system for documenting hours of experience. The sooner and better you understand, the more effective you will be in documenting the hours you need and avoid "missing" (not counting) hours you work to accrue.
- *Mandated Reporting:* Finally, it is worth mentioning that you should familiarize yourself with state-mandated reporting requirements as they apply to supervisees. No doubt, in most states, you are a mandated reporter for child, elder, and dependent adult abuse, but you should also learn about how a supervisee is expected to report it, both at the state level and in the specific agency in which you work. You should also learn about reporting requirements for domestic violence, consensual sex between minors, suicidal and homicidal threats, and threats to property.

Join a Professional Organization

If you have not done so already, you should join a professional organization when you start seeing clients. Although another expense at a time when few people have extra resources, a professional organization—such as the American Counseling Association, American Association of Marriage and Family Therapy, National Association of Social Workers, or American Psychological Association—are a source of essential information that will shape your identity as an emerging professional. The benefits these organizations offer to new professionals include:

- *Identity:* Understanding what it means to be a "professional counselor," "family therapist," "social worker," or "psychologist." Your professors give you a particular definition or sense of it, but the larger organization provides a much more complete sense of what that means.

- *Identity Within Field of Mental Health:* Perhaps a more subtle and critical sense of identity they can provide is helping you to understand how your specific discipline fits and relates to the other mental health disciplines. Ideally, professional organizations can help you better understand the unique strengths of your specialty and how this will enable you to work on interdisciplinary intervention teams. Often, this helps impart a sense of pride, clarity of purpose, and focus for training.
- *Cutting-Edge Knowledge:* Living in the age of too much knowledge—both a blessing and a curse—professional organizations are more important than ever in helping competent professionals stay up-to-date. It is nearly impossible to do it by yourself: you'd be reading professional, journals, books, and websites day and night. Professional organizations have teams of folks who do the sorting for you and identify what you absolutely must know to stay current.
- *Best Conferences:* In general, professional organizations host the best conferences because this is the one place when the organization "comes alive," so to speak, and the members get to connect face-to-face. In my first year of graduate school, I had a professor tell me that the way he decided his professional orientation was to go to several different conferences and join the group he liked best. His approach may work for you, too.
- *Lobbying for Your Paycheck:* A critical role that professional organizations play in any professional's life is enhancing paychecks. Essentially, professional organizations exist to promote the professional lives of their members (while keeping the needs of clients and public in mind). In the case of mental health, that translates to lobbying at state and national levels to ensure that a given license (MSW, LMFT, LPC, Psych) is covered under different bills and by other third-party payers. They will often have political action campaigns (PACs) that they ask members to donate to, in order enhance their ability to lobby on behalf of the members. And let me say, these lobbyists are busy; each year seems to bring some new option to get paid or get written out of a bill that would get you paid. So, if you want to ensure that you will get paid by as many sources as possible once you get licensed, it is important to be involved with a professional organization that advocates for your license.
- *Liability Insurance and Legal Advice:* Finally, my favorite reason for joining a professional organization is to protect myself. You can rest assured that your professional organization has negotiated the best possible rates and terms of professional liability insurance (that is, what will protect you if clients sue you). Also, they offer free legal consultations. Given that the average lawyer charges $350 per hour, one call to the organization's lawyer can make your annual dues a hard-to-beat bargain.

Liability Insurance

As just noted, one of the benefits of joining a professional organization is getting a strong liability insurance policy. You will need this as long as you are a practicing professional counselor or psychotherapist. Sometimes an employer or agency may say, "You don't need to get a policy; we have one that covers all of our employees and volunteers." That may be true, but there are some potential loopholes that make the relatively nominal fee (especially for students) worth it. Some employer-paid polices have clauses that may say if the employee (or volunteer) did not follow the employer's policy, their policy will not cover the employee. Similarly, it is possible that various exclusionary actions, such as sexual misconduct with a client, may not be covered on the employer's policy. So, if you want to be safe, it is always best to have your own personal policy in case things don't go the way you predicted. These policies generally cover a certain amount of legal representation, and as you can imagine, it is best to have your own policy to have a lawyer who puts you first—not your employer.

Getting the Most out of Supervision

Skillful Questions

The most important skill to master as a supervisee is how to ask great questions. The quality of your questions directly affects the quality of your supervision. Although it is tempting to attribute "great supervision" to the skill of the supervisor, such a linear perspective misses the systemic and relational dynamics that are inherent to supervisory (and all) relationships (Lee & Nelson, 2014; also see Chapter 12). Thus, it is important for you to recognize that how *you* interact with your supervisors significantly impacts and shapes the quality of the supervision you receive—good news, indeed, if you are in the market for skilled supervision.

Given that most teacher-student relationships in our culture are hierarchical and conceptualized as unidirectional in terms of influence and control, most supervisees quickly slip into an overly passive and receptive role instead of seeing themselves as active participants who shape the process (Anderson, 1997). As mentioned above, becoming a proactive learner requires a shift in perspective and paradigm for most supervisees. The way that this proactive stance expresses itself is not through defiance or being directive with the supervisor (probably not a successful strategy), but through *skillful questions.*

What is a skillful question? It's one that helps the participants to focus on key issues and concerns in such a way that learning is optimally promoted. Perhaps it is best to illustrate with some poor questions, and yes, some questions really are less than intelligent.

Questions NOT to Ask in Supervision

Questions to avoid in supervision include:

- [Blow-by-blow account of session with client] followed by "What should I do?"
- [Blow-by-blow account of session with client] followed by "What do you think?"
- [Blow-by-blow account of session with client] followed by blank stare and shrug.

Questions such as these set up the stage for receiving poor (and possibly aggravating) supervision. First, launching into a blow-by-blow description of he-said/she-said of a given session does not provide supervisors with guidance as to the type of supervision you are needing. Instead, it leaves the conversation wide open for supervisors to focus on anything that catches their attention, which too often ends up with the supervisor focusing on issues that you do not find helpful. Sometimes, supervisors end up of going back and reassessing for crisis or other issues that have already been dealt with; other times, they may start focusing on an issue that you think is a secondary priority. Such questions by the supervisor may be irritating to the supervisee because (a) you may not have time for the actual but unstated question you really want help with, and (b) your supervisor may begin to question your competence at the end of it all. Similarly, asking broad, open questions—such as, what should I do?—may yield responses from your supervisor that are not useful to you at all, such as suggesting interventions you have tried or reassessing areas you have already covered. Instead of setting yourself up for less-than-ideal supervisory encounters, I recommend preparing for supervision so that you can effectively request the type of supervision you need and ask for it in a way that best enables your supervisor to help you.

Preparing for Supervision

Before your weekly supervision meeting, you should put some thought into what you need from your supervisor. One option is to keep a *supervision notebook*, to keep a list of questions and concerns that arise during the week (obviously, you must not include confidential information such as client names in such a book). In addition, you might want to use the following worksheet to help you think through your client situations and create a prioritized agenda for supervision.

Pre-Supervision Worksheet

Crisis Situations: Do I have any cases with crisis situations? ❑ Yes ❑ No

These should generally be presented first in supervision.

❑ Potential child, elder, or dependent adult abuse?

❑ Suicide, homicide, self-harm, other forms of harm to self or others?

❑ Domestic violence or other forms of violence or harassment?

❑ Eating disorders?

❑ Alcohol or substance abuse?

❑ Prejudice, harassment or other forms of social justice issues?

If so, what do I need to know from my supervisor?

❑ How to handle a crisis that was identified in session this week?

❑ How to continue assessing and/or check in after crisis?

❑ Review how crisis was handled this week.

Stuck: Do I feel stuck or lost with any client this week? Is there any client who is not progressing as I had hoped? Is there any client where I don't feel like I have a clear conceptualization or sense of what to focus on? ❑ Yes ❑ No

If so, what type of help do I need from my supervisor?

❑ Developing a case conceptualization: Identifying primary interpersonal and intrapersonal dynamics of the case to focus my treatment?

❑ Diagnosis and symptom management?

❑ Identifying interventions for next session to specifically intervene on what aspect of case dynamics (from case conceptualization)?

❑ How to address relational issues between client and me? (e.g., tension, distance, over-friendliness, etc.)

❑ Lack of progress or feeling stuck?

❑ How to manage session (e.g., end on time, focus the session, and such)

❑ How to implement theory of choice?

Personal Issues: Do I have any personal issues that are affecting my ability to be fully present with and nonjudgmental of my clients? How have I tried to handle this? Is it an appropriate issue that should be raised in supervision? ❑ Yes ❑ No

Administrative: Are there any administrative issues I should address in supervision:

❑ Hour logs?

❑ Paperwork?

❑ Agency policies and procedures?

❑ Interactions with other agency personnel?

Skillful Questions for Supervision

Once you have completed your notes in your supervision journal and the pre-supervision worksheet, you should have a good idea of what you need to discuss in supervision. Once you are in your supervision session, you should quickly outline the agenda at the beginning of the meeting so that your supervisor has a sense of how to budget the time. You and your supervisor can then carefully prioritize how to use the time. If you wait even ten minutes to do this, then it is more likely you will not attend to all the things you want to discuss.

Announcing Your Agenda/Needs at the Beginning

"[Supervisor], today, I would like to discuss ________ crisis situations, ________ client cases (generally keep to 1–3 per hour), ________ personal issues (if any), and ________ administrative issues.

Once you and your supervisor have agreed on an agenda, your next task is to present your question and client case concisely—yet with sufficient information for the supervisor to provide you with a useful response. The general formula for this is:

Efficient Case Presentation Formula

Specific Supervision Need

"Today, I would like to focus our supervision of [name case] on":

Specify ONE—maybe two—items:

- ❑ Crisis issues
- ❑ Case conceptualization and treatment plan
- ❑ Diagnosis
- ❑ Intervention for next session
- ❑ My personal reaction to client
- ❑ Lack of progress
- ❑ Session management
- ❑ Theory-of-choice

Briefly Identify Client

Depending on how many cases you see and your supervisor's memory, you may need to remind the supervisor of the client. Try to do this in *one sentence or less* using one or more of the following identifies:

- ❑ Age, gender, ethnicity, sexual orientation, and so on.
- ❑ Individual, couple, family
- ❑ Presenting problem(s) or diagnosis (in more clinical contexts)
- ❑ Significant crisis issue
- ❑ Significant strength or resource (for a more strength-oriented approach)
- ❑ One interesting idiosyncratic descriptor (e.g., "the popcorn family")

Present Three to Five Key Pieces of Information

Then, based on most recent developments with the client, list out three to five key pieces of information that the supervisor would need to know to help you with the case. Try not to launch into a full story unless the supervisor asks for it. Instead, think through the situation and identify what are the key issues, and then STOP. If the supervisor needs more information, he/she will ask. Examples of salient information include:

Crisis

- ❑ Risk factors
- ❑ Safety indicators and plan
- ❑ Facts of the situation: what, what, when, where, how
- ❑ Past history/incidents

(continued)

Conceptualization and Treatment Planning

❑ Presenting problem

❑ Theoretical orientation(s)

❑ Diagnosis

Diagnosis

❑ Symptoms and presenting problems

❑ Psychiatric history for client and family

Interventions for Next Session

❑ Specific problem to be addressed

❑ Specific intervention or theory you want to use

Reaction to Client

❑ Your conceptualization of dynamic/countertransference

❑ Specific way it is manifested in session/in your head

❑ Specific concerns about how it is affecting or may affect therapy

Lack of Progress

❑ Identify progress to date if any

❑ Identify general treatment plan and interventions used and client response

❑ Your hypothesis as to why progress is stalled

Session Management

❑ As for specific help: how to end/begin session, handle conflict, and others.

Theory of Choice

❑ Try to identify one specific area for help: case conceptualization, treatment planning, counseling relationship, interventions, and so on.

Using Supervision Time Wisely

Although you may have heard that there is no such thing as a dumb question, in professional training that is not entirely true. If a supervisee can find the answer to a question with a little effort, the supervisee is not making the best use of precious supervision time if he or she asks the supervisor for the answer, and the supervisee is also slowing his/her own growth and independence. So, although a question may not be dumb, asking one that you can answer yourself may not be the best use of your time.

The time you have with your supervisor is precious and should be used wisely. Although it might be easier to ask your supervisor questions about filing papers or logging hours than figuring it out yourself, it really is best to find the answer to those questions elsewhere. Even if your supervisor is happy to answer such questions, in the long run you will be better trained if you focus your questions to your supervisor on clinical matters, as much as possible. Counselors have to master multiple, complex forms of knowledge and practice in the early years of training—theory, law and ethics, diagnosis, intervention, crisis management, personal growth—no amount of supervision can adequately cover all of these areas. Thus, spending time on nonclinical matters only further reduces how much of these critical areas are covered.

What to Do When or If Things Get Bumpy

Signs of Trouble

Sometimes things between a supervisor and supervisee can get bumpy: one person or the other is unhappy with or concerned about the other. The discontent can range from minor irritation to significant conflict (Nelson & Friedlander, 2001). Most likely, before you get licensed, you will have a handful of supervisory relationships that have a few bumps along the way. So, it is probably wise to think about how you might reduce the potential for such struggles (Nelson, Barnes, Evans, & Triggiano, 2008).

As with most relationships, unspoken expectations are frequently an issue in supervisory relationships (Falender & Shafranske, 2012). A supervisee may expect a supervisor to be warm and friendly, or a supervisor may have assumptions of certain professional behaviors, such as dress, timing, and so on. Thus, a good place to begin when things get rocky is to openly discuss expectations related to what is going on—in addition to simply having each person share their experience and interpretation of what is going on (Nelson et al., 2008). For supervisees, this may mean asking supervisors about concerns in an open and engaging manner (Nelson & Friedlander, 2001). It may also mean avoiding jumping to conclusions; for example, just because your supervisor isn't lavish with praise does not mean the supervisor thinks you are incompetent.

Common Issues That Are Worth Addressing

- *"Feeling" Disliked:* I have known several supervisees who "feel" disliked by their supervisor but base feeling this on very limited evidence; often this is due to expecting a supervisor to be more complimentary or warm than is realistic. In fact, many excellent supervisors, especially experienced ones, have more formal, businesslike boundaries in supervision.
- *"Feeling" Incompetent:* Some supervisees interpret the vast amount of information and suggestions that the supervisor offers as evidence that the supervisees are incompetent, or at least that the supervisor thinks so. This is often more common in supervisees who have had successful careers in other areas and find themselves suddenly in the role of a beginner again. In most cases, it is worth having a conversation with the supervisor about this; often the key is to become comfortable with the very steep learning curve required to become a mental health professional.
- *Misunderstanding Requirements:* If you and your supervisor or other agent at the site are starting to have mixed communication about the actual requirements of the site—number of hours, days, trainings, and such—it is important to clear these matters up sooner rather than later. Being as cooperative as possible is important. If there is any miscommunication, it is generally best practice to put it all down in writing so that everyone is clear about what the expectations are.

Talking Directly to Your Supervisor

If for any reason you begin to have concerns about your relationship with your supervisor—either you are concerned about something or believe he/she is concerned about you—it is generally best to directly address the concern by talking to him/her about it, preferably before things get too serious (Falender & Shafranske, 2012; Nelson & Friedlander, 2001; Nelson et al., 2008). In such circumstances, I often hear students say, "I am too intimidated to talk directly to my supervisor." It is exceptionally rare that a supervisor is so vindictive and one-sided that such a conversation hurts a trainee. It is far more common for a supervisee to be uncomfortable having difficult conversations with a person in power and to dread such a talk. However, as counselors and therapists, we are in the business of having difficult conversations. We are also in the business of working with difficult personalities. So, being intimidated is generally not a good reason to avoid a difficult conversation. That said, if your supervisor has a widely recognized reputation for being unreasonable and difficult to work with, you may want to ask someone else in the organization about how best to approach the situation. Again, this situation is quite rare. If you are nervous about approaching your supervisor about a concern, here are some suggestions:

- *Acknowledge the Supervisor's Reality:* Wherever possible, acknowledge the limits, pressures, or other realities that your supervisor may be faced with. Such acknowledgments go a long way toward making the other person feel understood and reducing defensiveness.

- *Raise Concerns Tentatively and Separate Interpretation from Behavior/Words:* If you are raising concerns, be sure to do so tentatively and in a nonaccusing manner. For example, "I feel that you attack me in supervision" is not a gentle way to raise the subject. Instead, begin by (a) asking permission to discuss a difficult topic, (b) acknowledge that it is only your subjective interpretation and that you may be misperceiving, (c) cite some specific, concrete behavior or words (not vague impressions), and (d) ask for the supervisor's interpretation of the same event.
    - Example: "If you have a moment, I would like to discuss a concern with you. Is now an okay time for you? [ask permission]. Before I begin, I want to emphasize that I understand that my concern is based on my interpretation, so I want to talk it through with you to make sure we are on the same page [acknowledge subjective position]. My concern is that sometimes when I am describing what I said or did in session, you interrupt me and say something like, "Well, you should have said/done X instead." [concrete, behavioral example, not just reporting a vague feeling] When that happens, I feel like you are angry with me and/or feel as though I am not performing at the level you expect. Am I misperceiving things? Can you share some of your thoughts about this? [inviting supervisor to share his/her perspective]"
- *Embrace Learning:* Sometimes the lesson supervisees learn when they raise concerns with supervisors is that they are simply in the position of learner—they are trying to master an extremely complex skill that most agree requires at least five years of guided practice before one can be trusted to not hurt others (essentially the definition of a license). Thus, often the lesson is learning to accept that your supervisor's job is to correct you. Hopefully, this is done in a spirit of support and recognition of your strengths, but it won't always be. And that is okay. As long as you stay open to the learning process.
- *Identify Unsolvable Problems:* Sometimes, although quite rarely, a supervisor may have unrealistic expectations, an unfair bias, or rigidity that makes it impossible to resolve conflict within the supervisory relationship. This is a very difficult position for a supervisee to be in because the supervisee is in the position with less power. At this point, it is critical to involve useful others if you happen to have them—the most common being a university supervisor.

Keeping University Supervisors in the Loop

If you are still enrolled at a university, it is very important to keep your university supervisor in the loop about any potential problems with your on-site field site supervisor. It has been my experience that, too often, supervisees wait too long to tell their university supervisor (in this case, me) about troubles brewing at their site. Typically, by the time I hear something, the problem has grown to such an extent that it is very difficult to solve. On average, I would say students bring in concerns about two months too late.

Ideally, you can turn to your university supervisor for suggestions on how to handle the first signs of trouble at your site. In most cases, it is best to talk to the university supervisor about ideas on how to best approach the problem at a site. In some cases, supervisees have unrealistic expectations, and the university supervisor can quickly resolve the issue without even speaking to the off-site supervisor. In other cases, there may be significant legal or ethical issues that the university supervisor can help investigate or otherwise help guide the supervisee through. In most cases, it will be less bumpy with the university supervisor—who hopefully knows the personalities involved and who may be able to serve as some form of mediator—involved.

Legal Quagmires

Of particular importance are legal or ethical issues that may arise in supervision. These can be difficult to handle, especially if you and your supervisor are not on the same page. Some general guiding principles are:

- Always seek legal counsel if ever in doubt; your professional membership should allow you access to a lawyer for general legal advice.

- If in doubt, it is generally safest to take the more conservative route, even if it requires a bit more work on your part. Clinical practice is generally not a place to take significant risk.

Some common legal or ethical issues that supervisees may experience include the following:

Licensing Paperwork One of the more common areas of legal and/or ethical conflict between supervisors and supervisees is paperwork for licensure (Nelson & Friedlander, 2001). Supervisees often assume that their supervisor will guide them; in stark contrast, most supervisors expect supervisees to be up-to-date on the latest requirements for their discipline. In some cases, supervisors have their own ways of interpreting the policies for documenting hours toward licensure. Supervisees are expected to critically evaluate the supervisor's system for documenting hours and to make sure said documentation is clearly within the bounds allowed by the state licensing board. If it is not, you and your supervisor need to discuss the issue and reach a shared understanding, perhaps with the help of the licensing board. In the end, it is the *supervisee's responsibility*—not the job of the supervisor—to ensure that hours toward licensure are accrued and recorded properly.

Legal and Ethical Issues with Clients When a serious legal and/or ethical issue arises with a supervisee's clients, it is imperative that the supervisor and supervisee work collaboratively together to resolve the issue. In most states and cases, the supervisor is ultimately responsible for the client's care, and therefore, the supervisor will have the final say in how to handle a situation. That said, if the issue is with a supervisee's client, it is important for the supervisee to be mindful of what is said and documented and to take extra steps to ensure all legal and ethical issues are handled properly. This may involve contacting the state licensing board, legal counsel, and/or other resources.

When to Leave

Although it is quite rare, there are times when it is appropriate to leave a training site earlier than contracted. In general, it is considered *highly* unprofessional (and some consider it a serious ethical issue and a form of abandonment, depending on the context) for a trainee to leave a training site before fulfilling a contract, especially if it is for personal gain or convenience. It can impact a supervisee's ability to get hired in the future. Some sites will file a complaint with the ethics board. That said, there are a handful of circumstances in which it may be necessary. First, if you have worked hard with your supervisor at the site to get the hours needed for graduation and have a contract saying that the site will provide the needed hours, but after several months of sincerely trying but failing to meet said contract stipulations, it may be reasonable to leave. In such cases, the site should be relatively supportive and understanding. Second, although extremely rare, you may end up at a site where you believe that there are numerous ethical or legal issues that you have not been able to resolve with your supervisor and/or the site director. If no mutually acceptable resolution has been reached after a reasonably long period to resolve the issue, then you may need to leave. If you believe you are in such a situation, it is best to work with your university supervisor (if you have one) and/or a lawyer to ensure that your concerns are appropriate, and that you exit as gracefully and professionally as possible, minimizing harm to clients.

What to Look for When Applying for Field Sites

What to Expect

Your search for your first traineeship is essentially a job search, even if you will be volunteering (Hodges & Connelly, 2010). Thus, you should expect to print your resume on pretty paper, get an interview suit, and look your best. You should also expect to be carefully and thoroughly interviewed, often more than you have been for any other position in the past. For the site and supervisor hiring you, they typically want to be picky with selecting a new supervisee because it is a relatively intimate and highly committed relationship for all parties. For the trainee, you are searching for your first training position, which will be the first working template for how to be a counselor or psychotherapist; it will have a lasting impression (although it can always be corrected if things go poorly). On the side of the site and supervisor, they will be taking on a significant liability in trying to train someone to be a counselor for the first time. At worst, they can be dragged into long and expensive lawsuits due to a supervisee's negligence; more commonly, things go wrong by having to put hours and hours into handling a difficult supervisory relationship or having a supervisee who can't quite perform as needed at the agency.

Quality Supervision

When new counselors ask me what to look for in an internship site, my answer is always: quality supervision! Although it is tempting to focus on a specific theory, client population, or location, I believe that the thing that has the most significant implications for training is the quality of supervision. If you learn from a supervisor with high standards, who teaches good clinical habits—for example, completing your progress notes before the end of the day, properly assessing cases, taking the time to meaningful conceptualize cases, using a theoretical model—then you will begin your career in such a way that you will succeed no matter where you go. However, if you start with bad habits and without a solid foundation, even if you are getting experience with the population you want to specialize in, your chances of becoming a highly skilled clinician are slimmer. You will have to teach yourself much of what you need to learn, through books, continuing education, or finding a mentor or better supervisor down the road.

Time Requirements

As mentioned above, the most common conflicts and problems at field sites arise around the issue of hours. In some cases, these conflicts are difficult to avoid. However, many can be prevented with good communication in the beginning. Often a supervisee hears (and is told) something like, "We expect you to see eight to ten clients per week." To a novice, this sounds like only ten or so hours is required each week. The supervisee does not think to ask for more details, and the supervisor doesn't think it needs to be spelled out that; of course, there are three hours of supervision, two hours of staff meeting, four hours of documentation, and a monthly training each month. Those hour are obvious—once you've worked in agency for a couple of years—but not to those starting out.

Whether applying for your first training or paid position, it helps greatly to get specific information about how much time is required for each of the following:

- *Direct Client Service Hours:* How many hours of individual, couple, family, and group clients must you see? How long will it take to build these hours up? Do any of these have to be on a particular day of the week or time of day?
- *Supervision Hours:* How many hours of supervision are offered/required per week? Are these days and times the same each week? Can they be moved?
- *Staff Meetings and Trainings:* Are there other staff meetings or trainings that you must attend on a weekly, monthly, or annual basis? Is there an initial training, and how long does it last?
- *Documentation:* How much time is typically spent on documentation per week?
- *Intakes or Special Clinical Tasks:* Are you responsible for doing special initial intake interviews or other special clinical tasks, such as meeting with families or running a group?
- *Crisis and Other Phone Calls:* How are crisis and other calls handled? Are you expected to be available off-site to answer these?

Questions to Ask

Although you probably have a good sense of what to ask when you go for an interview for a training site, now that you have read this chapter (or at least I hope you have), it probably is useful to include a list here, too:

- *History and Context:* Can you tell me about the history of this agency? How did it begin? Who does it serve? Where is it going?
    - This gives you a sense of the agency's stability and culture.
- *Clients:* What type of clients will I be seeing? How do they pay for services? What types of problems are common? Describe client diversity.
    - Provides sense of who you will be working with
- *Supervision:* Describe the supervision process and requirements here. Is there individual versus group supervision? Is there live supervision: co-therapy, videotaping, or audiotaping? What are the qualifications of the supervisors? Will I have a choice of supervisors?
- *Theoretical Orientation:* Is the agency committed to a particular theoretical orientation? What theoretical orientations do specific supervisors use? To what degree can you use your own?
- *Requirements:* Bring a list of requirements from both (a) your university (if applicable) and (b) your licensing board(s). Do not expect the site or supervisor to know these for you. Ask about getting the exact requirements you need.
- *Hours:* What are the site requirements:
    - How many clients per week?
    - How many hours of supervision per week?
    - How many hours per week does it typically take to complete paperwork, including intake reports?
    - Are there required staff meetings, trainings, or other weekly, monthly, or annual events?
    - Is there an initial training period, and what does it entail?
    - How long will it take to build up a full caseload?
    - Do you need to be on-call for crisis or intakes?
    - Do you need to be on-site during scheduled hours, even if you don't have clients scheduled?
- *Crisis:* How are crisis situations handled? Will there be a licensed person that you can talk to, physically at your site, when you are seeing clients? If not, how do you reach a supervisor to discuss immediate crisis issues?
- *Vacation:* What are the expectations regarding time off? How do you negotiate time off for a vacation or similar situation?
- *Conflict:* If differences or conflicts become a problem between staff members and/or between a supervisor and supervisee, how are these typically handled? Does the site or supervisor have a preferred way of handling such issues?
- *Safety:* How are safety issues handled? Are the clients or site likely to have safety issues? Will the student be in an unsafe area or parking lot, and how is this handled? Is there a special training for safety issues?
- *Money:* Will you be paid, and if so, how much? If you are to be paid, will they hire you within regulations set forth by the licensing board? Do you need to pay for any training costs or supplies? If you travel to see clients, will you be reimbursed for mileage?

The Competent Supervisee

Becoming a competent supervisee is an often-overlooked step on the journey to becoming a competent counselor and psychotherapist. Competent supervisees know how to learn, regardless of the context, because they are proactive learners who bring out the best in their supervisors and training situations. By managing their anxieties and thinking before they ask a question, they quickly become resilient, resourceful, and confident. By taking responsibility for their half of the supervisory relationship, they are able to focus the supervision conversation in ways that quickly accelerates their learning and enables them to feel fully supported by most any supervisor. In many ways, being competent in *receiving* supervision is the key to learning all other counseling skills.

Questions for Personal Reflection and Class Discussion

1. What ideas in this chapter were most surprising to you? Why?
2. Which ideas from this chapter do you find most personally relevant? Why?
3. What hallmarks of a professional are you already proficient in? In what ways might you need to grow?
4. Do you think you will be comfortable taking on a proactive learner role? Why or why not?
5. How might your gender, ethnicity, race, age, native language, social class, or other diversity variable affect you and your supervisory relationships? What can you do to address these issues?
6. How might you react to direct feedback about needing to improve in a particular area? How might you best make use of constructive feedback?
7. What style of supervision or supervisor behaviors do you think you will find easiest to work with? Which most difficult?
8. What type of supervisor diversity might be difficult for you: age, gender, ethnicity/race, social class, professional status, religion, sexual orientation, and so on?
9. How are you most likely to respond to a supervisor with whom you are struggling? How might you best deal with such a situation?
10. What methods do you plan to use to manage your initial anxiety in seeing clients?

Online Resources

Free Online Meditations

Start with these and also try YouTube.
www.dianegehart.com
www.marc.ucla.edu
www.mindfulselfcompassion.org/meditations_downloads.php
www.tarabrach.com/audioarchives-guided-meditations.html

References

Aasheim, L. (2012). *Practical clinical supervision for counselors: An experiential guide.* New York: Springer.

Anderson, H. (1997). *Conversation, language, and possibilities: A postmodern approach to therapy.* New York: Basic Books.

Bernard, J. M., & Goodyear, R. K. (2009). *Fundamentals of clinical supervision* (4th ed.). New York: Pearson.

Bradley, L. J., & Ladany, N. (2010). *Counselor supervision: Principles, process, and practice* (3rd ed.). New York: Brunner-Routledge.

Campbell, J. M. (2000). *Becoming an effective supervisor: A workbook for counselors and psychotherapists.* Philadelphia, PA: Accelerated Development.

Eysenck, M. W. (2013). The impact of anxiety on cognitive performance. In S. Kreitler (Ed.), *Cognition and motivation: Forging an interdisciplinary perspective* (pp. 96–108). New York: Cambridge University Press.

Farber, E. W. (2012). Supervising humanistic-existential psychotherapy: Needs, possibilities. *Journal of Contemporary Psychotherapy, 42*(3), 173–182. doi:10.1007/s10879-011-9197-x

Falender, C. A., & Shafranske, E. P. (2012). *Getting the most out of clinical training and supervision: A guide for practicum students and interns.* Washington, DC: American Psychological Association.

Fernando, D. M. (2013). Supervision by doctoral students: A study of supervisee satisfaction and self-efficacy, and comparison with faculty supervision outcomes. *The Clinical Supervisor, 32*(1), 1–14. doi:10.1080/07325223.2013.778673

Gehart, D., & McCollum, E. (2008). Inviting therapeutic presence: A mindfulness-based approach. In S. Hicks and T. Bien (Eds.), *Mindfulness and the healing relationship* (pp. 176–194). New York: Guilford.

Gehart, D. R., & McCollum, E. E. (2007). Engaging suffering: Towards a mindful re-visioning of family therapy practice. *Journal of Marital and Family Therapy*, 33(2), 214–226. doi:10.1111/j.1752-0606.2007.00017.x

Hayes, S. C., & Smith, S. (2005). *Get out of your mind and into your life. Oakland*, CA: New Harbinger.

Harris, M., & Brockbank, A. (2011). *An integrative approach to therapy and supervision: A practical guide for counsellors and psychotherapists*. London: Jessica Kingsley Publishers.

Hsu, W. (2009). The components of the solution-focused supervision. *Bulletin of Educational Psychology*, *41*(2), 475–496.

Hodges, S., & Connelly, A. R. (2010). *A job search manual for counselors and counselor educators*. Alexandria, VA: American Counseling Association.

Lawrence, G. P., Cassell, V. E., Beattie, S., Woodman, T., Khan, M. A., Hardy, L., & Gottwald, V. M. (2013). Practice with anxiety improves performance, but only when anxious: Evidence for the specificity of practice hypothesis. *Psychological Research*. Advance online publication. doi:10.1007/s00426-013-0521-9

Lee, R. E., & Nelson, T. S. (2014). *The contemporary relational supervisor*. New York: Taylor & Francis.

McCollum, E. E., & Gehart, D. R. (2010). Using mindfulness meditation to teach beginning therapists therapeutic presence: A qualitative study. *Journal of Marital and Family Therapy*, 36(3), 347–360.

McMahon, H., & Fall, K. A. (2006). Adlerian group supervision: Concept, structure, and process. *The Journal of Individual Psychology*, *62*(2), 126–140.

Morgan, M., & Sprenkle, D. (2007). Towards a common-factors approach to supervision. *Journal of Marital and Family Therapy*, *33*, 1–17.

Nelson, M., & Friedlander, M. L. (2001). A close look at conflictual supervisory relationships: The trainee's perspective. *Journal of Counseling Psychology*, *48*(4), 384–395. doi:10.1037/0022-0167.48.4.384

Nelson, M., Barnes, K. L., Evans, A. L., & Triggiano, P. J. (2008). Working with conflict in clinical supervision: Wise supervisors' perspectives. *Journal of Counseling Psychology*, *55*(2), 172–184. doi:10.1037/0022-0167.55.2.172

Reifer, S. (2001). Dealing with the anxiety of beginning therapists in supervision. In S. Gill (Ed.), *The supervisory alliance: Facilitating the psychotherapist's learning experience* (pp. 67–74). Lanham, MD: Jason Aronson.

Reiser, R. P., & Milne, D. (2012). Supervising cognitive-behavioral psychotherapy: Pressing needs, impressing possibilities. *Journal of Contemporary Psychotherapy*, *42*(3), 161–171. doi:10.1007/s10879-011-9200-6

Rust, J., Raskin, J., & Hill, M. (2013). Problems of professional competence among counselor trainees: Programmatic issues and guidelines. *Counselor Education and Super vision*, *52*, 30–42. doi:10.1002/j.1556-6978.2013.00026.x

Siegel, D. J. (2010). *The mindful therapist: A clinician's guide to mindsight and neural integration*. New York: Norton.

Stahl, B., & Goldstein, B. (2010). *A mindfulness-based stress reduction workbook*. New York: New Harbinger.

Stoltenberg, C. D., McNeill, B. W., & Delworth, U. (2010). *IDM supervision: An integrative developmental model for supervising counselors and therapists* (3rd ed.). New York: Routledge/Taylor & Francis.

Thomas, J. T. (2007). Informed consent through contracting for supervision: Minimizing risks, enhancing benefits. *Professional Psychology: Research and Practice*, *38*, 221–231.

Tromski-Klingshirn, D. (2007). Should the clinical supervisor be the administrative supervisor? The ethics versus the reality. *The Clinical Supervisor*, *25*(1–2), 53–67. doi:10.1300/J001v25n01_05

Tsai, S. (2012). The critical factors in the development of supervisory working alliance: Perspectives of supervisors and supervisees. *Bulletin of Educational Psychology*, *43*(3), 547–566.

Ungar, M. (2006). Practicing as a postmodern supervisor. *Journal of Marital and Family Therapy*, *32*(1), 59–71. doi:10.1111/j.1752-0606.2006.tb01588.x

Watkins, C. R. (2013). The contemporary practice of effective psychoanalytic supervision. *Psychoanalytic Psychology*, *30*(2), 300–328. doi:10.1037/a0030896

Weimer, M. (2002). *Learner-centered teaching*. New York: Jossey Bass.

Index